Surgical Atlas *of* Sports Medicine

Surgical Atlas *of* Sports Medicine

Mark D. Miller, MD
Associate Professor of Orthopaedic Surgery
Co-Director of Sports Medicine
University of Virginia
Department of Orthopaedic Surgery
Charlottesville, Virginia

Richard F. Howard, DO
Orthopaedic Specialist, PC
Assistant Professor, St. Louis University
Assistant Professor, Uniformed Services for Health Sciences
Chief of Surgery, Des Peres Hospital
St. Louis, Missouri

Kevin D. Plancher, MD
Plancher Hand and Sports Medicine
Stamford, Connecticut

Artist
Suzanne Edmonds
Redondo Beach, California

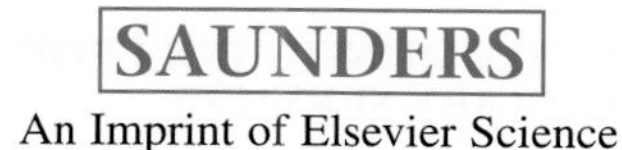

An Imprint of Elsevier Science

SAUNDERS
An Imprint of Elsevier Science (USA)

The Curtis Center
Independence Square West
Philadelphia, Pennsylvania 19106

SURGICAL ATLAS OF SPORTS MEDICINE ISBN 0-7216-7307-4

Notice

Sports Medicine is an ever-changing field. Standard safety precautions must be followed, but as new research and clinical experience broaden our knowledge, changes in treatment and drug therapy may become necessary or appropriate. Readers are advised to check the most current product information provided by the manufacturer of each drug to be administered to verify the recommended dose, the method and duration of administration, and contraindications. It is the responsibility of the treating physician, relying on experience and knowledge of the patient, to determine dosages and the best treatment for each individual patient. Neither the Publisher nor the author assumes any liability for any injury and/or damage to persons or property arising from this publication.

The Publisher

Library of Congress Cataloging-in-Publication Data

Miller, Mark D.
Surgical atlas of sports medicine / Mark D. Miller, Richard F. Howard, Kevin D. Plancher; artist, Suzanne Edmonds.
p. ; cm.
ISBN 0-7216-7307-4
1. Sports injuries—Surgery—Atlases. 2. Wounds and injuries—Surgery—Atlases. I. Howard, Richard F. II. Plancher, Kevin D. III. Title.
[DNLM: 1. Sports Medicine—Atlases. 2. Athletic Injuries—Atlases. QT 17 M649s 2003]
RD97 .M554 2003
617.1′027—dc21 2002075767

Acquisitions Editor: Richard Lampert
Assistant Editor: Hilarie Surrena
Project Manager: Amy Norwitz
Book Designer: Gene Harris

EH/DNP

Printed in Hong Kong

Last digit is the print number: 9 8 7 6 5 4 3 2 1

We dedicate this book to Sports Medicine surgeons and the athletes that we treat. The monkey bar gymnast, tetherball victor, college prospect, weekend warrior, Olympic champion, and professional athlete all deserve the best care possible from the greatest professionals on earth.

Preface

After years of searching for the best way to teach residents and colleagues surgical techniques, we developed the idea for a surgical atlas. The concept was to convert scribblings, technique articles and guides, lectures, clinical photos, radiographs, and arthroscopic photos into a single comprehensive resource. In order to ensure that both operative and nonoperative management were well covered, we chose to include history and physical examination, diagnostic imaging, nonoperative management, relevant anatomy, postoperative management, complications, and results, as well as detailed step-by-step illustrated techniques for each case. We envisioned that this work would be an excellent teaching tool for patients, medical students, primary care providers, orthopaedic residents, and orthopaedic surgeons alike.

We expected that this project could be finished in 1 year and take no more time than other projects we have been involved with. Over 3 years later, we finally delivered the manuscript for this mega-project to the publisher, unable to explain why it took so long to complete. We can now reflect with much better appreciation on the magnitude of the task that we had accepted and the diversity of care that we give to our patients.

We hope that you will find the format easy to follow, comprehensive, yet succinct for each procedure described. It is with great pride that we present what we hope will set a new standard for surgical atlases. We welcome you to join us in the surgical care of athletes.

Emperor Napoleon Bonaparte is credited with a now-common phrase that perhaps best sums up the utility of a surgical atlas: Un croquis vaut mieux qu'un long discours—a picture is worth a thousand words.

Mark D. Miller
Richard F. Howard
Kevin D. Plancher

Acknowledgments

We would be remiss if we did not first and foremost thank our families for letting us get submerged in yet another project, and more importantly for helping us to climb back to the banks afterwards. We also wish to recognize Dr. Mark Brinker for his ideas in the preliminary planning of this project, including many original thoughts regarding format and content. We also appreciate the patience, understanding, and sage counsel of our editor, Mr. Richard Lampert, at Elsevier Science. It was, indeed, a pleasure to work with our illustrator, Suzanne Edmonds, on this textbook. We believe that her work speaks for itself.

We would also like to recognize and acknowledge the many other illustrators who have contributed artwork to other Saunders texts that we have reproduced in this atlas. We have especially enjoyed the illustrations from J. W. Karapelou, who is the Chief Medical Illustrator for *Operative Techniques in Orthopedics*, which, along with its journal, *Operative Techniques in Sports Medicine*, was a wonderful resource for this book.

We also greatly appreciate the tremendous efforts of Jeannie Sanchez and Beth Williams, who contributed to the preparation of this manuscript.

Last, but by no means least, we owe a debt of gratitude to those surgeons that have taught us these techniques; specifically Drs. Freddie Fu, Chris Harner, J. P. Warner, Charles Rockwood, Jesse De Lee, Marv Royster, Dan Hinkin, and countless others who have influenced us, either directly or indirectly, through their work and dedication.

Contents

PART ONE. LOWER EXTREMITY

Section I. Knee

Section II. Leg, Ankle, and Foot

Section III. Thigh, Hip, and Pelvis

PART TWO. UPPER EXTREMITY

Section IV. Shoulder

Section V. Elbow

Section VI. Wrist and Hand

PART ONE

Lower Extremity

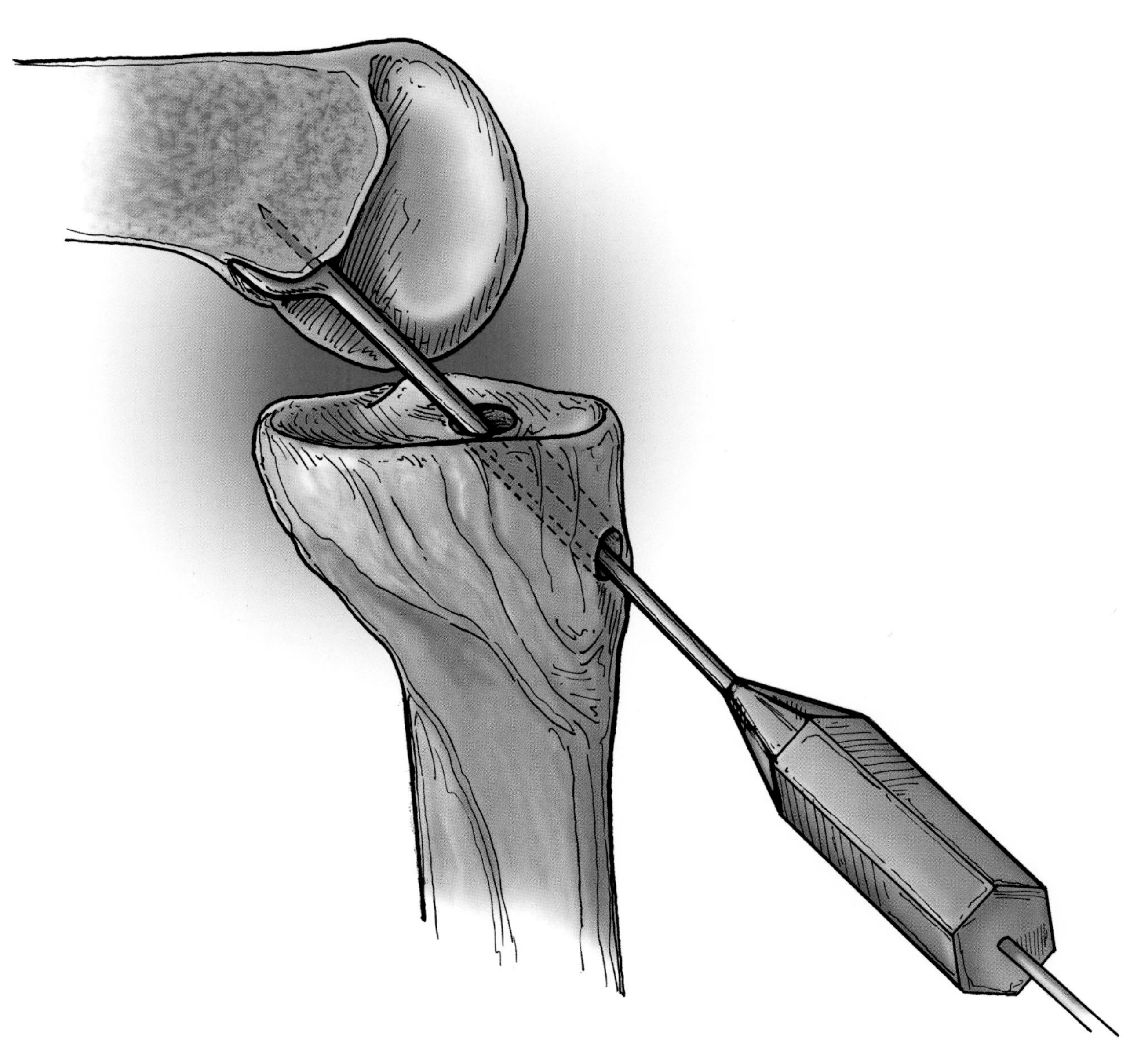

SECTION I

KNEE

CHAPTER 1

Knee Arthroscopy

INTRODUCTION

The arthroscope is a fundamental tool in sports medicine, especially in knee surgery. Indications vary and are related to different techniques described in this chapter.

POSITIONING

For most knee arthroscopic procedures, the patient is placed in the supine position with or without a table break at the thigh. Many surgeons prefer to place the well leg on a padded leg holder (carefully pad the fibular neck area to protect the peroneal nerve). The injured leg can be placed in a commercially available leg holder, or a post can be placed on the ipsilateral side (Fig. 1–1). A tourniquet is always placed, even if it is not planned to be used.

PORTALS

Arthroscopic portals for knee arthroscopy are shown in Figure 1–2. Standard portals include a superomedial or a superolateral portal for fluid inflow and outflow and inferomedial and inferolateral portals positioned just above the joint line on both sides of the patellar tendon for arthroscopy and instrumentation. The inferolateral portal is used most commonly for arthroscopic visualization. The inferomedial portal is used most commonly for instrumentation, although the instruments and arthroscope can be readily exchanged.

Accessory portals for the knee include the posteromedial and posterolateral, far medial and far lateral, proximal superomedial, and midpatellar portals. The posteromedial portal is helpful for visualizing the posterior cruciate ligament and the posterior horn of the medial meniscus. The posterolateral portal, located between the iliotibial band and the biceps tendon, is sometimes helpful, but extreme care should be taken to ensure that the portal is anterior to the biceps tendon to avoid injury to the peroneal nerve. The far medial and far lateral portals are rarely used but are sometimes helpful for instrument placement in hard-to-reach areas. The proximal superomedial portal, located 4 cm proximal to and in line with the medial edge of the patella, is useful for assessment of patellar tracking. The midpatellar portal sometimes is helpful when an additional portal is required for instrumentation (e.g., when removing a bucket-handle meniscal tear).

ARTHROSCOPIC ANATOMY

As with any joint, a systematic examination of the knee is appropriate. Before positioning of the patient, a complete examination under anesthesia is done to assess instability in all planes. An arthroscopic cannula is placed in the superomedial or superolateral portal for inflow and outflow, and the arthroscope is introduced into the inferolateral portal. Although many examination sequences are possible, it is important to visualize the suprapatellar pouch, patellofemoral joint, medial and lateral gutters, medial and lateral compartments (meniscus and articular cartilage), and intercondylar notch (cruciate ligaments) in all patients. Accessory viewing portals are established as necessary if other areas need to be evaluated. After a complete evaluation of the joint (Fig. 1–3), all surgical pathology is addressed.

COMPLICATIONS

Complications of knee arthroscopy are often procedure specific. General complications include inadvertent damage to intra-articular structures (especially articular

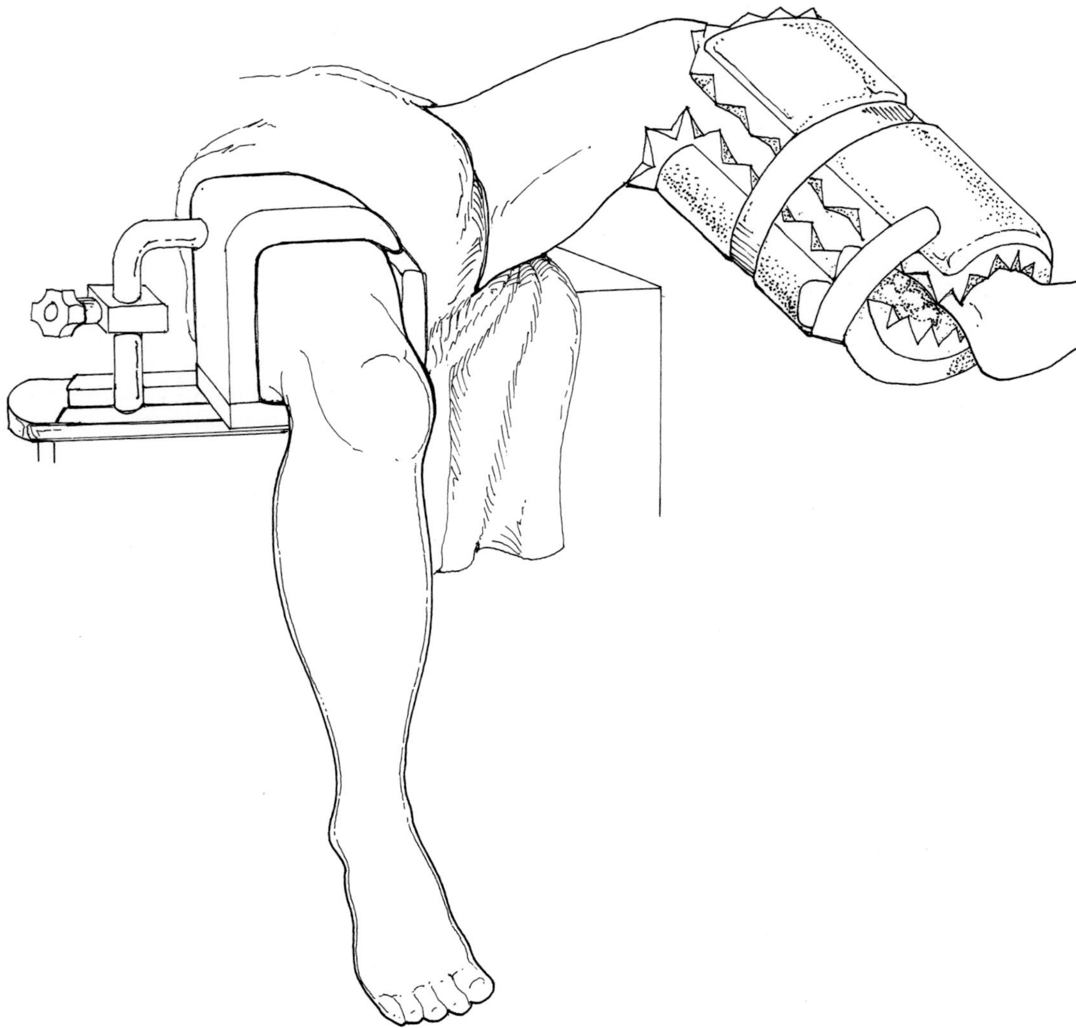

FIGURE 1–1. Setup for standard knee arthroscopy. The affected leg is positioned in a leg holder, and the opposite leg is placed in a well-padded leg holder (such as a GU leg holder).

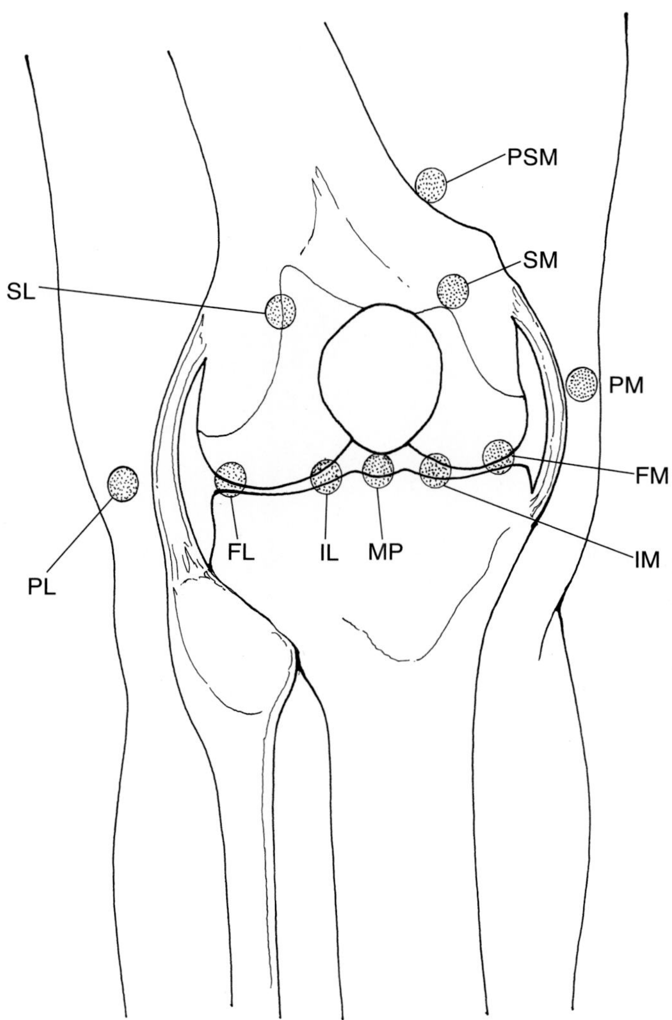

FIGURE 1–2. Arthroscopic knee portals. FL, far lateral; FM, far medial; IL, inferolateral; IM, inferomedial; MP, midpatellar; PL, posterolateral; PM, posteromedial; PSM, proximal superomedial; SL, superolateral; SM, superomedial.

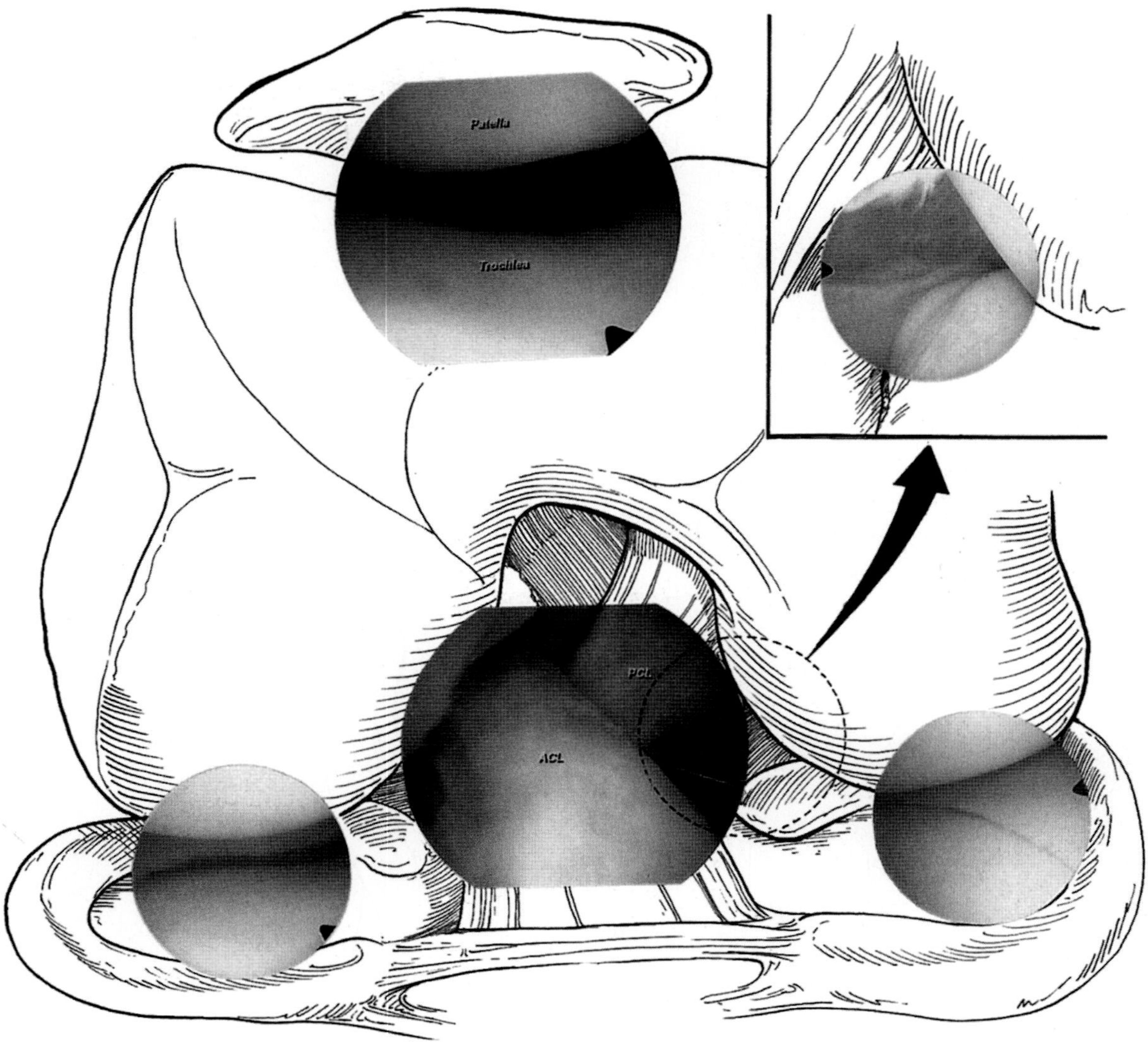

FIGURE 1–3. Normal arthroscopic anatomy of the knee. ACL, anterior cruciate ligament; PCL, posterior cruciate ligament. (From Miller MD, Osborne JR, Warner JJP, Fu FH: Knee arthroscopy. In MRI-Arthroscopy Correlative Atlas. Philadelphia, WB Saunders, 1997, pp 44–53.)

cartilage), instrument breakage, tourniquet problems, and extravasation of fluid. The last-mentioned occurs most commonly with the use of an arthroscopic pump but also may be a result of capsular injury. If fluid extravasation is suspected, the inflow should be turned off, and compartment pressures should be monitored. Most of these pressures spontaneously resolve with simple observation in a controlled environment. Other complications include synovial fistula (best treated with immobilization and antibiotics), hemarthrosis, neurovascular injuries, and other complications that are common with all knee procedures (e.g., deep venous thrombosis, infection, and reflex sympathetic dystrophy).

REFERENCES

DiGiovine NM, Bradley JP: Arthroscopic equipment and setup. In Fu FH, Harner CE, Vince KG (eds): Knee Surgery. Baltimore, Williams & Wilkins, 1994, pp 543–556.

Gold DL, Schaner PJ, Sapega AA: The posteromedial portal in knee arthroscopy: An analysis of diagnostic and surgical utility. Arthroscopy 11:139–145, 1995.

Jensen JE, Conn RR, Hazelrigg G, Hewell JE: Symptomatic evaluation of acute knee injuries. Clin Sports Med 4:295, 1985.

Miller MD, Osborne JR, Warner JJP, Fu FH: Knee arthroscopy. In MRI-Arthroscopy Correlative Atlas. Philadelphia, WB Saunders, 1997, pp 44–53.

CHAPTER 2

Partial Meniscectomy

INTRODUCTION

Treatment of meniscal pathology is a common application of arthroscopy. Meniscal tears represent approximately 50% of knee injuries that require surgery. The medial meniscus is involved most commonly. Classification of meniscal tears usually is based on the appearance and orientation of the tear (Fig. 2–1). Treatment of these injuries includes partial meniscectomy for central or degenerative tears and meniscal repair for peripheral tears (see Chapter 4).

HISTORY AND PHYSICAL EXAMINATION

It is helpful to consider patients with meniscal tears in two groups. The first group includes predominantly younger patients who sustain a twisting injury during sports with subsequent joint line pain. Swelling, loss of motion, catching with weight bearing, and other mechanical signs and symptoms are common. These patients often require surgical intervention and should be considered candidates for meniscal repair. The second group, consisting of an older population, may have a more insidious onset of pain with fewer mechanical symptoms. Patients in this second group are more likely to have degenerative tears that are less amenable to repair and may require partial meniscectomy.

Examination begins with evaluation for an effusion, evaluation of range of motion, checking for joint line tenderness, and assessment of ligamentous laxity. Meniscal cysts, which are associated most commonly with horizontal cleavage tears that are not repairable, sometimes can be palpated or seen by transillumination. Provocative (rotational) testing includes McMurray and Adson tests and duck-walking (Fig. 2–2).

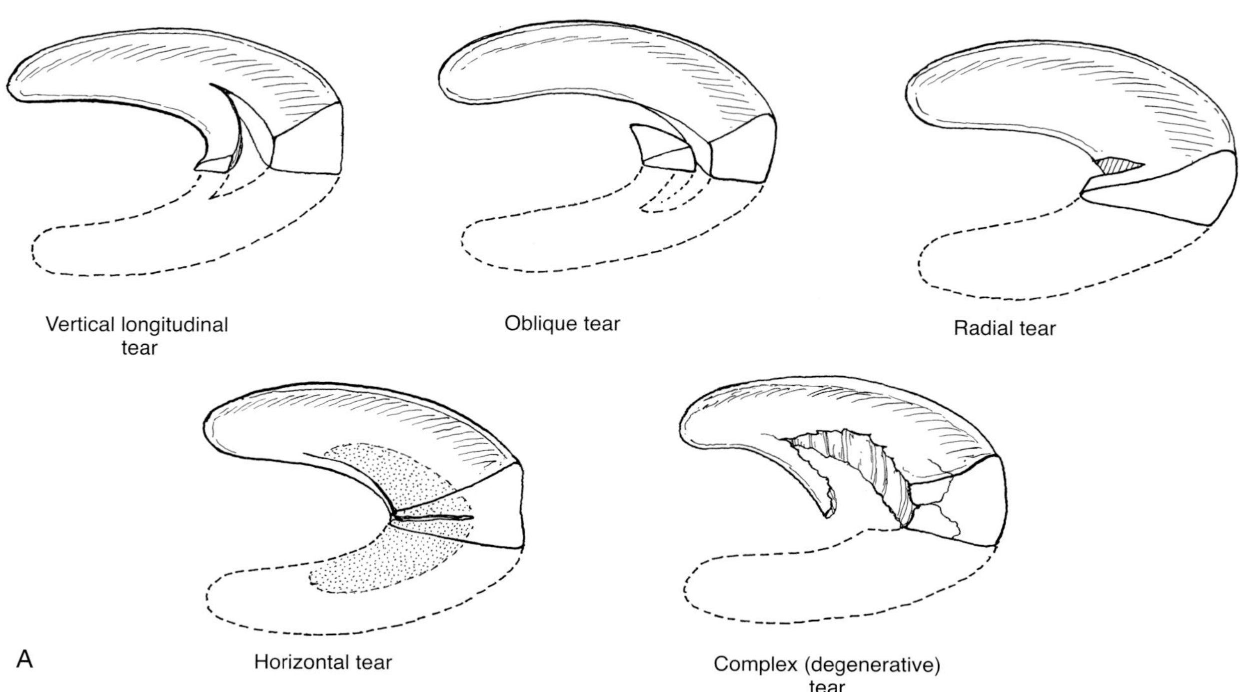

FIGURE 2–1. Tear nomenclature *(A)* and suggested resection *(B)*.

Illustration continued on following page

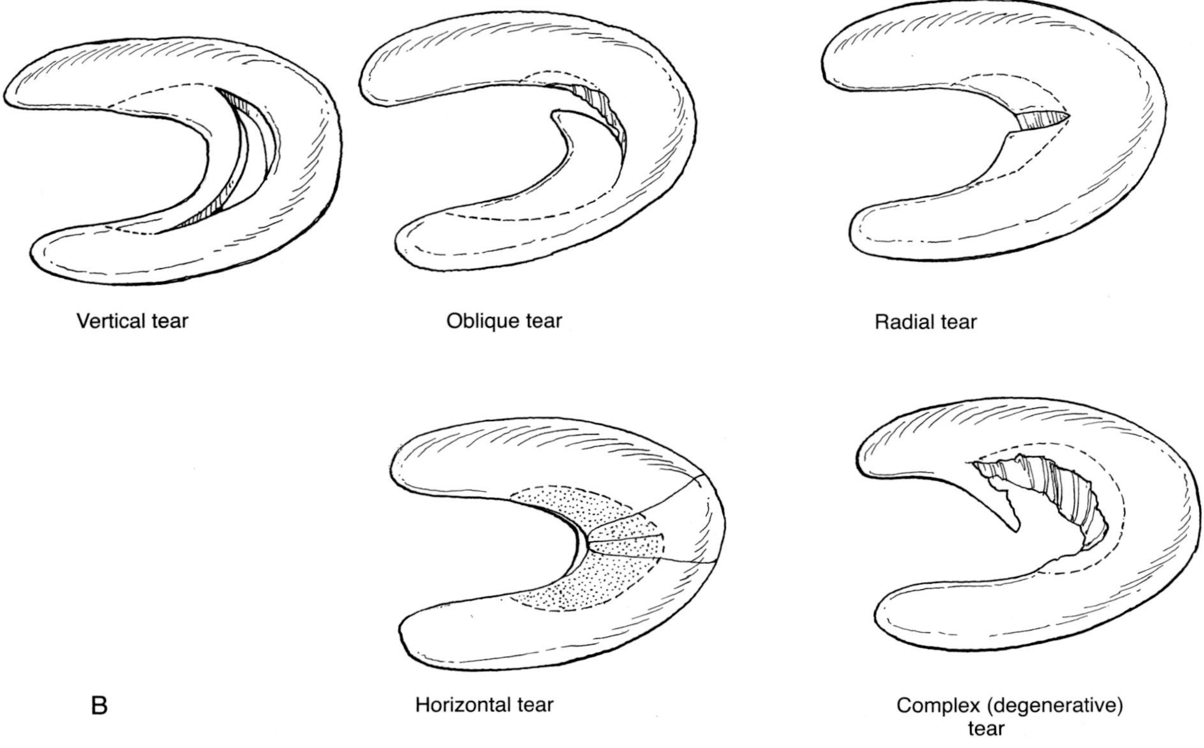

FIGURE 2–1 *Continued*

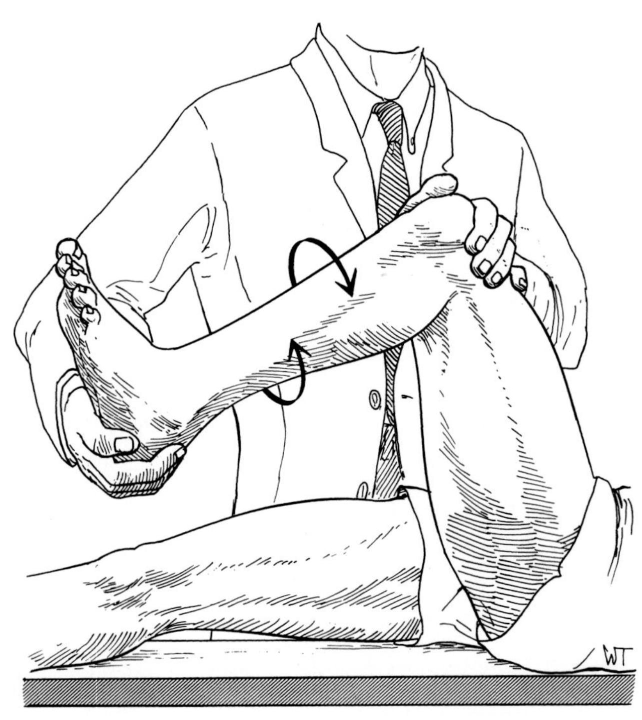

FIGURE 2–2. Provocative testing for meniscal tears. *A*, McMurray test. *B*, Apley compression test. *C*, Steinmann test. (From Insall JN: Examination of the knee. In Insall JN [ed]: Surgery of the Knee. New York, Churchill Livingstone, 1984, pp 55–72.)

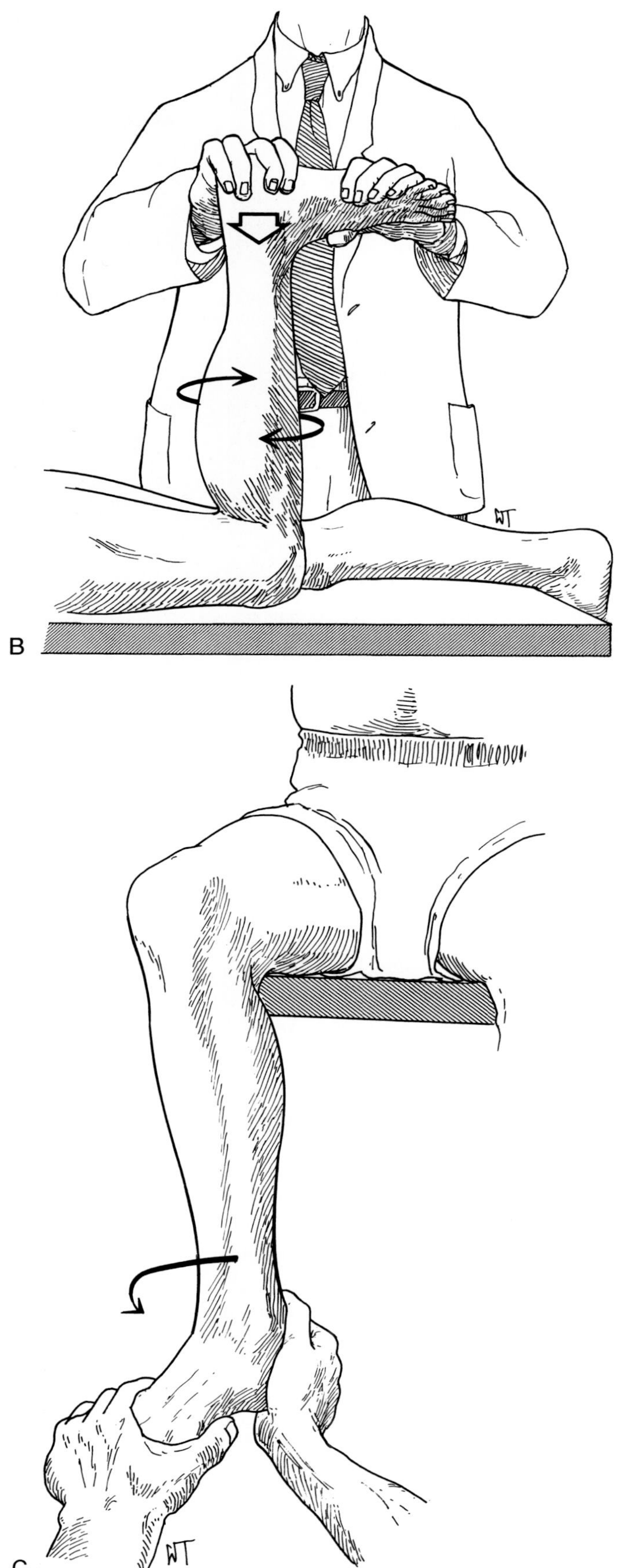

FIGURE 2–2 *Continued*

DIAGNOSTIC IMAGING

Plain radiographs are usually normal. The flexion posteroanterior weight-bearing radiograph (Rosenberg) (Fig. 2–3) is an important view, particularly in older patients with concomitant arthritis. Although its routine use is controversial, MRI is highly accurate in confirming the presence of meniscal tears (Fig. 2–4).

NONOPERATIVE MANAGEMENT

Many patients with clinically suspected meniscal tears improve with time. MRI of these injuries may reveal subchondral contusions, unsuspected collateral ligament injuries, or other problems. Although it is not clear why, small peripheral meniscal tears may heal spontaneously with nonoperative management. Degenerative tears, although not likely to heal, may become less symptomatic or asymptomatic with time. Most surgeons recommend a quadriceps-strengthening program and at least a brief period of nonoperative management before considering arthroscopy in patients with suspected meniscal tears. Ultimately, the patient must choose the final treatment plan.

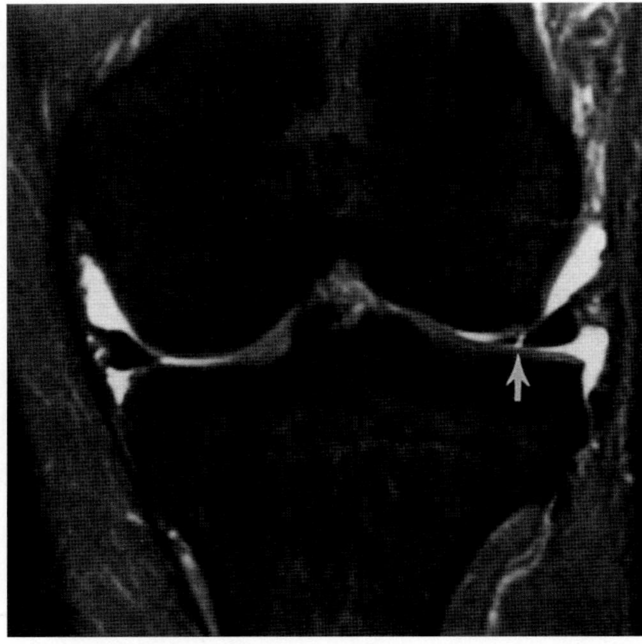

FIGURE 2–4. Coronal fat-suppressed proton-density fat-saturation echo MRI shows a radial tear *(arrow)* in the lateral meniscus. (From Osborne JR, Abraham WP, Forte MD: Magnetic resonance imaging of knee menisci: Diagnostic interpretation and pitfalls. Op Tech Orthop 5:10–19, 1995.)

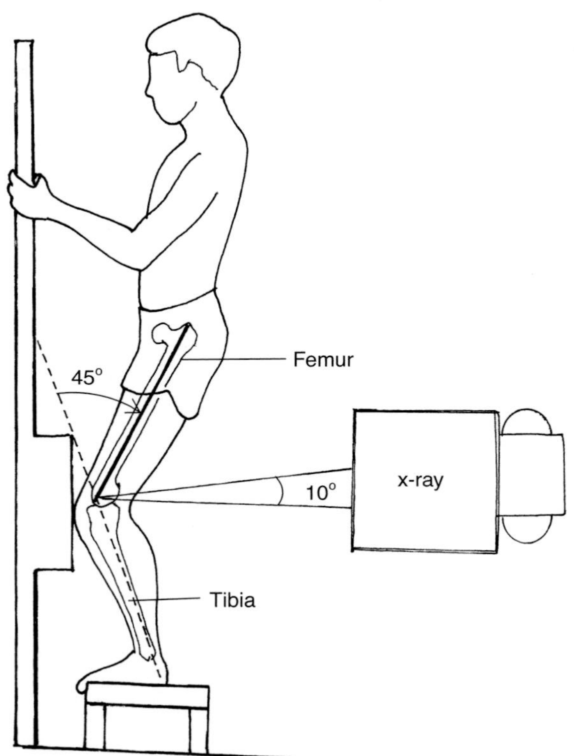

FIGURE 2–3. Flexion weight-bearing (Rosenberg) view for evaluating subtle knee arthritis.

RELEVANT ANATOMY

Standard arthroscopic portals are usually adequate for doing an arthroscopic partial meniscectomy. A posteromedial portal is helpful in evaluating peripheral tears of the posterior horn of the medial meniscus. Infrapatellar branches of the saphenous nerve can be injured during placement of anteromedial portals, but this is usually not a problem of clinical consequence.

SURGICAL *TECHNIQUE*

1. Positioning: The patient is positioned for knee arthroscopy. A tourniquet is applied but rarely inflated.
2. Diagnostic arthroscopy: Meniscal repair should be considered if possible (see Chapter 4). Certain tears are not repairable, however, and partial meniscectomy is required.
3. Partial meniscectomy: The technique varies based on the type of tear.
   a. Degenerative tears: Baskets and shavers are used to trim the meniscus back to a stable rim (Fig. 2–5). Yellowish tissue, which represents *mucoid degeneration* within the meniscus, may re-tear at a later date.

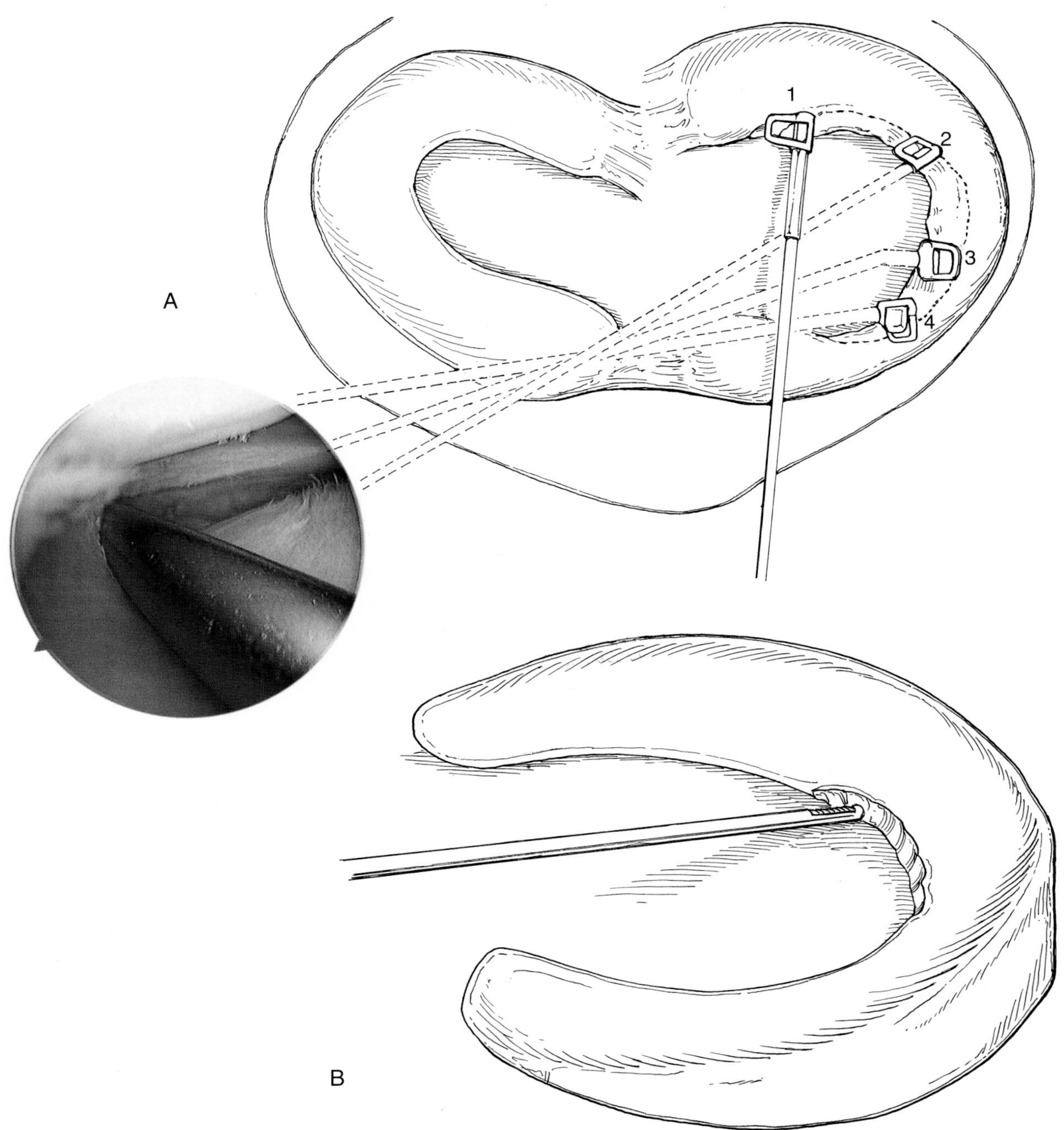

FIGURE 2–5. Arthroscopic resection of a degenerative tear. *A*, When the tear is characterized, different biters are used to resect the torn portion. Various angled biters and different portals should be used. *B*, The tear is smoothed with a 4.5-mm shaver, placed in direct opposition to the meniscus.

Illustration continued on following page

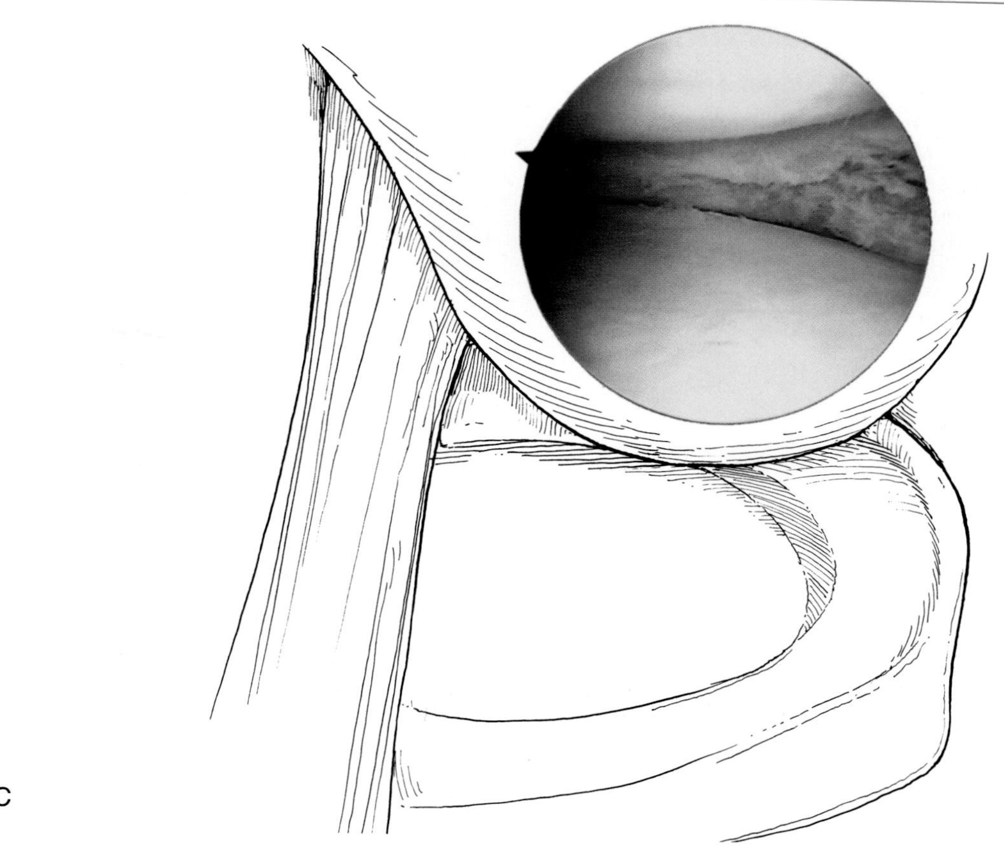

FIGURE 2–5 *Continued. C*, Final result.

b. Radial and flap tears: Baskets and shavers can be used to trim the affected area and allow for a smooth transition from torn to intact meniscus (Fig. 2–6).

c. Horizontal tears: Baskets and shavers can be used to trim these tears back to a stable rim. It is often possible to preserve one of the two *leaves* of the tear and remove the most degenerative or the

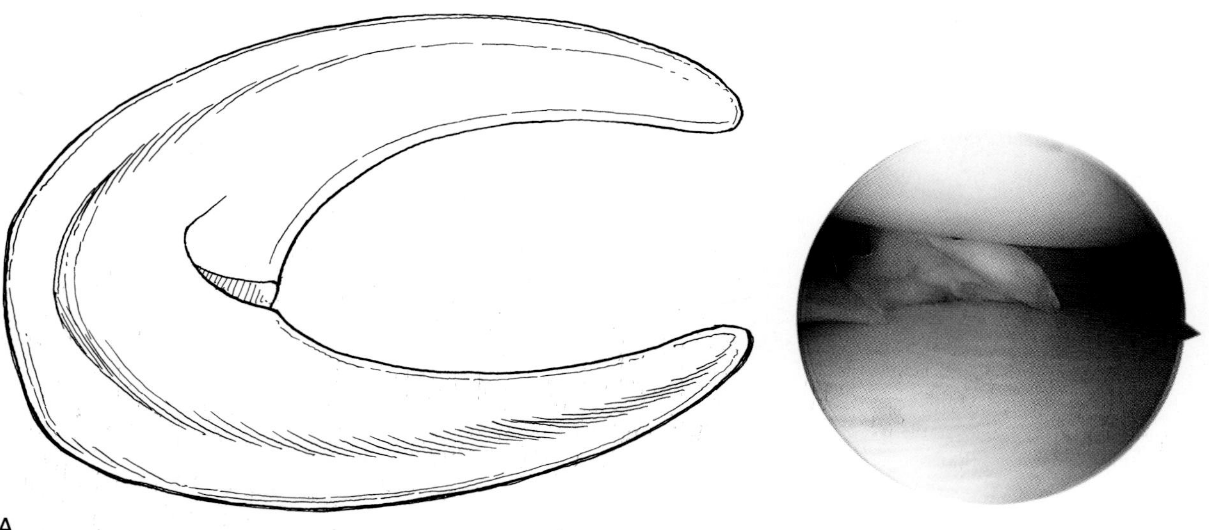

FIGURE 2–6. Arthroscopic resection of a radial/flap tear. *A*, Tear in situ.

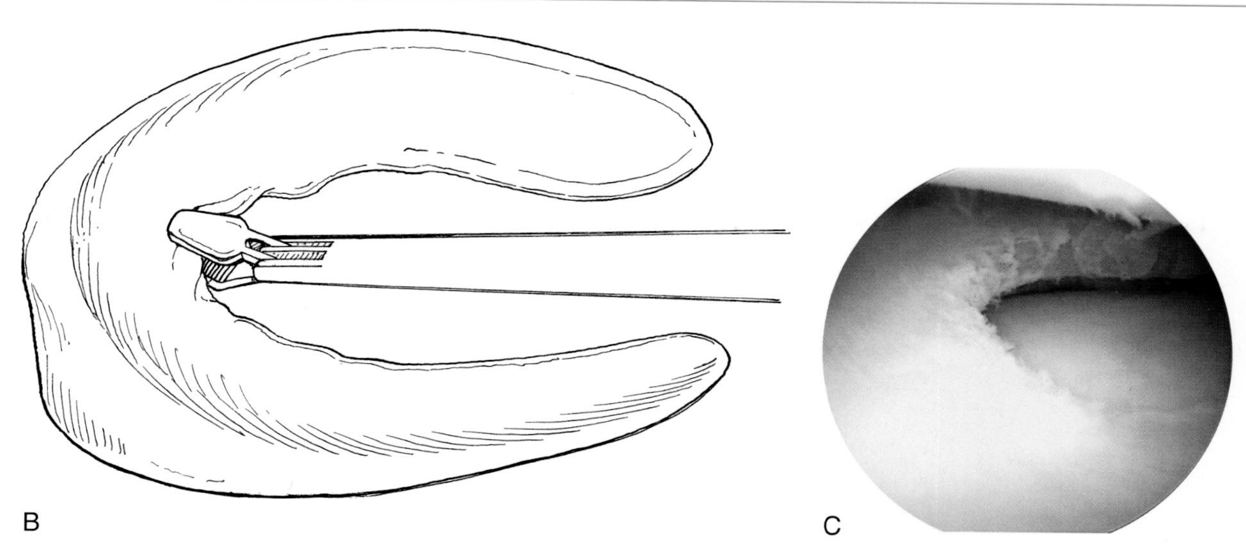

FIGURE 2–6 *Continued. B,* Initial resection. *C,* Arthroscopic image of final result.

smallest leaf. In patients with an associated meniscal cyst, the meniscus can be trimmed, and the cyst can be decompressed arthroscopically (Fig. 2–7).

d. Bucket-handle tears: These tears should be repaired whenever possible. For irreparable tears, one end of the tear is incised, leaving a small bridge of meniscus. The other end is completely incised, and a grabber is used to remove the meniscus by avulsing the bridge. The meniscus is trimmed with baskets and a shaver to allow for a smooth transition zone (Fig. 2–8).

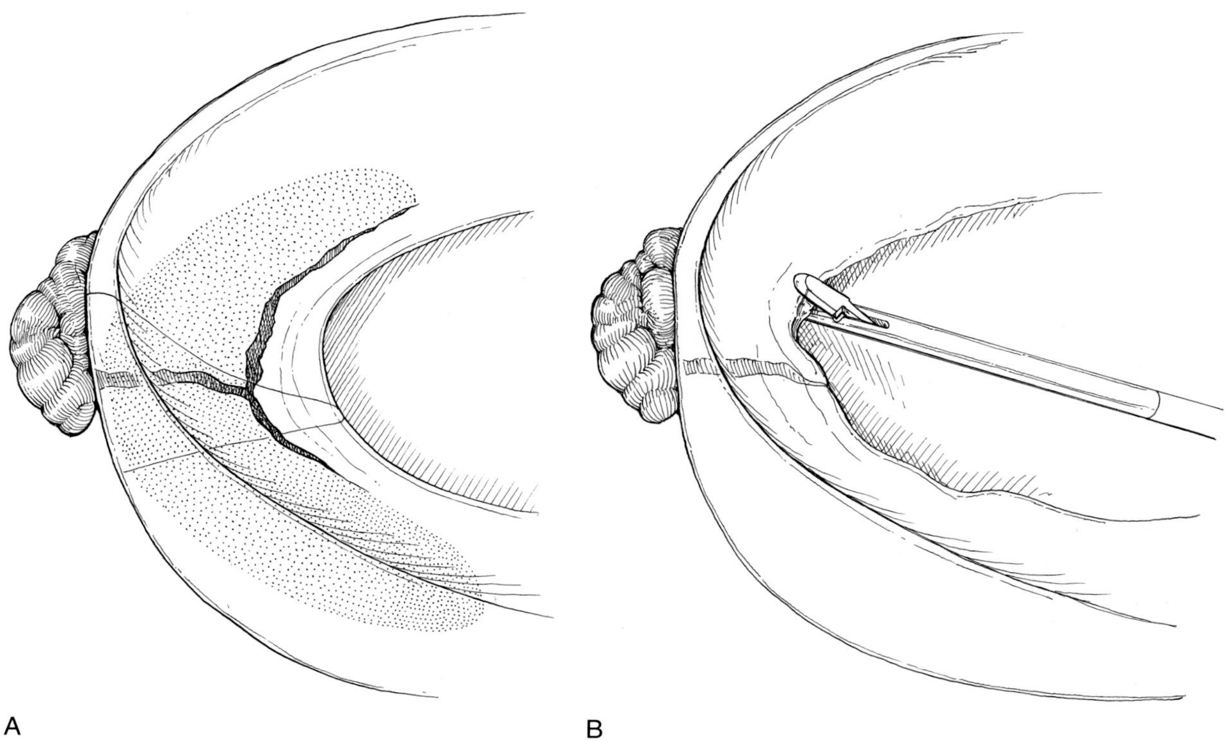

FIGURE 2–7. Arthroscopic resection and decompression of a meniscal cyst. *A,* Cyst in situ. *B,* Initial meniscectomy.

Illustration continued on following page

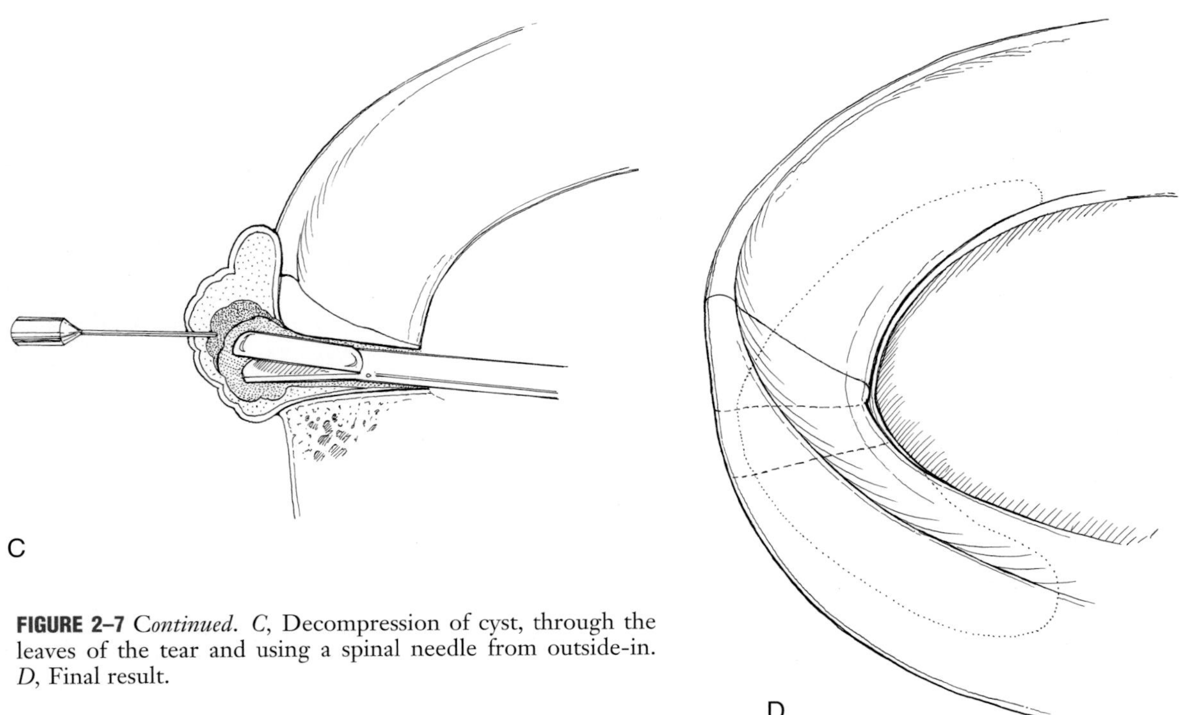

FIGURE 2–7 *Continued. C,* Decompression of cyst, through the leaves of the tear and using a spinal needle from outside-in. *D,* Final result.

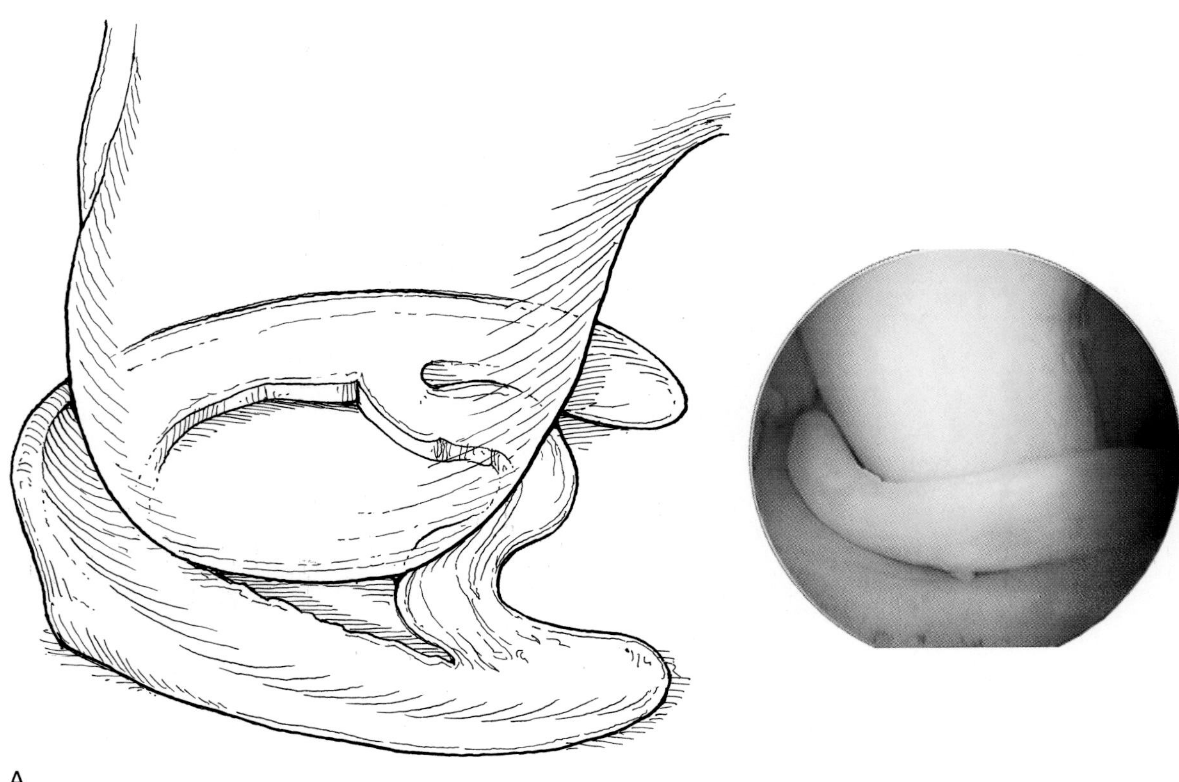

FIGURE 2–8. Arthroscopic partial meniscectomy of a bucket-handle tear of the meniscus. Most of these tears should be repaired. *A,* Tear displaced into the notch.

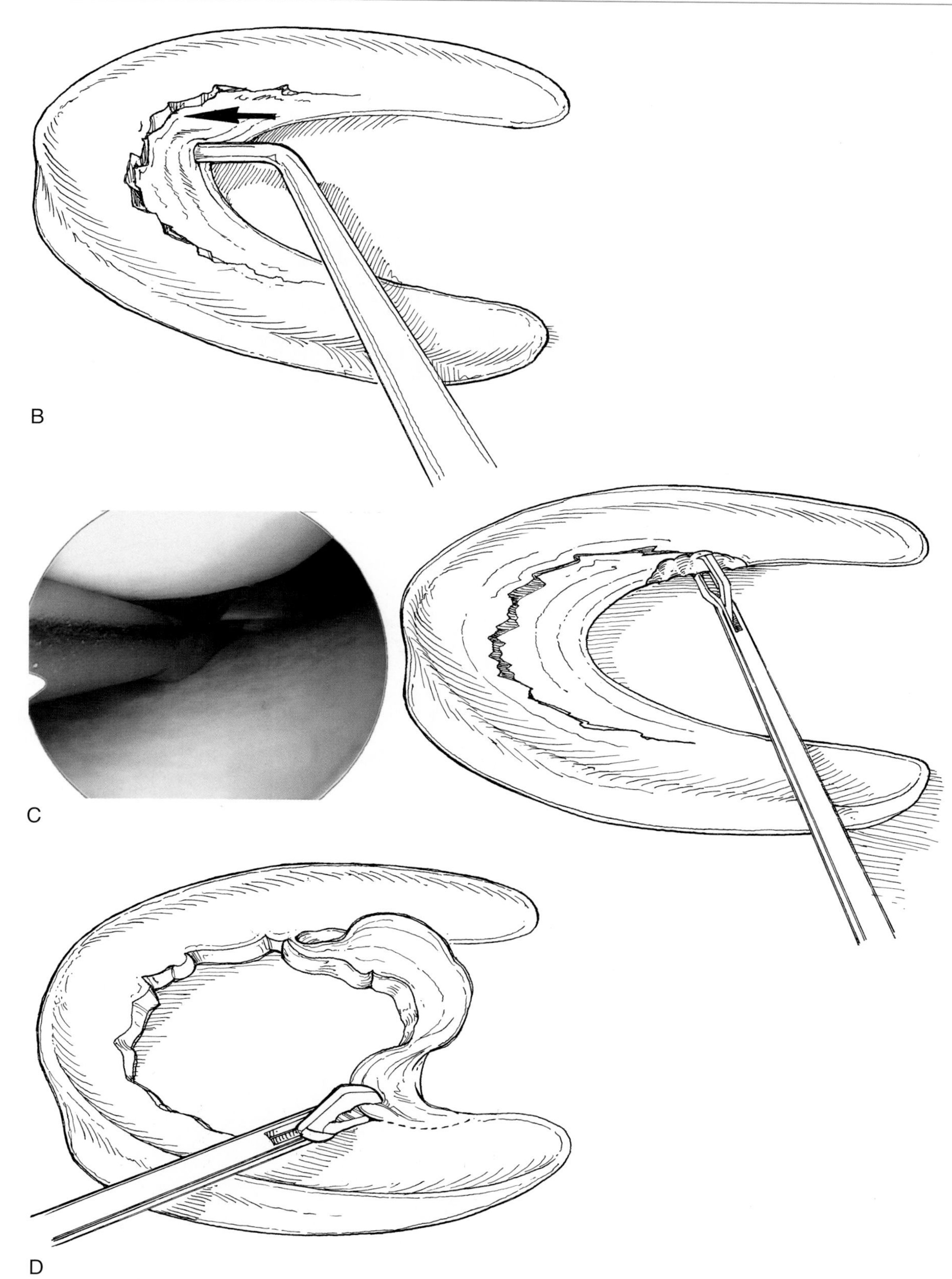

FIGURE 2–8 *Continued. B*, Reduction of tear. *C*, Initial resection of posterior portion of tear. *D*, Complete resection of anterior portion of tear.

Illustration continued on following page

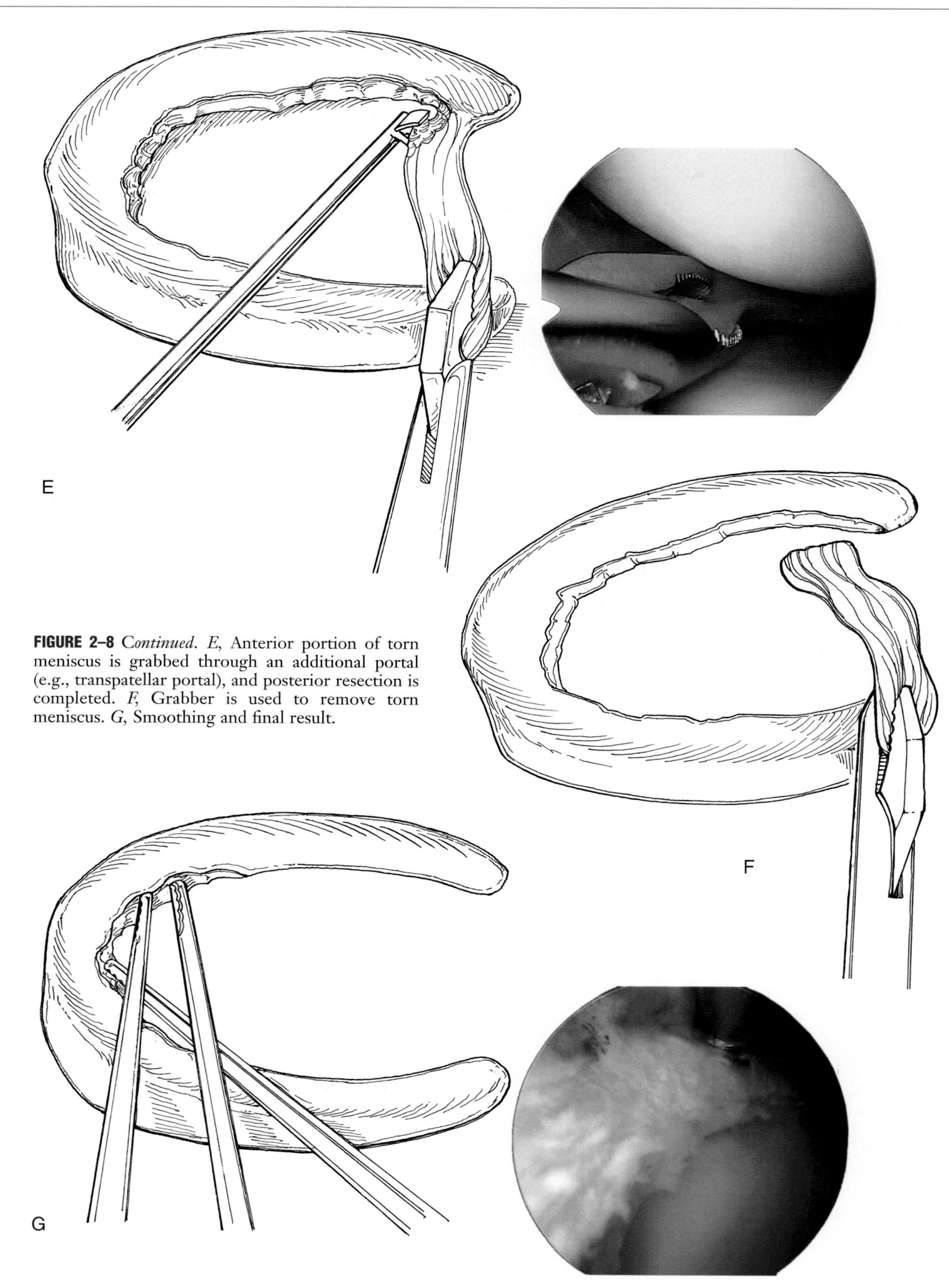

FIGURE 2–8 *Continued. E,* Anterior portion of torn meniscus is grabbed through an additional portal (e.g., transpatellar portal), and posterior resection is completed. *F,* Grabber is used to remove torn meniscus. *G,* Smoothing and final result.

POSTOPERATIVE MANAGEMENT

Postoperative management after partial meniscectomies usually involves application of a soft dressing (which can be changed to simple adhesive bandages [Band-Aids] after a couple of days) and crutches for comfort. Patients quickly advance their weight-bearing status as tolerated and begin a quadriceps rehabilitation program in the early postoperative period. The wounds are checked once during the first or second postoperative week, sutures are removed, and rehabilitation is continued. Sports are allowed when the knee has full range of motion, there is no effusion, and the quadriceps and hamstrings have normal strength.

COMPLICATIONS

Complications after arthroscopic partial meniscal removal are unusual. Infections are rare because of the large amount of fluid used during the procedure. Instruments occasionally can break during the procedure, necessitating removal of the broken pieces, but this too is unusual. Articular cartilage injury occurs commonly during insertion of arthroscopic equipment and instruments, and extreme care must be taken to avoid such injury. Intraoperative problems include fluid extravasation, which can be caused by malposition or soft tissue obstruction of the outflow cannula. Other postoperative complications, such as deep vein thrombosis, neurapraxias, fistulas, and other wound problems, also can occur.

RESULTS

Several studies showed improved short-term and intermediate-term results of arthroscopic partial meniscectomy compared with open total meniscectomy. Long-term results are still unknown but undoubtedly will be related to the amount of meniscus removed and the presence of other intra-articular pathology.

REFERENCES

Bardana DD, Burks RT: Meniscectomy: Is there still a role? Op Tech Orthop 10:183–193, 2000.

Bolano LE, Grana WA: Isolated arthroscopic partial meniscectomy: Functional radiographic evaluation at five years. Am J Sports Med 21:432–437, 1993.

Burks RT, Metcalf MH, Metcalf RW: Fifteen-year follow-up of arthroscopic partial meniscectomy. Arthroscopy 13:673–679, 1997.

Cicotti MG, Shields CL, El Attrache NS: Meniscectomy. In Fu FH, Harner CD, Vince KG (eds): Knee Surgery. Baltimore, Williams & Wilkins, 1994, pp 591–613.

Hinkin DT: Arthroscopic partial meniscectomy. Op Tech Orthop 5:28–38, 1995.

CHAPTER 3

Discoid Meniscus

INTRODUCTION

Discoid menisci are abnormally shaped and cover more of the surface of the tibial plateau than normal. They have been classified into three types: incomplete, complete, and the so-called Wrisberg variant (Fig. 3–1). The Wrisberg variant is perhaps better termed a *lateral meniscal variant* with absence of the posterior coronary ligament. This variant may be responsible for the so-called popping or snapping knee syndrome and is treated best with meniscal repair. It is not considered further in this chapter.

HISTORY AND PHYSICAL EXAMINATION

Most patients with complete and incomplete discoid menisci are asymptomatic. Torn discoid menisci present with signs, symptoms, and examination findings described in Chapter 2.

DIAGNOSTIC IMAGING

Plain radiographs may suggest the presence of a discoid meniscus with squaring of the lateral femoral condyle, joint space widening, cupping of the lateral aspect of the tibial plateau, a high fibular head, and hypoplasia of the lateral intercondylar spine, although these findings are unusual. MRI can be helpful in the diagnosis if three or more continuous 5-mm sagittal sections show continuity of the anterior and posterior horns of the meniscus (Fig. 3–2).

NONOPERATIVE MANAGEMENT

Nonoperative management is the treatment of choice for asymptomatic discoid menisci. If discoid menisci are discovered incidentally during arthroscopy and there is no associated tear, they should be left alone.

RELEVANT ANATOMY

Treatment of discoid menisci can be accomplished through standard arthroscopic portals.

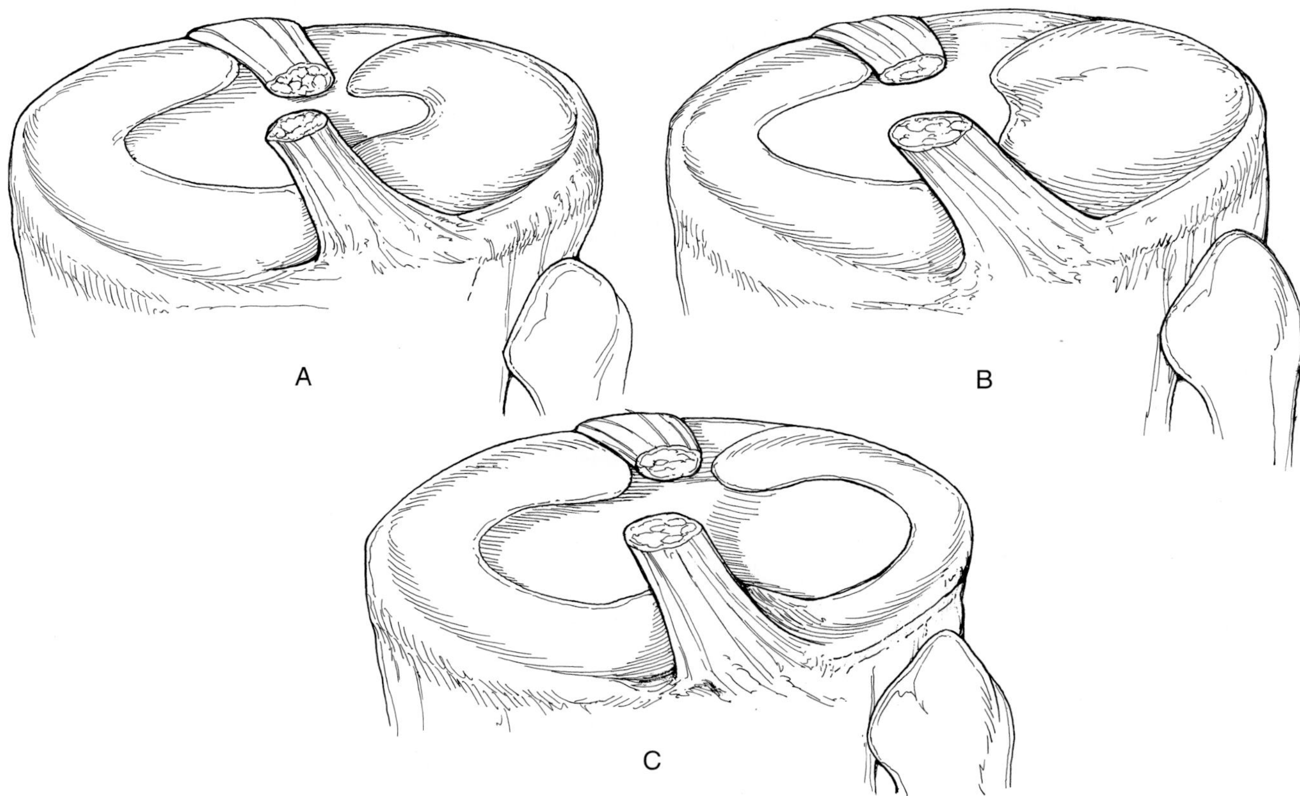

FIGURE 3–1. Classification of discoid menisci. *A*, Incomplete. *B*, Complete. *C*, Wrisberg variant (lateral meniscal variant with absence of the posterior coronary ligament).

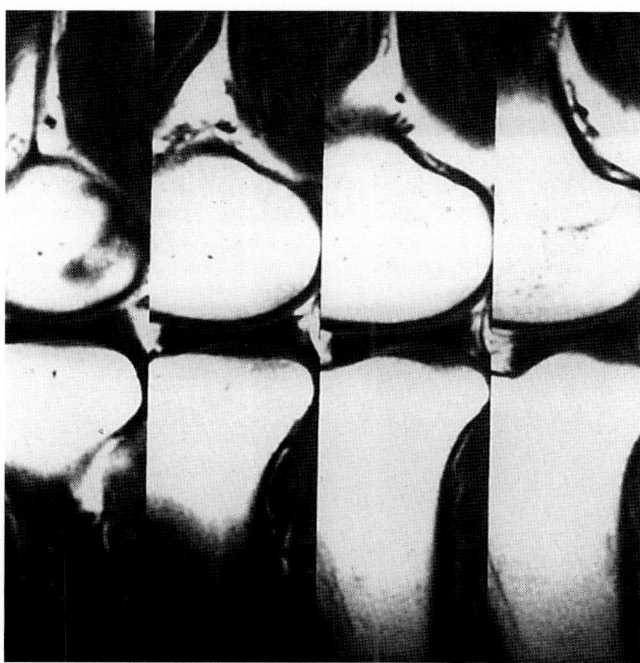

FIGURE 3–2. MRI of a discoid lateral meniscus. On the sagittal T1-weighted images, the lateral meniscus maintains the bow-tie configuration for three or more images. Images are from left to right, peripheral margin to free margin. (From Osborne JR, Abraham WP, Forte MD: Magnetic resonance imaging of knee menisci: Diagnostic interpretation and pitfalls. Op Tech Orthop 5:10–19, 1995.)

SURGICAL TECHNIQUE

Overview

Treatment options involve removal of torn fragments and repair of unstable menisci (Fig. 3–3).

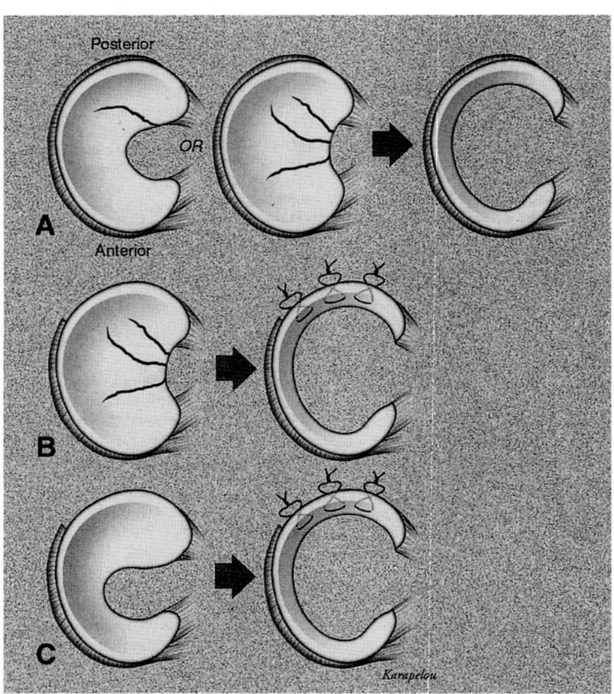

FIGURE 3–3. Surgical options. *A*, Partial excision of stable discoid meniscus. *B*, Partial excision and repair of unstable discoid meniscus. *C*, Partial excision of large posterior horn and repair of unstable discoid meniscus. (From Jordan MR: Lateral meniscus variants. Op Tech Orthop 10:234–244, 2000.)

Indications

Surgery is indicated for symptomatic tear of a discoid meniscus.

Technique

Recommended treatment for complete and incomplete discoid menisci with a tear is an arthroscopic partial meniscectomy, or *saucerization*. This can be accomplished with a one-piece excision or piecemeal.

One-Piece Excision

One-piece excision is done using an arthroscopic blade of scissors (Fig. 3–4). The anterior, middle, and posterior segments of the lateral meniscus are sequentially incised. The posterior attachment and the anterior horn are released, and the meniscus is removed with a grasper. The meniscus is contoured with baskets and an arthroscopic shaver.

Piecemeal Excision

Piecemeal excision is accomplished by first removing the anterior portion with a meniscal blade or a side-cutting basket. Various other baskets can be introduced from alternative portals to contour the meniscus (Fig. 3–5).

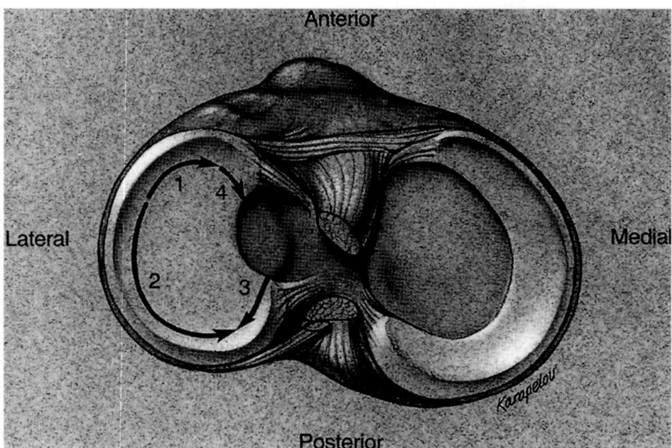

FIGURE 3–4. One-piece excision of a discoid lateral meniscus. Sequence of cuts is shown before removal of the entire fragment. (From Neuschwander DC: Discoid meniscus. Op Tech Orthop 5:78–87, 1995.)

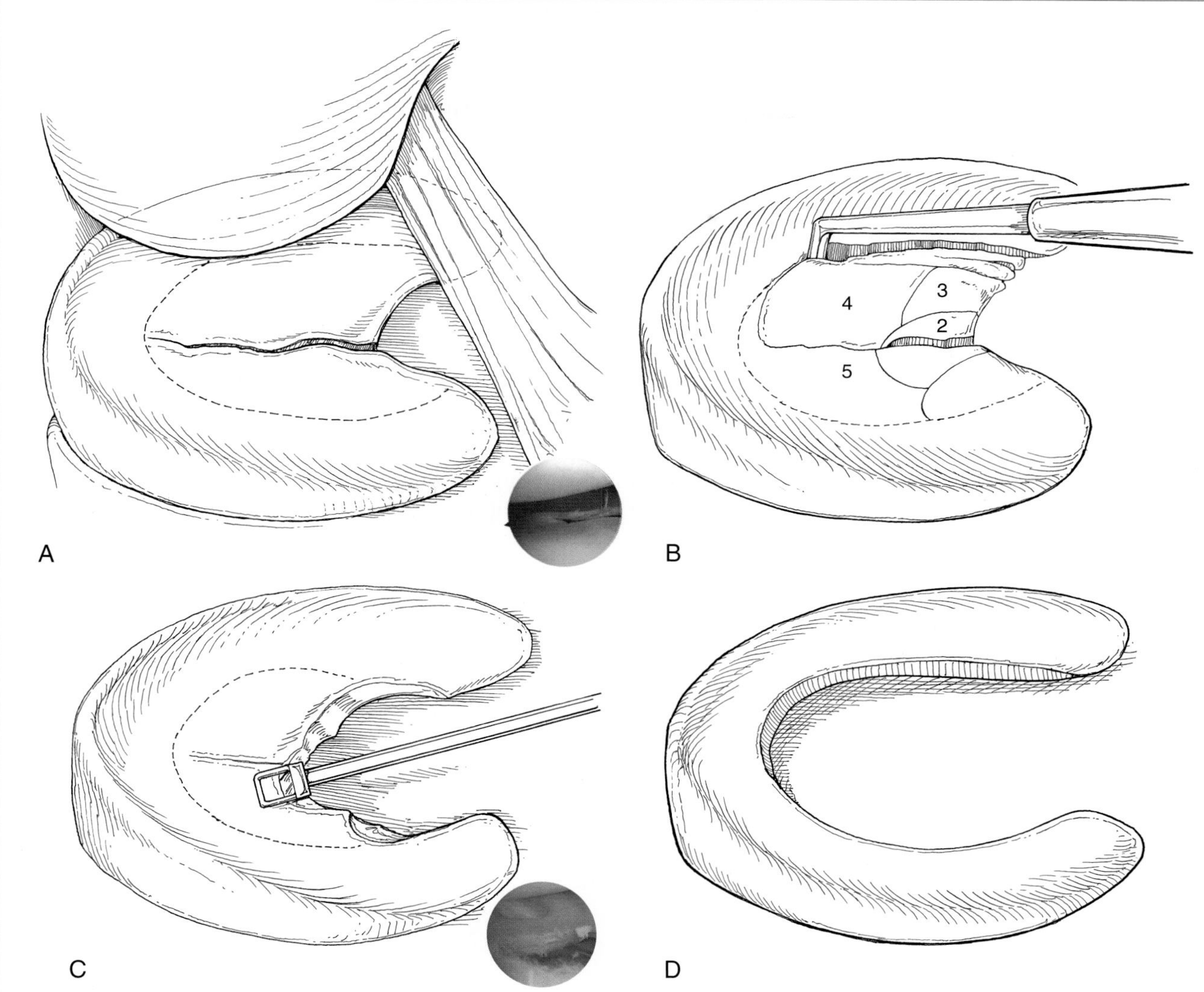

FIGURE 3–5. Piecemeal excision of torn discoid meniscus. *A*, Tear and planned resection. *B–D*, Resection using blade and baskets.

POSTOPERATIVE MANAGEMENT

Patients are allowed to progress quickly as in partial meniscectomy. Crutches, pain medications, and ice are helpful in early postoperative management.

COMPLICATIONS

Because there is limited space in a compartment filled with meniscus, additional care is required when inserting and using arthroscopic tools to avoid cartilage injury. Other complications are similar to those for partial meniscectomy.

RESULTS

Intermediate-term results with arthroscopic techniques are encouraging, but longer term results are needed. Open techniques had good early results, but long-term results were less satisfactory. It is hoped that arthroscopic techniques with preservation of intact menisci will yield better long-term results. Older patients with preexisting chondrosis have a worse prognosis.

REFERENCES

Dickhaut SC, DeLee JC: The discoid lateral-meniscus syndrome. J Bone Joint Surg [Am] 64:1068–1073, 1982.

Jordan MR: Lateral meniscal variants. Op Tech Orthop 10:234–244, 2000.

Neuschwander DC: Discoid meniscus. Op Tech Orthop 5:78–87, 1995.

Neuschwander DC, Drez D, Finney TP: Lateral meniscal variant with absence of the posterior coronary ligament. J Bone Joint Surg [Am] 74:1186–1190, 1992.

Vandermeer RD, Cunningham FK: Arthroscopic treatment of the discoid lateral meniscus: Results of long-term follow-up. Arthroscopy 5:101–109, 1989.

CHAPTER 4

Meniscus Repair

INTRODUCTION

Because of the predictable adverse consequences of meniscectomy, most notably late arthrosis, meniscus repair increasingly has been advocated. Several techniques have been developed for meniscus repair. The indications for repair have been expanded by many surgeons with a goal of saving the meniscus whenever possible.

HISTORY AND PHYSICAL EXAMINATION

The presentation and examination findings in patients with torn menisci are presented in Chapter 2. Peripheral meniscal tears, which are more amenable to repair, are more likely to have an associated hemarthrosis. These tears also are more likely to occur during sports (especially football, soccer, basketball, and wrestling) and usually involve the medial meniscus (except wrestling injuries, which more often are lateral). Associated tears of the anterior cruciate ligament (ACL) are common (and lateral meniscal tears are more common with acute ACL injuries).

DIAGNOSTIC IMAGING

Plain radiographs are usually unremarkable. MRI sometimes can be helpful in evaluating whether tears are repairable (Fig. 4–1). More peripheral tears without degenerative or stellate patterns are more suitable for repair. The addition of contrast material is helpful in evaluating menisci that were repaired previously because it can help determine if the tear is healed and the presence of new tears (Fig. 4–2).

NONOPERATIVE MANAGEMENT

Some smaller tears may heal spontaneously. Larger tears and particularly displaced bucket-handle tears should be treated with early operative intervention.

RELEVANT ANATOMY

It is crucial to appreciate the location of the common peroneal nerve (laterally) and branches of the saphenous nerve (medially) in relation to planned incision (Fig. 4–3).

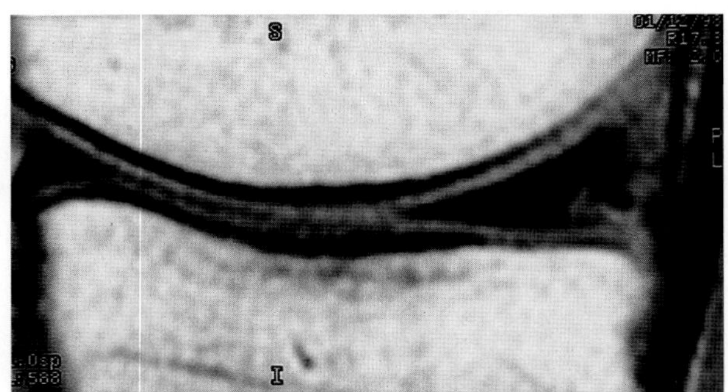

FIGURE 4–1. Sagittal proton-density MRI shows a peripheral meniscal tear that was confirmed arthroscopically.

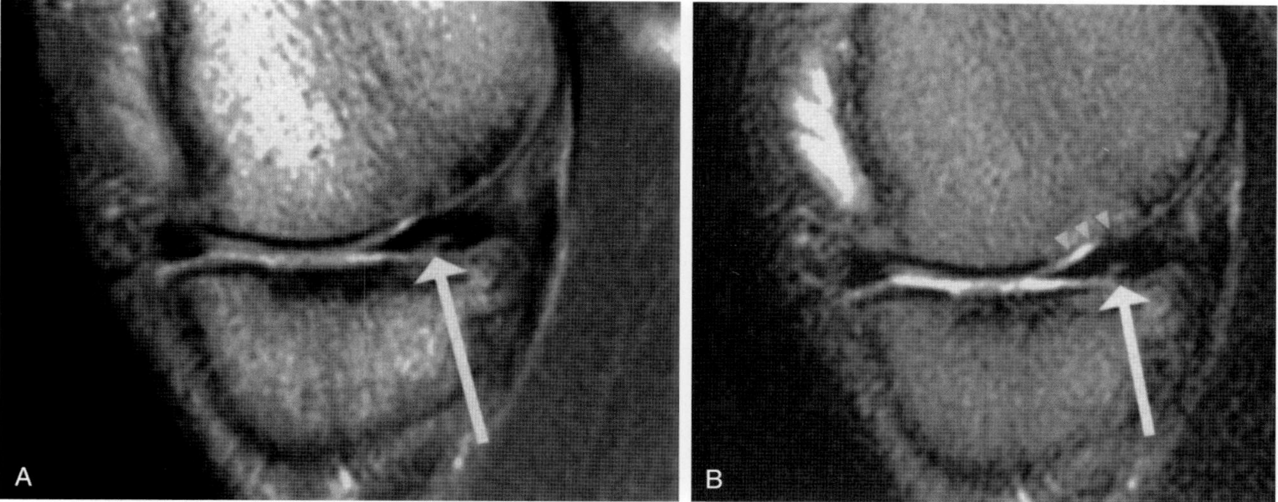

FIGURE 4–2. Administration of intra-articular gadolinium sometimes can be helpful in patients with previous meniscal surgery. *A*, Sagittal proton-density image of a patient status-post meniscal repair. This image was read as a re-tear *(arrow)*. *B*, Sagittal T2-weighted image of the same patient after intra-articular administration of gadolinium. The contrast material does not enter the repair site *(arrow)*, and this image was read correctly as a healed meniscus. This patient also has a full-thickness chondral defect *(arrowheads)*, which may have been responsible for recurrent symptoms. (From Sanders TG, Fults-Gary KA: Magnetic resonance imaging and knee menisci: Diagnostic interpretation and pitfalls. Op Tech Orthop 10:169–182, 2000.)

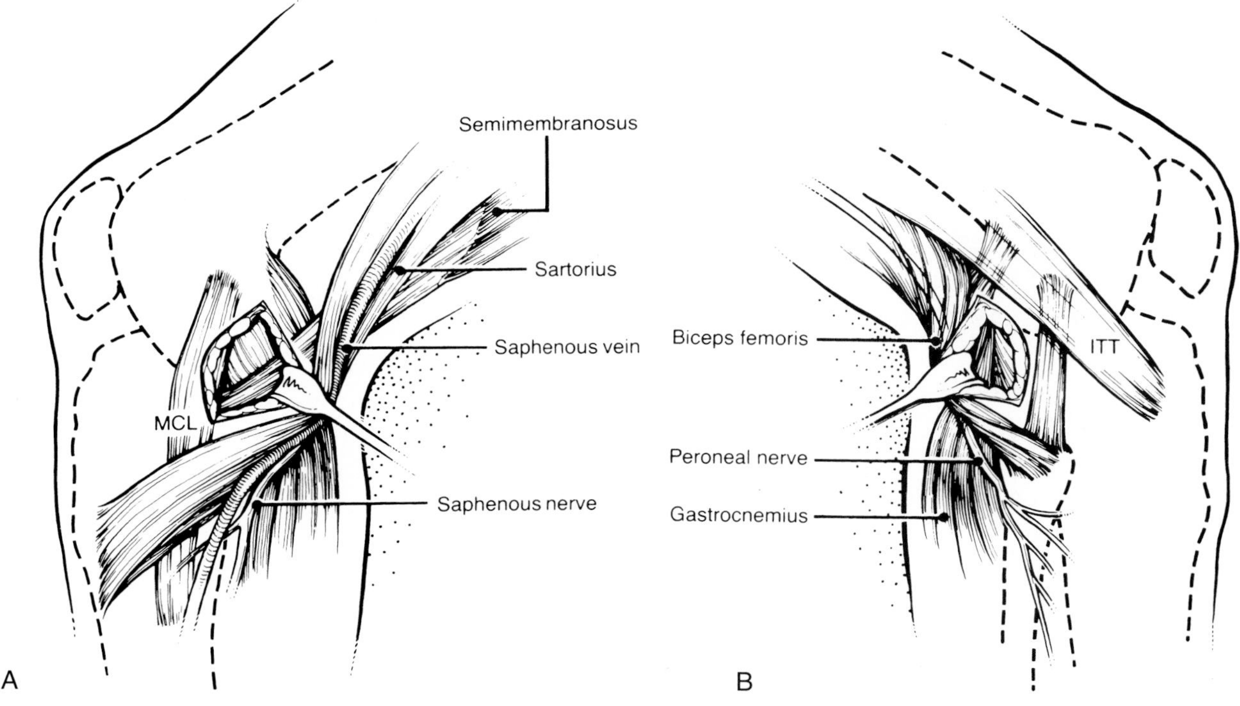

FIGURE 4–3. Anatomy of the medial and lateral knee in relation to incisions for meniscal repair. *A*, Lateral. *B*, Medial. ITT, iliotibial tract; MCL, medial collateral ligament. (From Scott WN [ed]: Arthroscopy of the Knee. Philadelphia, WB Saunders, 1990.)

SURGICAL *TECHNIQUE*

Indications

Meniscus repair has evolved over the years, and most arthroscopists should consider why they cannot repair a given meniscus tear rather than removing the damaged meniscus. The location of the tear (peripheral), type of tear (vertical), chronicity (acute), age of the patient (young), and presence of associated injuries (simultaneous ACL reconstruction) are important considerations in evaluating the repairability of a given tear.

Technique

Inside-Out Technique

1. Positioning: The patient is positioned for knee arthroscopy. A padded well-leg support and a commercially available leg holder or post are used. A tourniquet is applied but often is not necessary.
2. Diagnostic arthroscopy: Most often, the repairability of a meniscus tear is unknown before it is carefully evaluated arthroscopically. Standard superomedial or superolateral (inflow or outflow), inferomedial (instrumentation), and inferolateral (viewing) portals are used. A posteromedial portal is often helpful in the evaluation of peripheral tears of the medial meniscus.
3. Incisions
   a. Medial: A 2- to 3-cm vertical incision is made directly behind the medial collateral ligament. It is advisable to have most of the incision placed below the joint line. Care is taken during subcutaneous dissection to identify and protect any saphenous nerve branches. The sartorial fascia is incised, and a retractor is placed beneath this layer and under the medial head of the gastrocnemius.
   b. Lateral: A 2- to 3-cm vertical incision is made between the posterior border of the lateral collateral ligament and the biceps tendon. Most of the incision is made below the joint line. As long as the dissection stays anterior to the biceps tendon, the common peroneal nerve is protected. The iliotibial band/tract is incised, and a retractor is placed beneath this layer.
4. Suture placement: The arthroscope is placed in the ipsilateral portal, and a commercially available meniscus repair angled cannula is placed in the contralateral portal. The curve of the cannula should be away from the posterior structures. Beginning posteriorly and working anteriorly, sutures are placed sequentially (Fig. 4–4). Extreme care should be taken to avoid cutting previously placed sutures and to

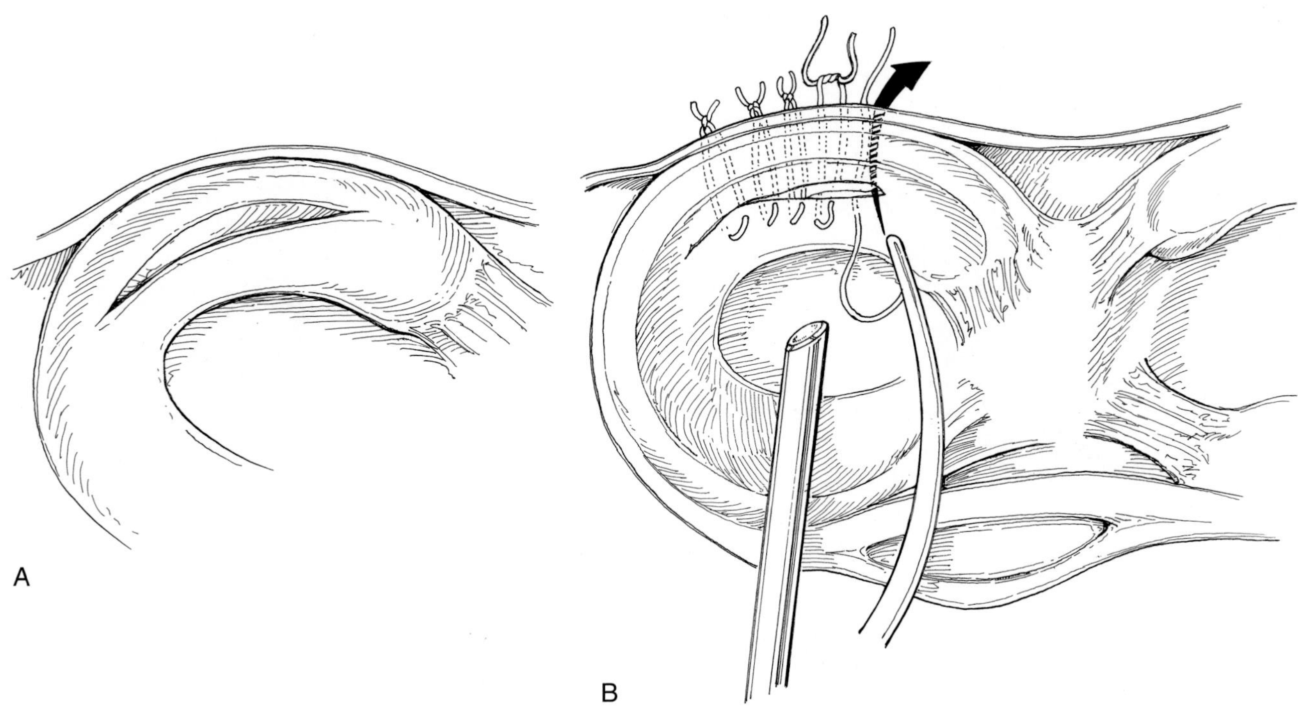

FIGURE 4–4. Inside-out technique for meniscal repair. *A*, Tear. *B*, Repair.

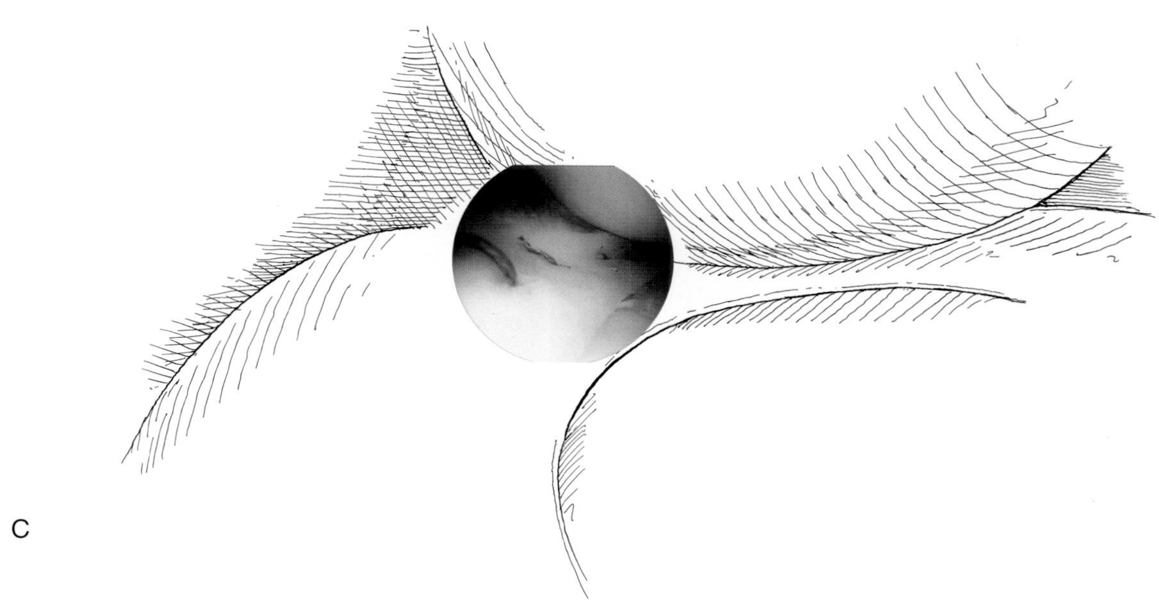

C

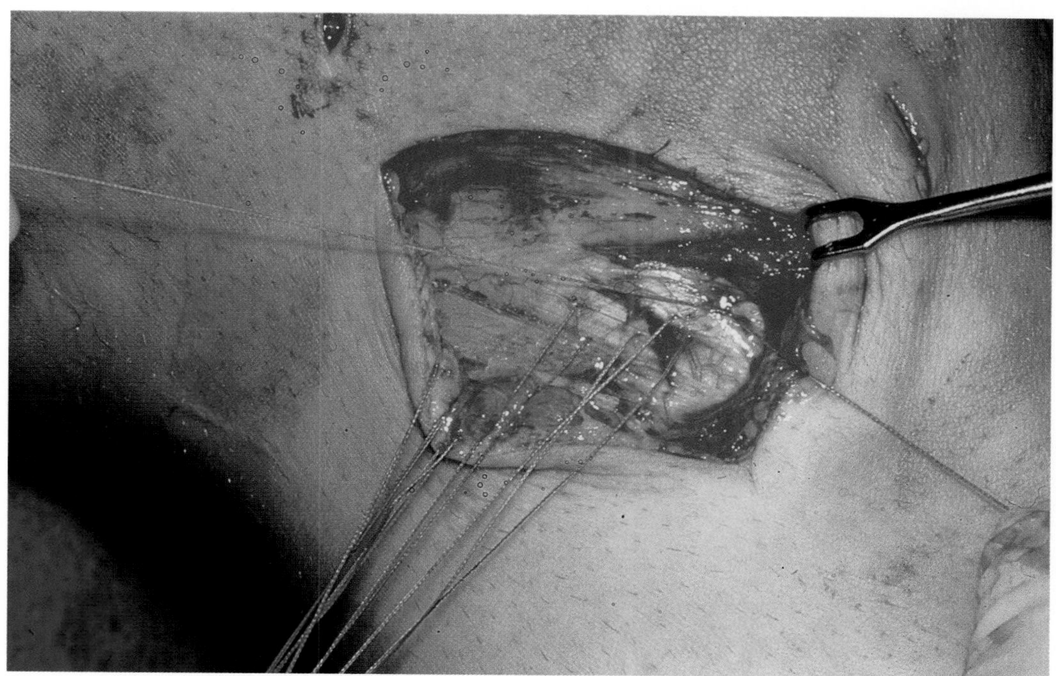

D

FIGURE 4–4 *Continued. C,* After repair. *D,* Sutures are retrieved through a 3-cm incision and tied directly over the capsule.

avoid needle sticks. Vertical suture placement is preferred. If sutures are placed horizontally, they should be placed on the top and on the bottom of the meniscus. A qualified assistant using a needle holder and a thimble (for palpation of the needles) retrieves sutures. The sutures are tagged and organized carefully as the repair continues; this can be done by collecting the finger holes of the snaps on an Allis clamp, which is clipped to the drapes.

5. Suture tying: This is best done after all other

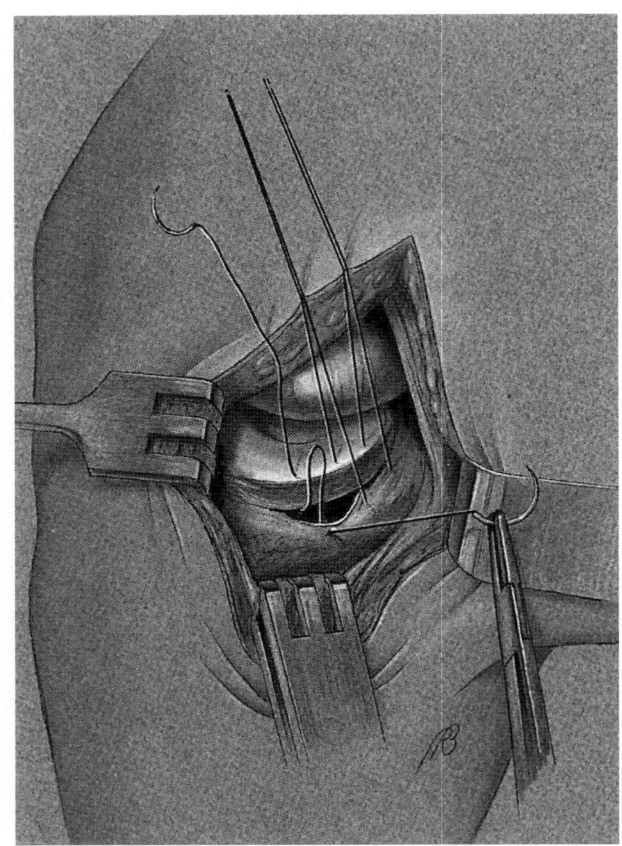

FIGURE 4–5. Open meniscal repair. (From Miller MD, Ritchie JR, Harner CD: Meniscus surgery: Indications for repair. Op Tech Sports Med 2:164–171, 1994.)

procedures are completed. The sutures should be tied directly over the capsule, and extreme care should be taken to avoid entrapping any nerve branches. It is helpful to use a fine-tipped hemostat to spread between the arms of the suture and, if necessary, to bring one end under any structures encountered. Although the sutures should be snug, it is easy to break these sutures during tying.

6. Wound closure: The fascia is closed with absorbable suture, and the subcutaneous tissues and skin are closed in standard fashion.

Other Techniques

Open Technique

A 3- to 5-cm incision is made directly over the joint line, and vertical sutures are placed from the capsule into the meniscus (Fig. 4–5). This technique is possible only for peripheral tears.

Outside-In Technique

Spinal needles are placed from outside the joint into the periphery of the meniscus, then through the tear (Fig. 4–6). Suture (usually 0 polypropylene) is passed through the needle, then the free end is either tied into a knot (Mulberry technique) or pulled back out through another spinal needle with a commercially available retriever. The sutures are tied over the capsule through separate small incisions.

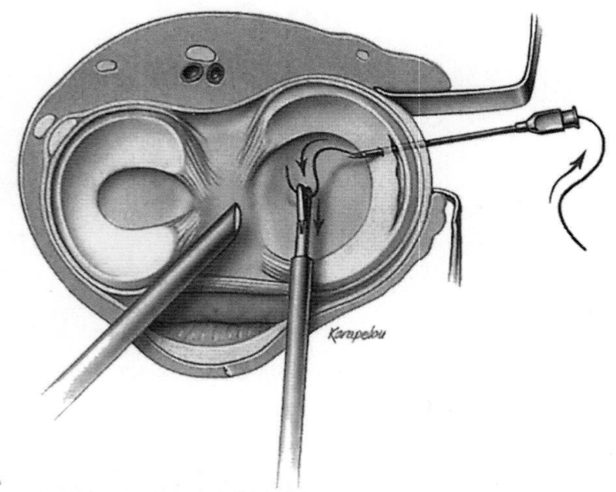

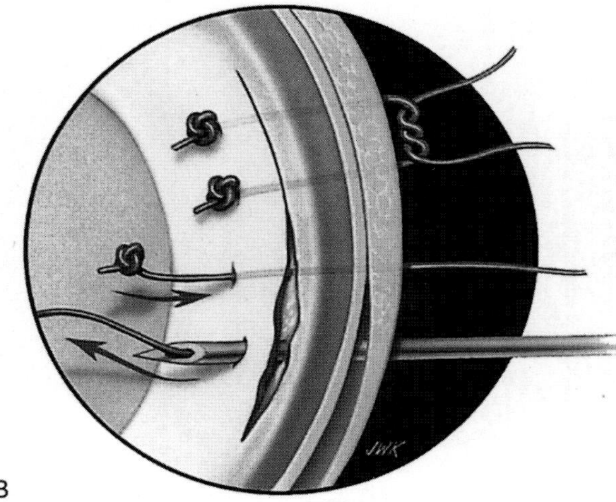

FIGURE 4–6. Outside-in mensical repair. *A,* Suture introduced through spinal needle from outside-in. *B,* Mulberry knot is tied, and suture is pulled back against the meniscus. Sutures are tied over capsule through a small incision. (From Miller MD: Atlas of meniscal repair. Op Tech Orthop 5:70–71, 1995.)

All-Inside Techniques

Several commercially available systems are available, including various arrows, barbed darts, and screws (Fig. 4–7). Each of these devices has instructions for insertion. The authors have found the cannulated systems to be easier to insert and more reliable. The problem with many of these new devices is that biomechanically they have not proved to be as strong as vertically oriented sutures.

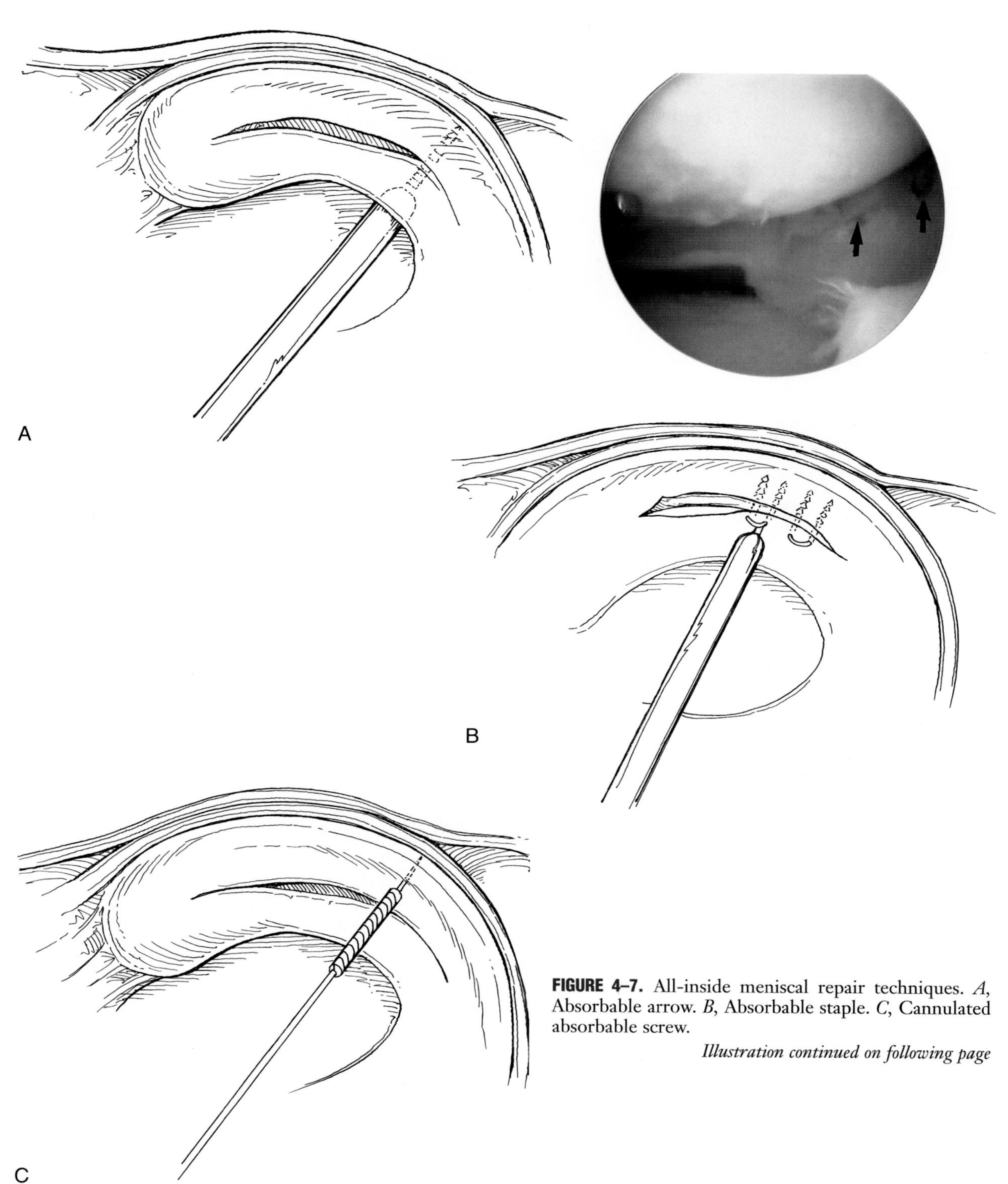

FIGURE 4–7. All-inside meniscal repair techniques. *A*, Absorbable arrow. *B*, Absorbable staple. *C*, Cannulated absorbable screw.

Illustration continued on following page

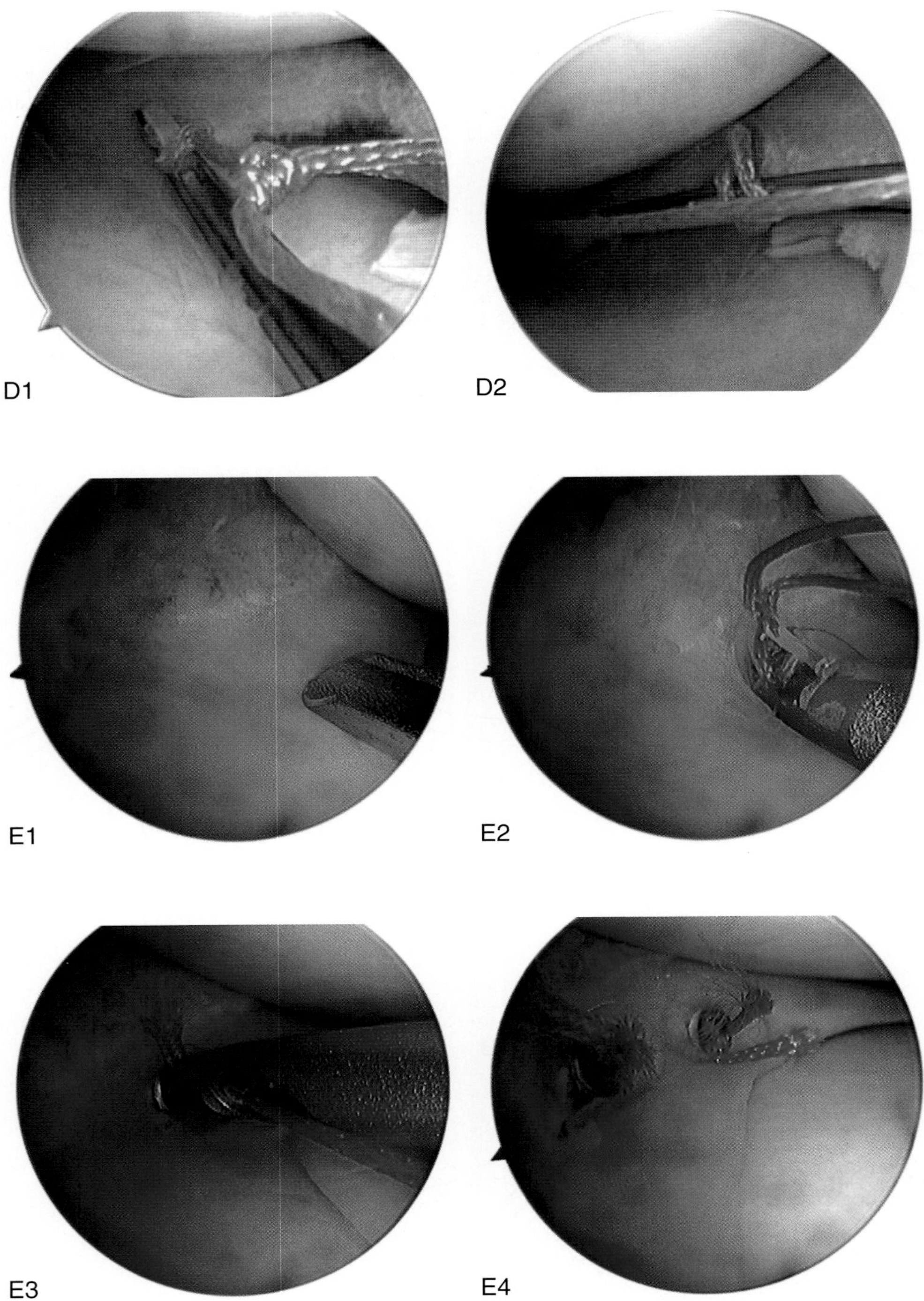

FIGURE 4–7 *Continued. D,* FasT-Fix (Smith & Nephew, Andover, MA): *1,* The first arm of the device is inserted. *2,* The second arm is inserted, and the device is tensioned with a knot pusher. *E,* Rapid Loc (Mitek, Westwood, MA): *1,* The point of the delivery gun pierces the meniscus. *2,* The device is pushed into the meniscus up to the silicone stop, and the trigger is fired. *3,* A knot pusher is used to advance the top hat and tension the repair. *4,* The implants are trimmed and examined.

POSTOPERATIVE MANAGEMENT

There are two considerations in the early rehabilitation of meniscus repairs: motion and weight-bearing status. At least theoretically, allowing motion beyond 90° would cause increased forces in the repair. Full weight bearing in the early postoperative period also may increase forces in the repaired meniscus. Many surgeons limit one or both of these factors for 4 to 6 weeks. More aggressive rehabilitation programs have been advocated, however, with early clinical success. Sports participation usually is allowed 3 to 6 months postoperatively.

COMPLICATIONS

The most significant complication with meniscus repair is neurovascular injury. Branches of the saphenous nerve are at risk with medial repairs, and the common peroneal nerve and popliteal artery are at risk laterally. Careful dissection and retraction during suture placement and when tying sutures can help reduce the incidence of these injuries. Other complications include needle sticks (again emphasizing the need for careful retraction and retrieval of needles), cartilage injury, loss of motion, instrument breakage, and infection. Failure of repair may be the most common complication, although expanding the indications for repair often is indicated in young athletic individuals. Preoperative counseling can be helpful in determining this issue before the case.

RESULTS

Follow-up studies revealed healing rates in the range of greater than 75%, based on the individual characteristics of the repair. Acute peripheral tear repair in young patients who undergo simultaneous ACL reconstruction has the best success rate.

REFERENCES

Arciero RA, Taylor DC: Inside-outside and all-inside meniscus repair: Indications, techniques, and results. Op Tech Orthop 5:58–69, 1995.

Cooper DE: Meniscal repair: Open and arthroscopic outside-in techniques. Op Tech Orthop 5:46–57, 1995.

McBride DG, Clancy WG Jr: Meniscus tears/repair. In Andrews JR, Timmerman LA (eds): Diagnostic and Operative Arthroscopy. Philadelphia, WB Saunders, 1997, pp 274–290.

Miller MD: Atlas of meniscal repair. Op Tech Orthop 5:70–71, 1995.

Miller MD, Warner JJP, Harner CD: Meniscal repair. In Fu FH, Harner CD, Vince KG (eds): Knee Surgery. Baltimore, Williams & Wilkins, 1994, pp 615–630.

CHAPTER 5

Meniscus Transplantation and Augmentation

INTRODUCTION

The development of techniques to replace the meniscus represents the end stage of the evolution from total meniscectomy to preservation (and reconstruction) of the meniscus. It is hoped that meniscus transplantation or replacement can retard the progressive joint deterioration following total or subtotal meniscectomy.

HISTORY AND PHYSICAL EXAMINATION

Patients who are candidates for a transplantation procedure usually have had an operative procedure to remove all or part of their own menisci. It is helpful to review operative notes and, ideally, arthroscopic images to appreciate the amount and quality of menisci remaining because the patients are typically poor historians. Symptoms of swelling, instability, and pain should be elicited. A complete knee examination should be done. Joint line tenderness may suggest a tear in the meniscal remnant or chondral damage. Persistent effusions may signify chondral injury. Ligamentous instability should be evaluated and addressed before or in conjunction with meniscus replacement.

DIAGNOSTIC IMAGING

Plain radiographs should be reviewed carefully. Weight-bearing studies should be evaluated carefully for joint space narrowing. Significant narrowing suggests advanced chondrosis and may imply that the patient is not a candidate for meniscus replacement. Lateral radiographs with markers to correct for magnification error typically are used for sizing. MRI (especially with contrast material) can be helpful in evaluating the meniscal remnant and looking for associated chondrosis. Some surgeons use MRI to size the meniscus.

NONOPERATIVE TREATMENT

Meniscus transplantation is an elective, investigational procedure, and nonoperative management is often appropriate. Patients should be encouraged to pursue low-impact conditioning exercises to delay the onset of arthritis, which is common in postmeniscectomy knees.

RELEVANT ANATOMY

It is crucial to understand the anatomy of the menisci and their anterior and posterior horns in particular when doing this procedure. Many surgeons believe that the key to successful meniscal transplantation is accurate restoration of the meniscal horns, usually with bony plugs or blocks. The lateral meniscus anterior and posterior horns are close to the tibial insertion of the anterior cruciate ligament (Fig. 5–1). The medial meniscal horns are widely separated.

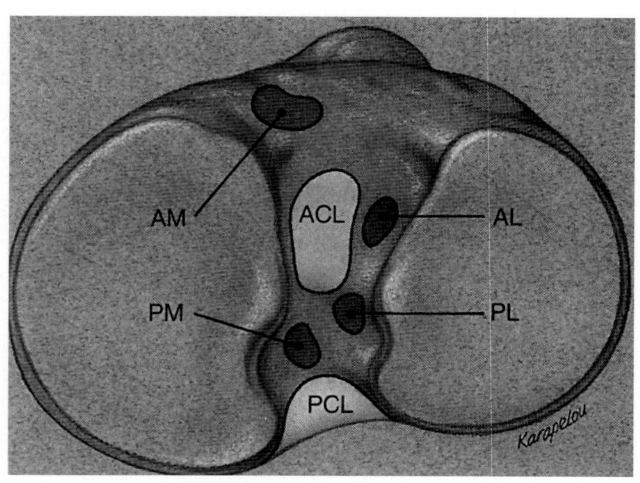

FIGURE 5–1. Insertion site anatomy of the medial and lateral menisci. ACL, anterior cruciate ligament; AL, anterior horn lateral meniscus; AM, anterior horn medial meniscus; PCL, posterior cruciate ligament; PL, posterior horn lateral meniscus; PM, posterior horn medial meniscus. (From Allen AA, Caldwell Jr GL, Fu FH: Anatomy and biomechanics of the meniscus. Op Tech Orthop 5:2–9, 1995.)

SURGICAL TECHNIQUE

Indications

The ideal candidate for meniscus transplantation should have documented evidence of a near-complete meniscectomy, ligamentous stability, early (grade I or II) chondrosis, no evidence of malalignment, and no articular incongruity as seen arthroscopically. Patients outside these parameters may have less successful results. Most patients with symptomatic postmeniscectomy knees already have developed advanced chondrosis.

Technique

1. Positioning: The patient is positioned for knee arthroscopy. A padded well-leg support and a commercially available leg holder or post are used. A tourniquet is applied but is usually not necessary.
2. Diagnostic arthroscopy: This is carried out through standard portals. A careful evaluation of the remaining meniscus, degree of chondrosis, and extent of other knee pathology is completed. Any remaining meniscus is trimmed back to its capsular insertion, and the surrounding synovium is shaved and rasped to promote vascular ingrowth (Fig. 5–2).
3. Graft preparation: The meniscal graft can be prepared using various techniques. Most surgeons prefer to preserve the bony insertions at the anterior and posterior horns of the menisci. This can be accomplished using bony plugs (medial meniscus) or by preserving a bony bridge (lateral meniscus) (Fig. 5–3).

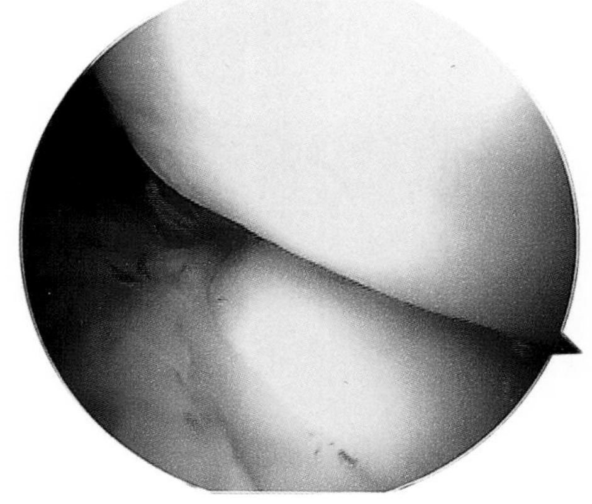

A

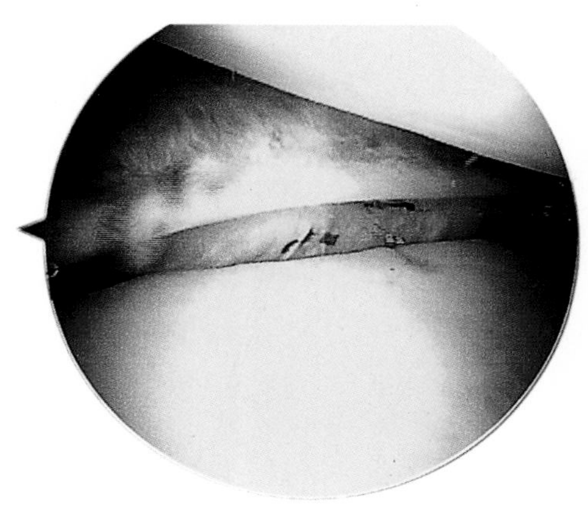

B

FIGURE 5–2. *A* and *B*, Débridement of meniscal remnant.

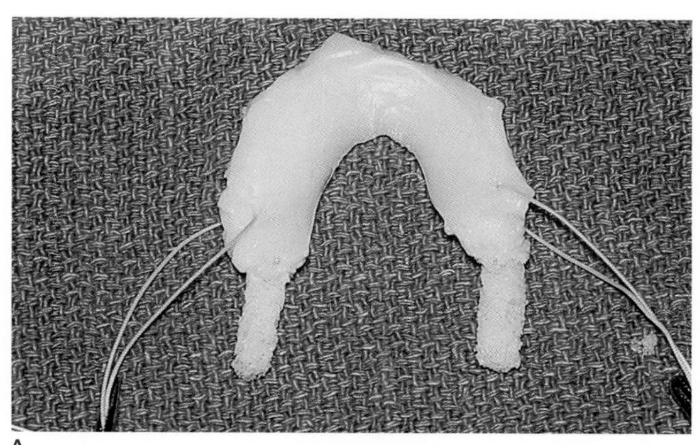

A

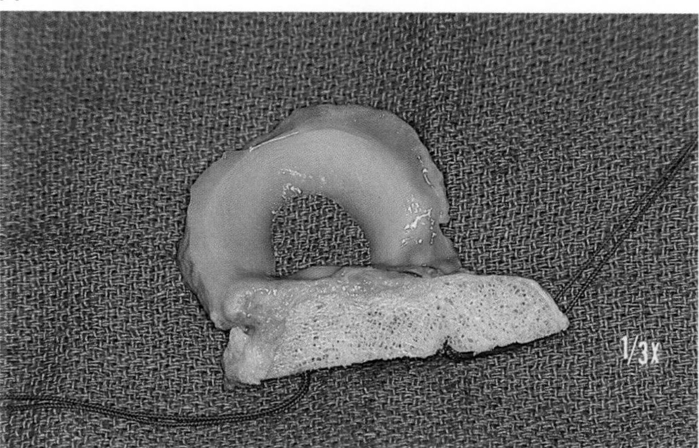

B

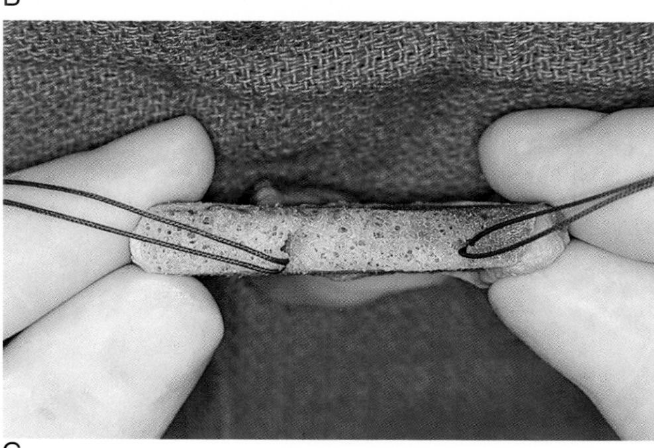

C

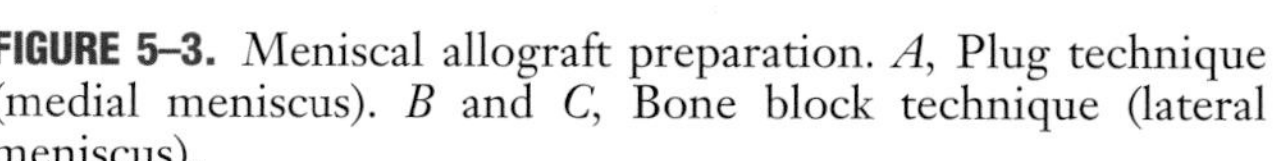

FIGURE 5–3. Meniscal allograft preparation. *A*, Plug technique (medial meniscus). *B* and *C*, Bone block technique (lateral meniscus).

When preparing bone plugs, a suture is placed through the plug and, in the meniscus itself, adjacent to the plug. The meniscal suture rather than the plug suture should be used for traction. Commercially available devices are available to preserve and tailor a bony bridge for insertion.

4. Medial meniscus: The medial meniscus usually is transplanted with bone plugs (6 to 8 mm) placed in bone tunnels. It is essential to understand the anatomy of the meniscal insertions. The posterior tunnel is placed between the anterior cruciate ligament and posterior cruciate ligament, and the anterior tunnel is very anterior. The meniscus can be delivered into the knee anteriorly or medially (Fig. 5–4). Extreme care must be taken when seating the bone plugs into the tunnel because the plugs can fracture easily.
5. Lateral meniscus: Because the anterior and posterior

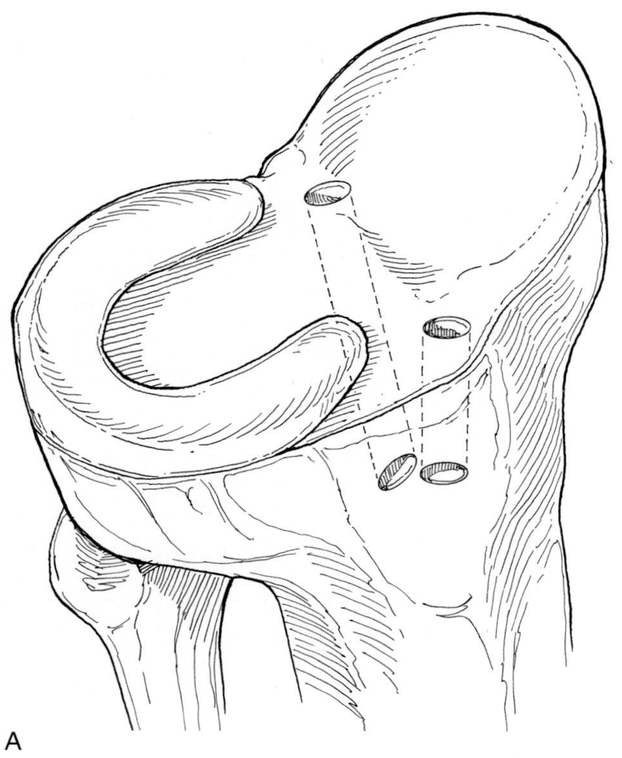

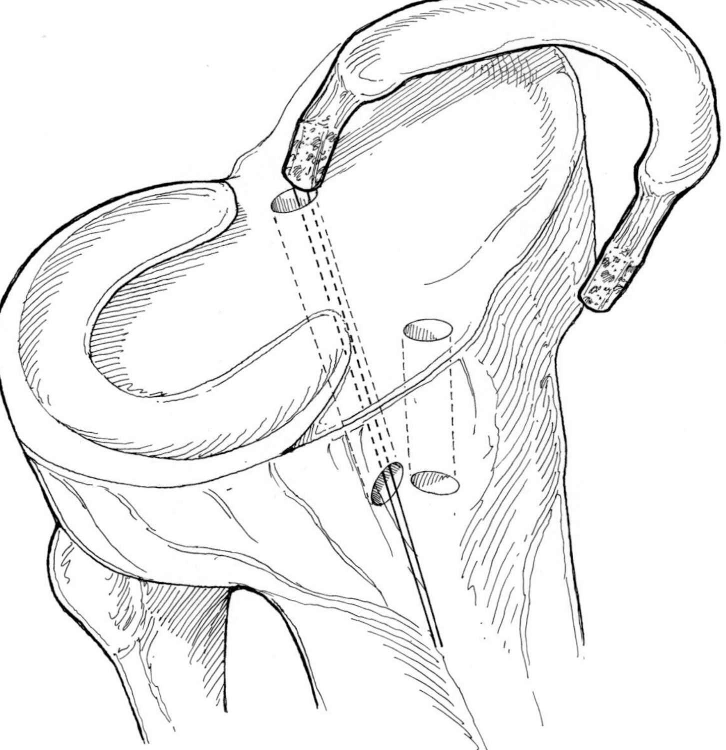

FIGURE 5–4. Medial meniscal transplantation. *A*, Tunnels are drilled in the anatomic position, and the posterior horn of the medial meniscus is first passed. *B*, The posterior bone plug is seated in the posterior tunnel.

FIGURE 5–4 *Continued. C*, The remaining meniscus is inserted into the knee. *D*, The anterior horn is passed.

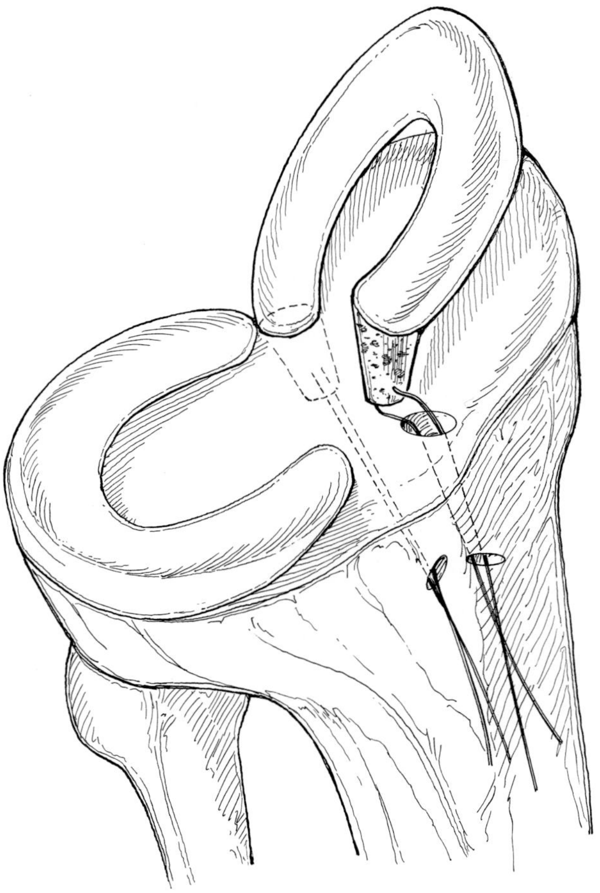

C

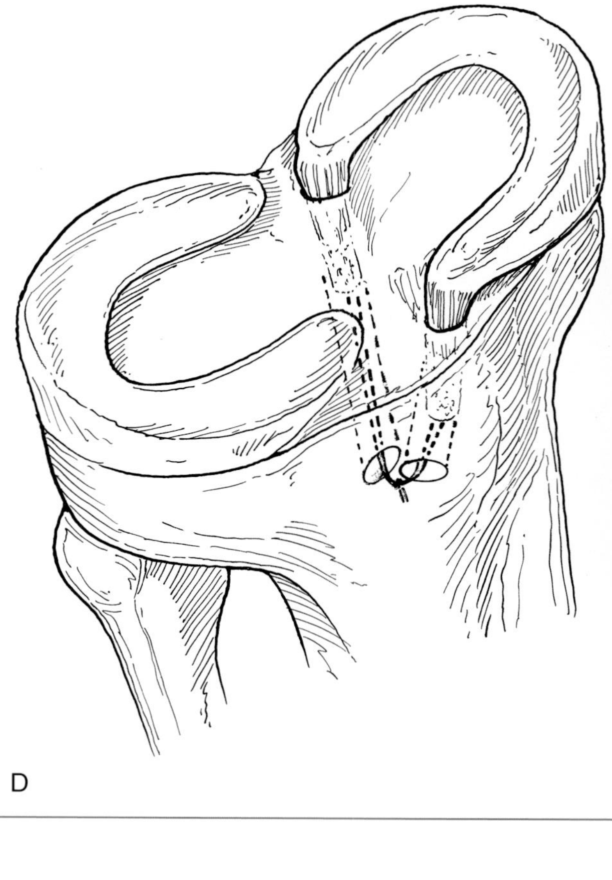

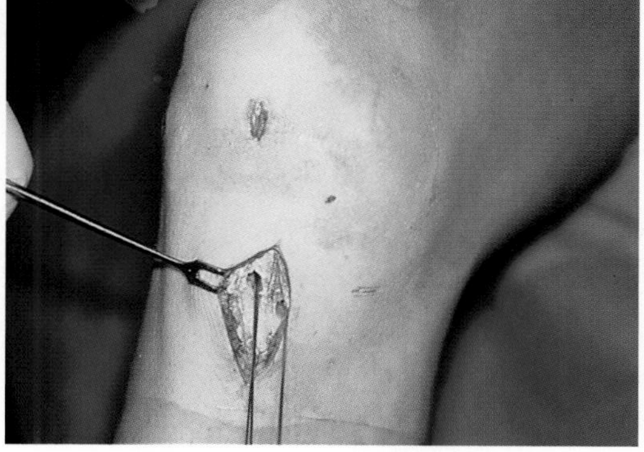

D

horns of the lateral meniscus are close to each other, it is better to preserve a bone bridge. The meniscus can be inserted from anterior to posterior with a *keyhole* technique or laterally and pulled into a trough that is fashioned freehand (Fig. 5–5).

6. Graft fixation: Sutures from the bone plugs are tied over a bony bridge, and the meniscus is sutured in place using standard meniscus repair techniques. The keyhole technique relies on a mechanical interference fit (Fig. 5–6).

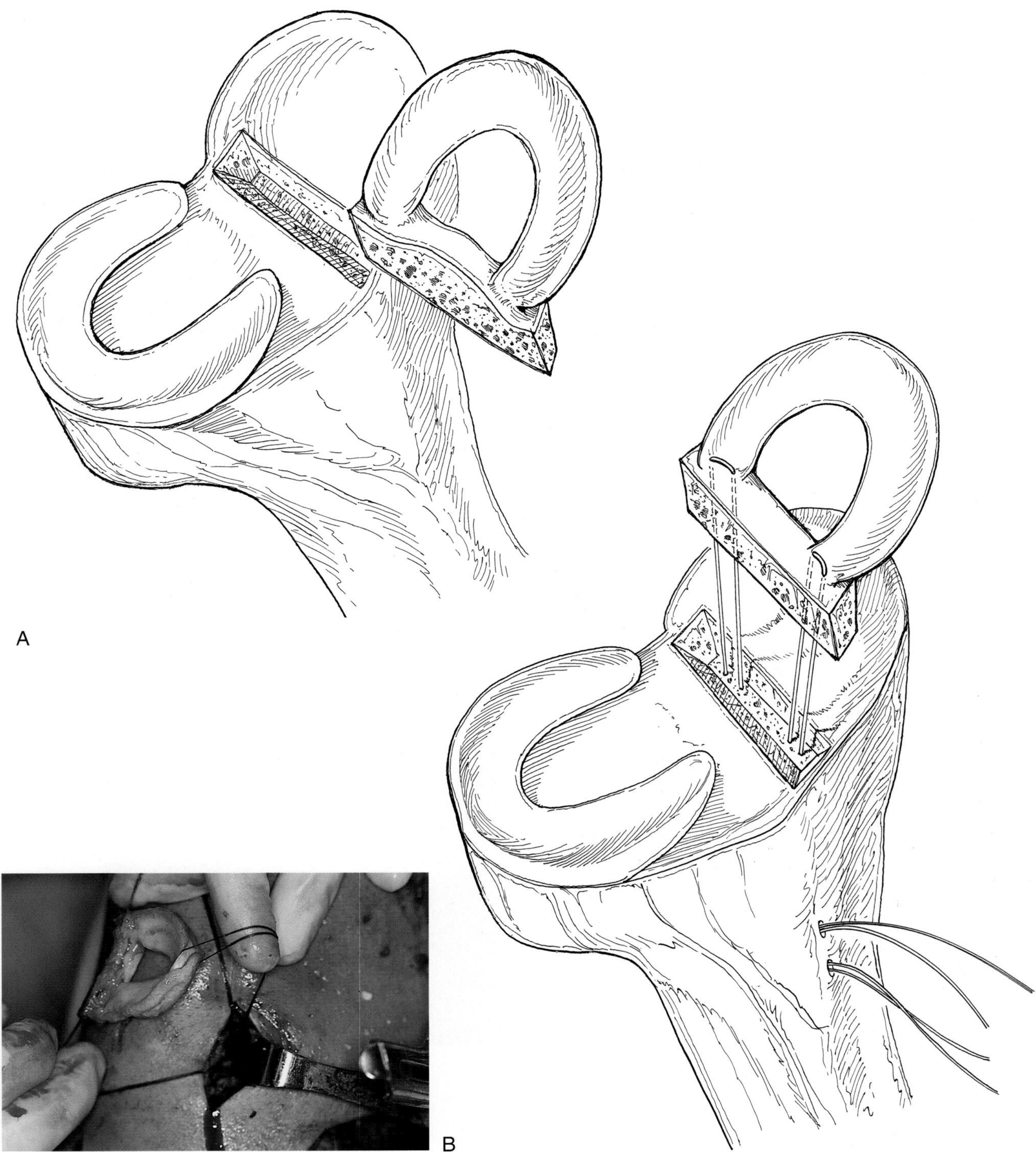

FIGURE 5–5. Lateral meniscal transplantation. *A*, Creation of trough to match bone block. *B*, Insertion of allograft meniscus.

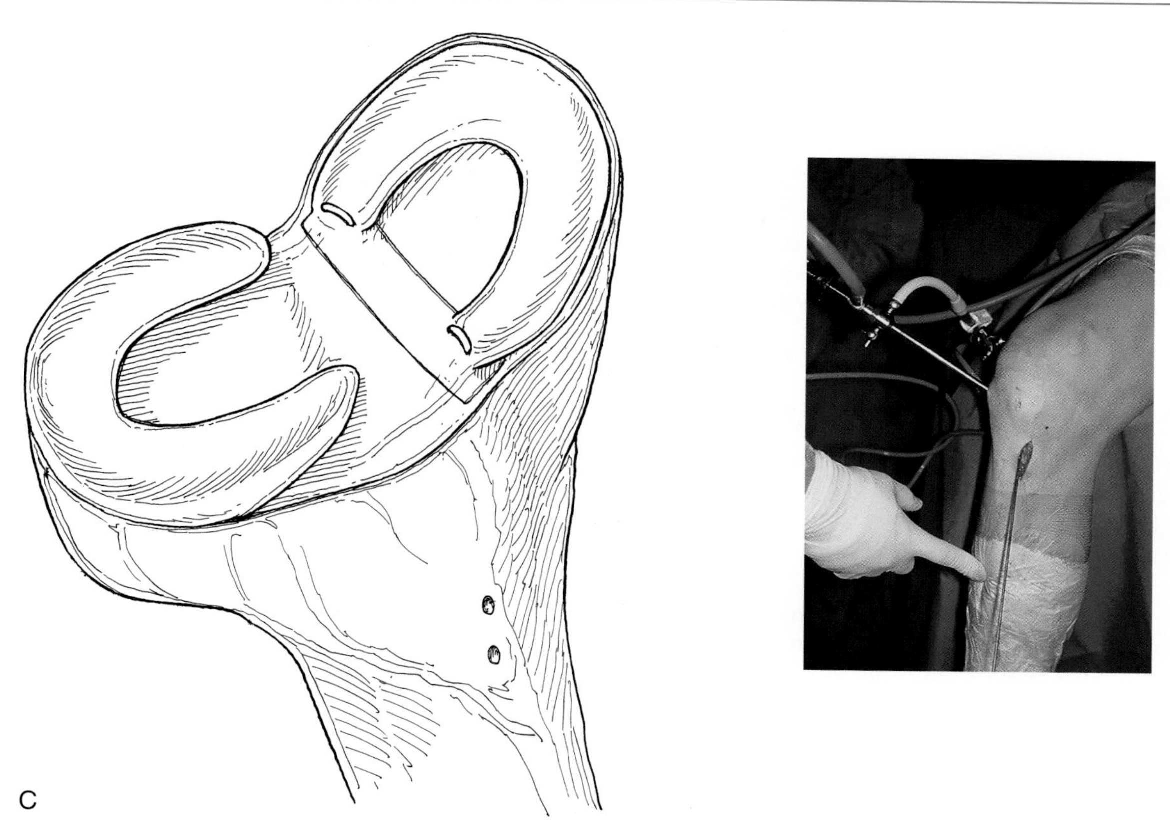

FIGURE 5–5 *Continued. C*, Fixation of bone block with sutures over bony cortex.

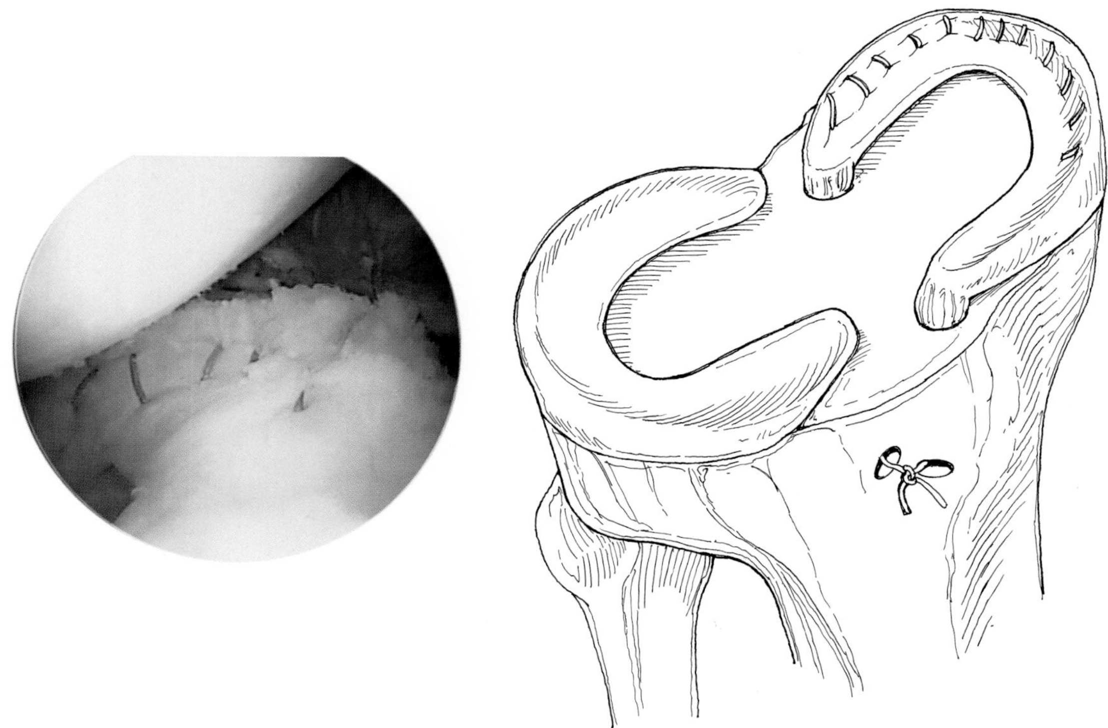

FIGURE 5–6. Suture repair of meniscus transplant.

POSTOPERATIVE MANAGEMENT

Postoperative management is identical to that for meniscus repair except that sports are not encouraged until 9 months to 1 year postoperatively.

COMPLICATIONS

Complications include loss of motion, nerve injury or neurapraxia, reinjury or damage to the meniscus, shrinkage of the meniscal graft, articular cartilage damage, and other complications described elsewhere.

RESULTS

Although preliminary, the results of this procedure, with careful patient selection, are encouraging. In one study, 20 of 23 patients had satisfactory results at 2 to 5 years' follow-up. Many second-look procedures have confirmed good incorporation of the grafts (Fig. 5–7). The key unanswered question is whether these transplants will function similar to the native meniscus, and only long-term studies will be able to resolve this issue.

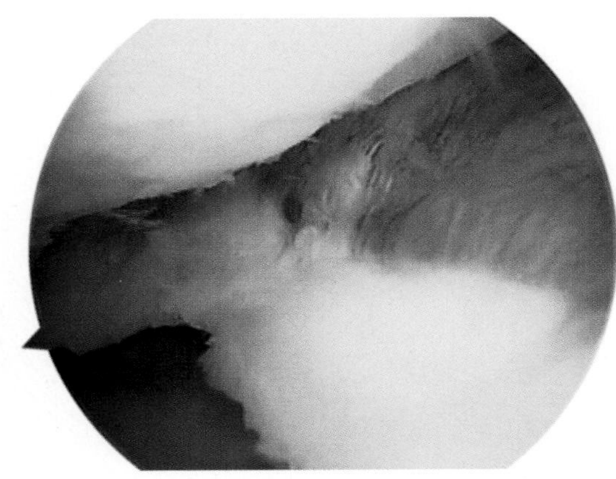

FIGURE 5–7. Arthroscopic view of second-look procedure 1 year postoperatively (same patient as in Figure 5–6).

REFERENCES

Goble EM: Meniscal allograft technique. Op Tech Orthop 10:220–226, 2000.

Johnson DL: Arthroscopically assisted technique for meniscal reconstruction using fresh frozen allograft. Op Tech Orthop 5:88–94, 1995.

Johnson DL, Swenson TM, Livesay GA, et al: Insertion-site anatomy of the human menisci: Gross, arthroscopic, and topographical anatomy as a basis for meniscal transplantation. Arthroscopy 11:386–394, 1995.

Van Arkel ER, de Boer HH: Human meniscal transplantation: Preliminary results at 2 to 5-year follow-up. J Bone Joint Surg [Br] 77:589–595, 1995.

CHAPTER 6

Arthroscopic Synovectomy

INTRODUCTION

Several synovial conditions have a predilection for the knee. Rheumatoid arthritis is one of the most common of these conditions. An aggressively destructive synovial proliferation called a *pannus* is responsible for articular cartilage damage characteristic of this disorder. Pigmented villonodular synovitis (PVNS), which presents 90% of the time in the knee, can be diffuse or local. Synovial chondromatosis represents a metaplasia of synovial tissue into multiple chondral or osteochondral loose bodies. Other conditions, such as intra-articular ganglia, synovial hemangioma, hemorrhagic disorders, and arthrofibrosis, also respond to arthroscopic synovectomy.

HISTORY AND PHYSICAL EXAMINATION

The history is often condition specific. Patients with synovitis associated with an underlying condition, such as rheumatoid arthritis, often are aware of their diagnosis on presentation. PVNS may present with an insidious onset in the 20s or 30s. Recurrent effusions and a multiple-year history of knee problems is common. Synovial chondromatosis may present with complaints of swelling and locking. Arthrofibrosis, although not a synovial disease per se, can follow cruciate ligament reconstruction, particularly procedures associated with poor technique or done acutely. Examination is notable for an effusion, loss of motion, and possibly warmth.

DIAGNOSTIC IMAGING

Rheumatoid arthritis has several characteristic findings on plain radiographs, including osteopenia and periarticular erosions. Calcification or ossification is characteristic of some disorders. MRI may be helpful in quantifying the extent of joint involvement (Fig. 6–1).

NONOPERATIVE TREATMENT

Medical treatment of rheumatoid arthritis is the first line of defense. Other disorders, such as PVNS and synovial chondromatosis, may respond to intra-articular injections but often require synovectomy.

RELEVANT ANATOMY

A good understanding of standard arthroscopic portals and accessory portals is essential to perform a complete arthroscopic meniscectomy. Proximal and posterior portals are required.

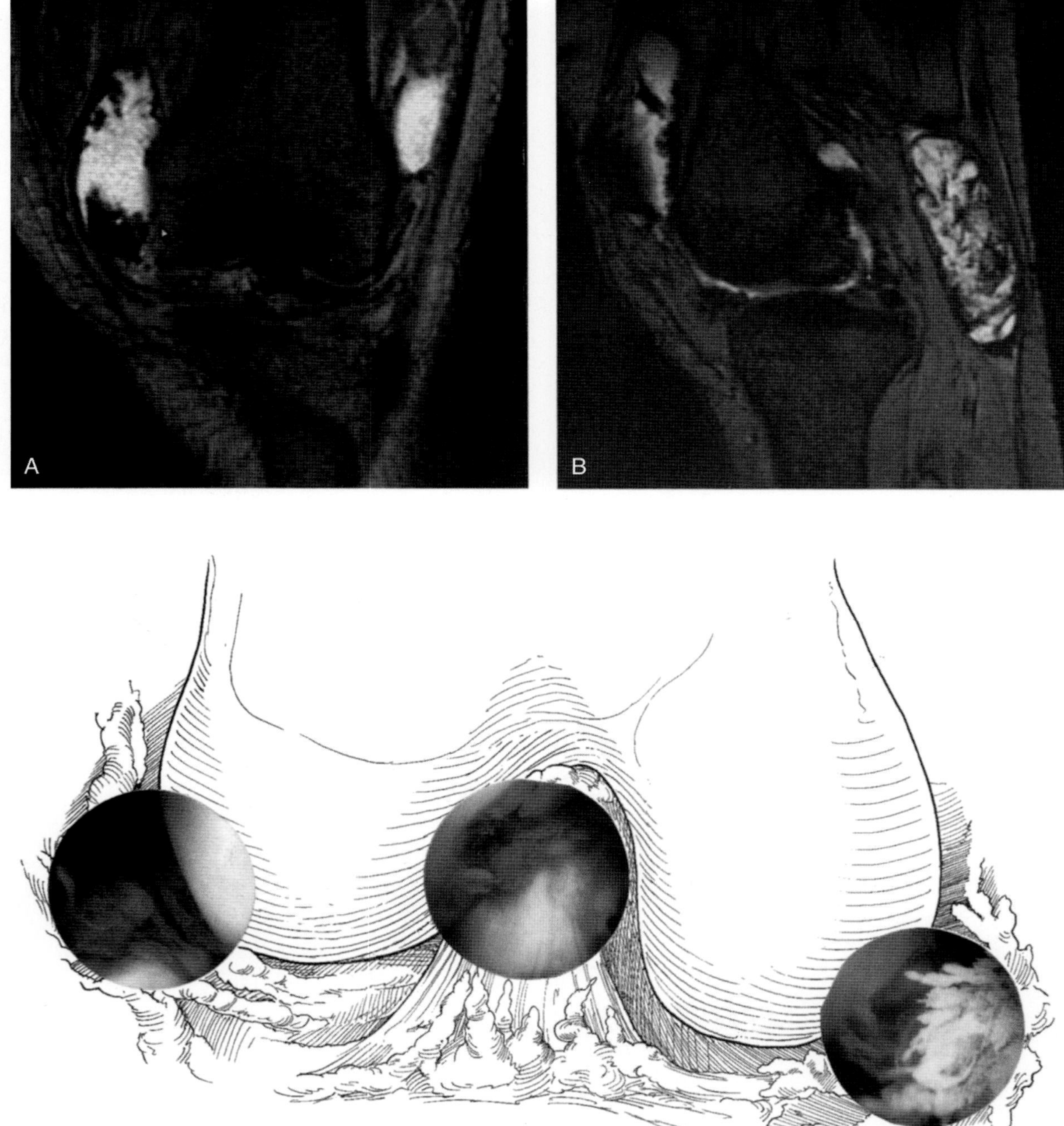

FIGURE 6–1. Pigmented villonodular synovitis (PVNS) *A*, Coronal GRE image shows multiple synovial deposits of diffuse dark signal intensity throughout the knee. *B*, Sagittal GRE image shows similar findings. *C*, Arthroscopic view shows proliferative PVNS throughout the knee. (From Miller MD, Osborne JR, Warner JJP, Fu FH: MRI-Arthroscopy Correlative Atlas. Philadelphia, WB Saunders, 1997, p 85.)

SURGICAL TECHNIQUE

Indications

For rheumatoid arthritis, arthroscopic synovectomy is indicated in patients who have failed medical management. Other conditions may cause enough symptoms that patients request the procedure. Occasionally, synovial biopsy is required to make or confirm a diagnosis. Lysis of adhesions in arthrofibrotic knees is required in patients who have not responded to extended physical therapy.

Technique

1. Positioning: The patient is positioned for knee arthroscopy. A padded well-leg support and a commercially available leg holder or post are used. A tourniquet is applied and may be required for certain synovial diseases.
2. Diagnostic arthroscopy: Standard portals are used, and complete visualization of the knee is accomplished. The extent of synovial involvement is characterized. A biopsy specimen can be obtained at this point.
3. Accessory portals: Using a combination of various portals, an arthroscopic shaver is used to remove all diseased synovium (Figs. 6–2 and 6–3). It is helpful to consider the procedure in five steps:

Step 1: The arthroscope is placed in the standard anterolateral portal and the shaver in the lateral suprapatellar portal, and synovium in the suprapatellar pouch and gutter is removed.

Step 2: With the arthroscope still in the anterolateral portal, the shaver is placed in the anteromedial portal, and the intercondylar notch, medial gutter, and menisci are cleared of synovium.

Step 3: The arthroscope is placed in the anteromedial portal, and the shaver is placed in the anterolateral portal. Remaining synovial tissue is removed completely from the notch, menisci, and lateral gutter.

Step 4: The arthroscope remains in the anteromedial portal, and the shaver is placed in the superomedial portal. The medial gutter and suprapatellar pouch is cleared.

Step 5: Posterior synovectomy is done. A posteromedial portal is made under direct visualization (from a modified Gillquist portal). A posterolateral portal also can be made, ensuring that the portal is anterior to the biceps tendon. The arthroscope and shaver are introduced through different portals until a complete synovectomy is done.

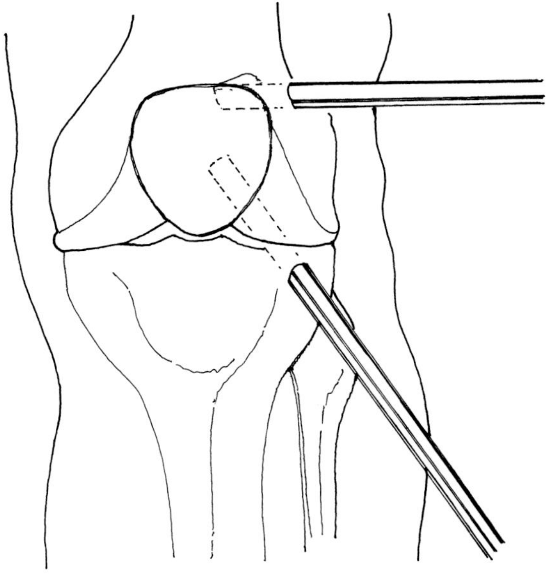

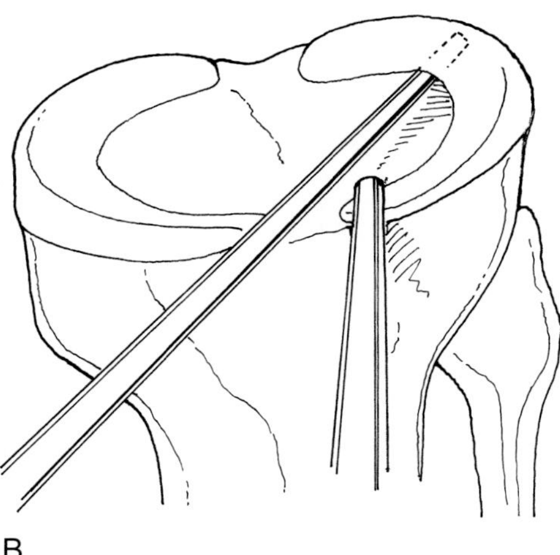

FIGURE 6–2. Sequential arthroscopic synovectomy. *A*, Suprapatellar pouch. *B*, Perimeniscal areas.

Illustration continued on following page

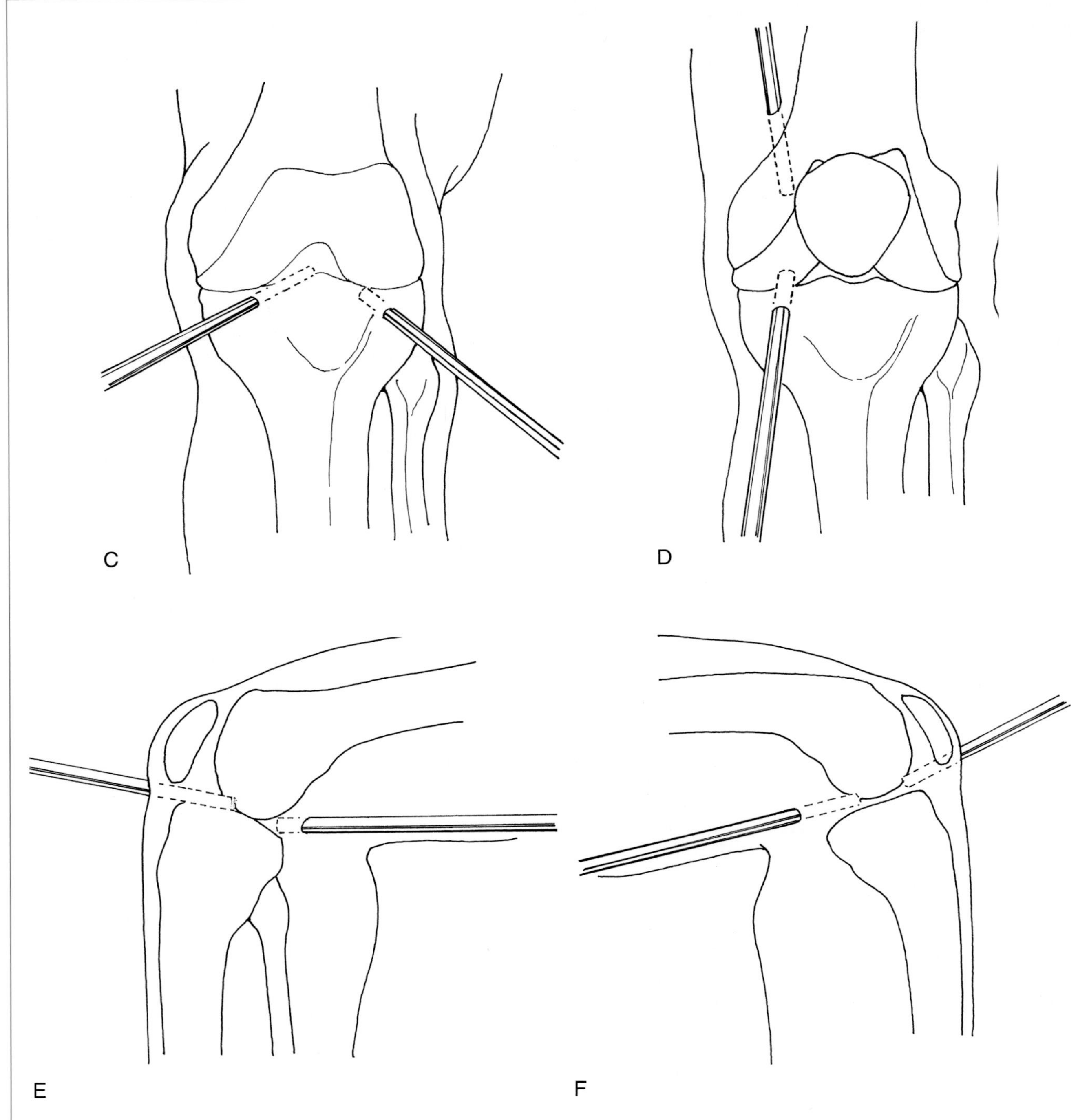

FIGURE 6–2 *Continued. C*, Notch. *D*, Switching portals. *E* and *F*, Posterolateral and posteromedial.

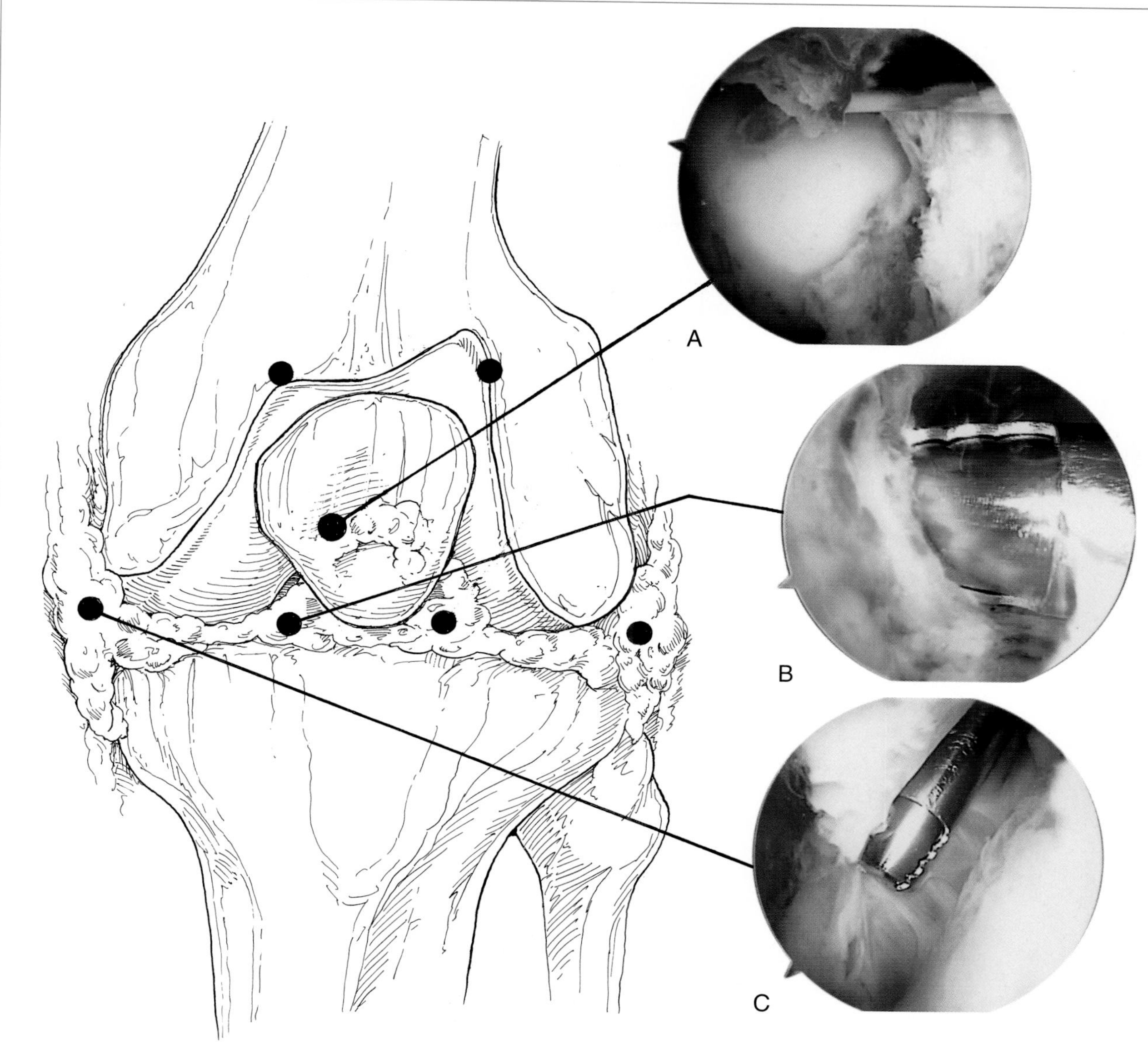

FIGURE 6–3. Arthroscopic view of synovectomy. *A*, Area in front of lateral femoral condyle. *B*, Notch. *C*, Medial gutter.

POSTOPERATIVE MANAGEMENT

A drain can be placed overnight if necessary, and range of motion is initiated early. Weight bearing is allowed as tolerated.

COMPLICATIONS

Complications include incomplete synovium removal (and recurrence), loss of motion, hemarthrosis, neurovascular injury (with posterior portal placement), and other complications mentioned for other arthroscopic procedures.

RESULTS

Results for arthroscopic treatment of rheumatoid arthritis is similar to open treatment. Good results can be expected for 5 years after the procedure, but eventually symptoms may recur. The results of synovectomy for PVNS are encouraging, but recurrence can occur in 10% to 20%. Results for other conditions are mixed.

REFERENCES

Andrews JR, Schluntz KC: Synovial lesions of the knee. In Andrews JR, Timmerman LA (eds): Diagnostic and Operative Arthroscopy. Philadelphia, WB Saunders, 1997, pp 347–354.

Klein W, Jensen K-U: Arthroscopic synovectomy of the knee joint: Indication, technique, and follow-up results. Arthroscopy 4:63–67, 1988.

Ogilvie-Harris DJ, Basinsi A: Arthroscopic synovectomy of the knee for rheumatoid arthritis. Arthroscopy 7:91–95, 1991.

Olgivie-Harris DJ, McLean J, Zarnett ME: Pigmented villonodular synovitis of the knee. J Bone Joint Surg [Am] 74:119–123, 1992.

CHAPTER 7

Anterior Cruciate Ligament Reconstruction

INTRODUCTION

Anterior cruciate ligament (ACL) reconstruction is one of the most popular procedures in orthopaedics today. Although there has been controversy regarding graft selection, most surgeons now recognize that there are probably two gold standards—the bone–patellar tendon–bone (BPTB) graft and the quadrupled hamstring (semitendinosus with or without gracilis) graft—and attempt to use a graft that is appropriate for the individual patient and situation.

HISTORY AND PHYSICAL EXAMINATION

The classic history for an ACL injury is an athlete who sustains a noncontact pivoting injury, feels or hears a pop, and has immediate swelling. If treatment is not sought, these patients may describe recurrent episodes of their knee's giving way. The key examination for ACL injury is the Lachman test, which is done in 20° to 30° of flexion (Fig. 7–1). The pivot shift or jerk test also can be helpful, particularly during examination under anesthesia. A complete knee examination should be done, and the presence of an effusion, joint line tenderness, and varus/valgus and posterior/posterolateral laxity should be considered.

DIAGNOSTIC IMAGING

As with most athletic injuries of the knee, plain radiographs are usually unremarkable. Occasionally a small fleck of bone adjacent to the lateral aspect of the tibia (Segond fracture) can be seen, and this is highly associated with an injury to the ACL. In pediatric patients, the tibial eminences should be evaluated carefully for the presence of an avulsion fracture. The use of MRI in the evaluation of ACL injuries is controversial; however, it is highly accurate in detecting the presence of concomitant injuries to the menisci and articular cartilage (Fig. 7–2).

NONOPERATIVE MANAGEMENT

Although nonoperative management is an extremely controversial issue, it is clear that patients with marked laxity (>5 to 7 mm of laxity compared with the opposite side) and patients who are active in pivoting sports should consider operative treatment. Patients who have less laxity and are less active may do well with nonoperative management. Nonoperative management is done in three phases, over a period of 10 to 14 weeks. In the initial phase, emphasis is placed on controlling the effusion and maintaining quadriceps tone. In the second phase, quadriceps strengthening is accomplished. In the third and final phase, sport-specific rehabilitation is accomplished. Patients may attempt to return to sports after their effusion has resolved, they have full range of motion, their quadriceps tone and strength have been restored (isokinetic testing is helpful), and they have no symptoms of instability (functional testing is useful).

RELEVANT ANATOMY

An understanding of the insertion site anatomy of the ACL is helpful. The tibial insertion of the ACL is broad and fanned out. It is impossible to recreate this large a "footprint," and most surgeons favor placing the graft in the posteromedial aspect of this footprint. The tibial guide wire should be (1) placed in the posteromedial aspect of the ACL footprint, (2) centered 7 mm in front of the crossing posterior cruciate (PCL), (3) along a line extended from the posterior border of the anterior horn of the lateral meniscus, and (4) adjacent to the medial eminence (Fig. 7–3*A*). Although there has been much discussion in previous literature regarding the so-called isometric position of the ACL femoral insertion, most authors recommend posterior tunnel placement with a 1- to 2-mm posterior cortex remaining after drilling. A 10- to 11-o'clock position (right knee) is favored (Fig. 7–3*B*). An understanding of the anatomy of the patellar tendon and the location of the hamstring tendons is important for graft harvesting.

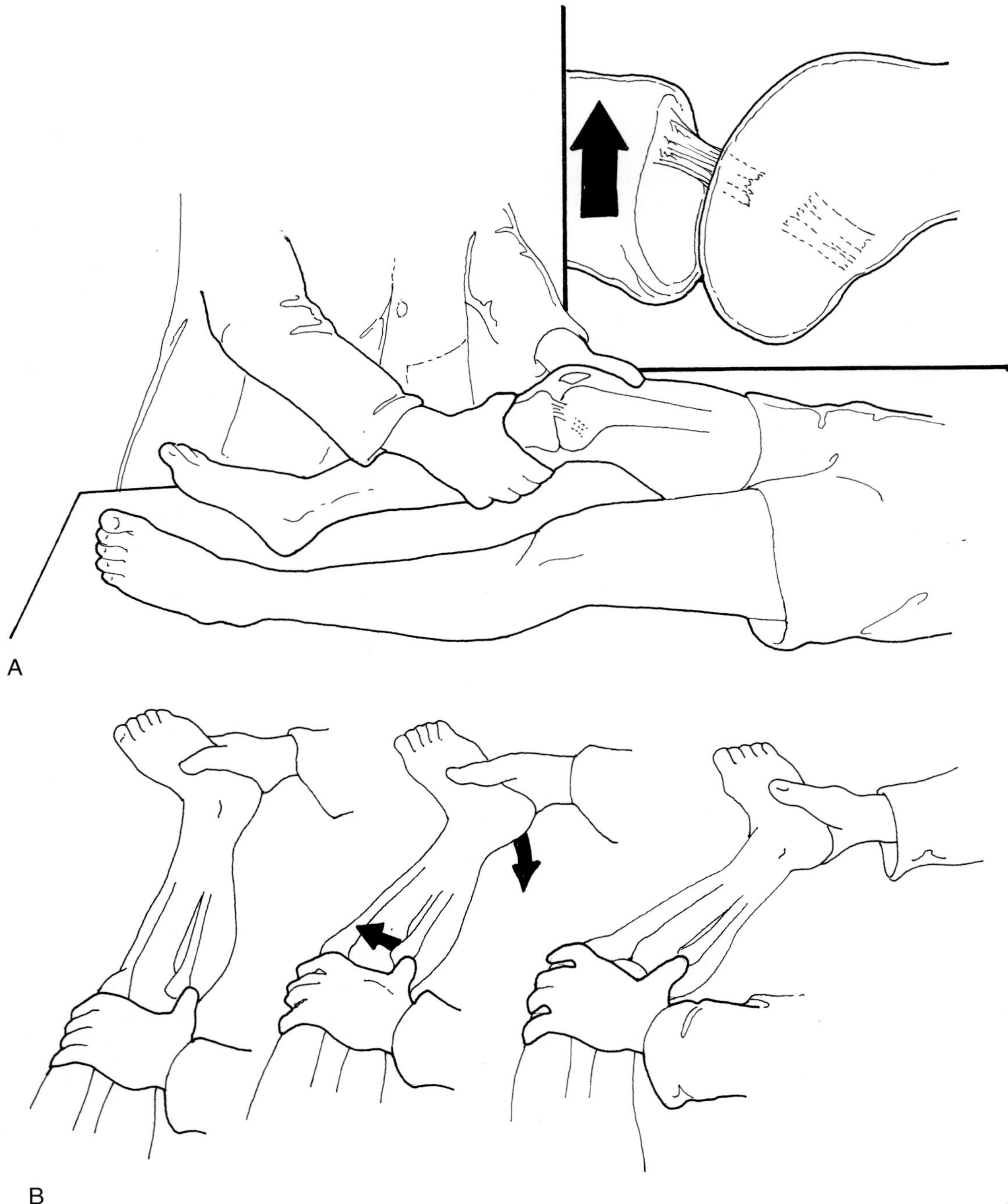

FIGURE 7–1. *A*, The Lachman test is the key examination for ACL deficiency. *B*, The pivot shift test is confirmatory and is especially good for examination under anesthesia.

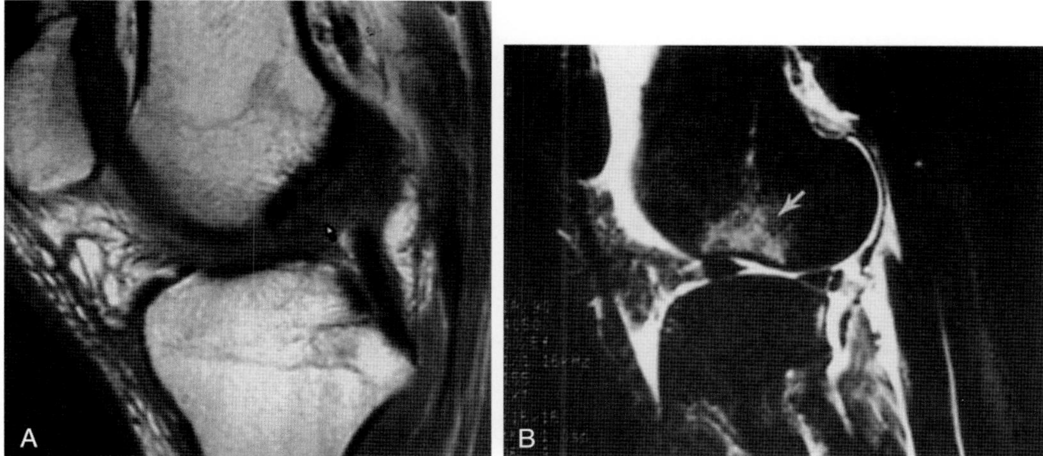

FIGURE 7–2. MRI of an ACL-injured knee. *A*, Sagittal T1-weighted spin-echo image shows mass effect, increased signal, and loss of continuity of the ACL *(arrow)*. *B*, Sagittal short-tau inversion recovery image with bright signal within the subchondral bone marrow consistent with a bone bruise *(arrow)*. (From Miller MD, Osborne JD, Warner JJP, Fu FH: MRI-Arthroscopy Correlative Atlas. Philadelphia, WB Saunders, 1997.)

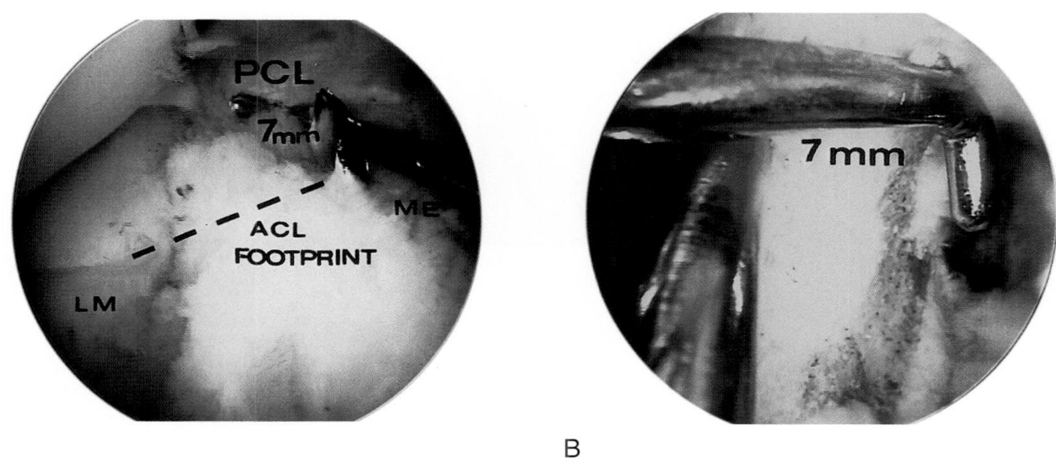

FIGURE 7–3. Landmarks for ACL tibial tunnel placement. *A*, Tibial tunnel. The guide wire is positioned in the posteromedial footprint, 7 mm anterior to the posterior cruciate ligament, adjacent to the medial eminence, and along a line extended from the posterior aspect of the anterior horn of the lateral meniscus. *B*, Femoral tunnel. The guide wire is placed 6 to 7 mm in front of the over-the-top position.

SURGICAL *TECHNIQUE*

Indications

Indications for surgery are controversial; however, most physiologically young athletic individuals with complete ACL tears should be offered ACL reconstruction. Although there is considerable debate regarding the risk of arthritis after ACL reconstruction, it is clear that recurrent giving-way episodes can cause additional meniscal and chondral injury.

Technique

1. Positioning: The patient is placed in a supine position, and anesthesia is administered. Examination under anesthesia should focus on the Lachman test and the pivot shift test. After examination, the patient is placed in a well-padded knee holder or a post for arthroscopy. ACL grafts can be obtained before or after diagnostic

arthroscopy based on examination under anesthesia and the surgeon's preference.

2. Graft harvesting: Techniques vary based on graft selection. There are three major autologous graft choices available: patellar tendon, hamstring tendons, and quadriceps tendon. Each graft has advantages and disadvantages. Patellar tendon grafts have been the gold standard for many years, but associated morbidity with graft harvesting and the incidence of anterior knee pain attributed to these grafts have made hamstring grafts more popular. Hamstring grafts have advantages such as low morbidity associated with graft harvesting and increased ultimate strength (with a quadriceps tendon construct); however, the initial fixation of these grafts is the weak link, and some surgeons believe they may stretch out slightly with time. Quadriceps tendon grafts have gained popularity only more recently. These grafts offer good strength and bony fixation but only on one end. Surgeons who do many ACL reconstructions, including revisions, should be familiar with all graft choices. Each graft harvesting technique is described.
    a. Patellar tendon: A central one third BPTB graft is harvested through a midline or paramedian incision (Fig. 7–4). The paratenon is dissected off

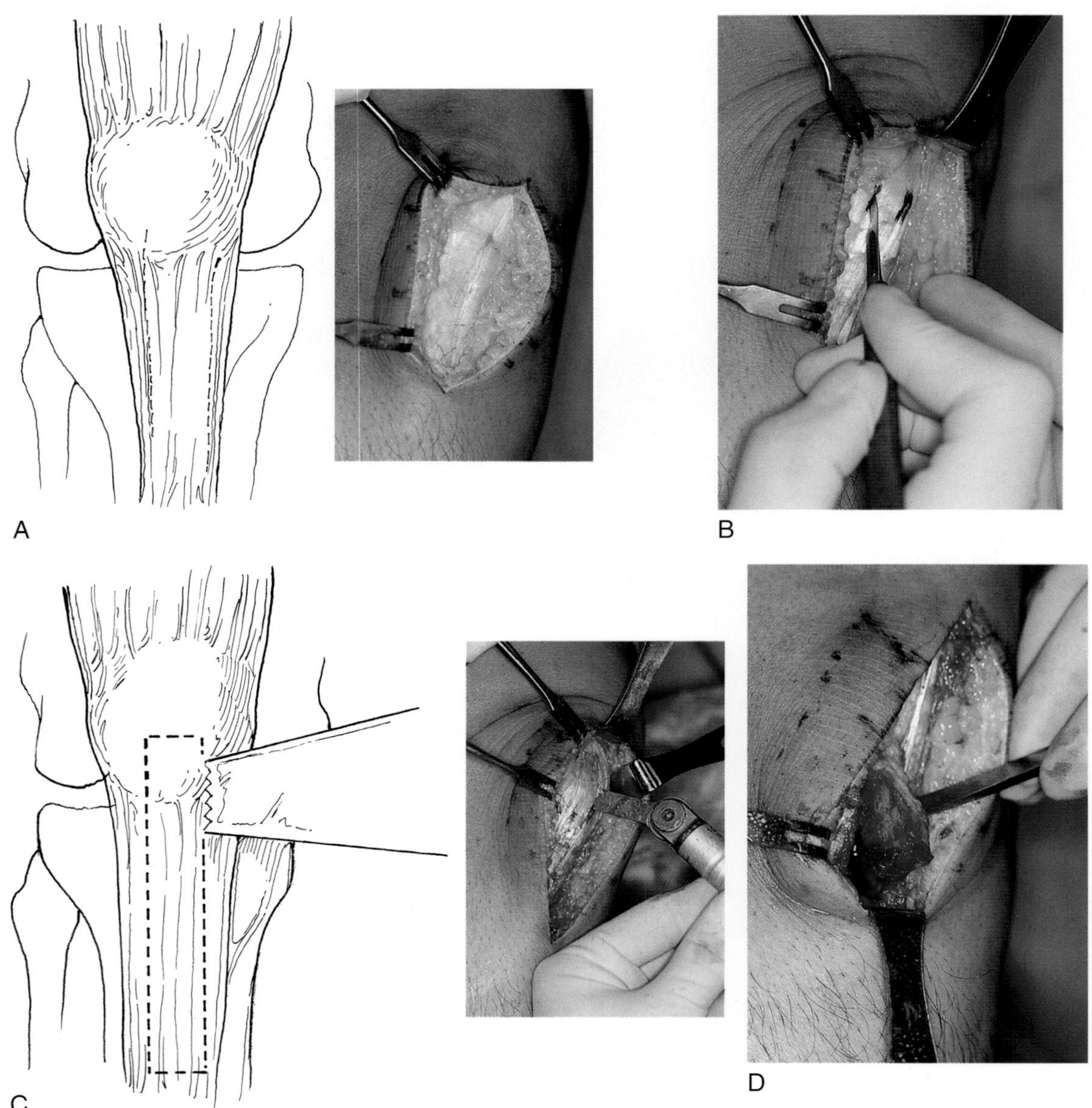

FIGURE 7–4. Bone patellar tendon bone graft harvest. *A*, The tendon is exposed, and the paratenon is incised. *B*, An appropriately sized graft is measured, and the tendon is incised parallel to its fibers. *C*, An oscillating saw is used to remove 25-mm bone blocks from the tibia and the patella. *D*, An osteotome is used to remove the bone blocks.

the tendon carefully to allow clear identification of the tendon fibers. Measurements are taken, and the graft is harvested. Care is taken to have parallel cuts that follow the same line as the tendon fibers. A 10- or 11-mm graft with 25-mm bone blocks is harvested.

b. Hamstring tendons: Most authors recommend harvesting the semitendinosus and gracilis tendons (Fig. 7–5). These tendons are harvested through a 3-cm vertical incision centered approximately 5 cm below the medial joint line, midway between the tibial tubercle and the posteromedial aspect of the tibia. The sartorial fascia is incised, and the tendons are identified and carefully freed from any attachments. A large band frequently runs from the semitendinosus to the medial head of the gastrocnemius, and it is crucial to release this band before harvesting the tendon. A whip stitch is placed in the tendon to control the end before detachment and for later fixation. The tendons are sharply removed from their insertions, and a tendon stripper is used for

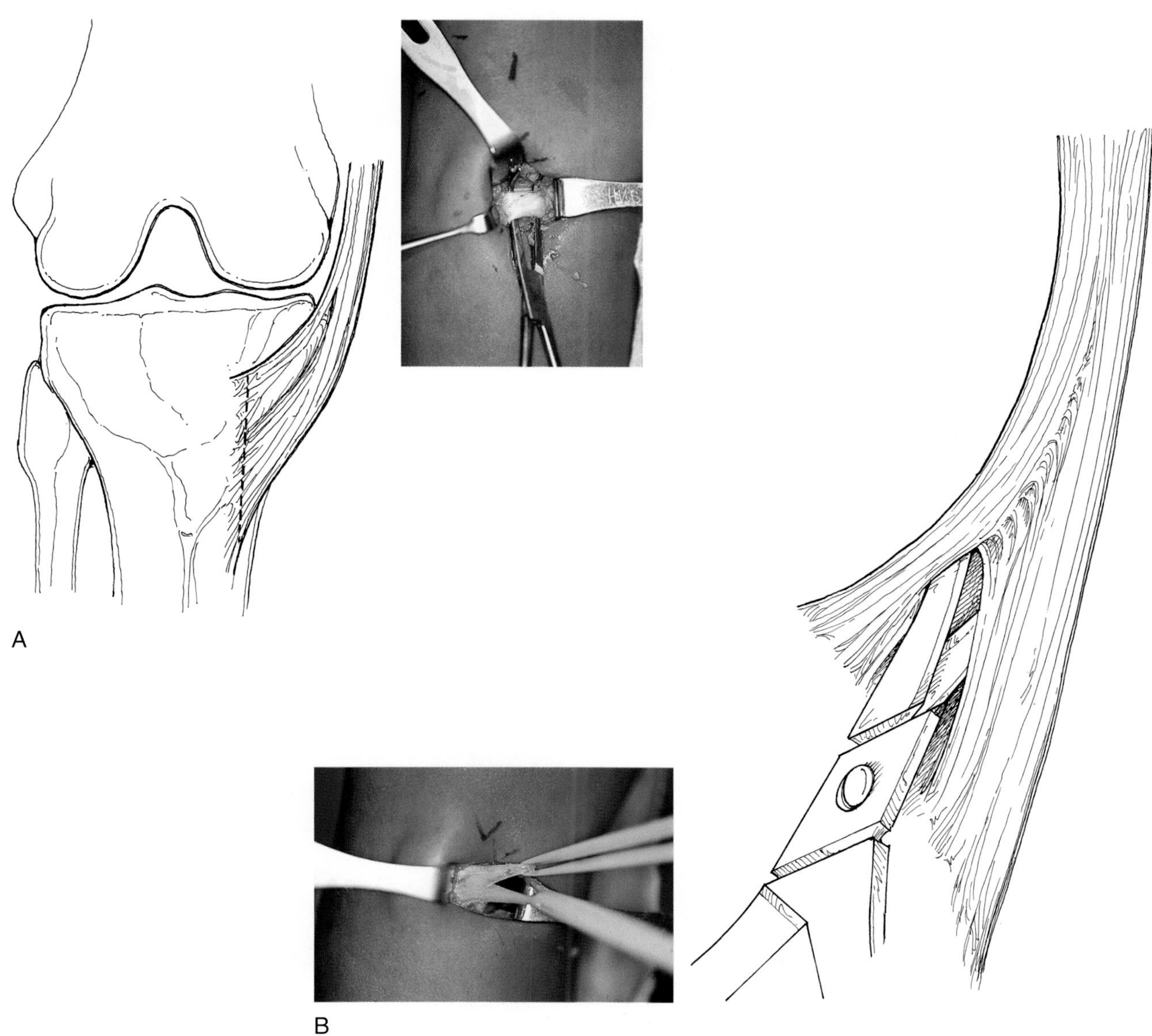

FIGURE 7–5. Hamstring graft harvest. *A* and *B*, Initial dissection beneath sartorial fascia and isolation of gracilis tendon (superior) and semitendinosus tendon (inferior).

Illustration continued on following page

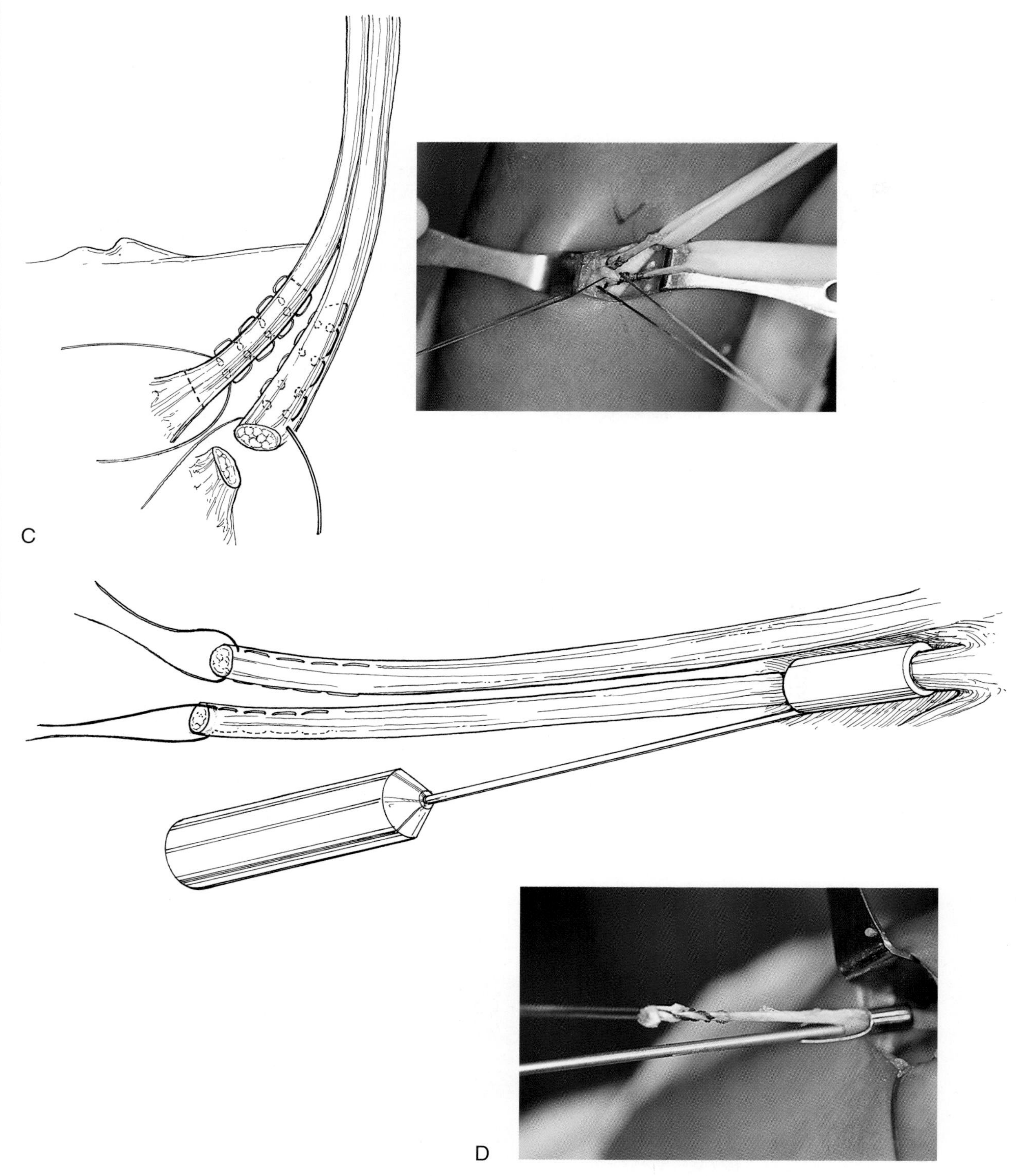

FIGURE 7–5 *Continued. C*, Sutures placed near insertion of each tendon with a whip stitch. D, Harvesting with a tendon stripper.

subcutaneous harvesting of the grafts. Extending the knee slightly when harvesting the graft may facilitate the harvesting of a better, longer graft.

c. Quadriceps tendon: This graft is harvested through a 5-cm midline incision superior to the patella (Fig. 7–6). A 20- to 25-mm patellar bone block is harvested, and a full-thickness or partial-thickness graft is harvested. It is usually possible to harvest a 7- to 8-cm strip of tendon.

3. Graft preparation: These techniques are discussed separately. Careful graft handling should be emphasized while working on all grafts. A qualified assistant should work on the graft in a well-lighted area away from the operative field. Scissors, suture,

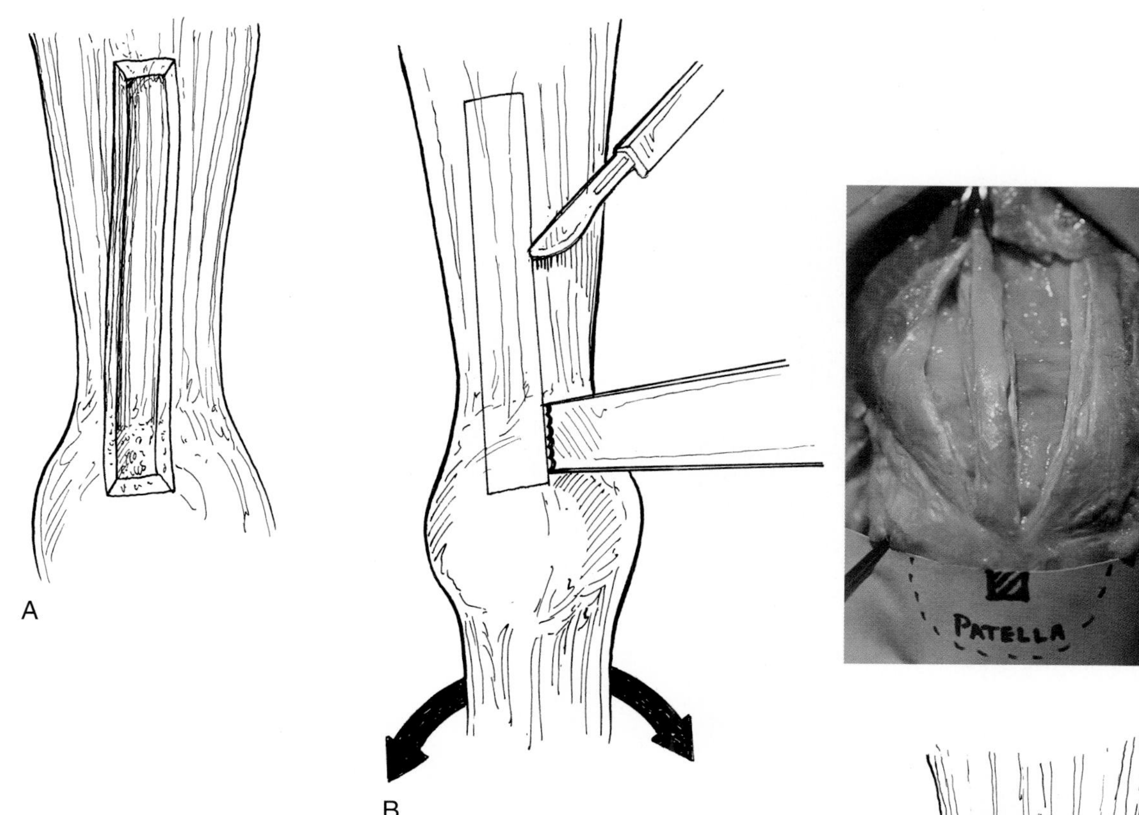

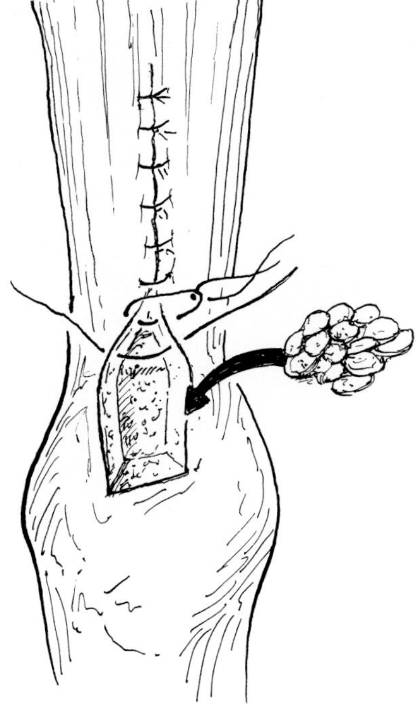

FIGURE 7–6. Quadriceps tendon graft harvest. *A*, Incision. *B*, Harvest of a 10-mm graft. *C*, Bone plug harvest. (*Inset B* from Fulkerson JP, Langeland RH: The central quadriceps tendon graft for cruciate ligament reconstruction. Op Tech Orthop 6:135–137, 1996.)

needle drivers, rongeurs, rasps, burr, drill, and curettes should be readily available. Special boards are available for working with hamstring grafts.

a. Patellar tendon: The surgeon should be careful to remove extra bone from the tibial side because there is frequently an overhang at the tibial tubercle that must be excised (Fig. 7–7). The graft is sculpted, and sizers are used to determine the appropriate tunnel diameter. The femoral bone block should be contoured to a bullet shape to allow easy passage. A rongeur, rasp, or burr can be used. A No. 5

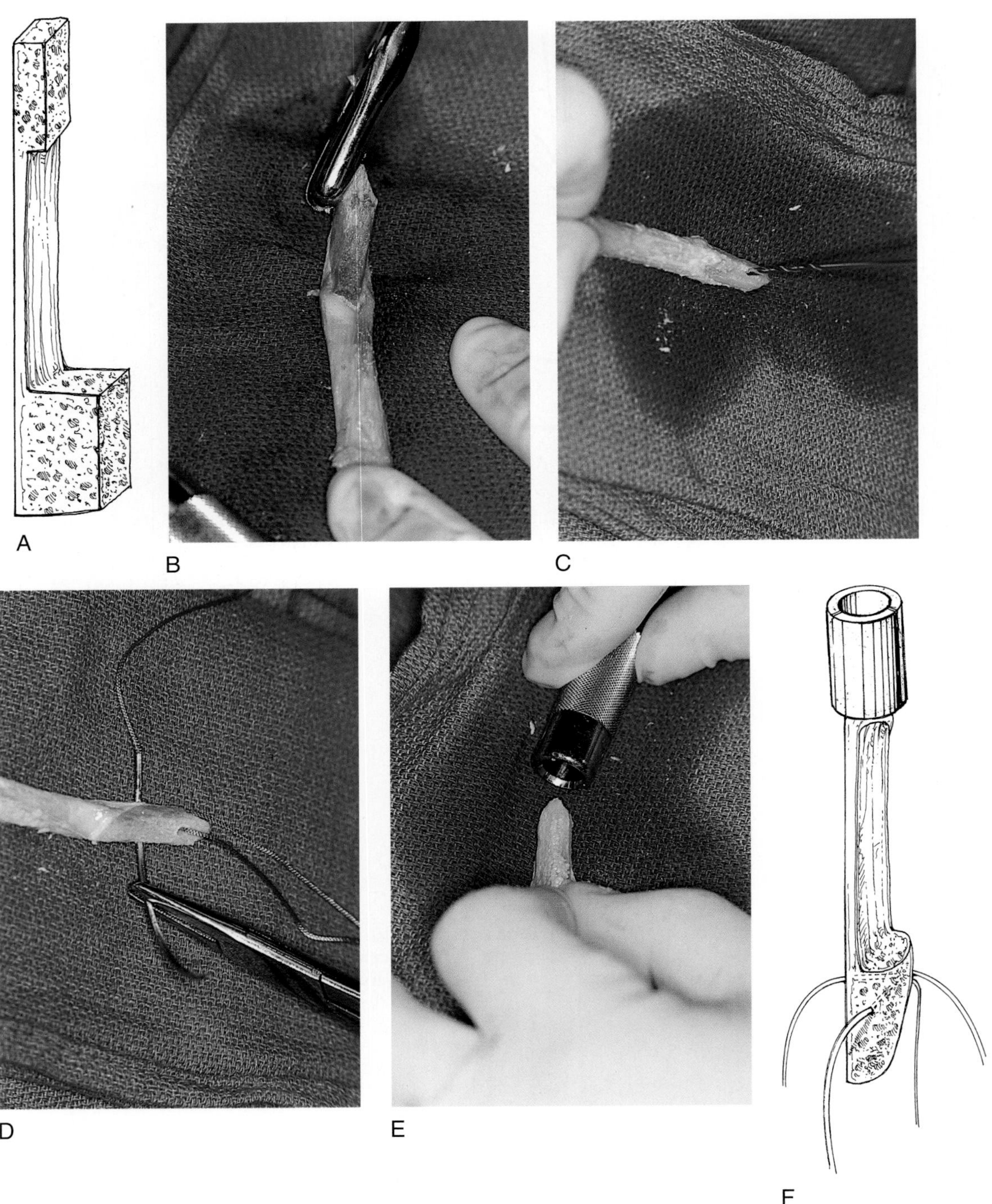

FIGURE 7–7. Bone patellar tendon bone graft preparation. *A*, Initial harvest with rectangular bone blocks. *B*, Graft is prepared with rongeur, file, or a burr. *C*, Drilling for suture placement. *D*, Suture placement. *E*, Graft is contoured to fit through appropriately sized tunnel. *F*, Final prepared graft. Note perpendicular placement of sutures in tibial bone block.

nonabsorbable suture is placed approximately 5 mm from the end of the side of the graft to be placed in the femoral tunnel (usually the tibial bone block), and two No. 5 nonabsorbable sutures are placed 10 and 15 mm from the end of the bone block that is planned for the tibial tunnel. These sutures can be placed perpendicular to each other to avoid suture *cutout*.

b. Hamstring tendons: The tendons are trimmed to an appropriate size (about 25 cm), muscle tissue is removed from the tendon with a curette, and this end is *tubularized* for easier graft passage (Fig. 7–8). After preparation, the grafts are folded in half over a 5-mm tape, and the size is determined (usually 8 to 9 mm). Final graft preparation depends on the fixation technique that is selected.

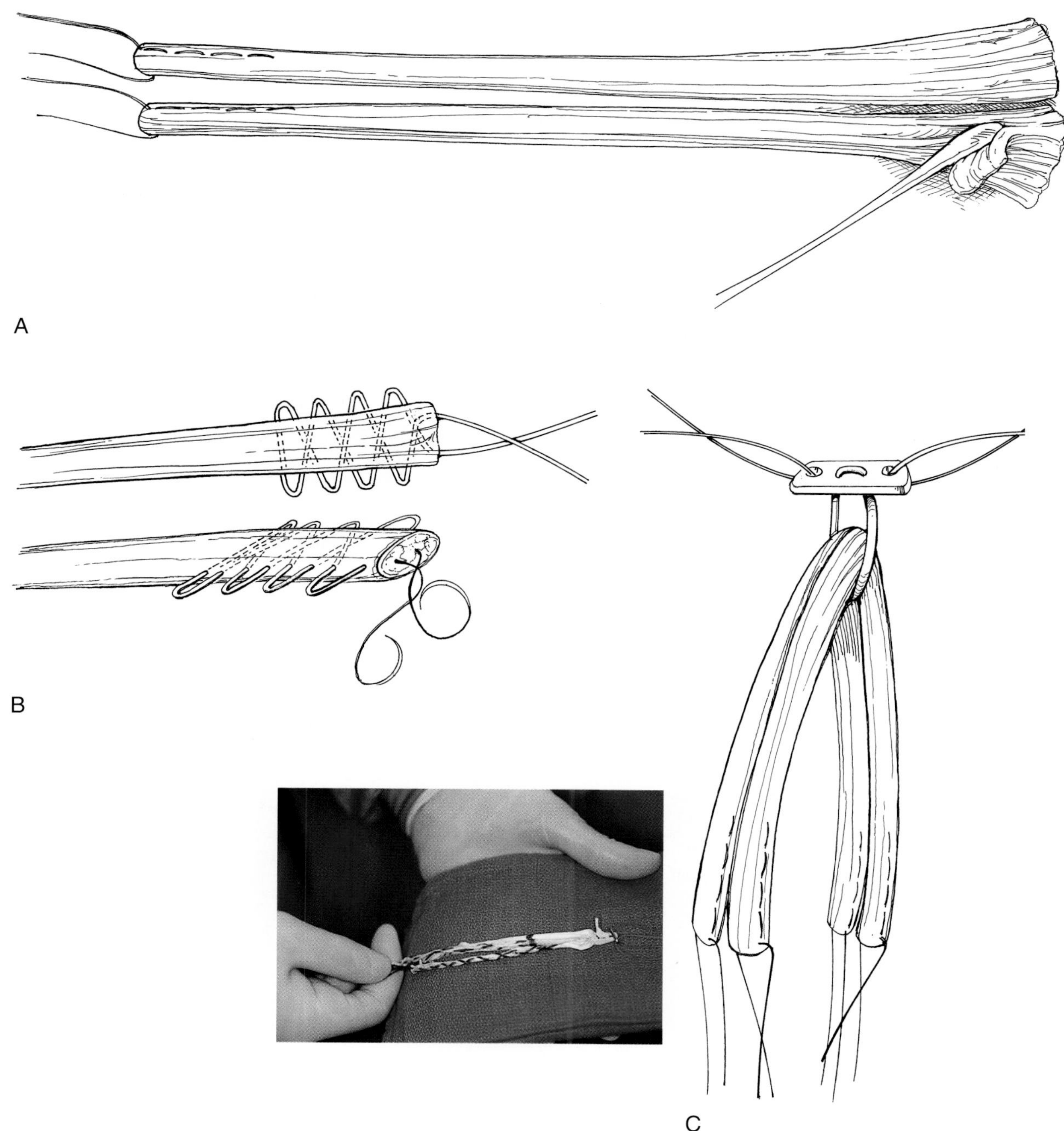

FIGURE 7–8. Hamstring graft preparation. *A*, Muscle is cleared off each tendon with a curette. *B*, Sutures are placed on the free ends of the grafts. *C*, A fixation device is prepared after graft has been sized.

c. Quadriceps tendon: The bony end is prepared as described for the patellar tendon graft previously (Fig. 7–9). The soft tissue end is prepared with a secure whip stitch.

4. Diagnostic arthroscopy: A thorough evaluation of the knee is done. The menisci are evaluated carefully. Meniscal tears are associated commonly with ACL injuries. Meniscus repair should be undertaken for any tear that possibly can be salvaged. Loose bodies are removed, articular cartilage lesions are identified and treated, and preparations are made for ACL reconstruction.

5. Débridement and notchplasty: The ACL stump is débrided, and fibrous tissue from the wall of the lateral femoral condyle is removed (Fig. 7–10). It is essential to be able to see the back of the notch to

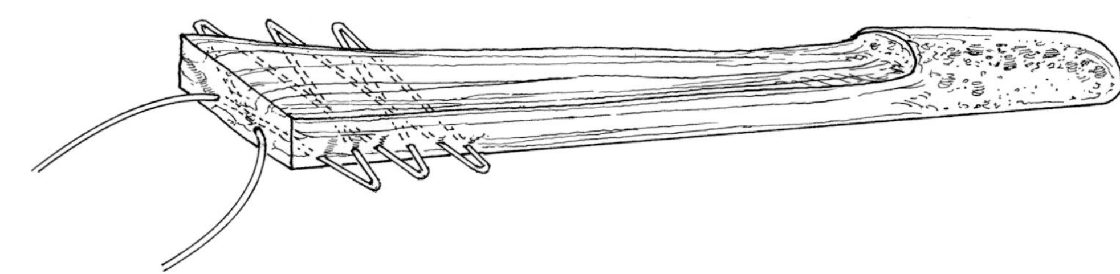

FIGURE 7–9. Preparation of the soft tissue end of the quadriceps graft. The bony end is prepared exactly like a bone patellar tendon bone graft.

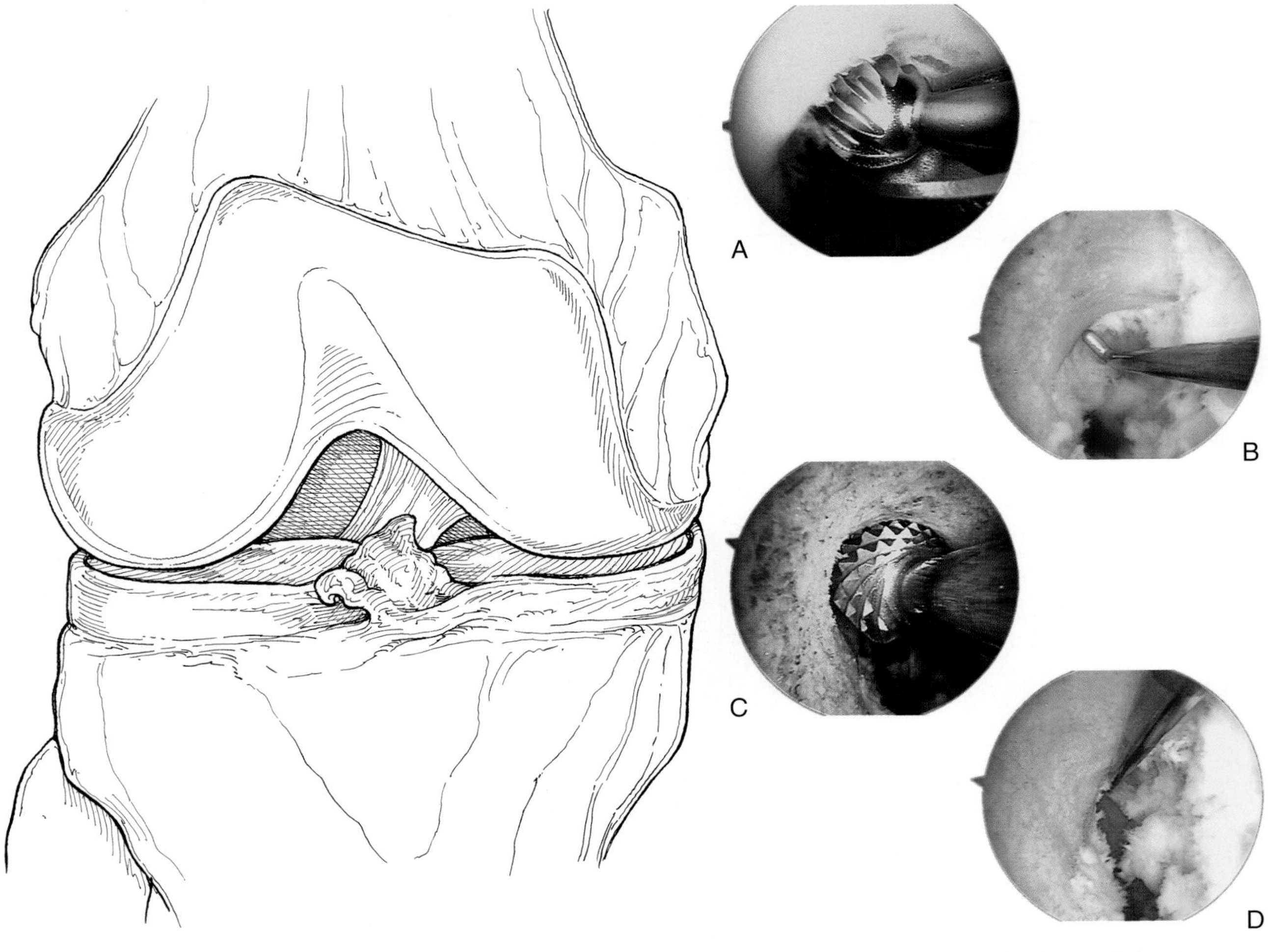

FIGURE 7–10. Notchplasty. *A*, Beginning at the articular margin, the notchplasty is initiated (the roof also is recessed). *B*, Resident's ridge is identified. *C*, All soft tissue is cleared. *D*, The over-the-top position is identified.

identify the over-the-top position. A notchplasty and a roofplasty can be done with the use of a motorized shaver and burr. The amount of notchplasty necessary is a controversial. Generally, it is necessary to do only enough to be able to see clearly the back of the notch and provide superior clearance for the graft. If the graft is placed more posteriorly, as is the current recommendation, the roofplasty does not need to be aggressive. Hamstring grafts usually require a more aggressive roofplasty.

6. Tibial tunnel placement: The tibial tunnel is placed in the posteromedial aspect of the tibial footprint and centered approximately 7 mm in front of the

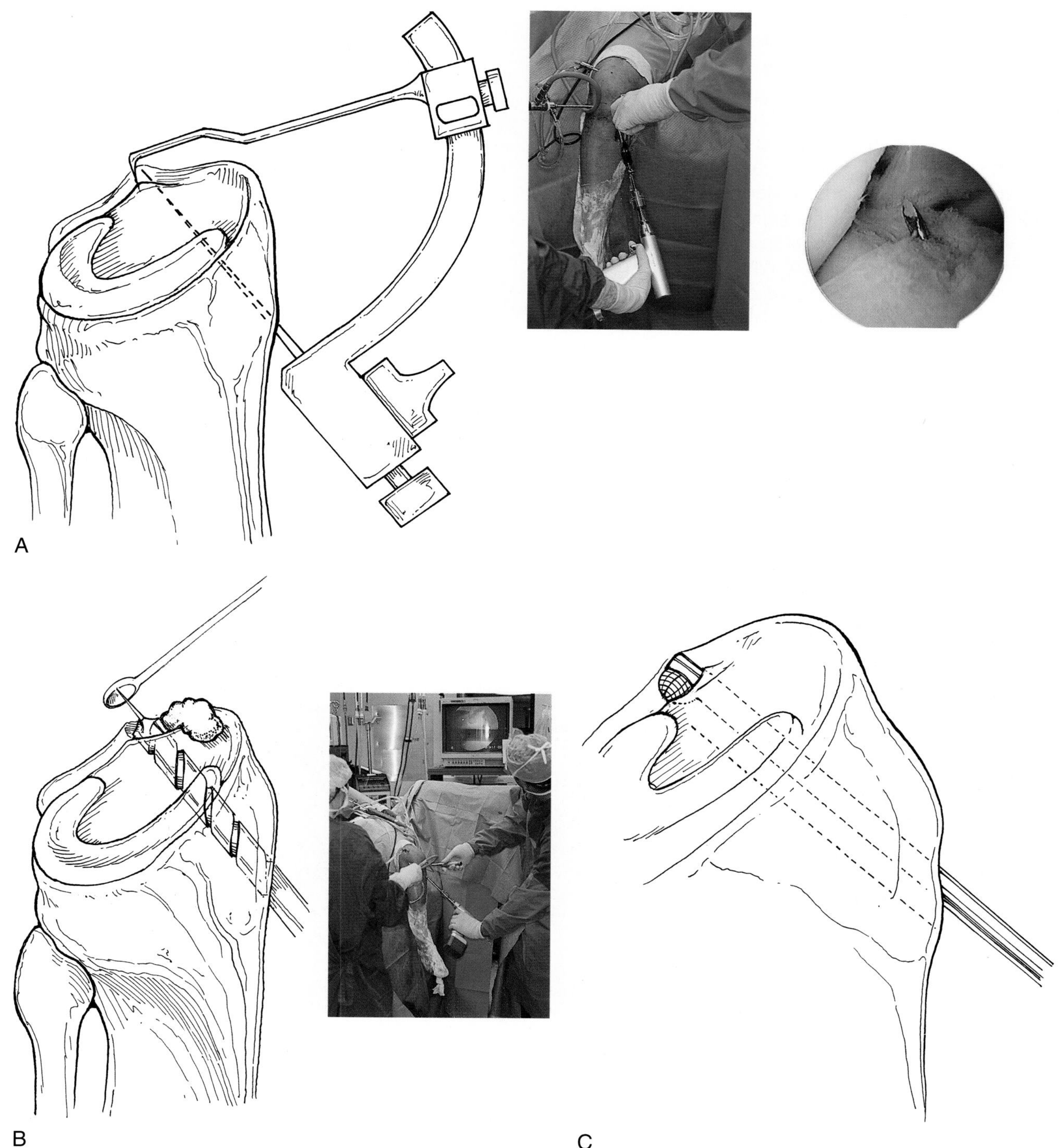

FIGURE 7–11. Tibial tunnel preparation. *A*, The guide wire is drilled using a tibial guide. *B*, When the position is accepted, the tunnel is overdrilled with an appropriately sized drill bit. *C*, The back edge of the tunnel is rasped.

crossing PCL fibers, adjacent to the medial eminence and along a line that extends from the anterior horn of the lateral meniscus (Fig. 7–11). Externally the guide is positioned midway betweenthe tibial tubercle and the posteromedial aspect of the tibia, and a guide wire is drilled into position and checked. Several recommendations for determining the length of the tibial tunnel or the ideal angle have been made. The *N + 7 rule* is a handy method to use as a preliminary setting for angled guides: Simply measure the distance between the bone plugs (patella tendon graft), add the number 7 to this value, and set the guide at this angle. After placing the guide, check the depth of the tunnel on the guide, and it should be about 1 to 2 mm more than the intertendinous distance. If it is not, the angle should be adjusted accordingly. It also is important that the arm of the guide be perpendicular to the tibia during drilling. When the guide pin has been drilled and its position checked, it is overdrilled with a fully threaded cannulated drill. Before entering the articular surface of the tibia, the drill can be retracted and bone graft collected from the flutes of the drill bit. The tunnel is drilled into the joint (a curette can be used to protect the PCL), and the edges are rasped to prevent graft abrasion.

7. Femoral tunnel placement: The femoral tunnel should be planned to leave a 1- to 2-mm posterior cortical rim (Fig. 7–12). For a 10- or 11-mm tunnel, the guide wire should be positioned 7 mm in front of the over-the-top position, and for an 8- or 9-mm tunnel, the guide wire should be placed 6 mm in front of the over-the-top position. Commercially available transtibial offset guides can be placed through the tibial tunnel and engage the posterior cortex, allowing accurate femoral tunnel placement. The tunnel is drilled to the appropriate depth (usually 5 mm longer than the femoral bone block), and the edges are rasped.
8. Final preparations: A Beath needle is passed through both tunnels, exiting the anterolateral thigh. Additional preparation usually is required for hamstring grafts. If an Endobutton (Smith & Nephew Dyonics, Mansfield, MA) is used, the femoral tunnel is drilled to the desired length (35 to 40 mm is usually possible), stopping short of the cortex, then the cortex is overdrilled with a 4.5-mm drill bit. A depth gauge is used to measure the length of the femoral tunnel (from the cortex to the intra-articular margin). The length of the 5-mm tape leader for the graft is tied using the following formula: Tape length = (overall tunnel length–depth drilled) + 6 mm (turning radius of the button). One of the criticisms of the Endobutton is that there can be some slippage at the knot in the tape. For this reason, the manufacturer currently is developing loops of various lengths that are preset without knots.

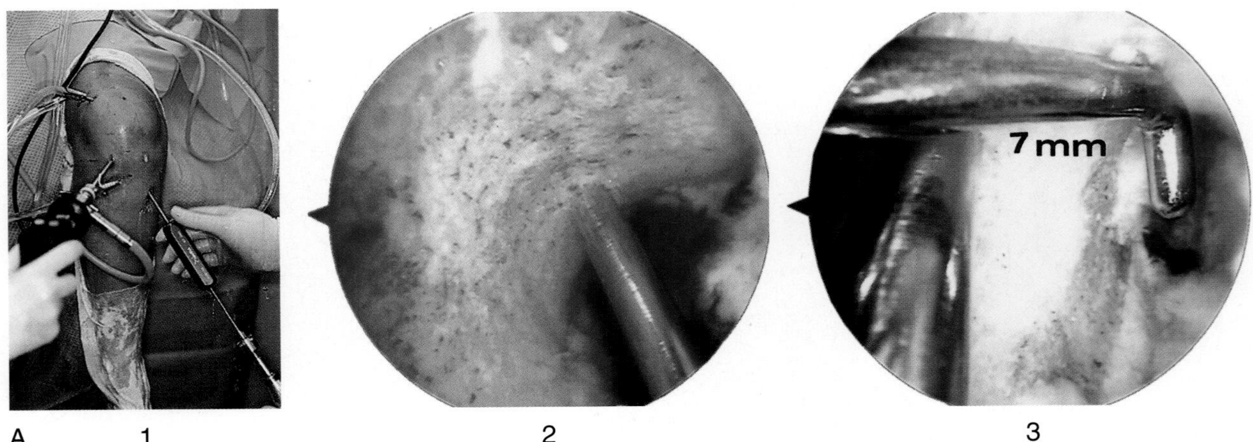

FIGURE 7–12. Femoral tunnel placement. *A1*, External view demonstrating use of the offset guide. *A2*, View from the inferolateral portal showing guide wire placement. *A3*, View from the inferomedial portal confirming that the guide pin is 7 mm from the over-the-top position.

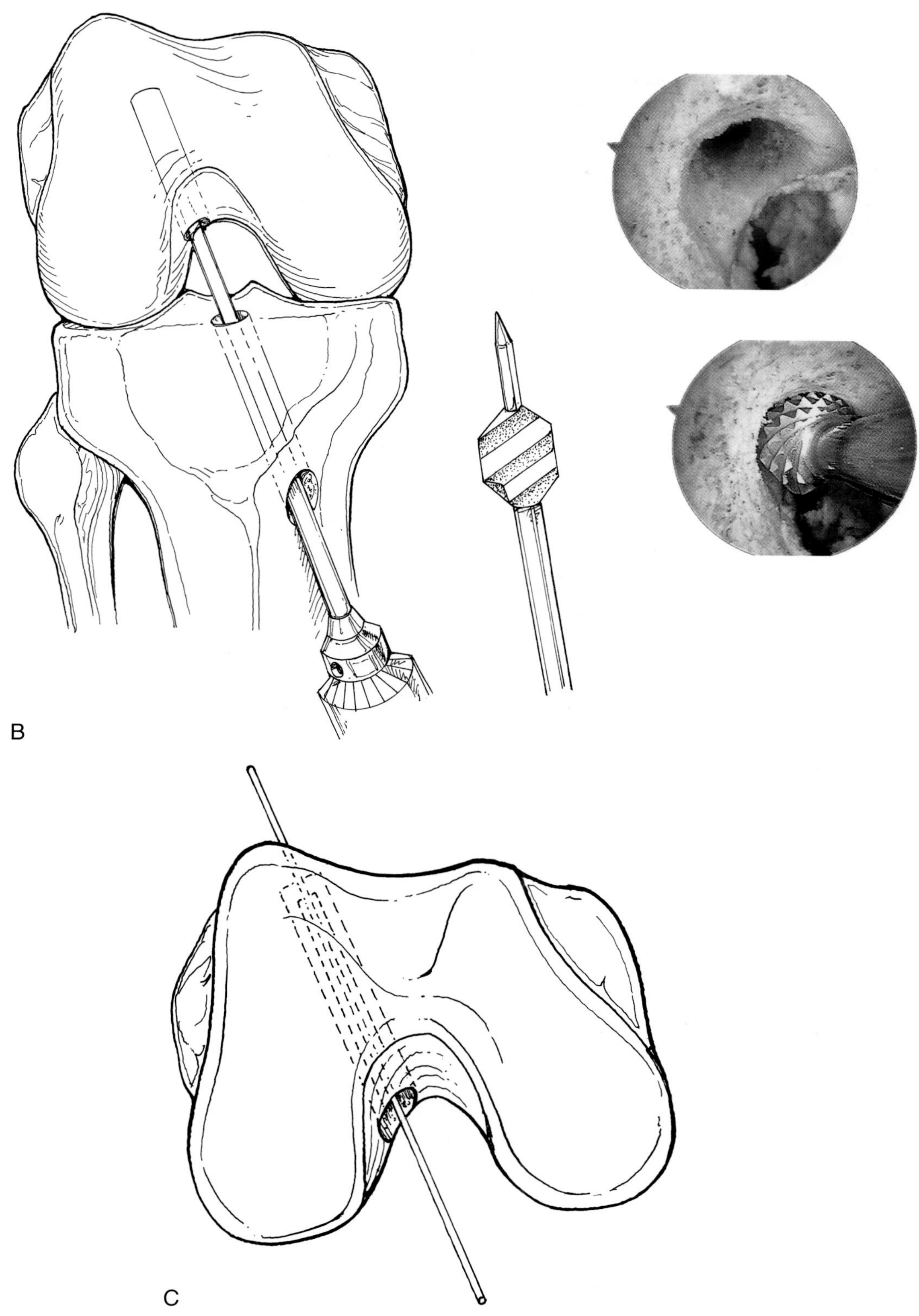

FIGURE 7–12 *Continued. B,* The tunnel is overdrilled with an appropriately sized, terminally threaded drill bit, and the front edge is rasped *(inset)*. *C,* Guide wire is left in place for graft passage.

9. Graft passage: Sutures (from the femoral bone plug or the Endobutton) are passed through both tunnels and exit the anterolateral thigh with the Beath needle and are used to pass the graft into the knee (Fig. 7–13).
10. Graft fixation
    a. Bone block fixation: The femoral bone block is fixed with a cannulated interference screw (Fig. 7–14). The screw guide wire is positioned on the anterior aspect of the bone block, as far away from the tendinous portion of the graft as possible. This positioning can be facilitated by laying the guide wire on the graft before pulling it into the knee. The interference screw (usually a 7 × 20 mm screw is adequate) is placed under arthroscopic visualization, and the guide wire is removed. It is important to flex the knee and to drop your hand toward the tibia when placing the screw. If there is any difficulty in placing the screw or if the guide wire rotates or disengages, the screw should be removed and the step repeated. The tibial side of the graft is secured with a cannulated interference screw (usually 9 × 20 mm).

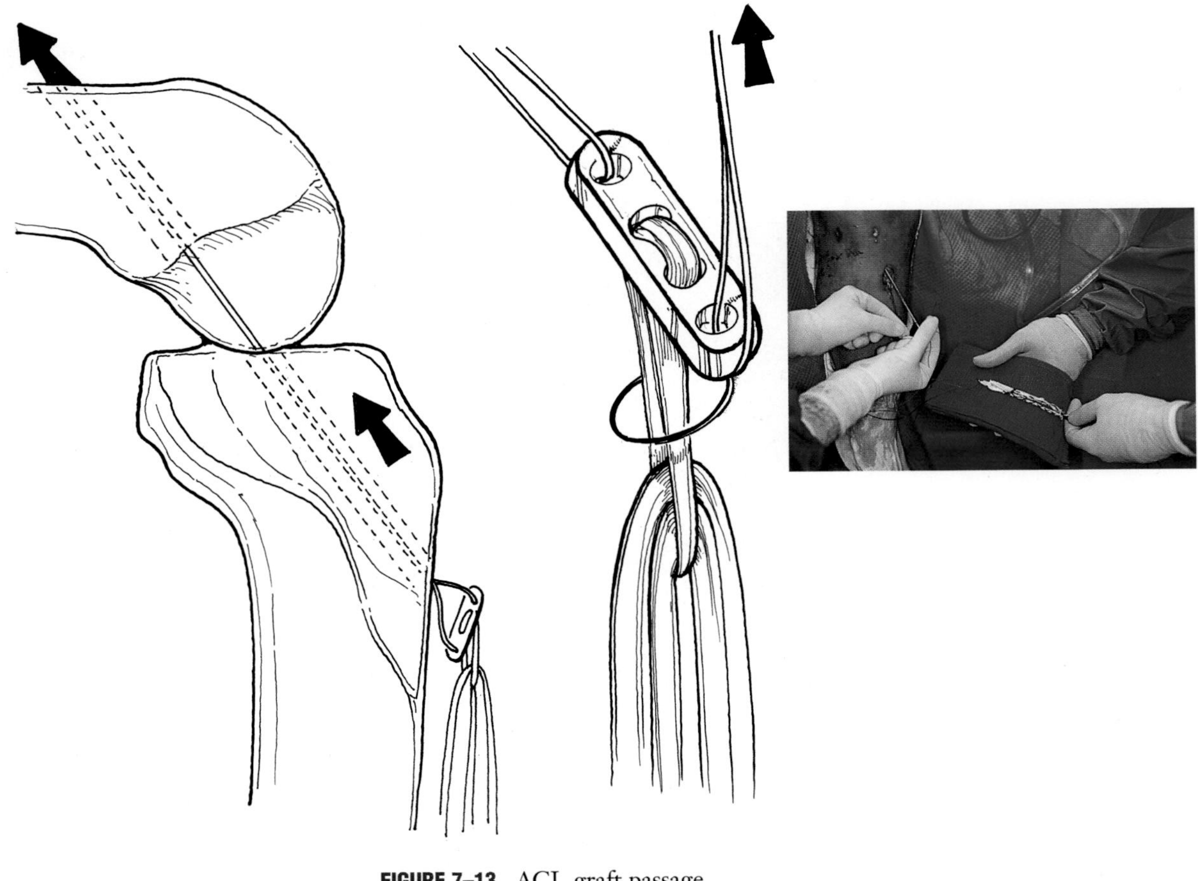

FIGURE 7–13. ACL graft passage.

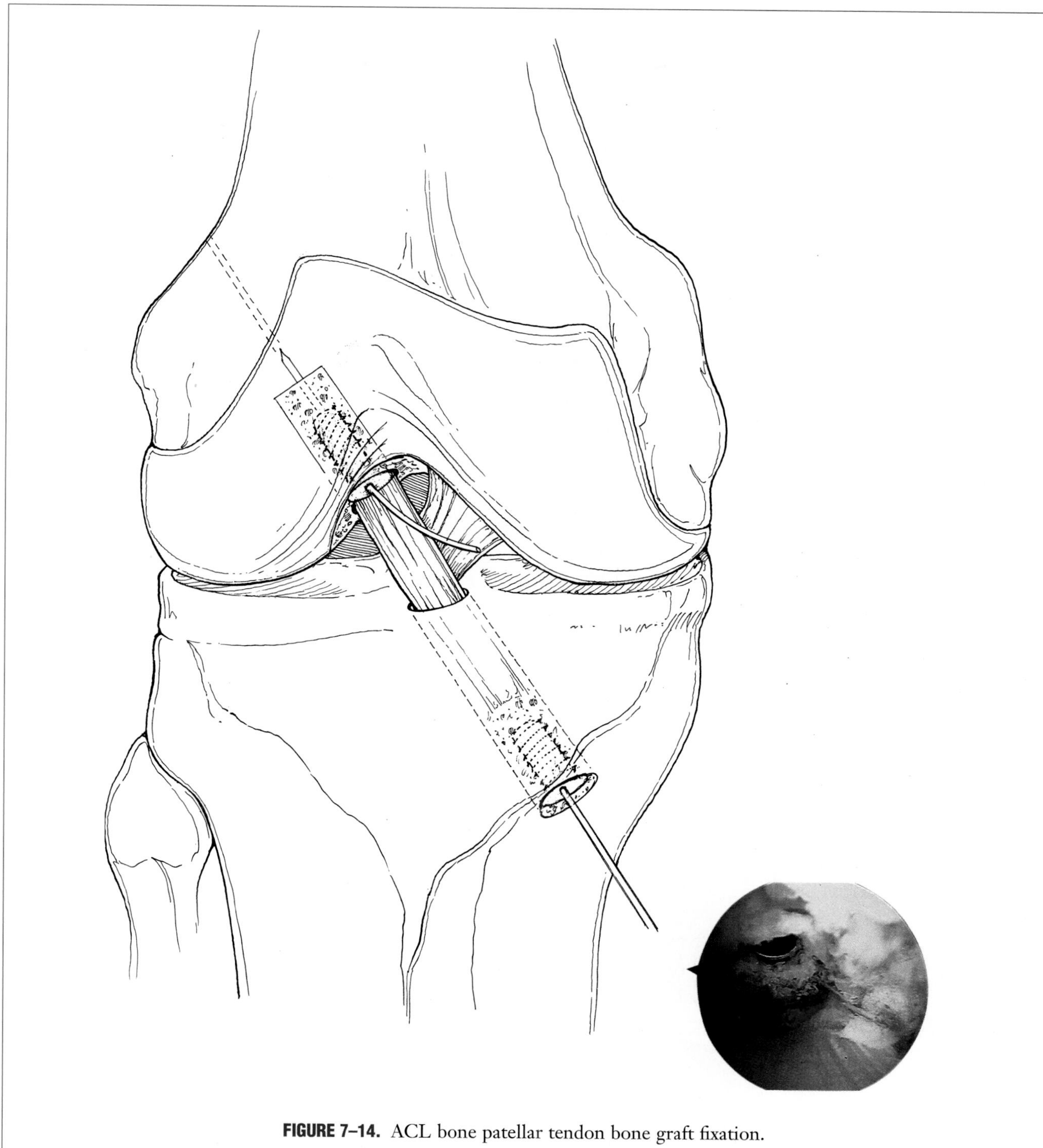

FIGURE 7–14. ACL bone patellar tendon bone graft fixation.

b. Hamstring fixation: If an Endobutton is used, it is prepared so that the two middle holes of the button are filled with the 5-mm leader tape, and the two outer holes are filled with a No. 2 and a No. 5 nonabsorbable suture (Fig. 7–15). Both of these sutures are passed through the tunnels and exit the anterolateral thigh. The number 5 suture is tensioned and allows the graft to pass up the femoral tunnel. When the graft reaches the maximal extent of the tunnel (premeasured and marked on the graft), the No. 2 suture is used to deploy the button. The graft is secured by placing tension on the free ends of the graft. The tibial side of the graft can be secured with a variety of techniques (e.g., screw over post, screw and soft tissue washer, staple).

11. Wound closure: The wound is closed in anatomic layers. A drain is placed if necessary.

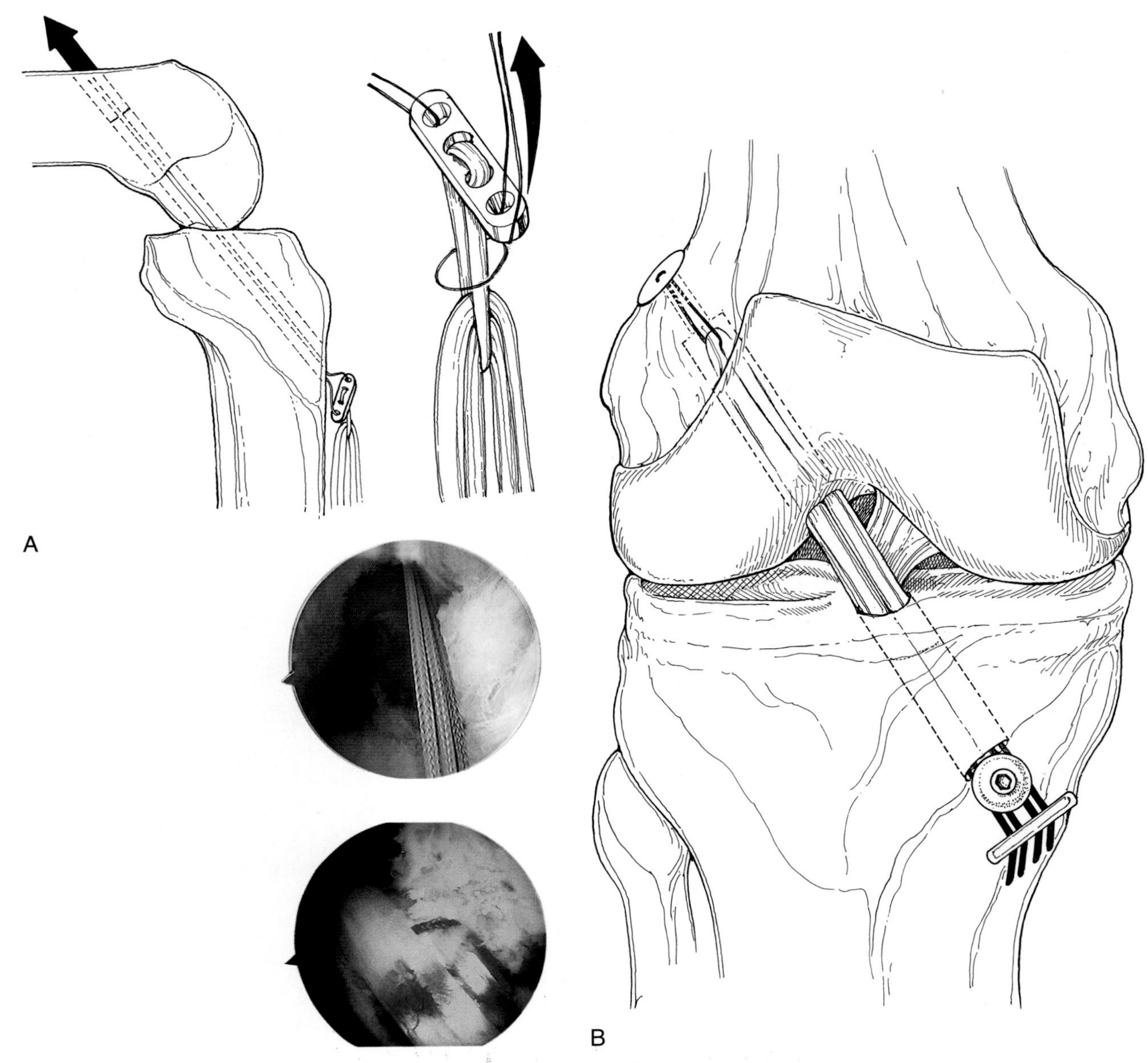

FIGURE 7–15. ACL hamstring graft passage *(A)* and fixation *(B)*.

POSTOPERATIVE MANAGEMENT

Patients are kept in a knee brace in full extension. Early range of motion is encouraged. Quadriceps isometric exercises and stimulation are started shortly after surgery. Crutch ambulation is allowed with weight bearing as tolerated on the first postoperative day. The patient is allowed to return to full activities if full range of motion has been achieved, the knee is stable, and the strength of the operative leg is equal to the opposite side, usually at about 6 months postoperatively.

COMPLICATIONS

There are numerous technical steps with this procedure, and a failure of any step can result in a complication. Careful padding and judicious tourniquet use can limit neurapraxias. Graft harvesting can cause patellar fractures (BPTB and quadriceps tendon) or saphenous nerve injury (hamstrings). Instrument breakage, hardware problems, errant tunnels, and other problems can be avoided with careful technique. Postoperative problems include patellofemoral problems (especially with BPTB grafts), loss of motion, effusion, late laxity, and other complications.

RESULTS

With experience and careful technique, excellent results can be expected in 80% to 90% of ACL reconstructions.

REFERENCES

Frank CB, Jackson DW: The science of reconstruction of the anterior cruciate ligament: Current concepts review. J Bone Joint Surg [Am] 79:1556–1576, 1997.

Larson RL: Anterior cruciate ligament reconstruction with hamstring tendons. Op Tech Orthop 6:138–146, 1996.

Larson RL, Taillon M: Anterior cruciate ligament insufficiency: Principles of treatment. J Am Acad Orthop Surg 2:26–35, 1994.

Palmeri M, Bartolozzi AR: Arthroscopic anterior cruciate ligament reconstruction with patellar tendon. Op Tech Orthop 6:126–134, 1996.

CHAPTER 8

Pediatric Anterior Cruciate Ligament Reconstruction

INTRODUCTION

Because of the early emphasis on sports in the United States, anterior cruciate ligament (ACL) injuries in children are occurring with increasing frequency. Some of these injuries involve avulsion of the tibial eminence, and primary repair is possible. As in adults, most of these injuries are midsubstance. Because of the presence of the physis, ACL reconstruction techniques, especially in younger children, must be modified.

HISTORY AND PHYSICAL EXAMINATION

Findings are similar to the adult knee. Hip range of motion and tenderness should be checked to ensure that other conditions, such as Legg-Calvé-Perthes syndrome or slipped capital femoral epiphysis, are not causing referred knee pain. An attempt to determine the amount of growth remaining is important if operative treatment is being considered.

DIAGNOSTIC IMAGING

Plain radiographs should be evaluated carefully. Physeal injuries, osteochondral fragments, and bony avulsions should be sought out (Fig. 8–1). The width of the physis is measured, and anticipated growth remaining is considered. If there is any associated collateral ligament laxity, stress radiographs should be obtained to rule out physeal injury. MRI can be helpful in evaluating the ligament and the physis.

NONOPERATIVE MANAGEMENT

Because reconstruction techniques that avoid the growth plates are not as successful as procedures in the adult, most surgeons advocate initial nonoperative treatment of midsubstance ACL injuries in children. Temporary immobilization, progressive range of motion, quadriceps strengthening, functional bracing, and activity modification are the mainstays of this approach. Often the plan is to wait for the child to reach skeletal maturity and then consider ACL reconstruction. This approach is often unsuccessful, and recurrent injuries can result in meniscal and chondral injury. Minimally displaced tibial eminence fractures can be reduced and held in extension. There is almost universal support for operative repair of displaced avulsion fractures of the tibial eminence.

RELEVANT ANATOMY

It is crucial that the surgeon have a good understanding of the location and orientation of the tibial and the femoral growth plates (Fig. 8–2). Particular care should be taken around the tibial tubercle physis, which is sensitive to injury.

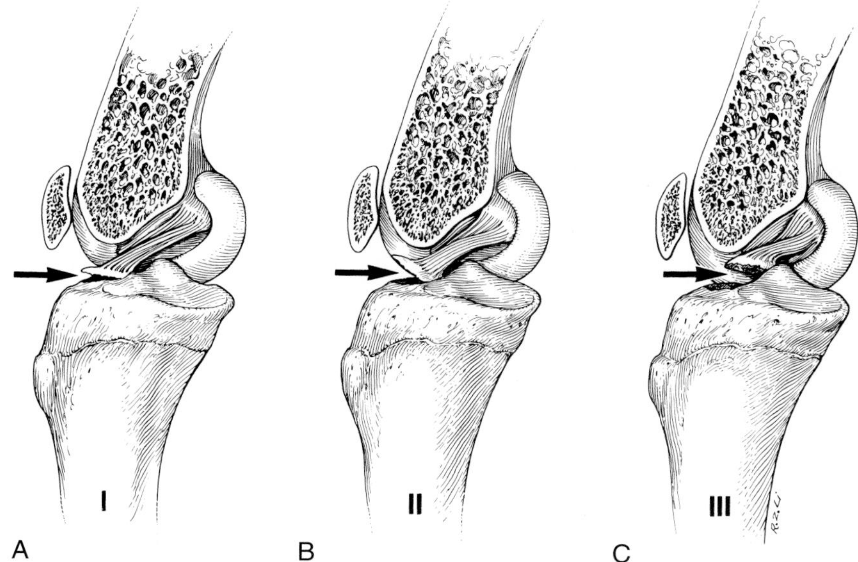

FIGURE 8–1. Tibial eminence fractures have been classified by Meyers and McKeever. *A*, Type I nondisplaced fracture. *B*, Type II fracture with elevation of the anterior portion only. *C*, Type III, completely displaced fracture. (From Tria AJ, Klein KS: An Illustrated Guide to the Knee. New York, Churchill Livingstone, 1992.)

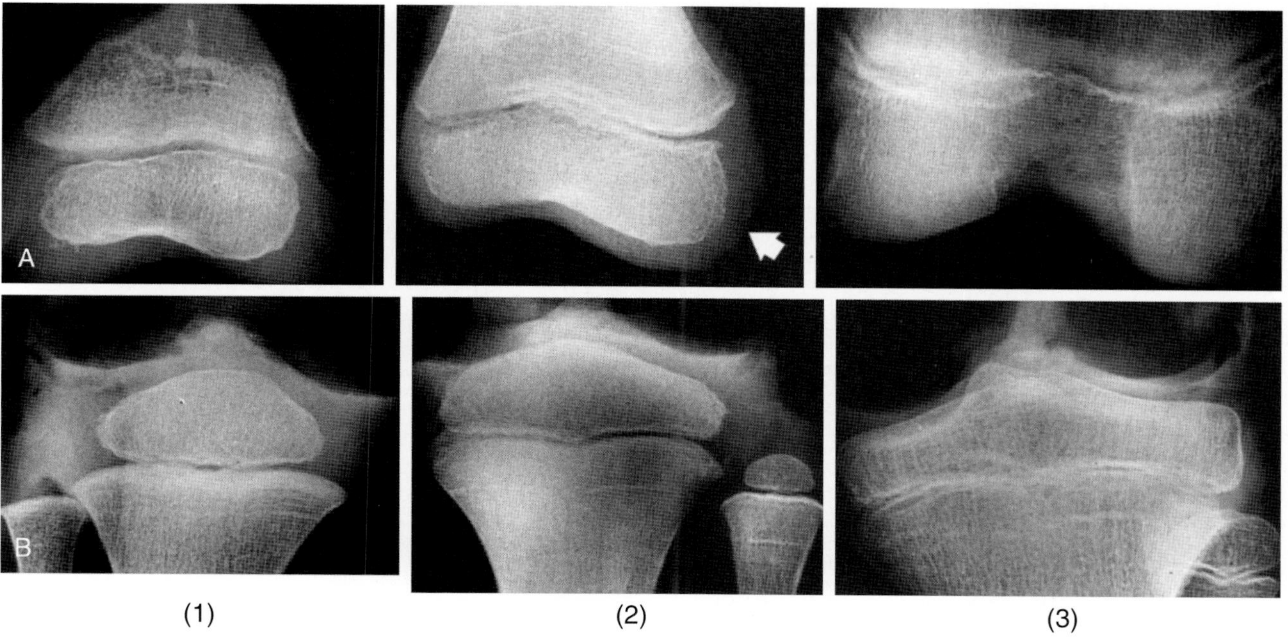

FIGURE 8–2. Femoral and tibial growth plate anatomy. *A*, Distal femoral physis radiograph in *(1)* a 3-year-old child, *(2)* a 7-year-old child, and *(3)* a 15-year-old child. *B*, Proximal tibial physis in *(1)* a 2-year-old child, *(2)* a 5-year-old child, and *(3)* an 11-year-old child. (From Ogden JA: Skeletal Injury in the Child, 2nd ed. Philadelphia, WB Saunders, 1990.)

SURGICAL *TECHNIQUE*

Indications

Indications for surgery include displaced tibial eminence fractures, tibial eminence fractures that do not reduce in extension, and midsubstance ACL tears that have failed nonoperative management. An algorithm is helpful in considering appropriate treatment for pediatric ACL deficiency (Fig. 8–3).

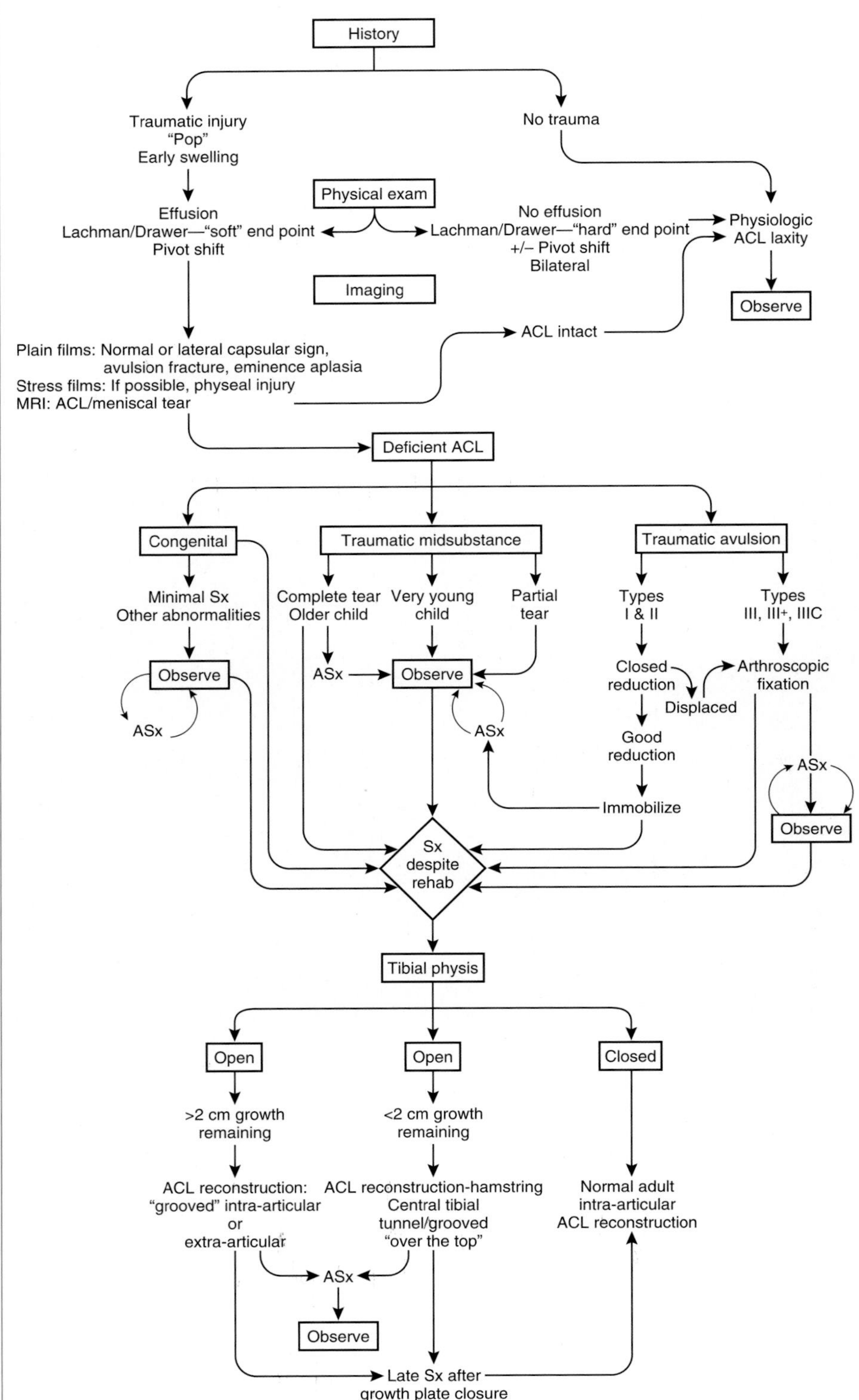

FIGURE 8–3. Algorithm for the treatment of ACL deficiency in the skeletally immature individual. (From Miller MD, Eilert RE: Management of anterior cruciate ligament deficiency in the skeletally immature individual. Op Tech Orthop 5:254–260, 1995.)

Technique

Tibial eminence fractures are repaired primarily with arthroscopically assisted techniques (Fig. 8–4). A Bunnell-type suture is placed in the ligament and brought out through drill holes that are tied over a bony bridge avoiding the physis.

Midsubstance tears can be addressed with reconstructions that avoid the physis (Figs. 8–5 and 8–6). Many surgeons suggest that except in very young patients, a small tibial tunnel can be drilled centrally without disruption of the tibial growth plate, and the technique can be modified accordingly. The femoral physis should be avoided except in adolescents who are near skeletal maturity.

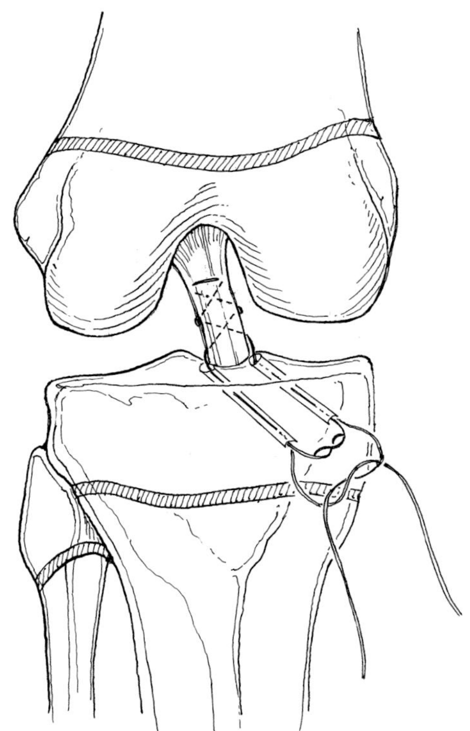

FIGURE 8–4. Operative management of a tibial eminence fracture.

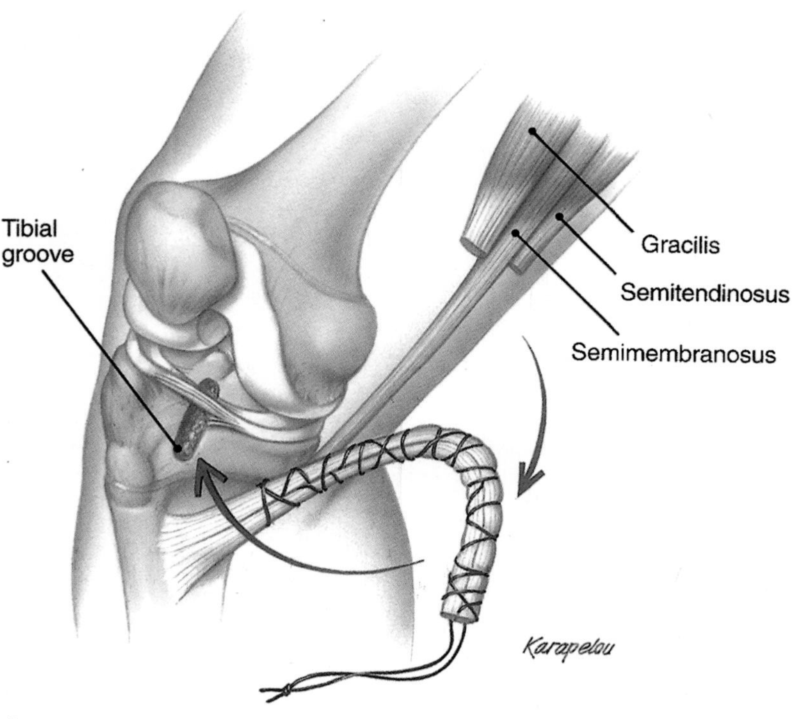

FIGURE 8–5. Technique of intra-articular ACL reconstruction using hamstring tendons and avoiding both growth plates. In most adolescents, a central tibial tunnel is probably acceptable. *A*, Semitendinosus and gracilis tendons are harvested leaving distal insertion intact.

Illustration continued on following page

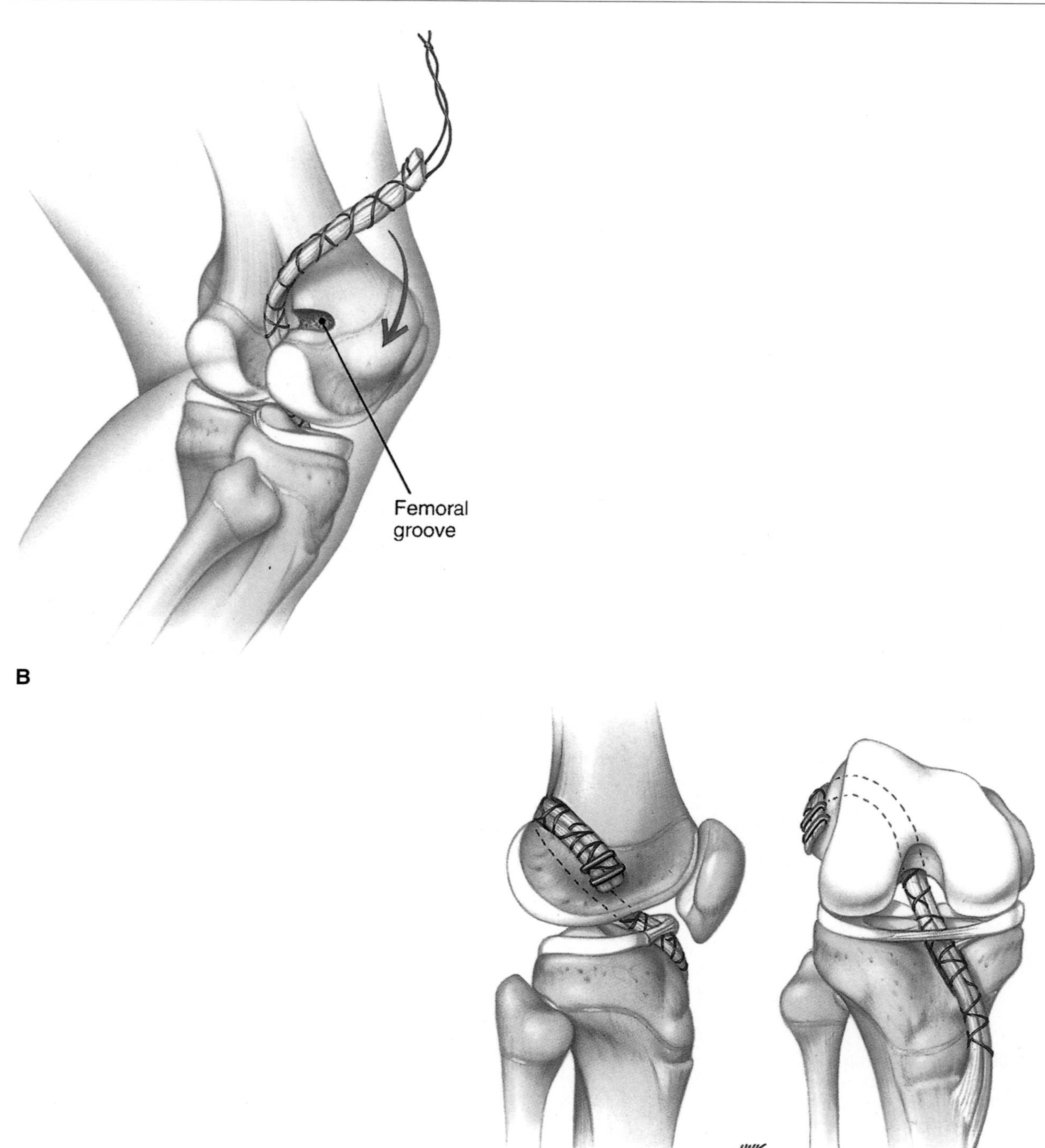

FIGURE 8–5 *Continued. B,* Graft is passed over the top. *C* and *D,* Final fixation. (From Miller MD, Eilert RE: Management of anterior cruciate ligament deficiency in the skeletally immature individual. Op Tech Orthop 5:254–260, 1995.)

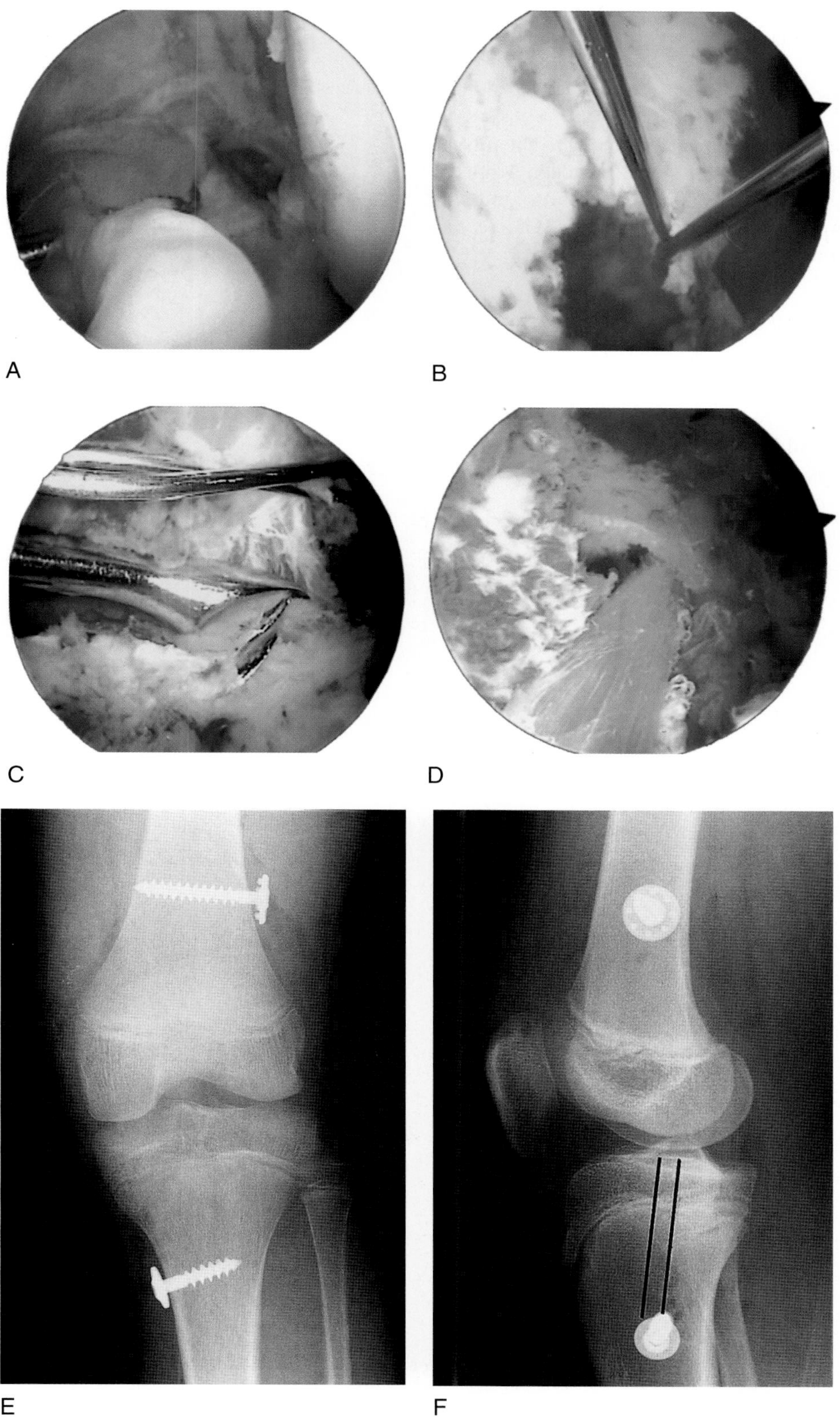

FIGURE 8–6. A 12-year-old boy with a complete ACL tear and recurrent instability treated with a vertically placed tibial tunnel and passage of the graft over the top. *A*, Torn ACL stump. *B*, Passing wire passed over the top. *C*, Tibial tunnel guide wire. *D*, Graft after passage from tibial tunnel and over the top. *E* and *F*, Anteroposterior and lateral radiographs after reconstruction.

POSTOPERATIVE MANAGEMENT

Rehabilitation is similar to that in an adult.

COMPLICATIONS

The complication of most concern is injury to the physis. Growth arrest, although uncommon, has been reported after ACL reconstruction in skeletally immature individuals. Other complications associated with ACL reconstruction also occur.

RESULTS

Early results with these procedures and with reconstructions that use central tibial tunnels are encouraging. Even if the reconstruction serves only to prevent recurrent reinjury until the child reaches skeletal maturity, the procedure can be considered a success.

REFERENCES

Lo IKY, Bell DM, Fowler PJ: Anterior cruciate ligament injuries in the skeletally immature patient. Instr Course Lect 47:351–359, 1998.

Miller MD, Eilert RE: Management of anterior cruciate ligament deficiency in the skeletally immature individual. Op Tech Orthop 5:254–260, 1995.

Parker AW, Drez D Jr, Cooper JL: Anterior cruciate ligament injuries in patients with open physes. Am J Sports Med 22:44–47, 1994.

Stanistki CL: Anterior cruciate ligament injury in the skeletally immature patient: Diagnosis and treatment. J Am Acad Orthop Surg 3:146–158, 1995.

Van Loon T, Marti RK: A fracture of the intercondylar eminence of the tibia treated by arthroscopic fixation. Arthroscopy 7:385–388, 1991.

CHAPTER 9

Revision Anterior Cruciate Ligament Reconstruction

INTRODUCTION

Anterior cruciate ligament (ACL) reconstruction is a popular procedure. Although most orthopaedic surgeons believe they can perform reconstruction successfully, surgeons who do this procedure only occasionally may not be familiar with the numerous technical pitfalls that can occur. Technical errors account for most failures of ACL reconstruction. Most of these errors are caused by nonanatomic tunnel placement.

HISTORY AND PHYSICAL EXAMINATION

It is helpful to ascertain whether the patient ever felt that his or her knee returned to normal after the index ACL reconstruction. Occasionally, traumatic reinjury may be responsible for failure. Most often, however, patients cannot recall a specific event but note gradual onset of laxity as they increase their activities. Examination must include a careful evaluation of range of motion (arthrofibrosis can limit motion) and laxity (evaluation of the end point with the Lachman test is important) and consideration of meniscal and cartilage injury.

DIAGNOSTIC IMAGING

Plain radiographs should be studied carefully with attention to prior graft placement and hardware. Posteroanterior flexion weight-bearing radiographs should be obtained to evaluate joint space narrowing. A lateral hyperextension radiograph should be obtained and tunnel placement evaluated as described by Howell (Fig. 9–1). MRI is useful in evaluating failed ACL reconstructions (Fig. 9–2).

NONOPERATIVE MANAGEMENT

Patients who are less active or do not experience significant instability despite graft failure can be managed with aggressive quadriceps rehabilitation and activity modification. Although there is no basic science to support its use, functional bracing sometimes can be helpful in this setting.

RELEVANT ANATOMY

Although the anatomy is similar to primary reconstruction, there are several considerations. Additional scarring extra-articularly and intra-articularly can be anticipated. Tunnel enlargement must be considered, and if it could affect tunnel placement (i.e., if the new tunnel would encroach on this area), a two-staged procedure must be planned. Incisions should be planned to allow skin bridges of 5 to 7 cm. Graft choice is limited by prior procedures, and alternative choices often are required. Hardware removal must be preplanned. A revision notchplasty often is required.

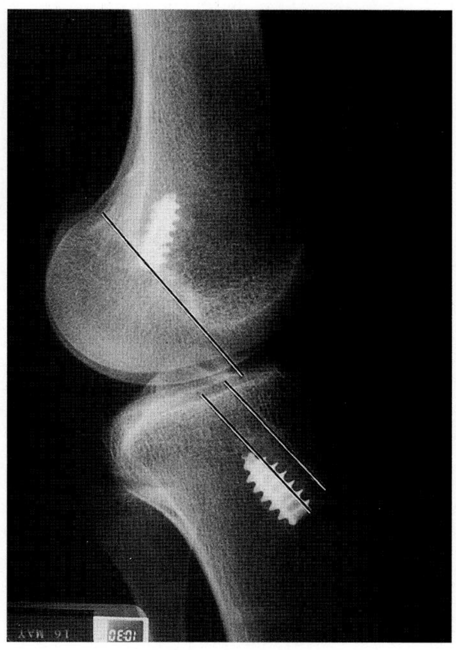

FIGURE 9–1. Tibial tunnel evaluation on lateral hyperextension radiograph as described by Howell. The tibial tunnel should fall entirely behind the intercondylar line (as it is in this case) to be unimpinged.

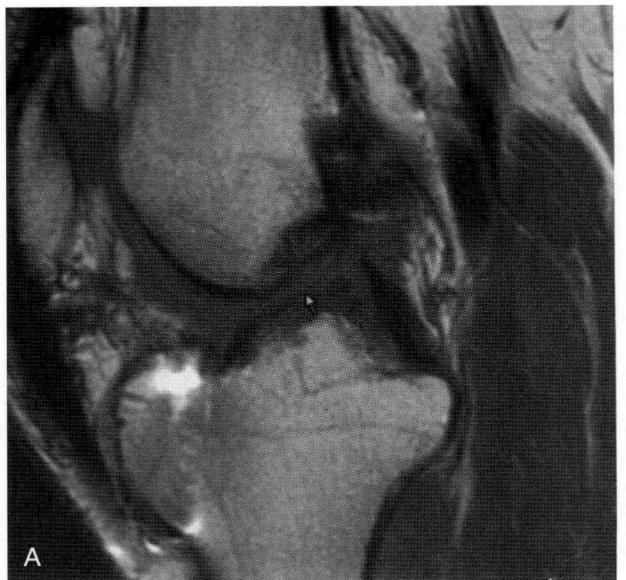

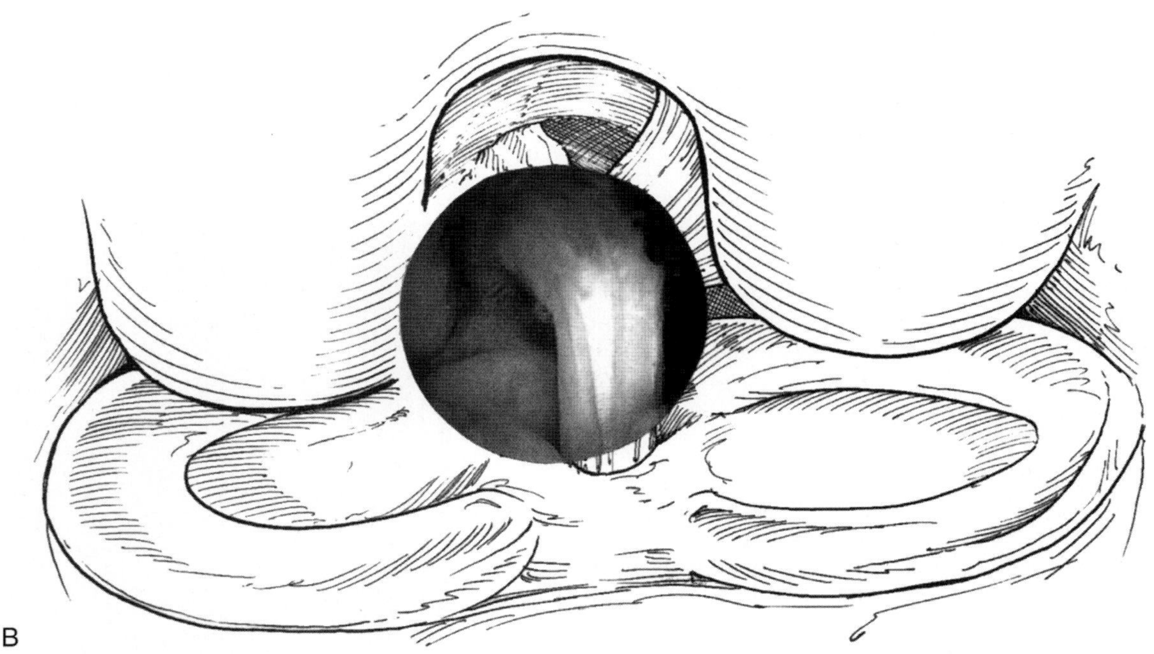

FIGURE 9–2. Failed ACL reconstruction. *A*, Sagittal T1-weighted spin-echo image shows marked attenuation of ACL graft *(arrow)*. *B*, Arthroscopic view of lax ACL graft with poor vascularity and attenuation. (From Miller MD, Osborne JR, Warner JJP, Fu FH: MRI-Arthroscopy Correlative Atlas. Philadelphia, WB Saunders, 1997.)

SURGICAL TECHNIQUE

Indications

Revision reconstruction is indicated for symptomatic ACL reconstruction failure.

Technique

Although techniques vary, a typical example case is shown in Figure 9–3. A variety of techniques may be required based on the characteristics of the case.

1. Enlarged tunnels that will affect graft placement or fixation or both: The defect is repaired with bone graft, and a two-step procedure with the steps separated by several months is done (Fig. 9–4).
2. Anterior tunnel placement: The tunnels are drilled in the correct position, and the previous tunnels and hardware are ignored (Fig. 9–5).
3. Posterior femoral tunnel blowout: The procedure is converted to over-the-top fixation (Fig. 9–6).

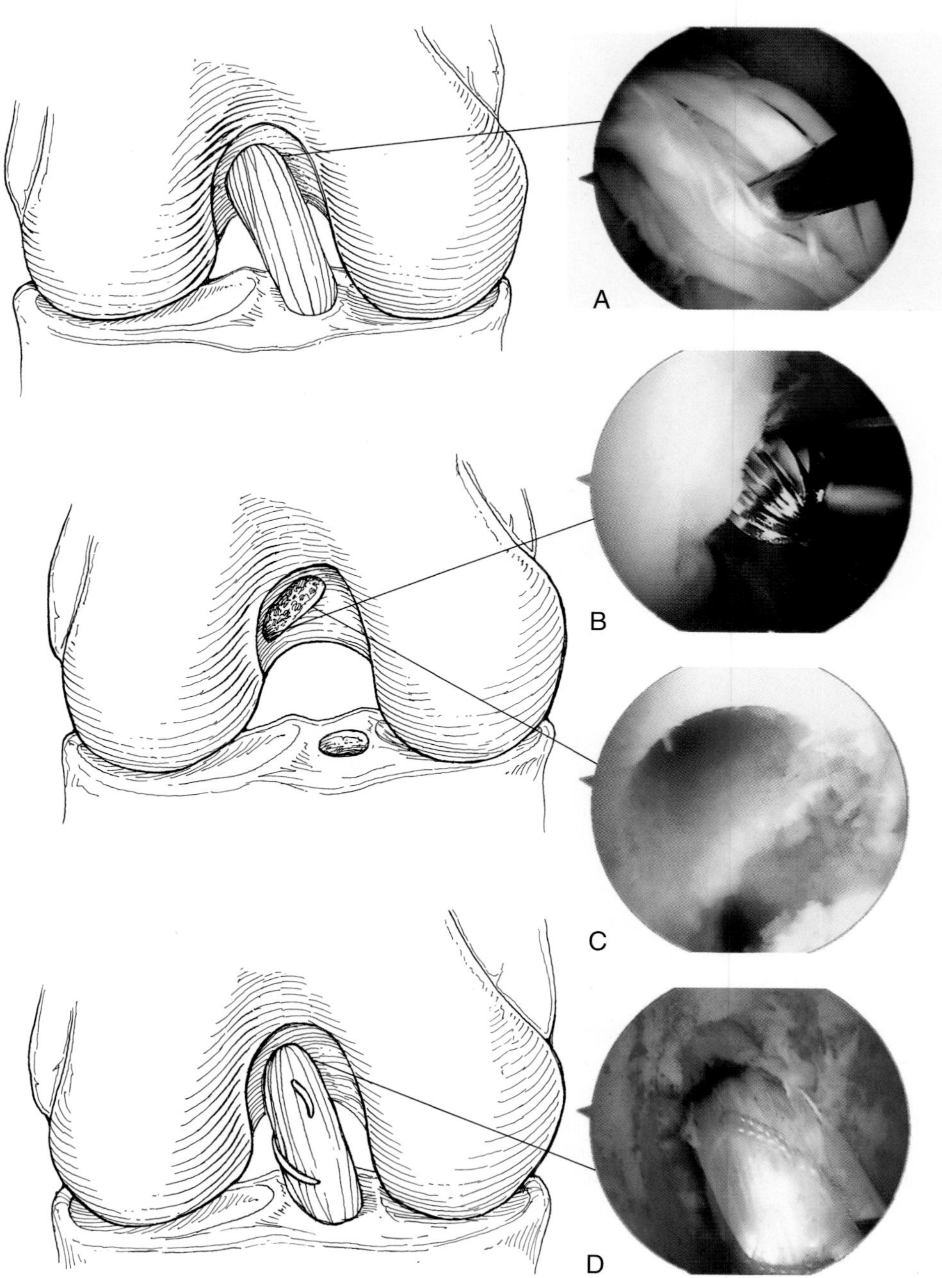

FIGURE 9–3. *Top*, Failed ACL graft. Note avascular graft. *Middle*, Revision notchplasty (note overgrowth) and femoral tunnel placement. *Bottom*, Final graft placement.

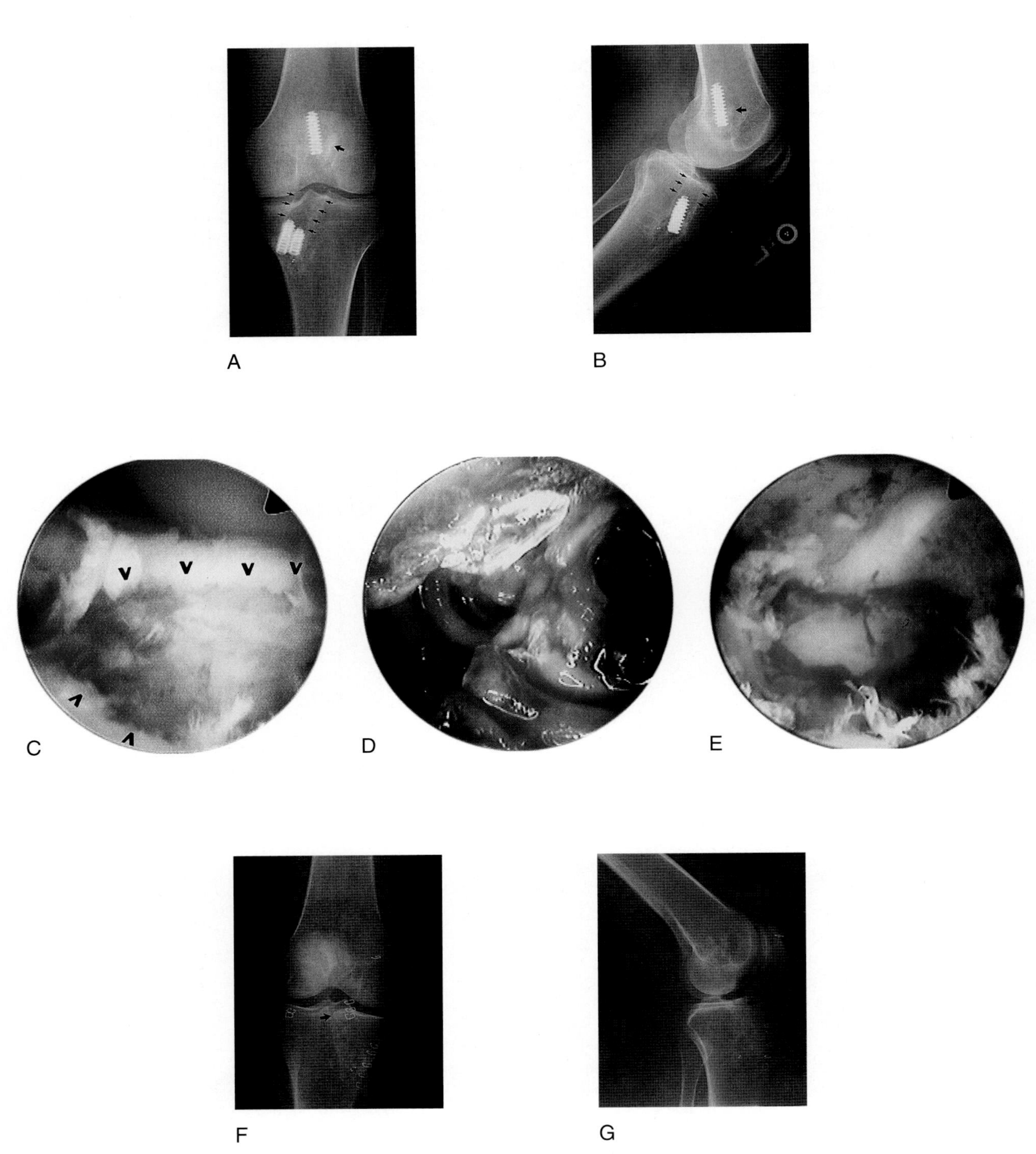

FIGURE 9–4. Two-stage ACL reconstruction. *A* and *B*, Anteroposterior and lateral radiographs at presentation. Note tunnel enlargement, especially of the tibia. *C*, Arthroscopic view after tibial tunnel débridement. *D*, Arthroscopic view of the expanded tunnel. *E*, Arthroscopic view after bone grafting of the tibial tunnel. *F* and *G*, Anteroposterior and lateral radiographs after bone grafting.

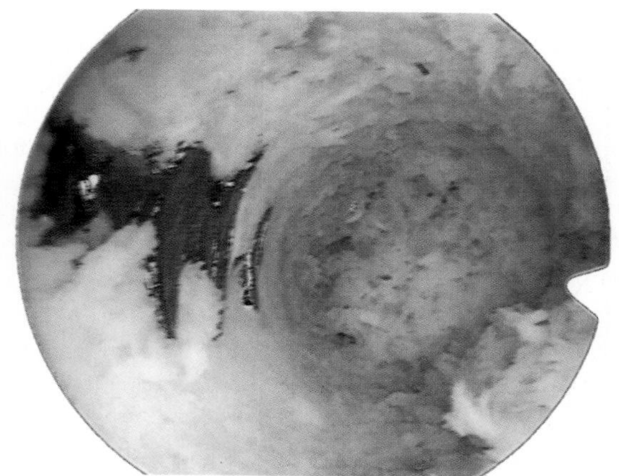

FIGURE 9–5. Arthroscopic view with the scope through the tibial tunnel and into the femoral tunnel shows femoral tunnel placement behind the previous interference screw. The drill contacted and *smoothed* the threads on the screw.

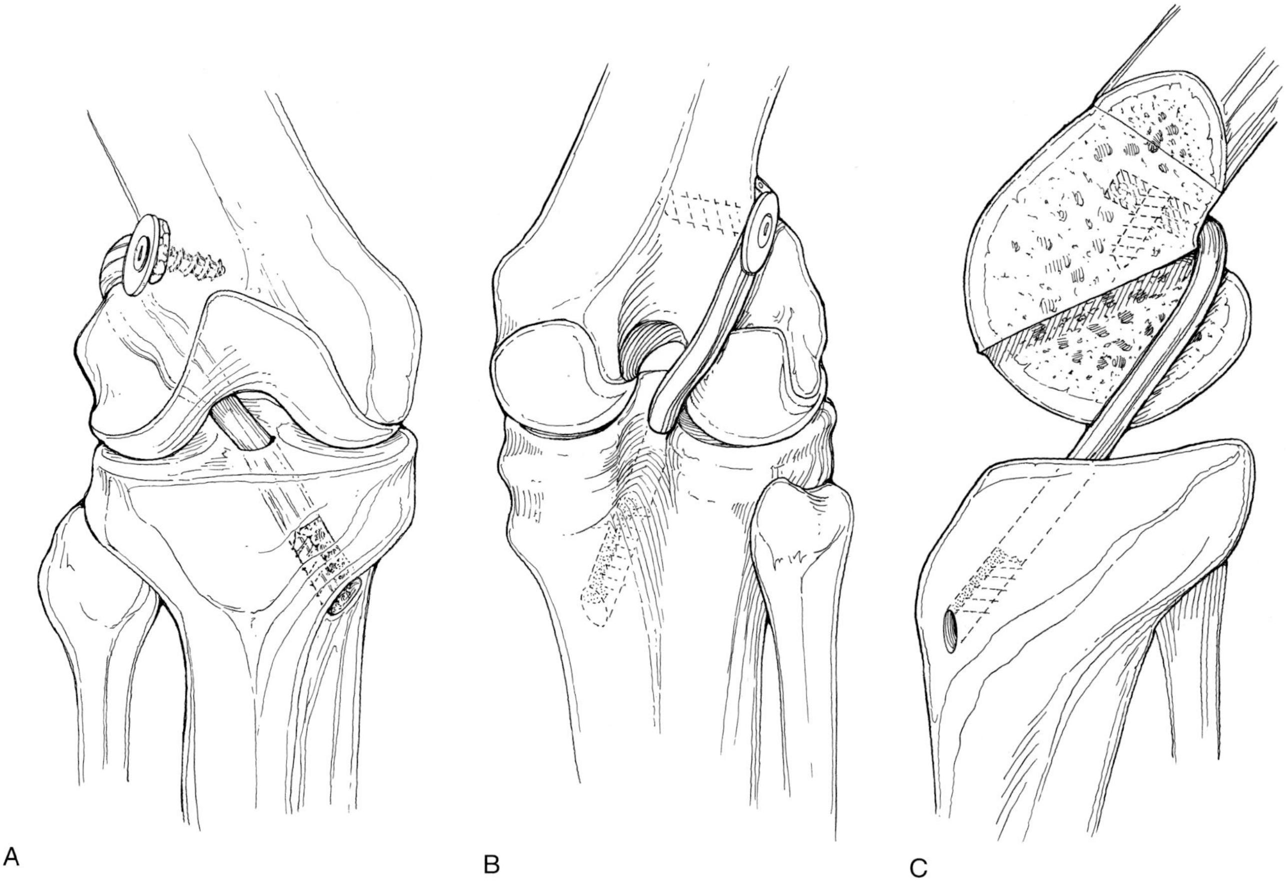

A B C

FIGURE 9–6. Over-the-top technique. Anterior *(A)*, posterior *(B)*, and sagittal *(C)* views.

Other techniques that may apply include removing the previous hardware and, if the position is in a good location for the tunnel, incorporating this defect into the new tunnel. To some degree, the angle or location of the tunnel can be altered to accommodate a new tunnel. Larger bone blocks can be created (especially with allografts) to fill expanded or eccentric tunnels. Different graft fixation techniques (e.g., the Endobutton [Smith & Nephew Dyonics, Mansfield, MA]) can be used in some settings. Simultaneous bone grafting and ACL revision sometimes can be done. Different techniques (e.g., one incision versus two incisions, arthroscopic versus open) also can be employed (Fig. 9–7).

Some patients may have additional injuries that may have contributed to the failure. Meniscal tears, posterolateral instability, and other problems must be addressed.

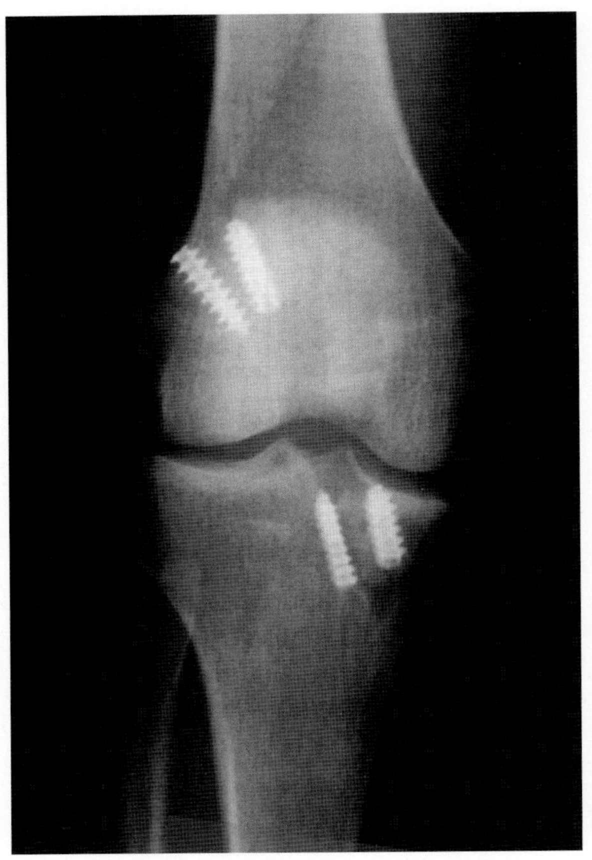

FIGURE 9–7. Endoscopic revision of a two-incision ACL reconstruction with retention of original hardware. (From Wetzler MJ, Bartolozzi AR, Gillespie MJ, et al: Revision anterior cruciate ligament reconstruction. Op Tech Orthop 6:181–189, 1996.)

POSTOPERATIVE MANAGEMENT

Accelerated or aggressive rehabilitation, which is popular after primary ACL reconstruction, is not appropriate after revision ACL reconstruction. Fixation is often less than ideal, and grafts may need additional time to heal. Early range of motion (especially extension) is emphasized, but a delay in return to running and sports is appropriate. Patients should be advised that revision ACL reconstruction is often a salvage procedure and is not intended to return the competitive athlete to the same level of competition.

COMPLICATIONS

Complications are similar to those resulting from primary reconstruction. There is an increased risk for graft failure.

RESULTS

It is important for the surgeon and patient to recognize that results are not as good as in primary ACL reconstruction. Most patients can return to activities of daily living successfully, including recreational sports. Return to competitive sports is unlikely, however. The procedure is best considered a salvage operation.

REFERENCES

Carson EW, Simonian PT, Wickiewicz TL, et al: Revision anterior cruciate ligament reconstruction. Instr Course Lect 47:361–368, 1998.

Greis PE, Johnson DL, Fu FH: Revision anterior cruciate ligament surgery: Causes of graft failure and technical considerations of revision surgery. Clin Sports Med 12:839–853, 1993.

Howell SM, Taylor MA: Failure of reconstruction of the anterior cruciate ligament due to impingement by the intercondylar roof. J Bone Joint Surg [Am] 75:1044–1055, 1993.

Miller MD, Harner CD: Revision anterior cruciate ligament surgery. In Chow JCY (ed): Advanced Arthroscopy. New York, Springer Verlag, 2001, pp 471–488.

Wetzler MJ, Bartolozzi AR, Gillespie MJ, et al: Revision anterior cruciate ligament reconstruction. Op Tech Orthop 6:181–189, 1996.

CHAPTER 10

Posterior Cruciate Ligament Reconstruction

INTRODUCTION

Posterior cruciate ligament (PCL) injuries and their treatment are controversial. The diagnosis, which often has been missed in the past, is being made with increasing accuracy as a result of improved recognition of the injury, better examination skills, and enhanced diagnostic imaging tools.

HISTORY AND PHYSICAL EXAMINATION

Patients most commonly relate a history of a blow to the anterior tibia. Hyperflexion and hyperextension injuries also can injure the PCL. Patients may not complain of frank instability but commonly relate vague symptoms of discomfort, swelling, or a sensation that something is "not right" with their knee. The key examination is the posterior drawer test. In performing this test, it is crucial to palpate the medial tibial plateau and appreciate its position relative to the medial femoral condyle (Fig. 10–1).

DIAGNOSTIC IMAGING

Plain radiographs are usually normal but may show a bony avulsion, which should be fixed primarily. A bone scan may be useful in chronic cases to characterize cartilage injury (medial femoral condyle and patella), which can occur in PCL-deficient knees. MRI is highly sensitive and specific in evaluating PCL injuries (Fig. 10–2).

NONOPERATIVE TREATMENT

Aggressive quadriceps rehabilitation is the mainstay of nonoperative treatment of PCL injuries. Newer braces that attempt to prevent posterior tibial translation are available, but their clinical efficacy has not been proved. Studies have suggested that prolonged nonoperative management of PCL injuries may lead to chondrosis of the medial femoral condyle and patella as a result of altered contact pressures.

RELEVANT ANATOMY

The PCL origin is a comma-shaped area on the medial femoral condyle. Its insertion is located in an oval midline shallow sulcus below the articular surface of the tibia. Two components (bundles) of the PCL are commonly recognized: a thicker, stronger anterolateral portion that is tight in flexion and a smaller posteromedial portion that is tight in extension. Two variable meniscofemoral ligaments (Humphrey's and Wrisberg's)

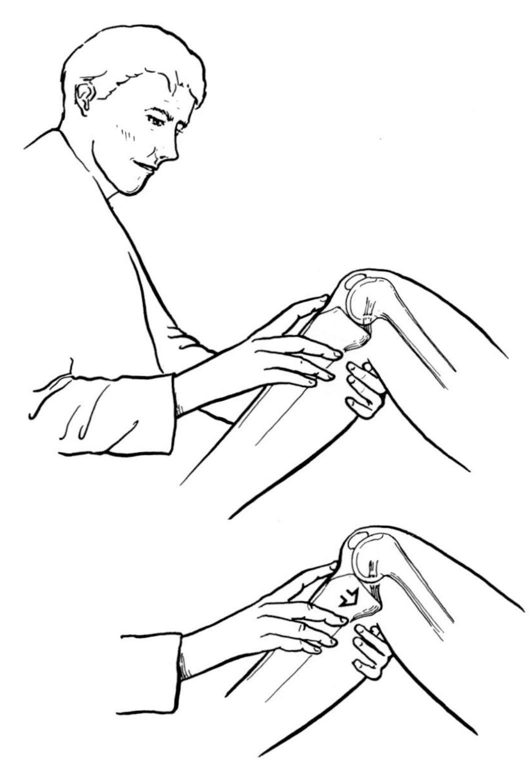

FIGURE 10–1. Posterior drawer examination. It is important to assess the normal starting point of the medial tibial plateau in relation to the medial femoral condyle. (From St. Pierre P, Miller MD: Posterior cruciate ligament injuries. Clin Sports Med 18:199–221, 1999.)

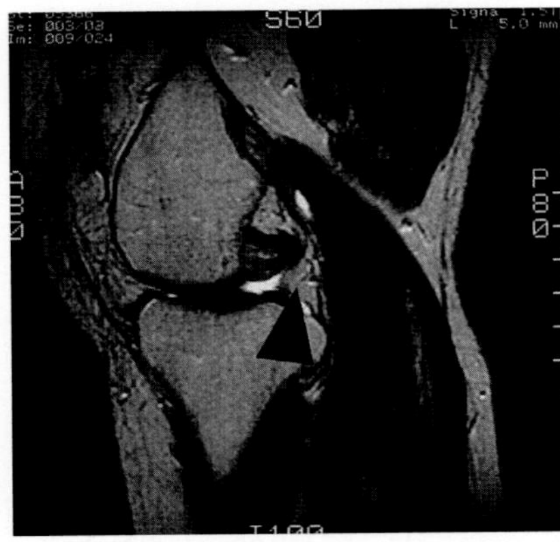

FIGURE 10–2. Sagittal MRI shows complete disruption of the PCL *(arrowhead)*.

originate from the posterior horn of the lateral meniscus and insert in the front (Humphrey's ligament) and back (Wrisberg's ligament) of the PCL. The femoral origin of the PCL can be seen arthroscopically through the anterolateral portal, and the tibial insertion can be seen if the arthroscope is placed into the posterior aspect of the joint (modified Gillquist portal) or through a posteromedial arthroscopic portal (Fig. 10–3). The popliteal artery is located immediately posterior to the PCL insertion and capsule. It is crucial to consider the location of the artery when doing PCL reconstruction procedures. The normal ACL may appear sloppy or loose in a PCL-deficient knee. Placing an anterior drawer force on the knee restores the normal integrity of the ACL. This pseudolaxity should not be misinterpreted as true laxity.

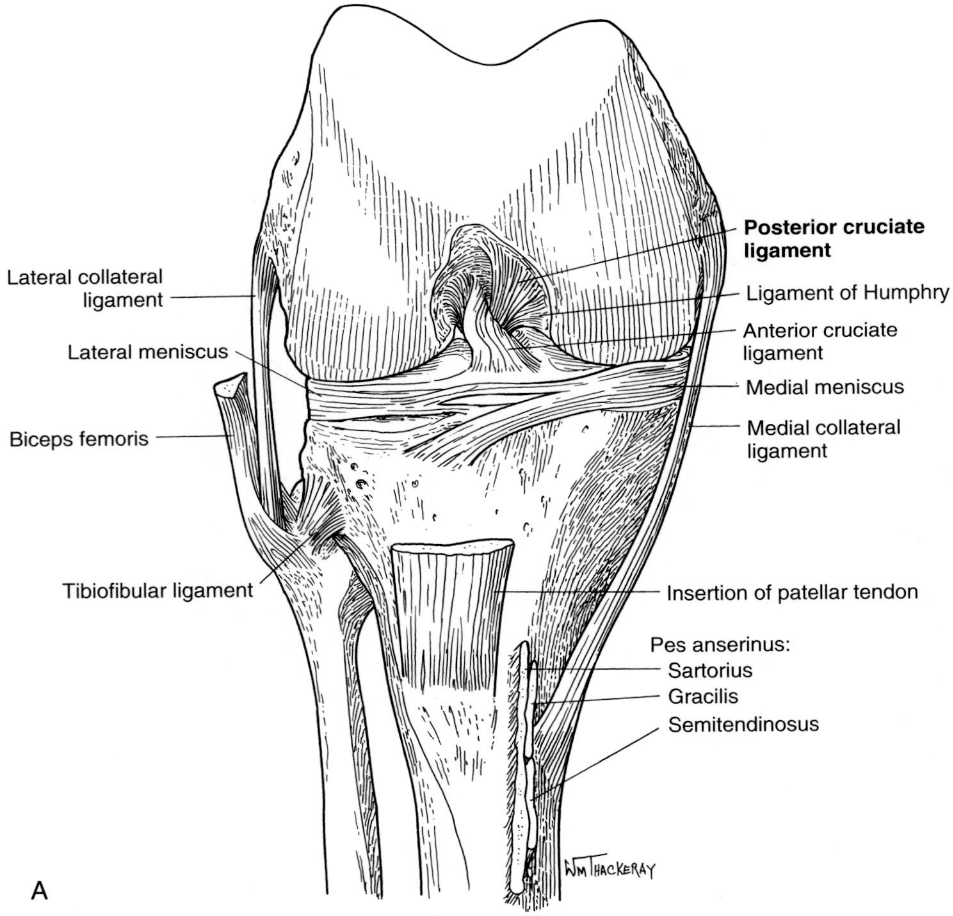

Lateral collateral ligament
Lateral meniscus
Biceps femoris
Tibiofibular ligament
Posterior cruciate ligament
Ligament of Humphry
Anterior cruciate ligament
Medial meniscus
Medial collateral ligament
Insertion of patellar tendon
Pes anserinus:
Sartorius
Gracilis
Semitendinosus
WM THACKERAY
A

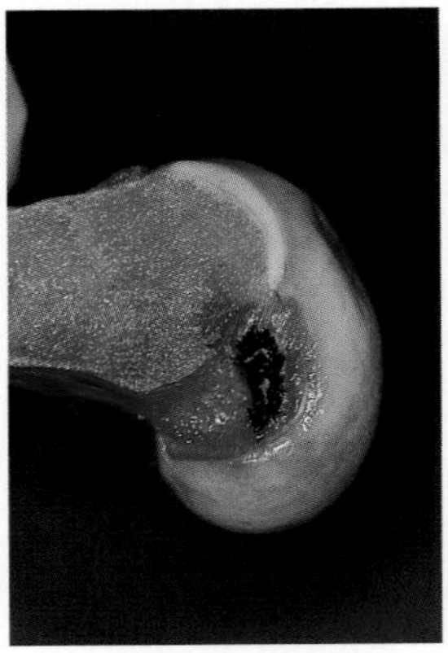

FIGURE 10–3. Insertion site anatomy of the PCL. *A*, Anterior view shows broad insertion of the PCL on the medial femoral condyle. *Inset*, Cadaver dissection shows insertion site anatomy.

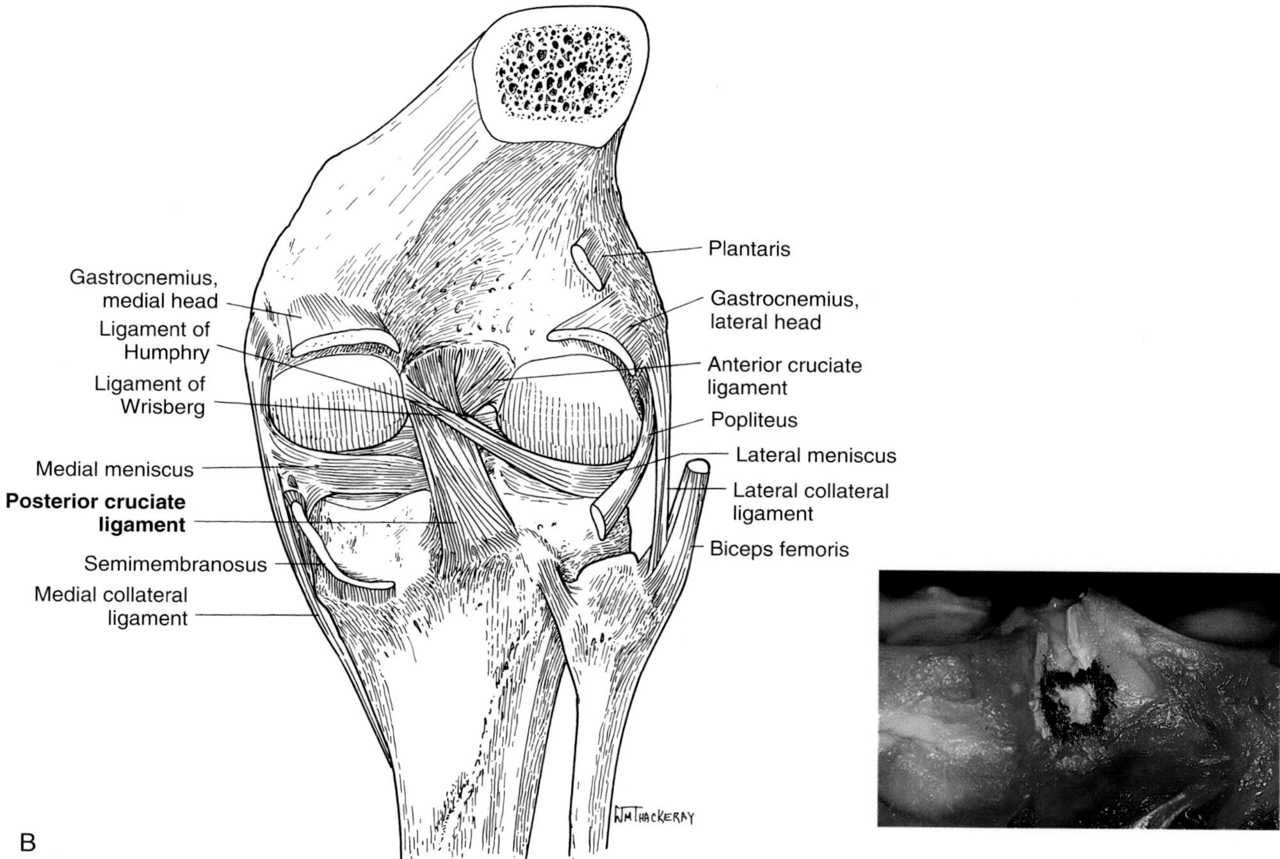

FIGURE 10–3 *Continued. B,* Posterior view shows insertion of the PCL distal to the joint line. *Inset,* Cadaver dissection shows insertion site anatomy. (*A* and *B* From Insall JN: Anatomy of the knee. In Insall JN [ed]: Surgery of the Knee. New York, Churchill Livingstone, 1984.)

SURGICAL *TECHNIQUE*

Isolated Posterior Cruciate Ligament Reconstruction

Indications

Early PCL reconstruction should be considered for patients with grade 3 laxity, other (combined) ligament injuries (including posterolateral corner injuries), associated meniscal or chondral injuries, and all bony avulsions. Chronic grade 2 or 3 injuries that are refractory to extended (>6 months) physical therapy also should be considered for operative treatment.

Techniques

Historical procedures that substituted muscles or other structures for the PCL in a nonanatomic fashion have not been successful over time. Three different current techniques commonly are used: (1) arthroscopic (anterior) procedures, (2) tibial inlay reconstruction, and (3) two-bundle techniques that can be combined with either arthroscopic or inlay procedures. Each technique is outlined. Examination under anesthesia should be done before positioning with each technique.

Arthroscopic Technique

1. Positioning: The patient is positioned supine as for standard arthroscopy. A padded well-leg holder and an operative leg holder or post are applied. A tourniquet is placed on the patient and is used if needed.
2. Graft harvesting and preparation: Autografts that can be used for PCL reconstruction include patellar tendon, quadriceps tendon, and hamstrings. Hamstring use is not popular because historically these results have been less encouraging. The reader is referred to Chapter 7 for details on graft harvesting and preparation. Allografts commonly used for PCL reconstruction include patellar tendon and Achilles tendon. Allograft preparation is similar to autograft preparation except that more tendon usually can be

included in the graft by *tubularizing* the extra tissue. The Achilles allograft is prepared in the same fashion as the quadriceps tendon. Care must be taken not to *banana* the bone plug of this graft.

3. Arthroscopy: Standard arthroscopy is carried out, the injured PCL is visualized anteriorly and posteriorly, and it is débrided. A 70° arthroscope placed in the back of the knee and a posteromedial portal are helpful. Curved curettes, elevators, and rasps are available to assist in débridement.
4. Tibial tunnel placement: The tibial drill guide is placed through the notch and into the back of the knee (Fig. 10–4). The position of the guide must be seen arthroscopically through the posteromedial portal. The guide is placed through the anteromedial portal and is placed on the anteromedial tibial cortex externally. The guide is placed on the skin to determine its location. A 3-cm vertical skin incision is made down to the periosteum of the tibia. The pes insertion should not be disrupted. Extreme care must be taken while drilling guide wires and drills from anterior to posterior. Some surgeons recommend that this portal be enlarged so that the surgeon's finger can be inserted into it to allow for palpation and protection when drilling the guide wire and drill into the back of the tibia. After the guide wire is placed, an intraoperative image should be taken to confirm its location before proceeding with drilling. The tip of the guide wire should be protected with a large curette or similar instrument when drilling. Some surgeons recommend completing the final drilling by hand to avoid plunging the drill into the back of the knee. Fluoroscopy also can be used during tunnel drilling.
5. Femoral tunnel placement: A small incision is made at

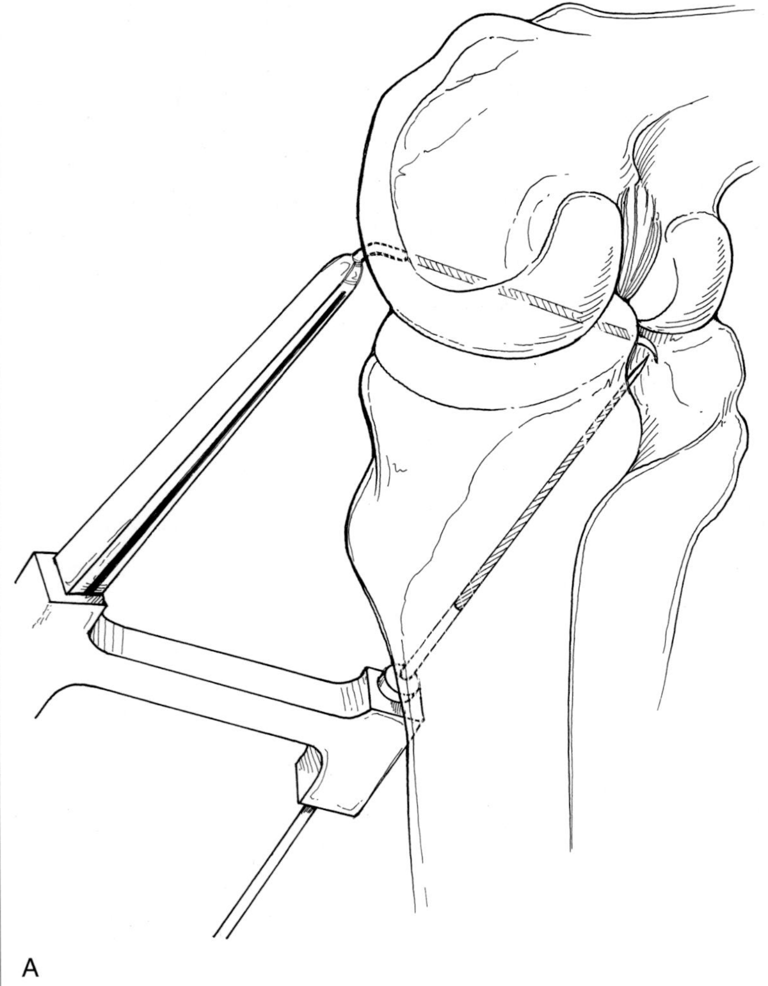

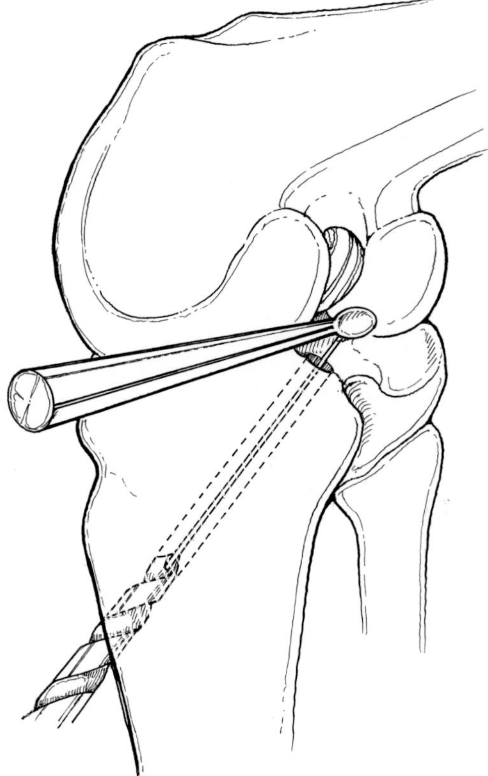

FIGURE 10–4. Arthroscopic (transtibial) technique for PCL reconstruction. *A* and *B*, Tibial tunnel placement.

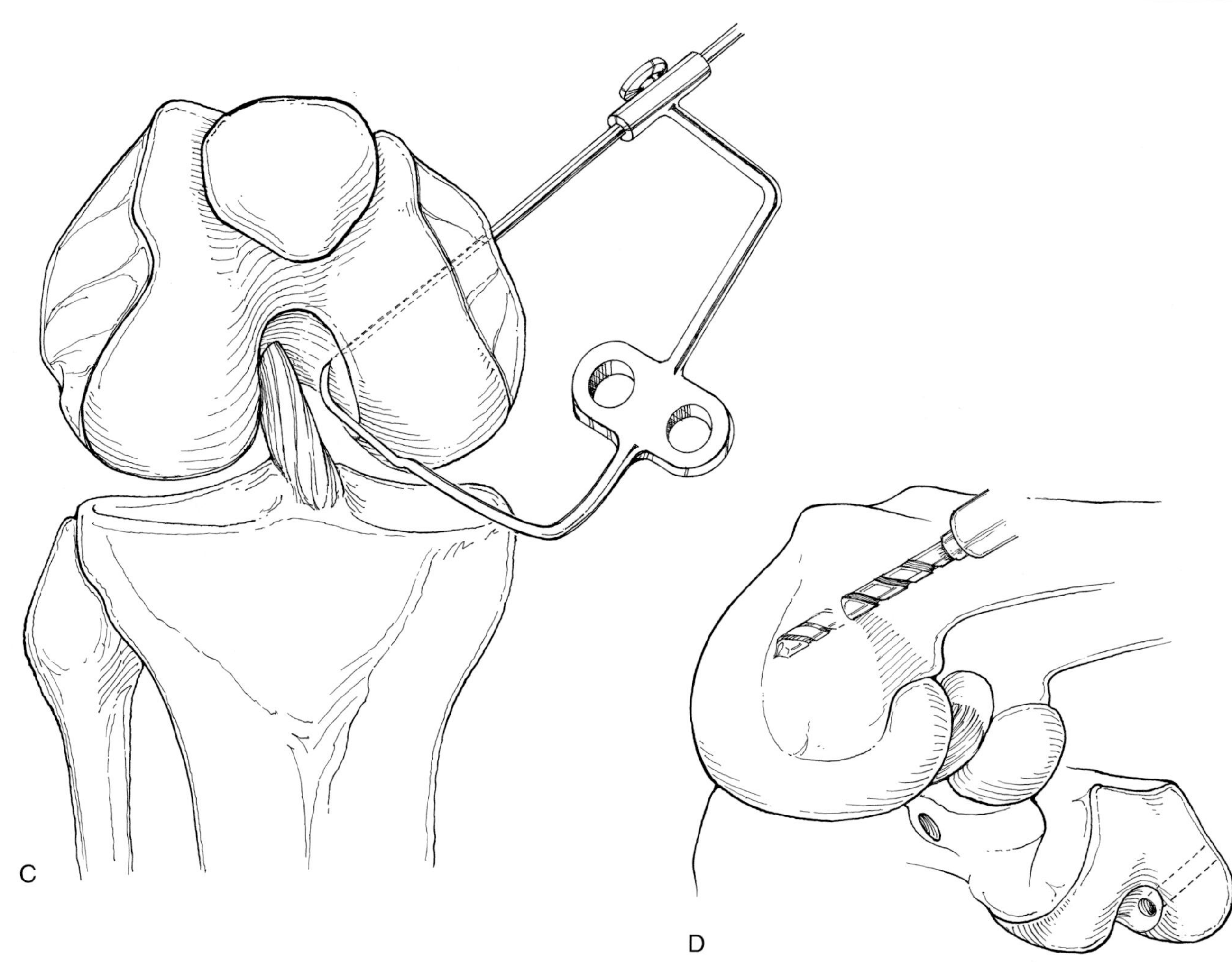

FIGURE 10–4 *Continued. C* and *D*, Femoral tunnel placement.

Illustration continued on following page

the superomedial border of the patella, the vastus medialis obliquus (VMO) muscle fibers are split, and the external tunnel guide is positioned away from the articular surface of the medial femoral condyle. The internal arm of the guide is placed in the anterior and superior aspect of the PCL footprint, approximately 8 to 10 mm behind the articular margin. The edges of the tunnels are rasped to smooth the edges and prevent graft abrasion, and debris is removed from the knee.

6. Graft passage: A looped 18-gauge wire is passed from one of the tunnels into the other to facilitate graft passage. For grafts with only one bony end (Achilles and quadriceps grafts), two options are possible. Conventionally the bony end is placed into the femoral tunnel, and the soft tissue end of the graft is passed through the femoral tunnel and into the tibial tunnel. It can be secured onto the anteromedial cortex of the tibia with a variety of techniques. Some surgeons suggested that this technique requires the graft to negotiate a turn in excess of 90°, which may lead to late laxity of the construct. Alternatives include tibial inlay reconstruction (discussed subsequently) or *retrograde* graft passage, leaving the bony end of the graft in the tibial tunnel (ideally just at the articular margin of the tibial tunnel). In either case, graft passage can be difficult. It can be facilitated by using commercially available *graft passers,* using various *smoothers* (care must be taken not to be too aggressive because these devices can expand the tibial tunnel anteriorly), and placing an instrument through the posterior portal to serve as a fulcrum or pulley for graft passage.
7. Graft fixation: The bony side of the graft usually is fixed first using an interference screw. The knee is cycled many times to ensure that the graft is not kinked. An anterior drawer force is applied to the knee, and the soft tissue side is fixed over a post. Supplemental fixation with a screw and soft tissue

washer or a staple is accomplished. The graft is checked arthroscopically before closure.

8. Wound closure: The wounds and portals are closed in standard fashion. A hinged knee brace, initially locked in extension, is applied to the knee after dressings are in place.

Tibial Inlay Technique

1. Positioning: The patient is placed in the lateral decubitus position with the injured leg up. The leg can be externally rotated and positioned for arthroscopy or abducted and placed on a Mayo stand for a posterior approach.
2. Graft harvesting: A paramedian incision is used to harvest a central one third bone–patella tendon–bone autograft. Care is taken to obtain a rectangular rather than a triangular tibial bone block.
3. Graft preparation: The tibial bone block is prepared for placement in the posterior tibial trough. A 3.2-mm hole is predrilled in the center of the bone block for later fixation. The patellar bone block is prepared for passing into a 10- to 11-mm femoral tunnel. The leading edge of the graft is fashioned into a bullet shape, and sutures are placed perpendicularly to avoid cutting both sutures with the interference screw.
4. Arthroscopy: The knee is positioned for arthroscopy, and injury to the PCL is confirmed. (If there is any doubt regarding the diagnosis, the knee can be examined arthroscopically before graft harvesting.) The torn PCL is débrided, leaving a footprint to assist in tunnel placement.

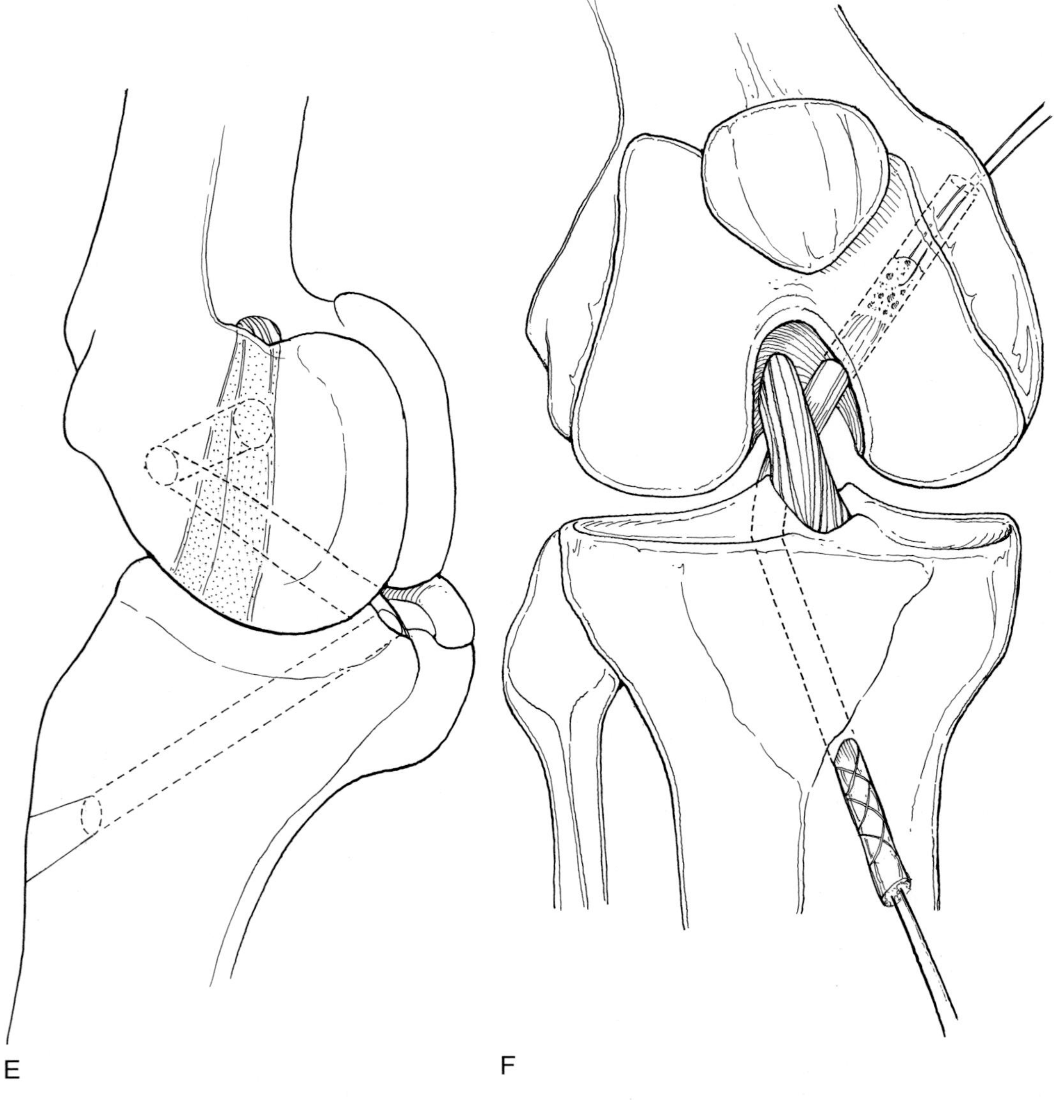

FIGURE 10–4 *Continued. E,* Final tunnel locations. *F,* Graft passage.

5. Femoral tunnel placement: A small incision is made at the superomedial border of the patella, the VMO muscle fibers are split, and the external tunnel guide is positioned away from the articular surface of the medial femoral condyle (Fig. 10–5). The internal arm of the guide is placed in the anterior and superior aspect of the PCL footprint, approximately 8 to 10 mm behind the articular margin. The edges of the tunnel are chamfered and rasped, debris is removed from the knee, and a looped 18-gauge guide wire is

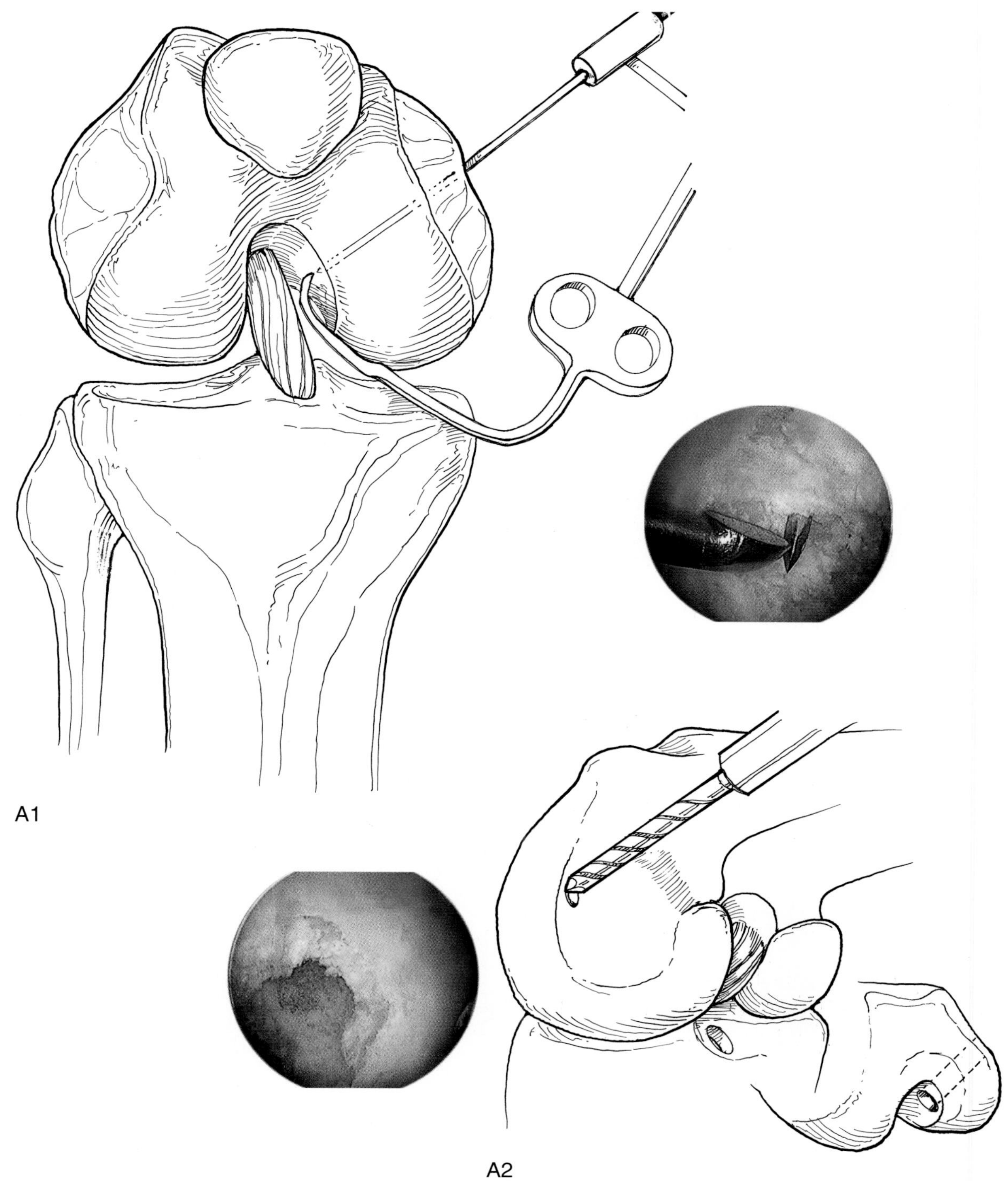

FIGURE 10–5. PCL tibial inlay technique. *A*, Femoral guide wire placement.

Illustration continued on following page

placed through the tunnel into the back of the knee. It is held in place with a tunnel plug.

6. Posterior approach: The leg is extended and placed on a padded Mayo stand, and a posteromedial *hockey stick* incision is made. The fascia overlying the medial head of the gastrocnemius is split, the interval between the gastrocnemius and semimembranosus is developed, and the medial head of the gastrocnemius is mobilized past midline. Its muscle belly protects the neurovascular structures, which need not be visualized. Several 5/64-inch Steinmann pins can be drilled into the tibia from posterior to anterior and bent laterally to retract the muscle.

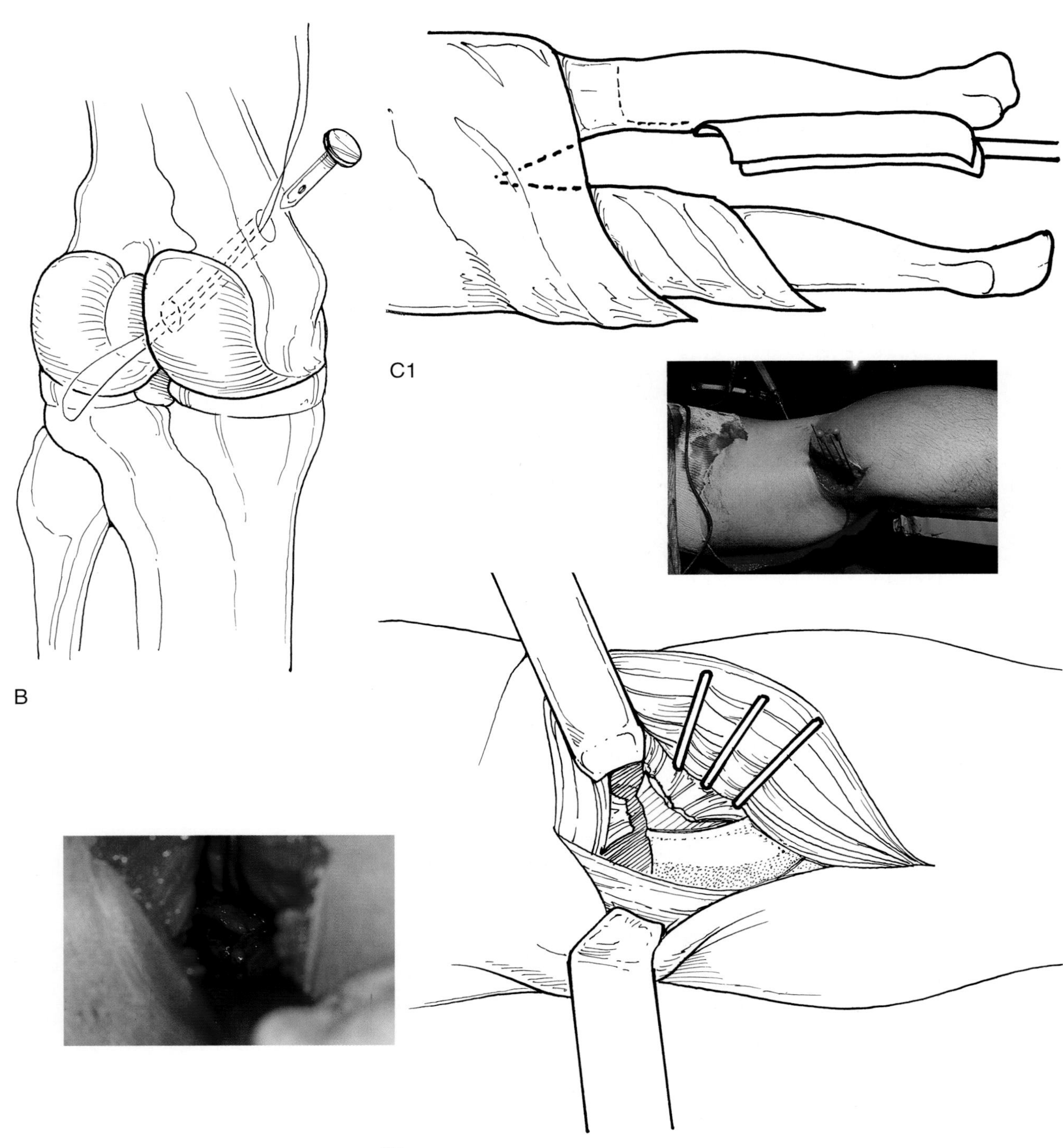

FIGURE 10–5 *Continued. B*, Femoral tunnel drilling and placement of a passing wire. *C*, Tibial inlay approach and creation of a bone trough.

7. Posterior trough and preliminary graft fixation: Using an osteotome, burr, and bone tamp, a cortical window is created in the posterior tibial sulcus, below the articular surface, to match the prepared bone graft. The graft is brought onto the field and provisionally fixed with a Steinmann pin or a staple.
8. Graft passage: A small posterior arthrotomy is made, and the preplaced guide wire is retrieved. The sutures that were placed on the patellar side of the graft are pulled into the femoral tunnel, and the graft is advanced into the tunnel. Its position is checked arthroscopically.
9. Graft fixation: The knee is repositioned on the Mayo stand, and the tibial bone block is secured with a bicortical screw and washer. A staple can be used to supplement the fixation. The knee is externally rotated, and an anterior drawer force is placed on the knee to reproduce the normal stepoff. The graft is tensioned, and the femoral side is fixed with an interference screw placed on the nonarticular side of the graft. The knee is examined to ensure that the posterior drawer has normalized.
10. Wound closure: The posterior capsule is closed, a drain is placed above the capsule, and all wounds are closed in anatomic layers.

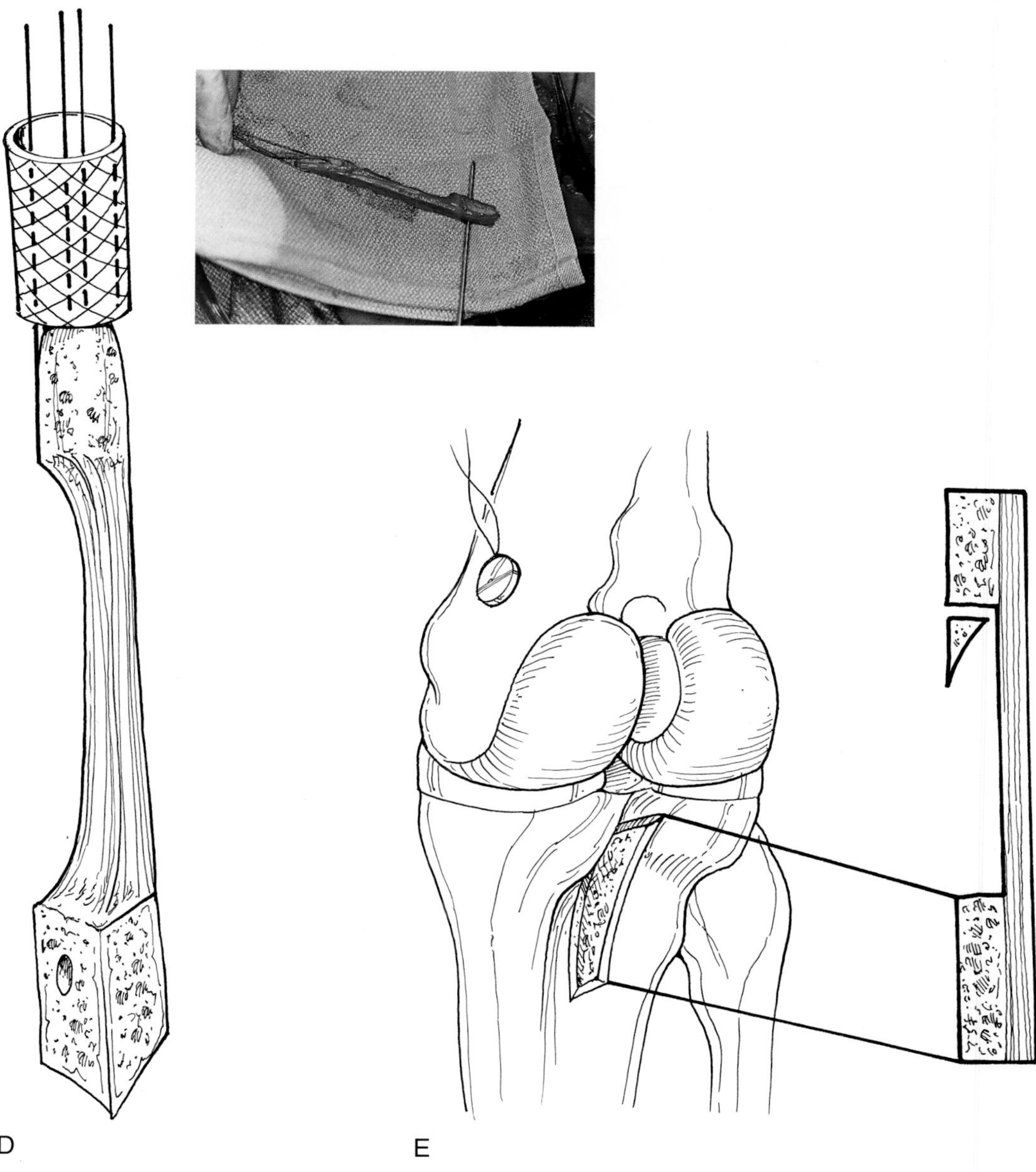

FIGURE 10–5 *Continued. D*, Graft preparation. *E*, Inlay.

Illustration continued on following page

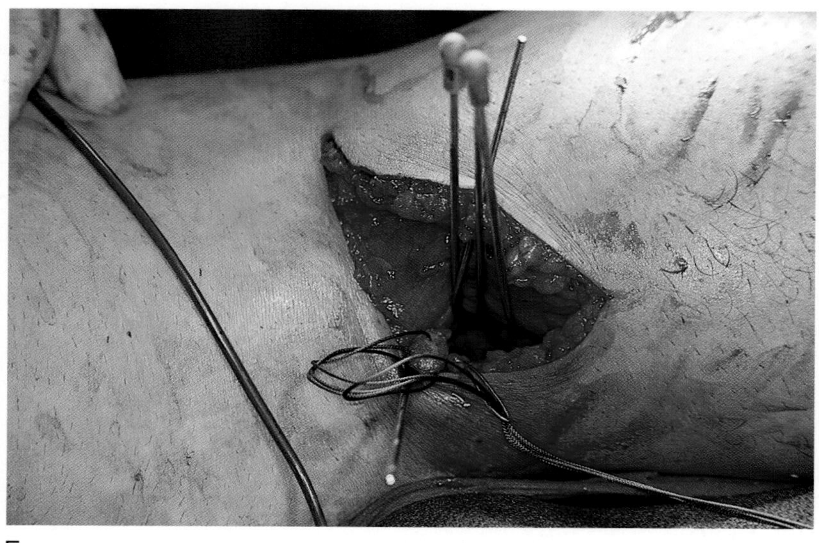

F

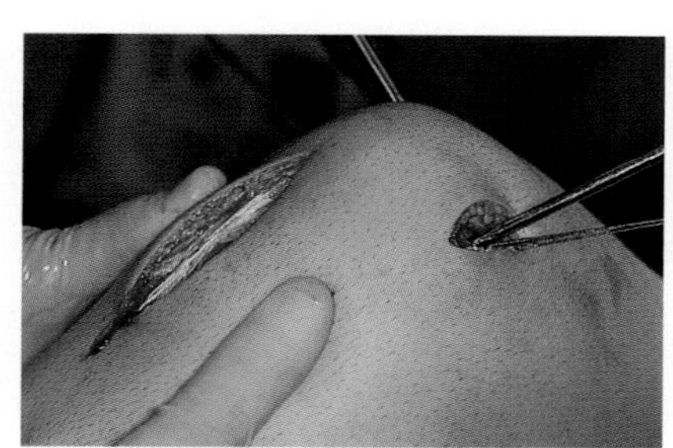

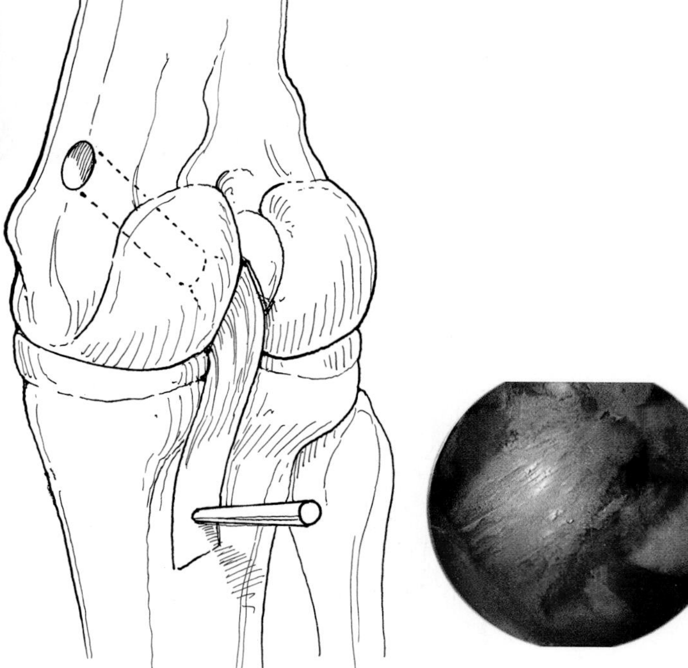

G

FIGURE 10–5 *Continued. F,* Graft passage. *G,* Final fixation.

Two-Bundle Technique

The only difference with the two-bundle technique is that two separate grafts or a *split-tail* graft is used, and two separate femoral tunnels are drilled in the medial femoral condyle (Fig. 10–6). It is important to leave a bone bridge of several millimeters between the two tunnels. The anterolateral portion of the graft is fixed with the knee in flexion and the posteromedial portion of the graft with the knee in extension. It is unclear whether the theoretical advantage of reconstructing both bundles is a clinical advantage.

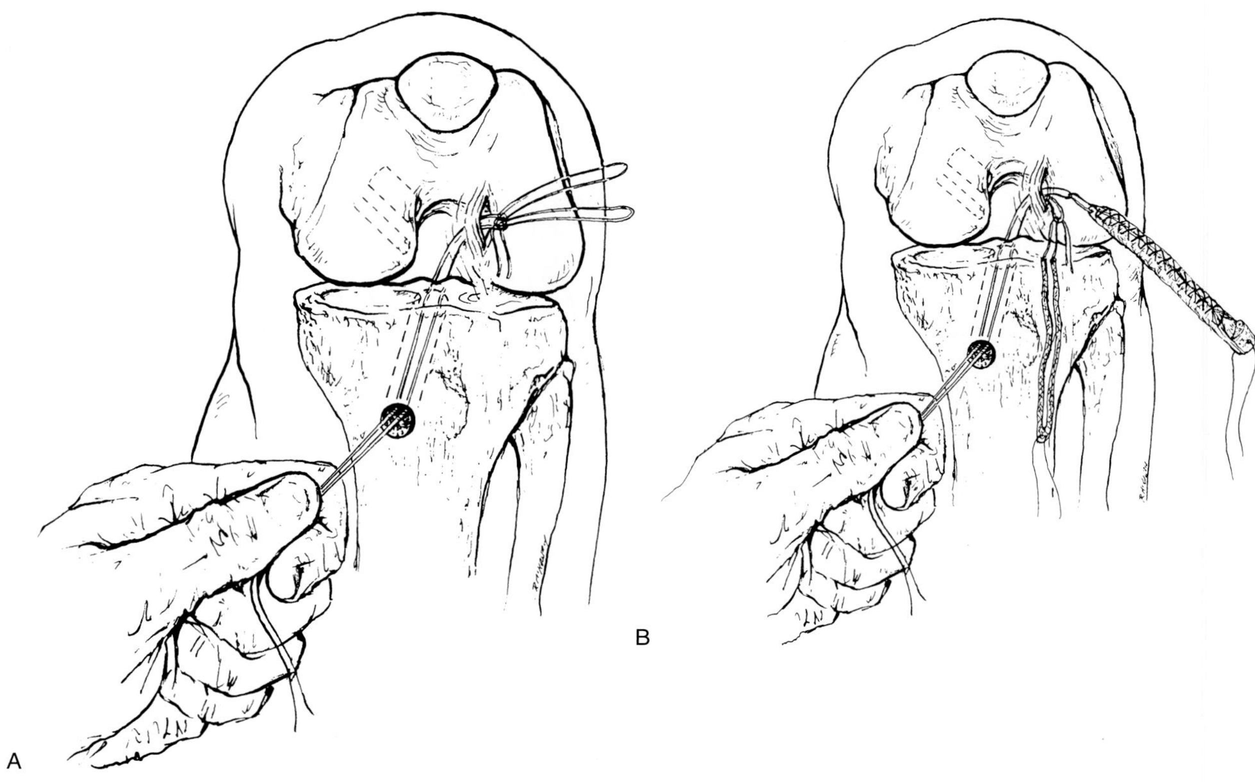

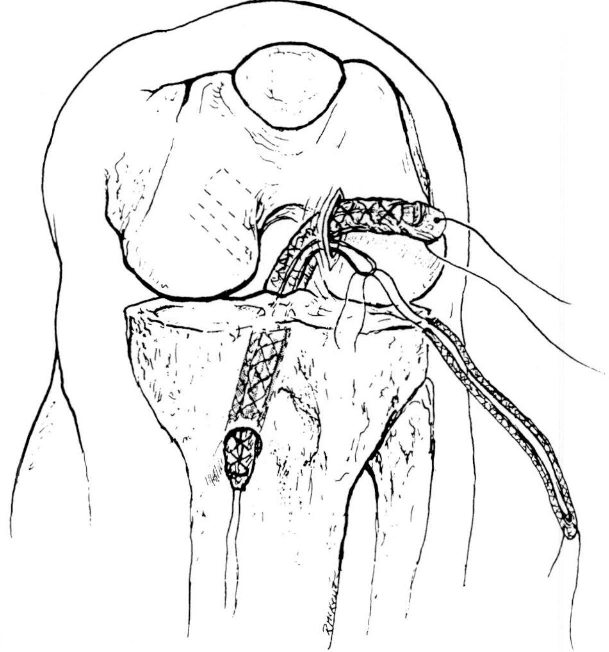

FIGURE 10–6. Two-bundle technique. Tunnels are drilled using a technique similar to that described for the single-bundle arthroscopic technique, except that a smaller tunnel also is drilled posterior and distal to the femoral tunnel for a double-strand semitendinosis graft. *A*, An 18-gauge wire is placed into the tibial tunnel, exiting the anterolateral portal, and two passing sutures are retrieved. *B*, Using one set of the two passing sutures, sutures are passed from the soft tissue end of Achilles tendon graft into the tibial tunnel. *C*, Achilles tendon allograft is pulled into and out of the tibial tunnel distally. Sutures from the free end of the looped semitendinosus are passed into the tibial tunnel using the other preplaced passing suture.

Illustration continued on following page

Revision Posterior Cruciate Ligament Reconstruction

A revision procedure requires many of the same considerations for revision ACL reconstruction and primary PCL reconstruction. When possible, existing asymptomatic hardware can be retained. It is relatively easy to revise a previous arthroscopic procedure into an inlay technique, but not vice versa. Fluoroscopy is useful in revision cruciate ligament surgery. In cases with expanded tunnels, it may be necessary to fill the existing tunnels with bone graft and do the procedure in two steps.

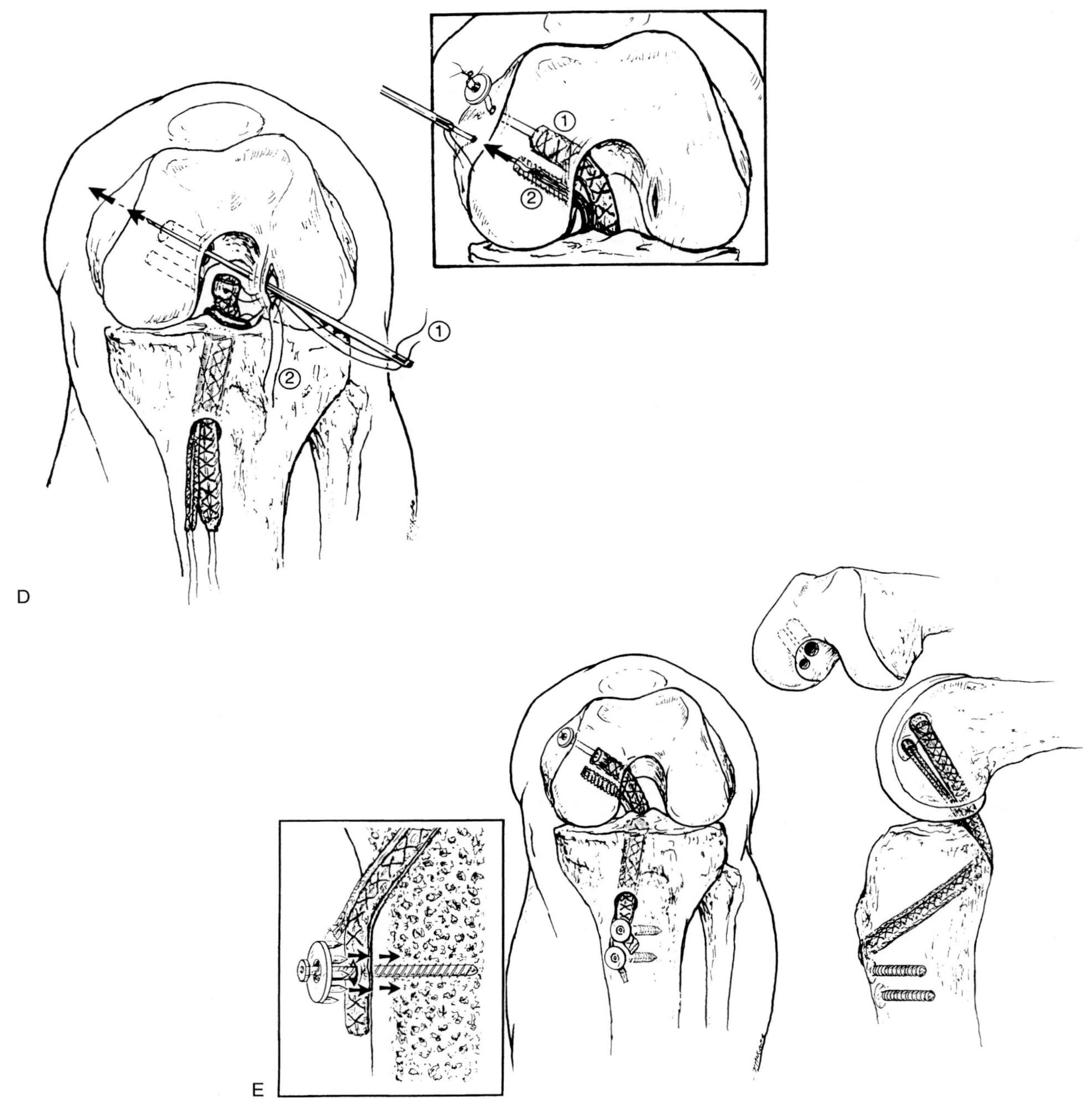

FIGURE 10–6 *Continued. D,* A Beath needle is drilled from the anterolateral portal into the larger anterolateral tunnel. A second Beath needle is drilled into the smaller posteromedial tunnel. Using the Beath needles, the Achilles tendon graft is passed into the anterolateral tunnel, and the semitendinosus graft is passed into the posteromedial tunnel. *E,* The grafts are fixed using a variety of methods. A plastic button (shown here for the Achilles graft), endobutton, or interference screw (bioabsorbable screw shown here for the semitendinosis graft) can be used on the femoral side, and screws and soft tissue washers can be used on the tibial side. (From Petrie RS, Harner CD: Double bundle posterior cruciate ligament reconstruction technique: University of Pittsburgh approach. Op Tech Sports Med 7:118–126, 1999.)

POSTOPERATIVE MANAGEMENT

Patients are kept in a knee brace in full extension. The posterior tibia is supported during assistive range of motion to prevent posterior translation. Continuous passive motion, straight-leg raising, and quadriceps isometric exercises are started shortly after surgery. Crutch ambulation is allowed with weight bearing as tolerated on the first postoperative day. In the early rehabilitation period, gravity-assisted flexion exercises to 90° and closed-chain exercises emphasizing quadriceps strengthening are encouraged. At 9 to 12 months postoperatively, the patient is allowed to return to full activities if full range of motion has been achieved, the knee is stable, and the strength of the operative leg is equal to that on the opposite side.

COMPLICATIONS

The most common complication after PCL reconstruction is loss of motion. It can take 1 year to regain full flexion. Other reported complications include osteonecrosis of the medial femoral condyle from femoral tunnel placement, neurovascular injury, and loss of fixation.

RESULTS

Although results are preliminary, the inlay (and possibly the modified arthroscopic) procedure seems to restore the normal tension in the PCL better than transtibial techniques. The graft is not required to negotiate a hairpin turn at the tibial side of the graft, as it does with arthroscopic procedures.

REFERENCES

Berg EE: Posterior cruciate ligament tibial inlay reconstruction. Arthroscopy 11:69–75, 1995.

Burks RT, Schaffer JJ: A simplified approach to the tibial attachment of the posterior cruciate ligament. Clin Orthop 254:259–270, 1990.

Keller PM, Shelbourne KD, McCarroll JR, Rettig AC: Nonoperatively treated isolated posterior cruciate ligament injuries. Am J Sports Med 21:132–136, 1993.

Klimkiewicz JJ, Harner CD, Fu FH: Single bundle posterior cruciate ligament reconstruction: University of Pittsburgh approach. Op Tech Orthop 7:105–109, 1999.

Miller MD, Gordon WR: Posterior cruciate ligament: Tibial inlay technique. Op Tech Orthop 9:289–297, 1999.

Miller MD, Olszewski AD: Posterior cruciate ligament injuries: New treatment options. Knee Surg 8:145–154, 1995.

Petrie RS, Harner CD: Double bundle posterior cruciate ligament reconstruction technique: University of Pittsburgh approach. Op Tech Sports Med 7:118–126, 1999.

CHAPTER 11

Posterolateral Corner Reconstruction

INTRODUCTION

Injuries to the posterolateral corner (PLC) of the knee previously have been overlooked or underappreciated. Failure to address this crucial injury probably has contributed to several anterior cruciate ligament (ACL) and posterior cruciate ligament (PCL) reconstruction failures. Many techniques have been developed to address this injury, and there continues to be much speculation and research into the best method for repair.

HISTORY AND PHYSICAL EXAMINATION

Isolated injury to the PLC is rare. PLC injuries most often are associated with concurrent PCL injury and occasionally with ACL injury. PLC injury is caused by a blow to the anteromedial aspect of the proximal tibia, usually with the knee in extension or hyperextension. Patients may complain of localized pain or swelling or a feeling of giving way with the knee in extension. The key examination is external rotation asymmetry (>10° to 15°) of the feet with the knee flexed 30° (Fig. 11–1). Varus stress testing and palpation of the lateral collateral ligament (LCL) by placing the knee in a figure-four position are helpful in evaluating the LCL. Asymmetry that is also present at 90° may signify concurrent PCL injury. A variety of other tests, including external rotation recurvatum, posterolateral drawer, reverse pivot shift, and other confirmatory tests, also have been described.

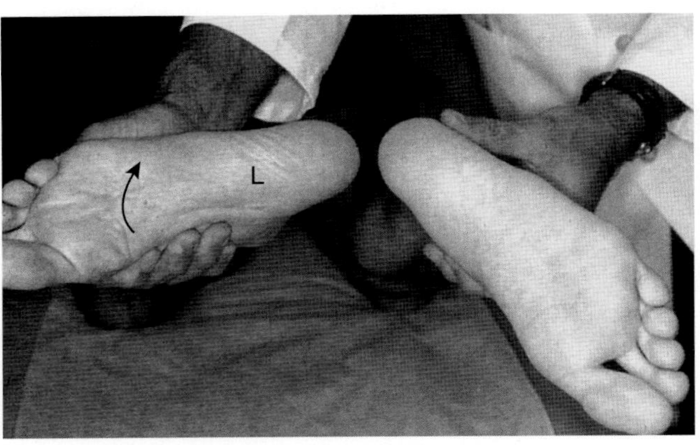

FIGURE 11–1. External rotation asymmetry associated with PLC injury. The patient is prone, and the injured left lower extremity (L) rotates externally *(arrow)* farther than the uninjured right side. (From Miller MD, Gordon WT: Posterior cruciate ligament reconstruction: Tibial inlay technique: Principles and procedure. Op Tech Sports Med 7:127–133, 1999.)

DIAGNOSTIC IMAGING

Plain radiographs are usually normal; however, occasionally an avulsion fracture of the proximal fibula can be seen with acute injuries. Primary repair of these fractures, which usually have the LCL and biceps still attached, is successful (Fig. 11–2*A*). MRI evaluation of PLC injuries is evolving (Fig. 11–2*B*).

NONOPERATIVE TREATMENT

Because these injuries frequently are not recognized acutely, the natural history of PLC injuries is not good. Early operative intervention may avoid some of these problems.

RELEVANT ANATOMY

The important PLC structures include the popliteus tendon, the iliotibial band/tract, the biceps tendon, the lateral collateral ligament, the capsule/arcuate ligament complex, and the more recently recognized popliteal fibular ligament (Fig. 11–3). Occasionally, injuries to the popliteus can be recognized arthroscopically. More commonly, injury can be suspected with excessive opening of the lateral compartment during arthroscopy.

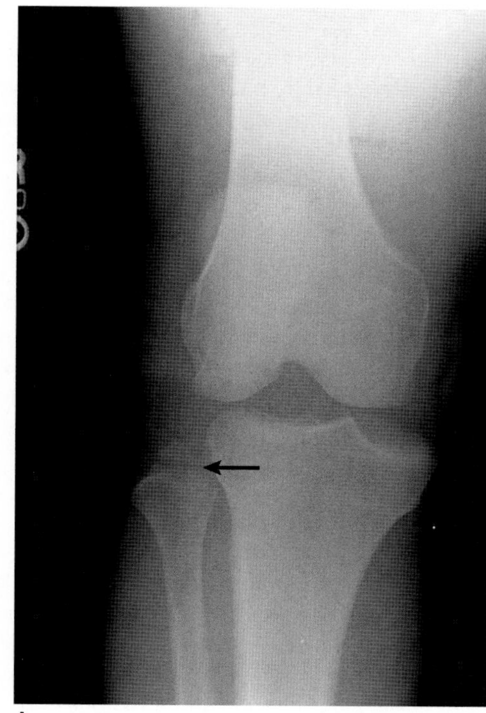

A

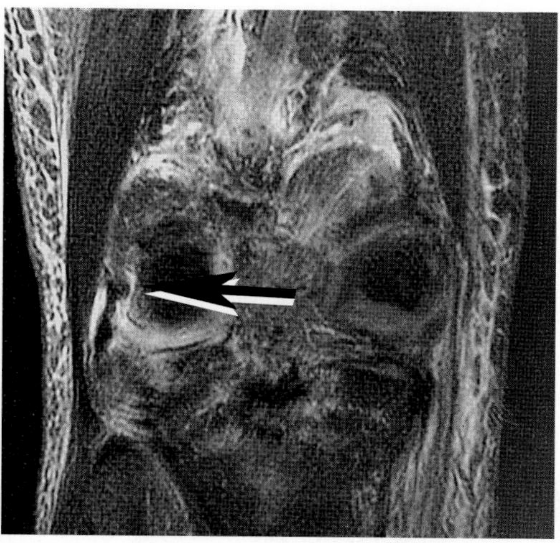

B

FIGURE 11–2. *A*, Anteroposterior radiograph shows avulsion fracture of the fibular head *(arrow)*. *B*, Coronal MRI shows avulsion of the popliteus off the lateral femoral condyle *(arrow)*.

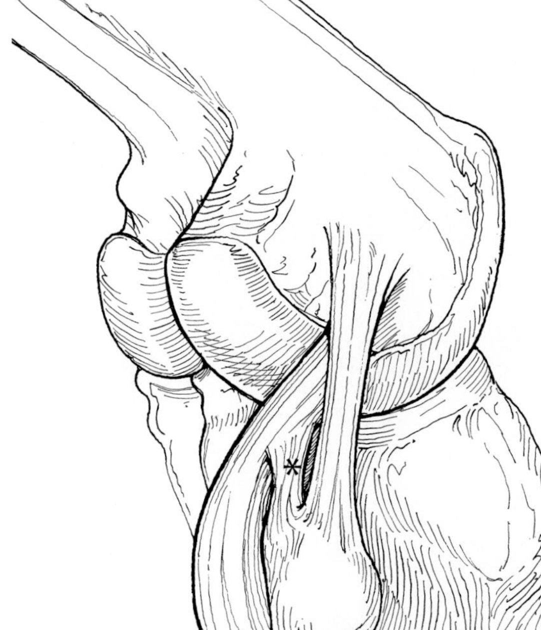

FIGURE 11–3. Diagram of popliteal fibular ligament (*).

SURGICAL *TECHNIQUE*

Indications

Primary repair of acute PLC injuries is recommended by most authors. More often than not, these injuries are not recognized in the acute setting. Patients may present with posterolateral pain, buckling in hyperextension with weight bearing, and instability with stair climbing. Patients also may have a varus thrust (which may be addressed better with an upper tibial osteotomy).

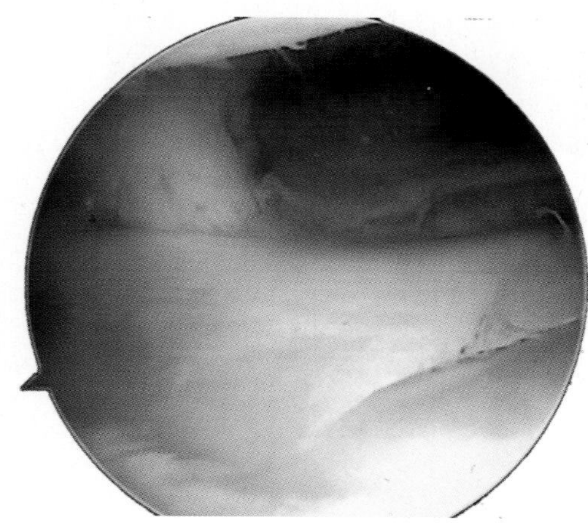

FIGURE 11–4. Arthroscopic view shows widening of the lateral compartment in a patient with a PLC injury (drive-through sign).

Technique

1. Positioning: The patient is positioned in the lateral decubitus position with the injured leg up. Because these injuries often are associated with cruciate ligament tears, combined procedures are common. If concurrent cruciate ligament surgery is planned, the leg can be externally rotated to allow for anterior procedures without repositioning of the patient. Diagnostic arthroscopy is often helpful. If the lateral compartment opens widely (Fig. 11–4), a posterolateral injury can be confirmed.
2. Surgical approach: A lateral approach is used, beginning 10 cm proximal to the joint line and extending 4 to 5 cm distal to it. The incision is midway between the patella and fibular head and extends to Gerdy's tubercle. The interval between the iliotibial band and biceps femoris is dissected, and the peroneal nerve is identified and protected. The LCL, popliteus tendon, and popliteal fibular ligament are identified carefully. For acute repairs, it may be possible to recreate the normal anatomy by reattaching injured or avulsed structures (Fig. 11–5).

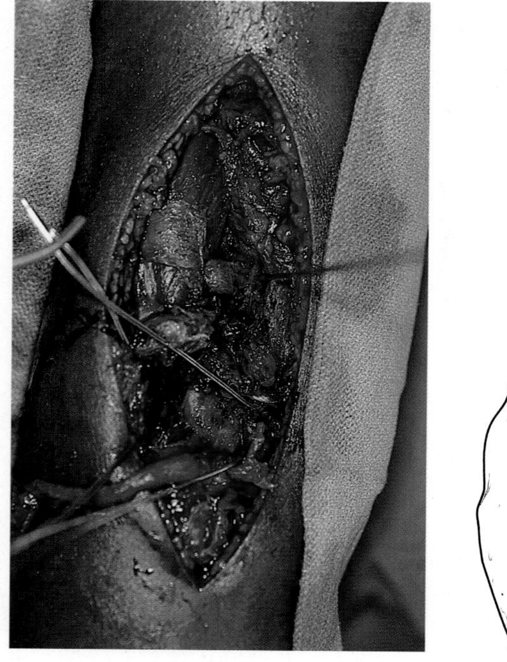

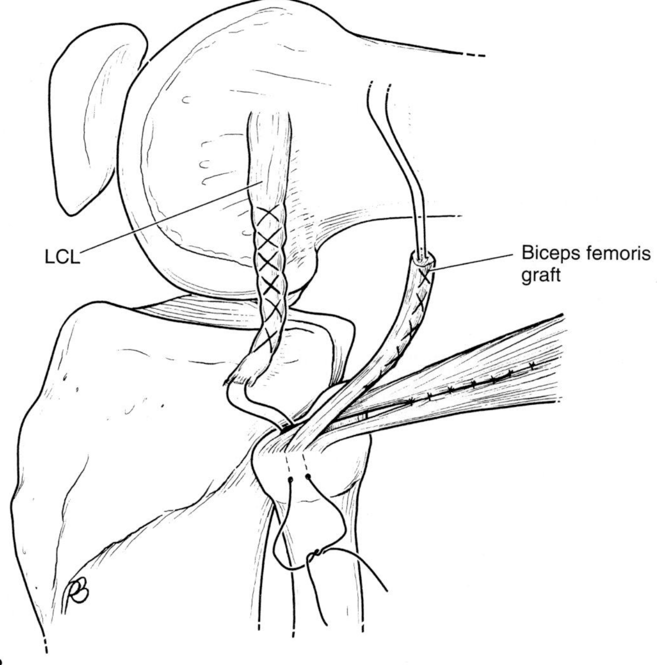

FIGURE 11–5. *A*, Acute PLC injury. Note complete avulsion of biceps, rupture of peroneal nerve, and severe capsular stripping. Guide wires are placed for two-tailed graft reinforcement after primary repair. *B*, Primary repairs can be supplemented with local tissues. LCL, lateral collateral ligament. (*B* from Cooper DE: Treatment of combined posterior cruciate ligament and posterolateral injuries of the knee. Op Tech Sports Med 7:135–142, 1999.)

3. Graft harvesting: If reconstruction or augmentation of torn structures is required, hamstring tendons can be used. The knee can be externally rotated, and a combined semitendinosus–gracilis tendon graft can be harvested from a medial incision, approximately 4 to 6 cm below the joint line. Alternatively an allograft Achilles tendon can be used.
4. Graft preparation: The hamstring graft is prepared by combining the two tendons with an absorbable stitch after the ends are *tubularized*. Tapered needles and atraumatic technique are used. If an Achilles tendon allograft is used, a two-tailed graft is fashioned, with an 8- to 10-mm bone block.
5. Tibial tunnel placement: The tibial tunnel is drilled from directly superior to Gerdy's tubercle to the musculotendinous junction of the popliteus (Fig. 11–6). Some techniques do not use this tunnel

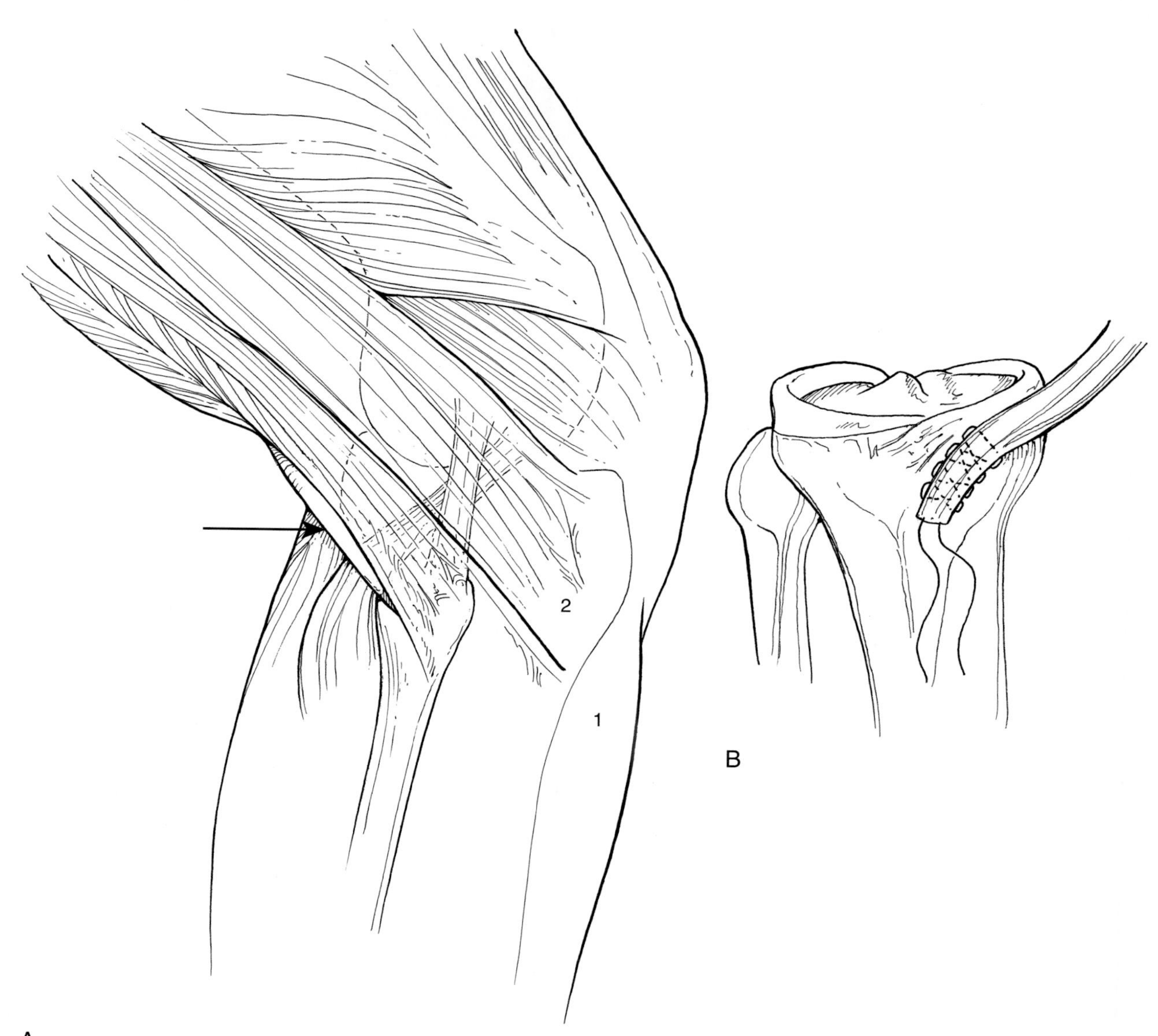

FIGURE 11–6. PLC reconstruction using a two-tailed graft. *A*, Incision with dissection (1) between the iliotibial tract and biceps and (2) between the iliotibial band and tract. *B*, Hamstring tendon harvest for free graft.

Illustration continued on following page

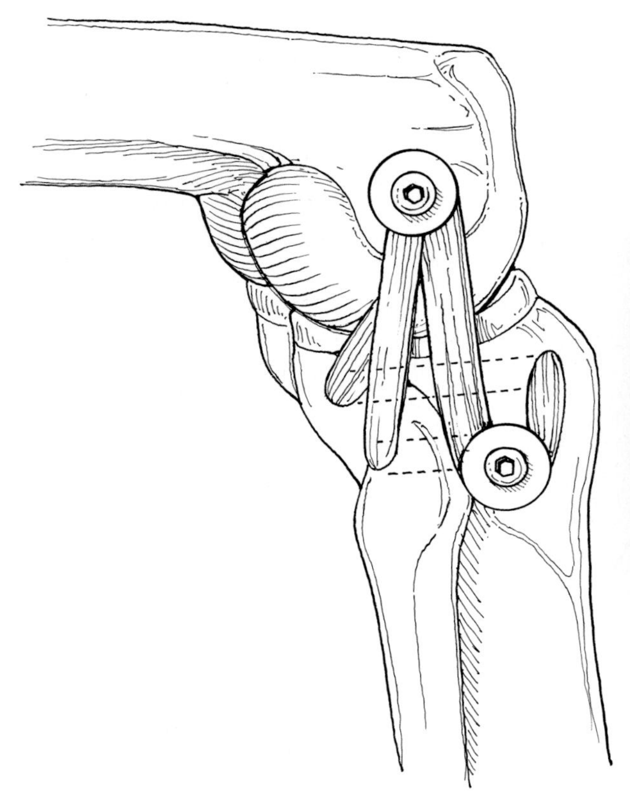

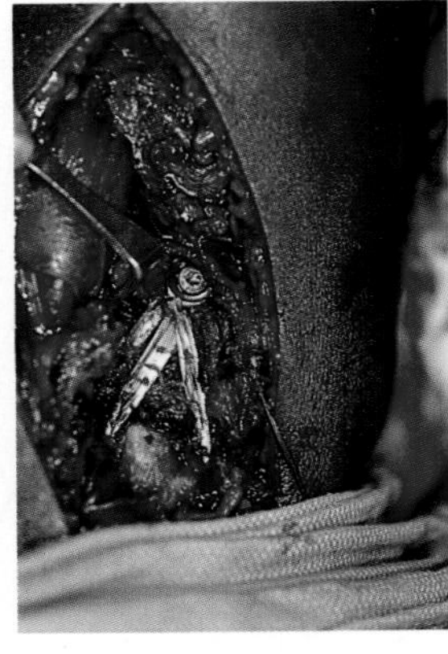

FIGURE 11–6 *Continued.* *C*, Final graft placement.

but employ a figure-eight graft between the fibular neck and the lateral femoral epicondyle (Fig. 11–7).

6. Fibular tunnel placement: The fibular tunnel is drilled from anterior to posterior, across the fibular neck. It is crucial to protect the peroneal nerve during drilling.
7. Femoral fixation: A tunnel, trough, or screw is placed in the lateral femoral condyle between the LCL and popliteus tendon insertions. Bone blocks can be fixed with an interference screw or tied over a button. Alternatively the graft can be fixed with an inlay technique. Soft tissue grafts can be looped over a post or fixed with suture anchors.
8. Graft passage: The two arms of the graft are passed under the iliotibial band, then passed from posterior to anterior through the two tunnels.
9. Graft fixation: The femoral side of the graft is secured first by tightening the screw and soft tissue washer for the hamstring graft or by securing the bone block before graft passage for the Achilles tendon graft. The two tails of the graft are secured on the anterolateral tibia by suturing the free ends to the periosteum or tying the ends over a post.
10. Wound closure: The wound is closed in anatomic layers. A drain is placed if necessary.

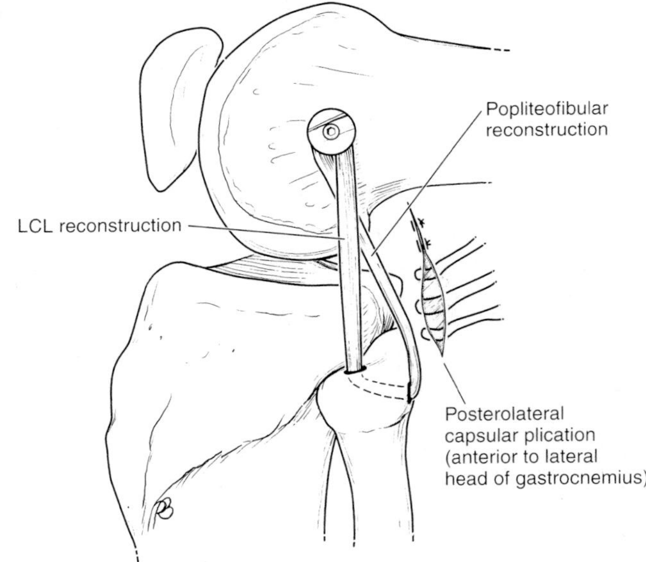

FIGURE 11–7. PLC reconstruction using a figure-eight approach combined with posterolateral capsular plication. LCL, lateral collateral ligament. (From Cooper DE: Treatment of combined posterior cruciate ligament and posterolateral injuries of the knee. Op Tech Sports Med 7:135–142, 1999.)

POSTOPERATIVE MANAGEMENT

Patients are kept in a knee brace in full extension. Early range of motion in the brace is encouraged. External rotation is limited in the early postoperative period. Continuous passive motion, straight-leg raising, and quadriceps isometric exercises are started shortly after surgery. Crutch ambulation is allowed with weight bearing as tolerated on the first postoperative day. The patient is allowed to return to full activities when full range of motion has been achieved, the knee is stable, and the strength of the operative leg is equal to the opposite side, usually at about 6 months postoperatively.

COMPLICATIONS

Our experience with other posterolateral reconstructions is that they have a tendency to *stretch out* with time. Our early experience with the two-tailed reconstruction suggests that the graft remains stable and prevents excessive external rotation. Extreme care must be taken to isolate and protect the peroneal nerve with this operation. Peroneal nerve injury from traction or direct trauma can be devastating. Other potential complications include hardware loosening, loss of motion, and infection. Hardware loosening or *backing out* can be related to excessive stress on the graft or lack of isometric positioning (Fig. 11–8).

RESULTS

Although results are preliminary, this procedure seems to be better at restoring the normal tension in the PLC. Restoration of the popliteal fibular ligament, an important concept of this procedure, may be the key to reconstruction of the PLC of the knee.

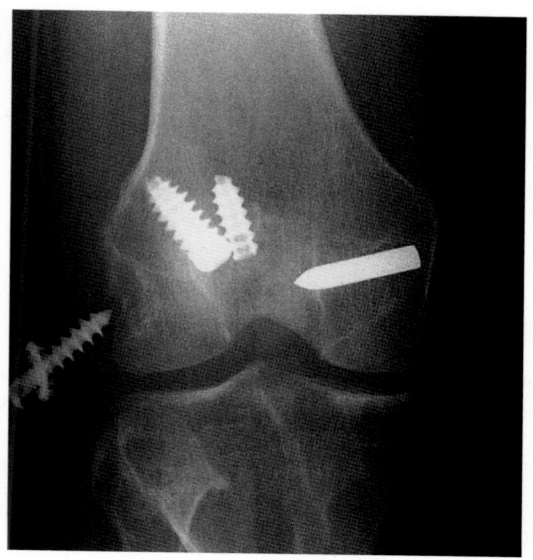

FIGURE 11–8. Failure of PLC reconstruction as a result of poor isometric placement of the femoral screw.

REFERENCES

Cooper DE: Tests for posterolateral instability of the knee in normal subjects: Results of examination under anesthesia. J Bone Joint Surg [Am] 73:30–36, 1991.

Cooper DE: Treatment of combined posterior cruciate ligament and posterolateral injuries of the knee. Op Tech Sports Med 7:135–142, 1999.

Miller MD, Olszewski AD: Posterior cruciate ligament injuries: New treatment options. Knee Surg 8:145–154, 1995.

Terry GC, LaPrade RF: The posterolateral aspect of the knee: Anatomy and surgical approach. Am J Sports Med 24:2–8, 1996.

Veltri DM, Warren RF: Posterolateral instability of the knee. Instr Course Lect 44:441–453, 1995.

CHAPTER 12

Medial Collateral Ligament Repair

INTRODUCTION

Although primary repair of complete medial collateral ligament (MCL) tears was advocated at some centers, the opinion now is almost universal that the initial management of isolated MCL tears should be nonoperative. MCL reconstruction may be necessary in patients with multiple ligament injuries and chronic MCL tears that do not heal with nonoperative management.

HISTORY AND PHYSICAL EXAMINATION

Typically, patients sustain a valgus contact injury and may hear a pop. Unlike in anterior cruciate ligament injuries, a large effusion is unusual (localized swelling is more common). The key examination finding is opening (>10 mm for a complete injury) with valgus stress with the knee flexed approximately 30° (Fig. 12–1). If the knee also opens in full extension, there is likely a second ligamentous injury (usually to the posterior cruciate ligament).

DIAGNOSTIC IMAGING

As with other soft tissue injuries, plain radiographs are often normal. Chronic MCL injuries off the femoral side may have an area of calcification or ossification adjacent to the femoral epicondyle (the Pellegrini-Stieda lesion) (Fig. 12–2*A*). MRI is usually not necessary, but it may show the origin of the tear, bone contusions (usually on the lateral side of the knee), and other associated injuries (Fig. 12–2*B*).

NONOPERATIVE TREATMENT

As mentioned earlier, nonoperative treatment is the treatment of choice for all isolated MCL injuries. Typically, 6 to 8 weeks in a hinged knee brace is appropriate. Most orthopaedists limit motion in the brace (30° to 60°) for the initial 3 to 4 weeks of treatment, then allow unrestricted motion for the remaining period. There is some evidence that a hinged knee brace may have a prophylactic effect for MCL injuries, especially with football interior linemen.

RELEVANT ANATOMY

It is helpful to consider the medial side of the knee in layers (Fig. 12–3). Dissection through the sartorial fascia (layer 1) allows exposure of the superficial MCL (layer 2). The deep MCL (layer 3) is a thickening in the knee capsule. The MCL attaches to the medial epicondyle (the most frequent site of injury), perpendicular to the attachment of the medial patellofemoral ligament.

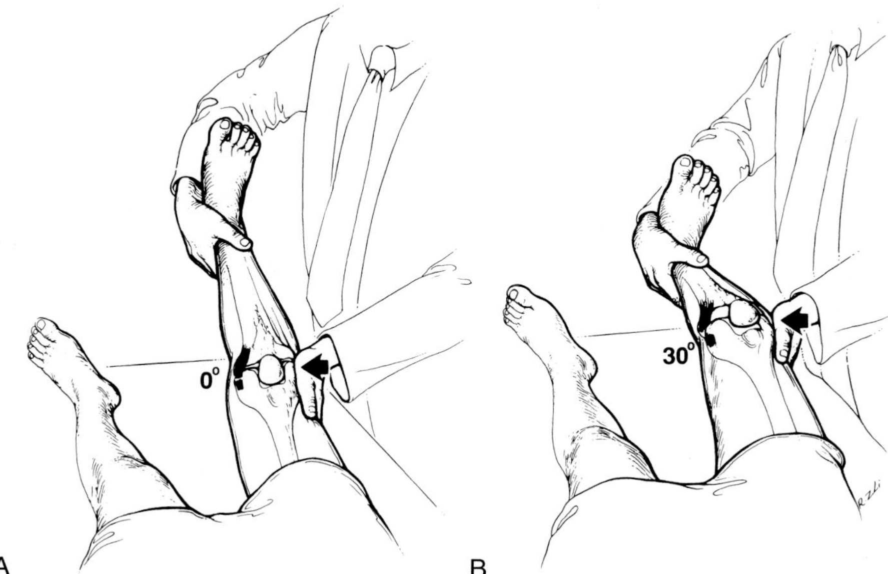

FIGURE 12–1. Valgus stress test. *A*, Test in extension (0°) is normal with isolated MCL injuries. Opening in extension usually is associated with concomitant cruciate ligament injuries. *B*, Test in 30° flexion should result in medial opening in MCL-injured knees. (From Tria AJ, Klein KS: An Illustrated Guide to the Knee. New York, Churchill Livingstone, 1992.)

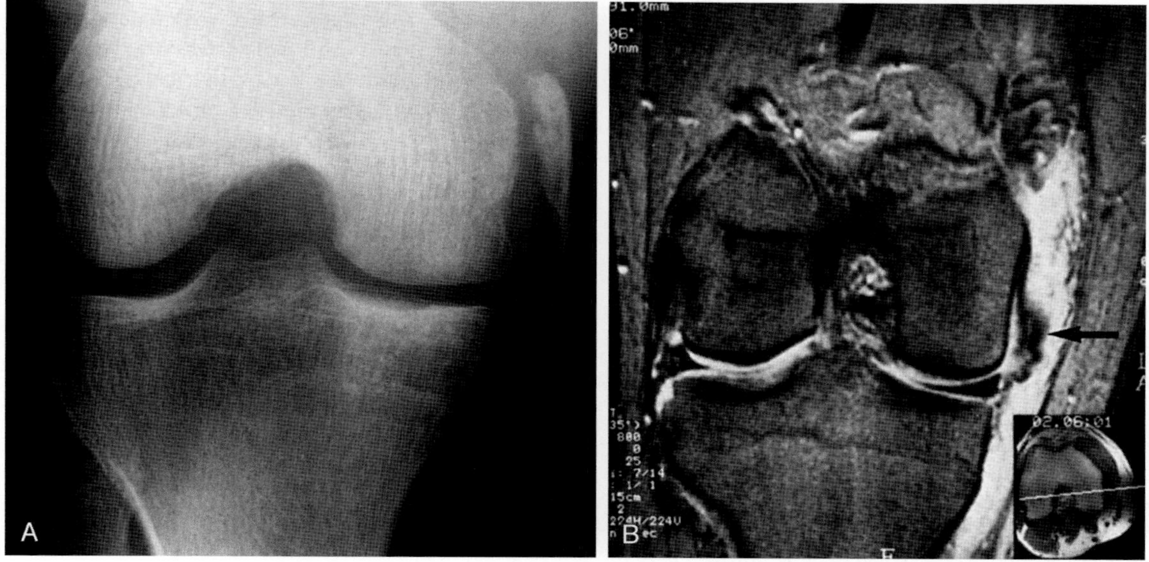

FIGURE 12–2. *A*, Anteroposterior radiograph of a large Pellegrini-Stieda lesion associated with a chronic MCL injury. *B*, Coronal MRI shows MCL injury *(arrow)*. (From Linton RC, Indelicato PA: Medial ligament injuries. In DeLee JC, Drez Jr D [eds]: Orthopaedic Sports Medicine: Principles and Practice. Philadelphia, WB Saunders, 1994, pp 1261–1274.)

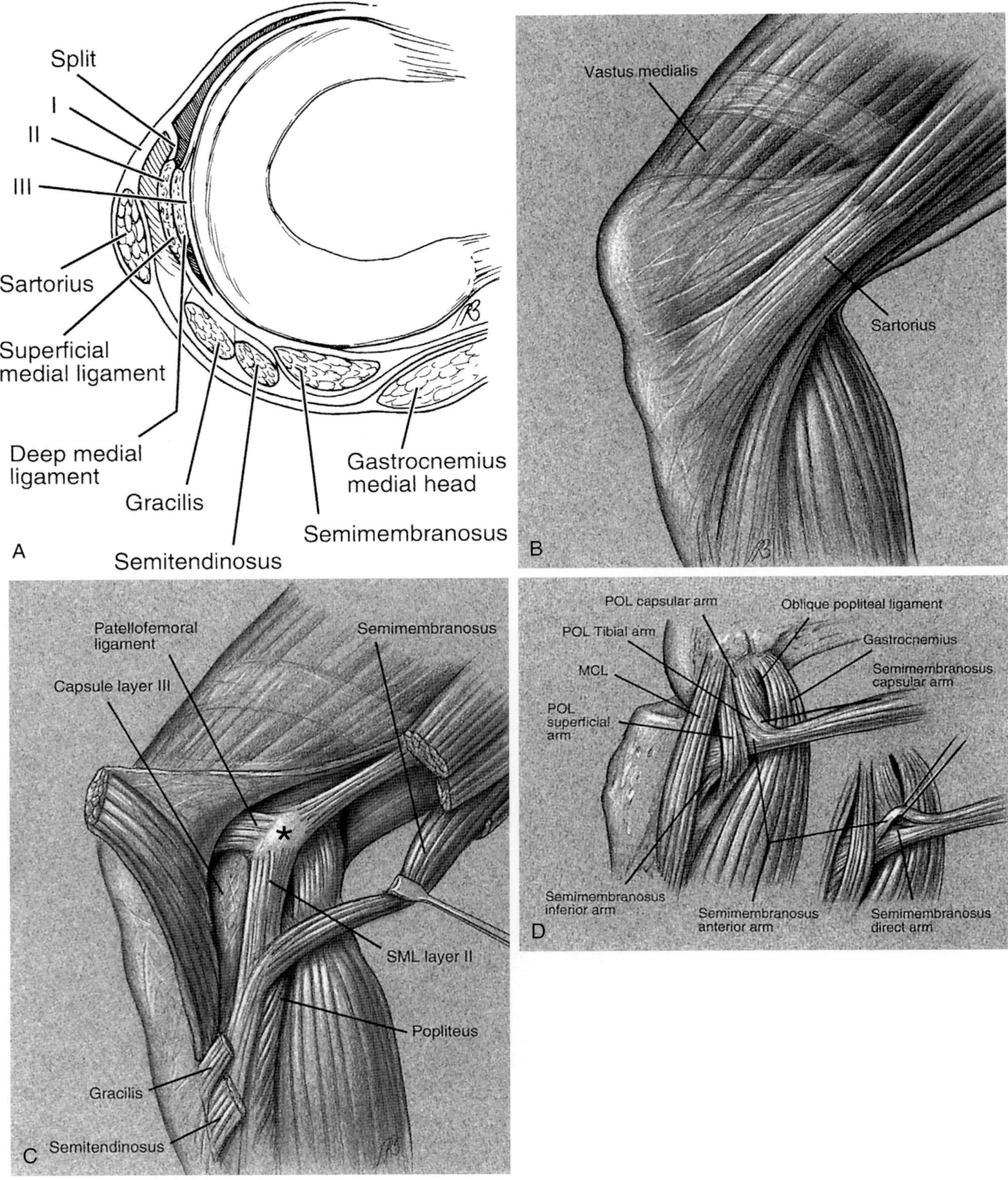

FIGURE 12–3. Layers of the medial side of the knee. *A*, Cross section shows the three layers. The superficial MCL represents layer II, and the deep MCL represents layer III. *B*, Layer I consists primarily of the sartorius and its fascia. *C*, Layers II and III lie deep to this fascia. Note the medial femoral epicondyle (asterisk) and attachments of the medial patellofemoral ligament and superficial MCL (SML) *D*, Relationship of the posterior oblique ligament (POL) to the MCL. (From Satterwhite Y: The anatomy and biomechanics of the medial structures of the knee. Op Tech Sports Med 4:134–140, 1996.)

SURGICAL *TECHNIQUE*

Indications

Surgery is indicated for chronic isolated MCL injuries that have failed nonoperative management and for acute combined injuries.

Technique

1. Positioning: The patient is positioned supine on the table. A tourniquet is placed, but inflation is usually not necessary.
2. Diagnostic arthroscopy: Diagnostic arthroscopy may be beneficial to rule out concurrent meniscus pathology. It also is often possible to get an impression of whether the injury is off the femoral (more commonly) or the tibial side by evaluating the knee when it is stressed. The injured side separates further from the medial meniscus with stress.
3. Incision: A 10- to 15-cm *hockey stick* incision is made centered on the joint line (Fig. 12–4). The incision is vertical with the knee extended. The sartorial fascia is incised. Alternatively an L-shaped incision in the fascia can be made, which allows a flap to be raised for later repair. The superficial and deep layers of the MCL are identified.
4. Tibial dissection: If the injury is believed to have occurred on the tibial side, it is important to ensure that the tibial arm of the semimembranosus is intact. If not, additional repair of this structure is required.

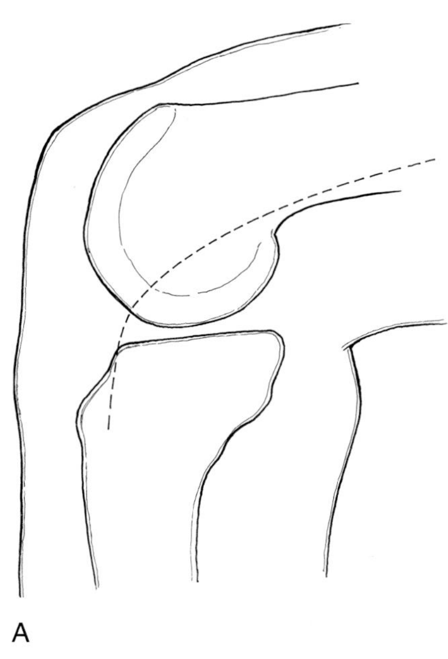
A

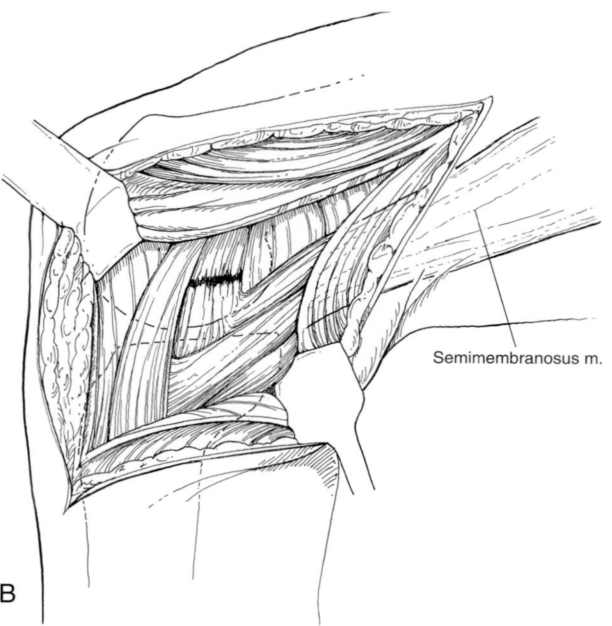

B

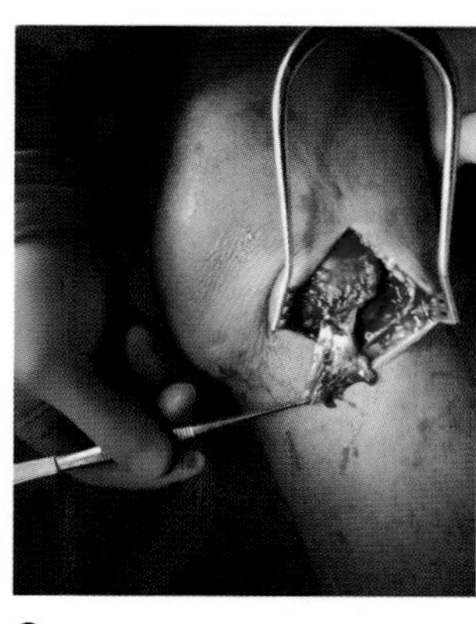
C

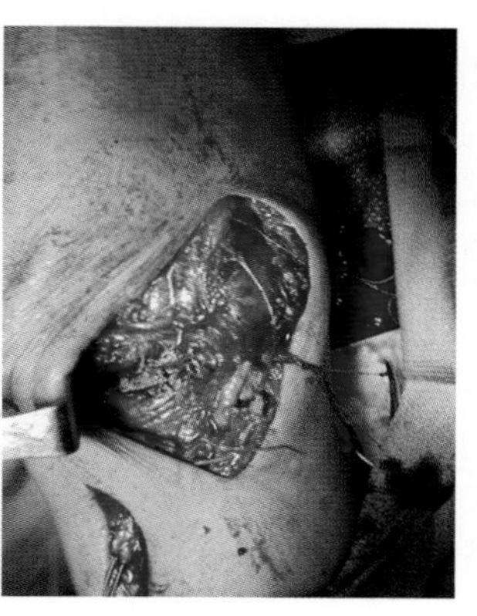
D

FIGURE 12–4. Incision and initial dissection. *A*, Skin incision. *B*, Dissection. *C*, Clinical example of ruptured MCL. *D*, Primary repair.

5. Advancement: The MCL is advanced proximally on the femoral side (Fig. 12–5). This advancement can be accomplished by subperiosteally dissecting the ligament and advancing proximally onto roughened cortical bone or by including a thin corticocancellous block with the ligament. When advanced, the MCL (with or without bone block) usually is secured with a screw and washer. The posterior oblique ligament is imbricated in a pants-over-vest fashion into the posterior border of the MCL.

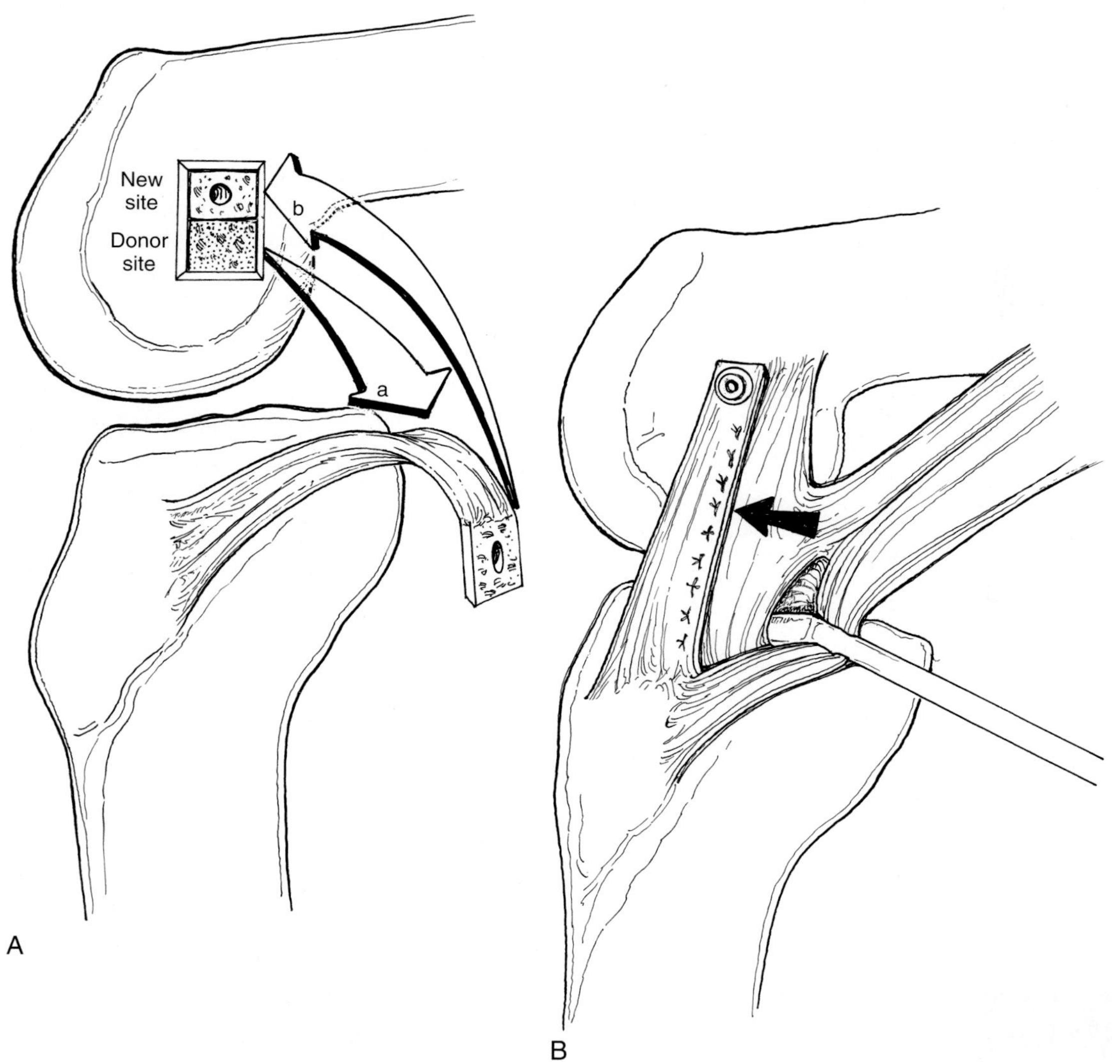

FIGURE 12–5. MCL advancement and plication of the posterior oblique ligament. *A*, Attenuated MCL is detached with a bone block from the medial femoral condyle (a), and the trough is extended superiorly (b). *B*, The MCL bone block is advanced superiorly and fixed in its new location. The posterior oblique ligament is advanced anteriorly and imbricated.

6. Reinforcement: The MCL can be reinforced with the semitendinosus in a technique credited to Bosworth (Fig. 12–6). The distal attachment of the semitendinosus is left intact, and the proximal end is harvested with an open-end tendon stripper (a closed-end stripper requires that the end of the tendon be inserted into the opening). The proximal end is trimmed, débrided, and tubularized. It is then looped over the same screw and soft tissue washer used to secure the bone block, and sutured to itself.
7. Wound closure: The sartorial fascia is sutured carefully, and the remaining layers are closed in standard fashion.

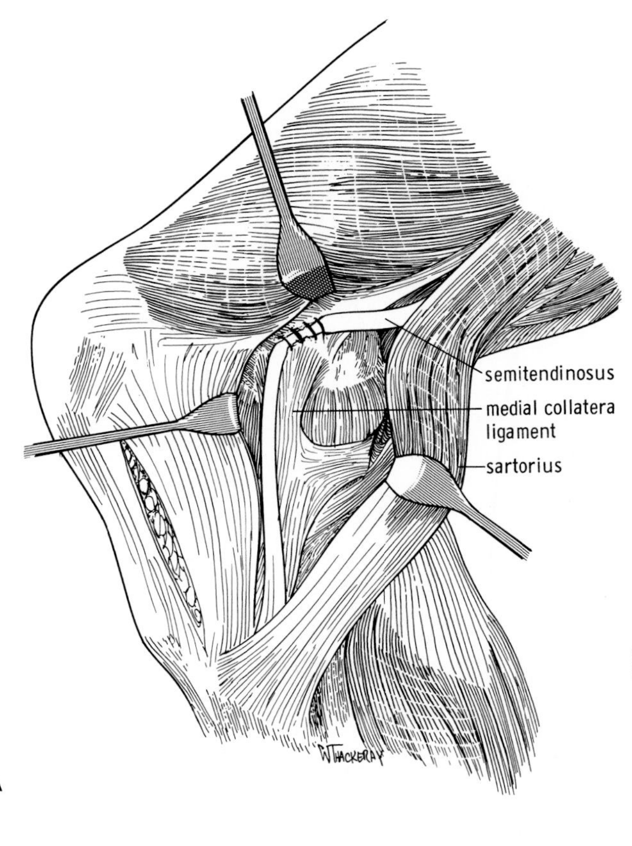

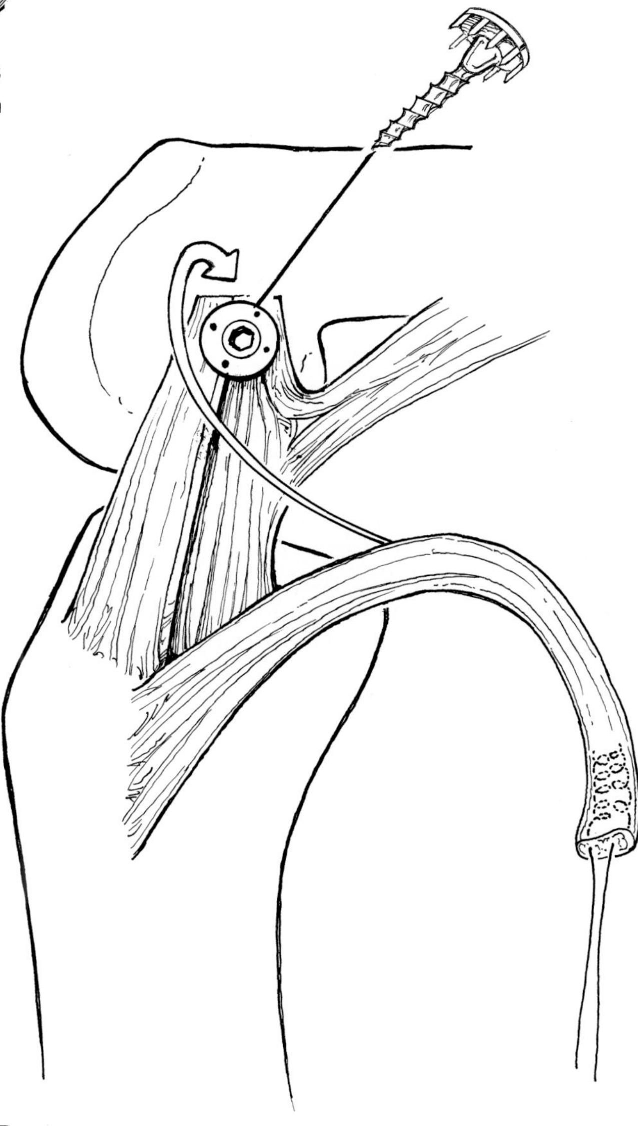

FIGURE 12–6. Harvesting the semitendinosus and augmentation of the MCL repair. *A*, Original description of repair (Bosworth). *B* and *C*, Modification with placement of semitendinosus over screw and soft tissue washer construct. (*A* From Warren RF: Acute ligament injuries. In Insall JN [ed]: Knee Surgery. New York, Churchill Livingstone, 1984, pp 261–294.)

Illustration continued on following page

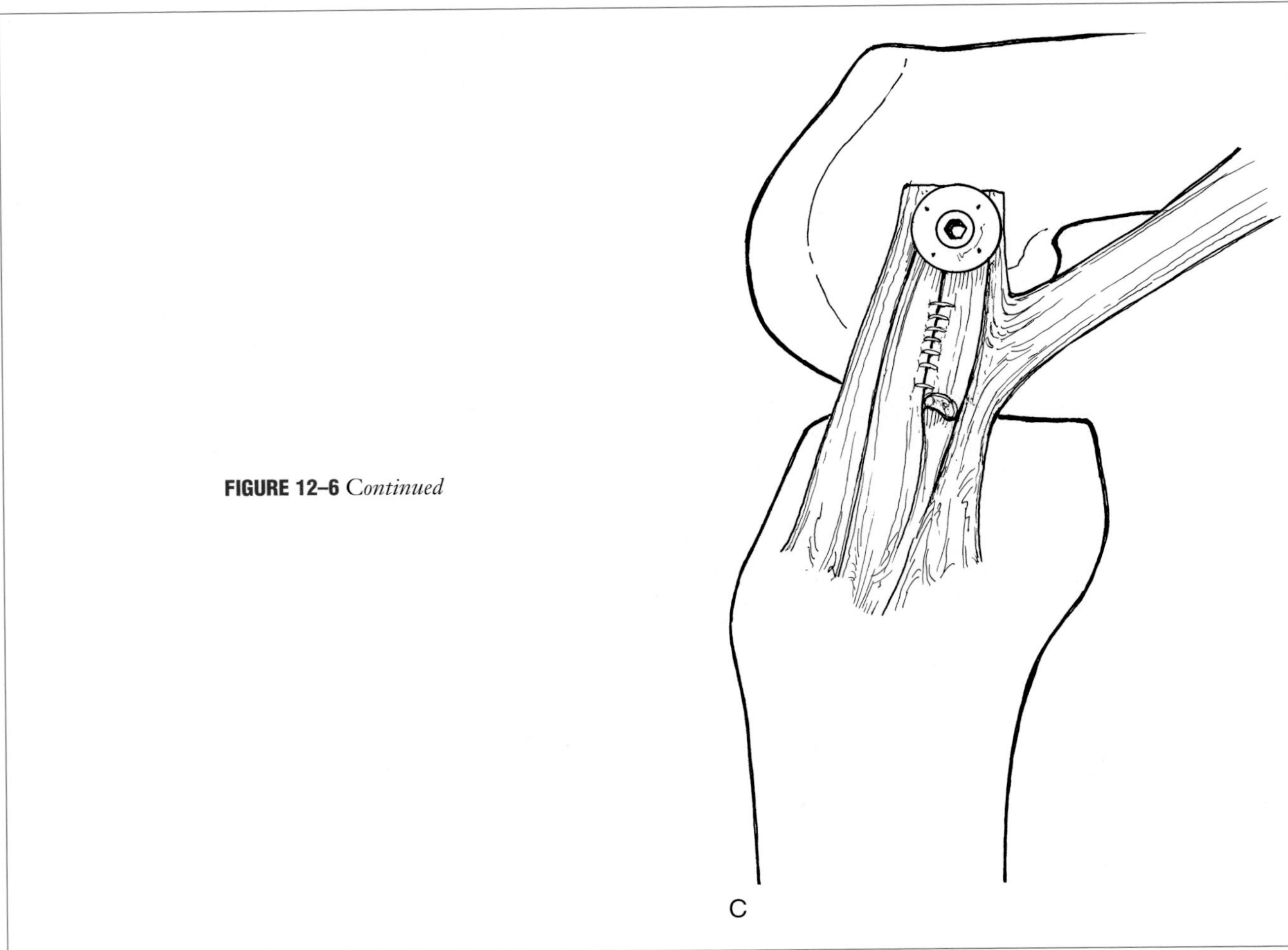

FIGURE 12–6 *Continued*

POSTOPERATIVE MANAGEMENT

Postoperative management is similar to nonoperative management of acute injuries. Prolonged use of a hinged brace is encouraged. Full weight bearing and conditioning should begin 2 to 3 months postoperatively. With combined injuries, rehabilitation of the cruciate ligaments should take priority.

COMPLICATIONS

Complications are similar to other procedures about the knee. Late laxity can occur, especially if bracing is not encouraged in the early postoperative period. Residual pain, usually around the femoral epicondyle, also occasionally can be a problem. Loss of motion, bleeding, infection, and other complications can occur.

RESULTS

Most authors report a greater than 90% success rate with nonoperative treatment of acute isolated MCL tears. The operative technique described in this chapter is successful in most other cases. In our experience, MCL repair is more successful than lateral or posterolateral procedures.

REFERENCES

Baker CL, Shalvoy RM: Treatment of acute and chronic injuries to the medial structures of the knee. Op Tech Orthop 4:166–173, 1996.

Indelicato PA: Non-operative treatment of complete tears of the medial collateral ligament of the knee. J Bone Joint Surg [Am] 65:323–329, 1983.

Indelicato PA: Isolated medial collateral ligament injuries in the knee. J Am Acad Orthop Surg 3:9–14, 1995.

Warren LF, Marshall JL: The supporting structures and layers on the medial side of the knee: An anatomical analysis. J Bone Joint Surg [Am] 61:56–62, 1979.

CHAPTER 13

Treatment of Multiple Knee Ligament Injuries

INTRODUCTION

Injury to more than one knee ligament can occur with severe trauma. This injury may or may not be associated with a knee dislocation, and this distinction is not always obvious because the knee may reduce spontaneously. It is crucial to assess the neurovascular status of the patient after these injuries because associated injuries to the popliteal artery and peroneal nerve are common. An arteriogram should be considered if there is any question (Fig. 13–1).

HISTORY AND PHYSICAL EXAMINATION

Typically, multiple knee ligament injuries are associated with major trauma from sports or motor vehicle accidents. Occasionally, even seemingly minor injuries can result in knee dislocation. Examination is notable for marked effusion, instability in more than one plane, and other findings (discussed for each ligament injury; see previous chapters). A thorough neurovascular examination, with reevaluation of the pulses at regular intervals, is crucial.

DIAGNOSTIC IMAGING

Plain films of knee dislocations allow classification of the injury (Fig. 13–2). The injury is classified based on the direction of the tibia. MRI can be helpful in the evaluation of the multiple ligament–injured knee (Fig. 13–3).

NONOPERATIVE TREATMENT

Historically, nonoperative treatment has been the treatment of choice. The knee is immobilized in a cast or external fixator, usually in full extension, for several weeks. Some patients, especially those who are less active, do satisfactorily with this treatment. Occasionally, treatment of vascular injuries or other associated injuries mandates nonoperative management of multiple ligament injuries of the knee.

RELEVANT ANATOMY

The reader is referred to discussions of individual ligaments in preceding chapters.

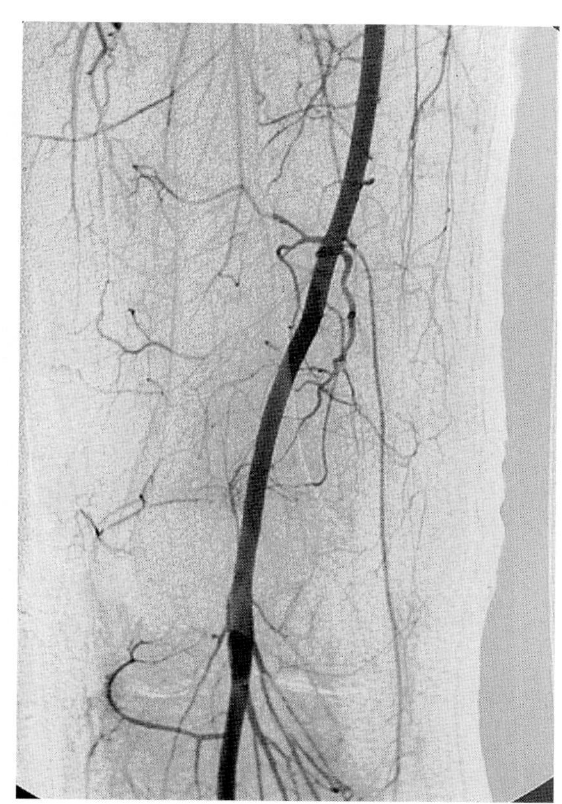

FIGURE 13–1. Normal arteriogram in a patient with a knee dislocation.

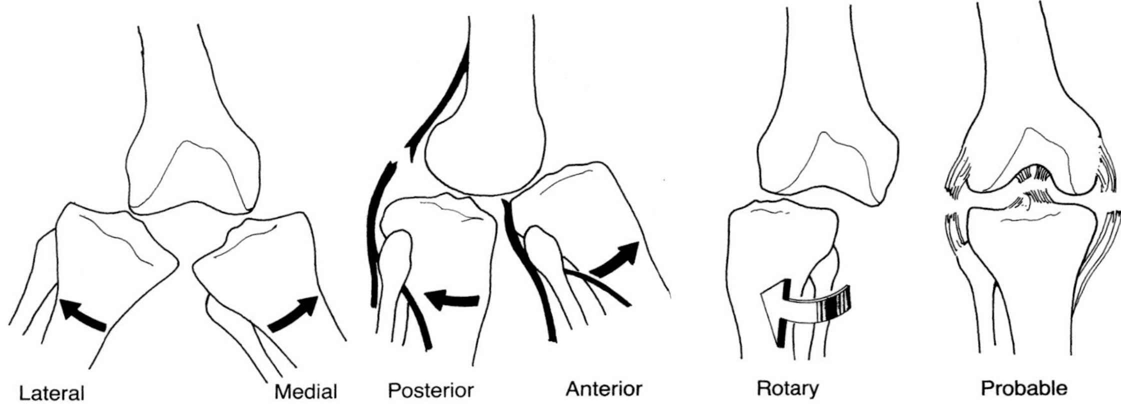

FIGURE 13–2. Classification of knee dislocations. (From Miller MD, Cooper DE, Warner JJP: Review of Sports Medicine and Arthroscopy, 2nd ed. Philadelphia, WB Saunders, 2002.)

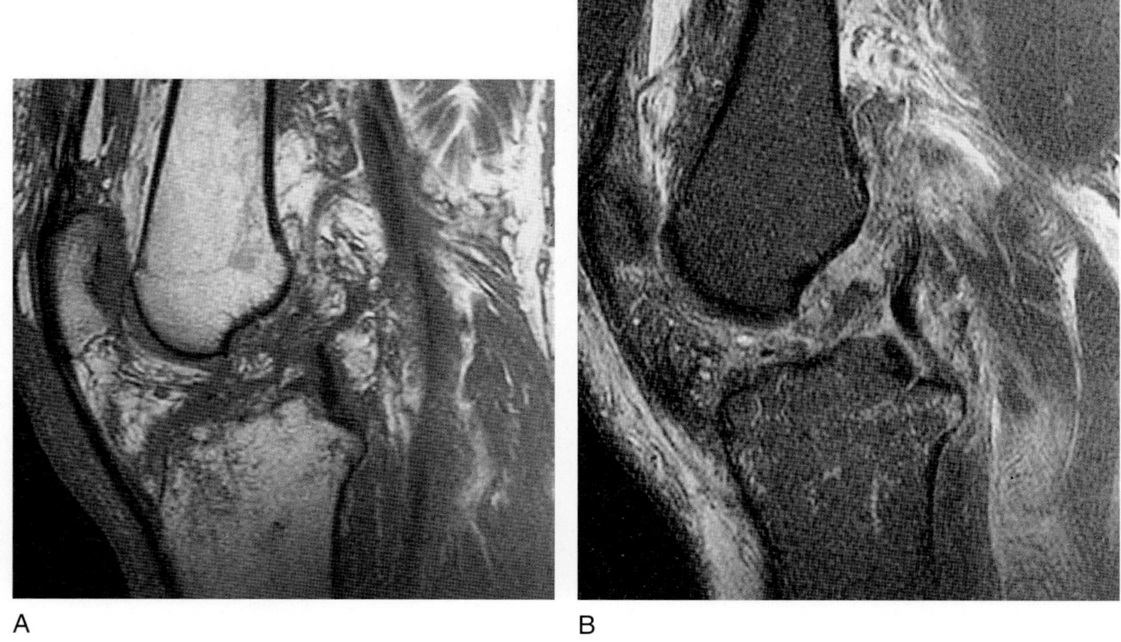

FIGURE 13–3. T1-weighted *(A)* and T2-weighted *(B)* images of a patient with a combined ACL-PCL injury.

SURGICAL TECHNIQUE

Indications

Although there is some debate regarding the treatment and timing of operative treatment of multiple ligament injuries, most knee surgeons currently favor reconstruction of all injured ligaments 10 to 14 days after the injury. Primary repair is favored whenever possible, especially for the collateral ligaments. Cruciate ligament injuries, unless they involve a bony avulsion, usually require reconstruction. Some surgeons favor the use of allografts or ligaments from the contralateral knee to avoid additional injury to the dislocated knee.

Technique

Each ligament is addressed using techniques described previously. When both cruciate ligaments are reconstructed, we recommend passing both grafts before final fixation (Fig. 13–4). The posterior cruciate

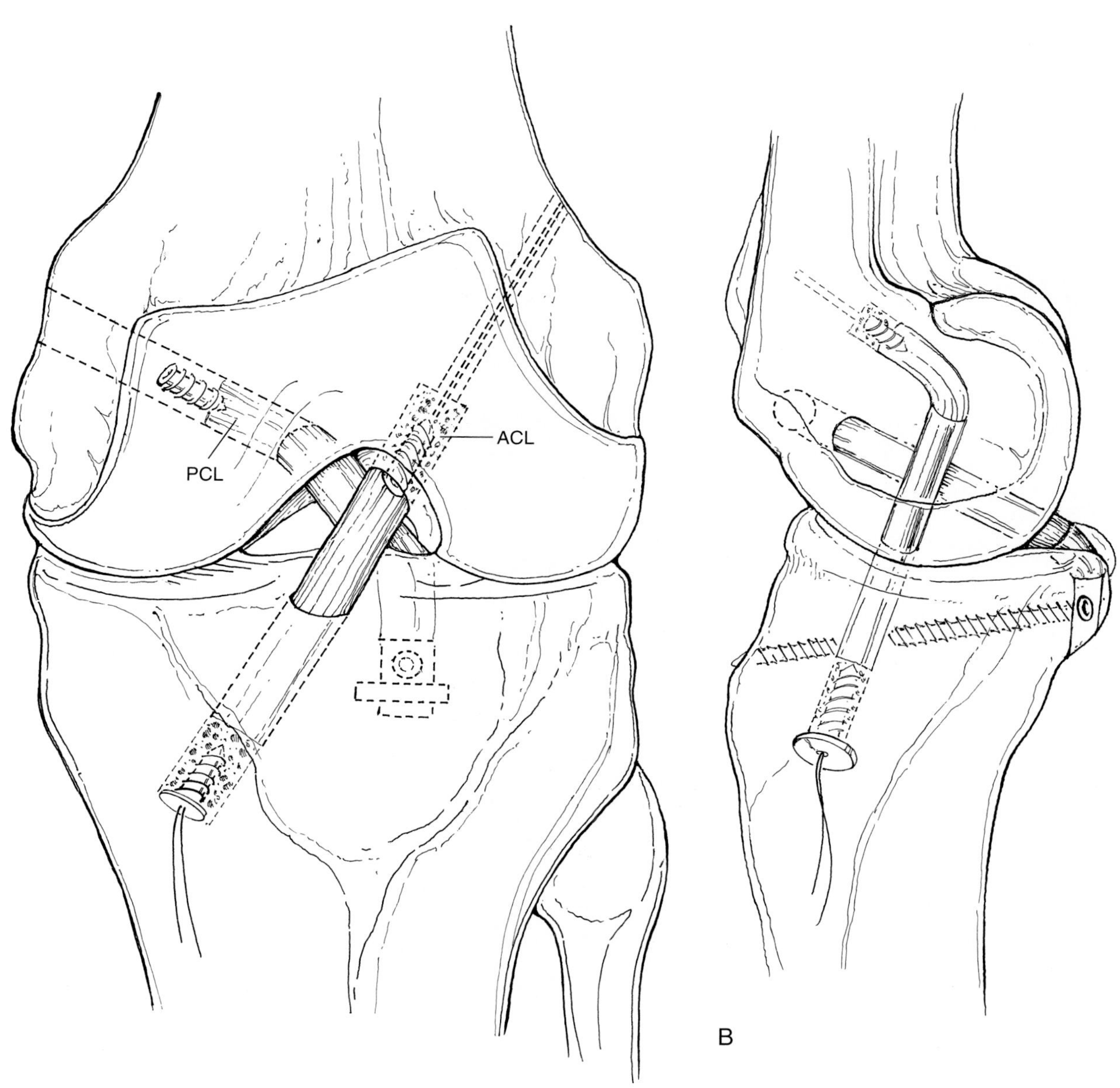

FIGURE 13–4. Combined ACL-PCL reconstruction. *A*, Anteroposterior view. *B*, Lateral view.

Illustration continued on following page

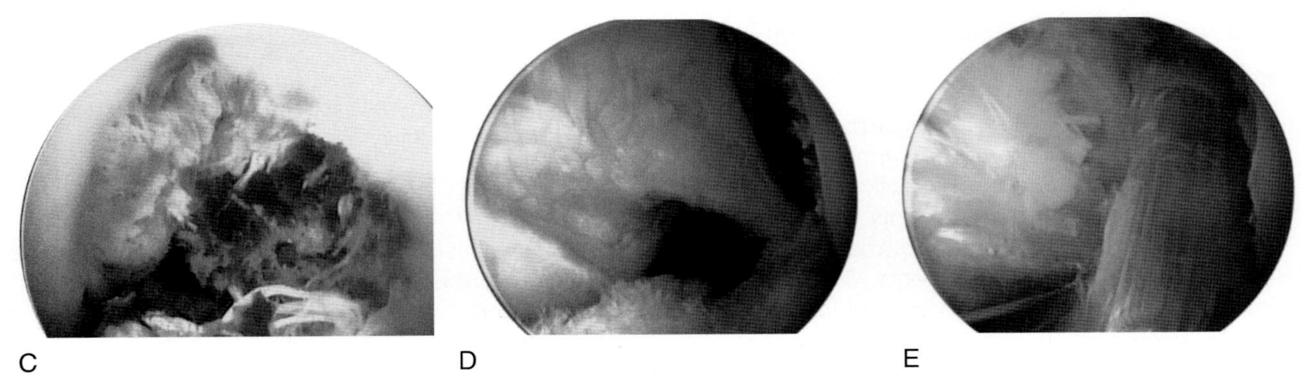

FIGURE 13–4 *Continued. C,* Arthroscopic view of combined ACL-PCL injury. *D,* Arthroscopic view of combined ACL-PCL injury after débridement; note ligament of Wrisberg is still present. *E,* Arthroscopic view of ACL-PCL injury (same patient as in *D*) after ligamentous reconstruction.

ligament is tensioned and fixed first, recreating the normal medial stepoff of the medial tibia. The anterior cruciate ligament can be fixed with the knee in extension. Collateral ligament injuries are addressed next, with an emphasis on primary repair (Fig. 13–5). Augmentation with local tissue is favored when possible.

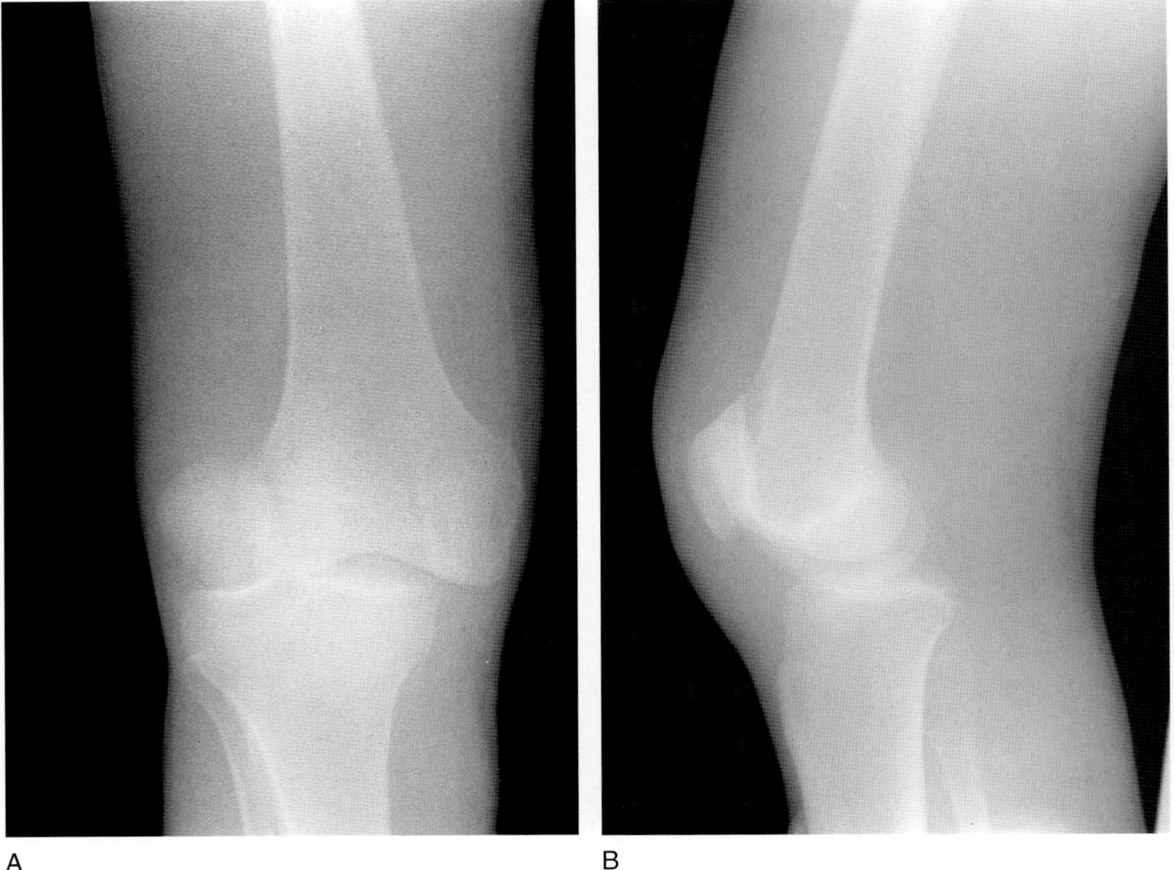

FIGURE 13–5. ACL and PCL reconstruction. *A,* Anteroposterior radiograph. *B,* Lateral radiograph. *A* and *B* show a posterolateral knee dislocation.

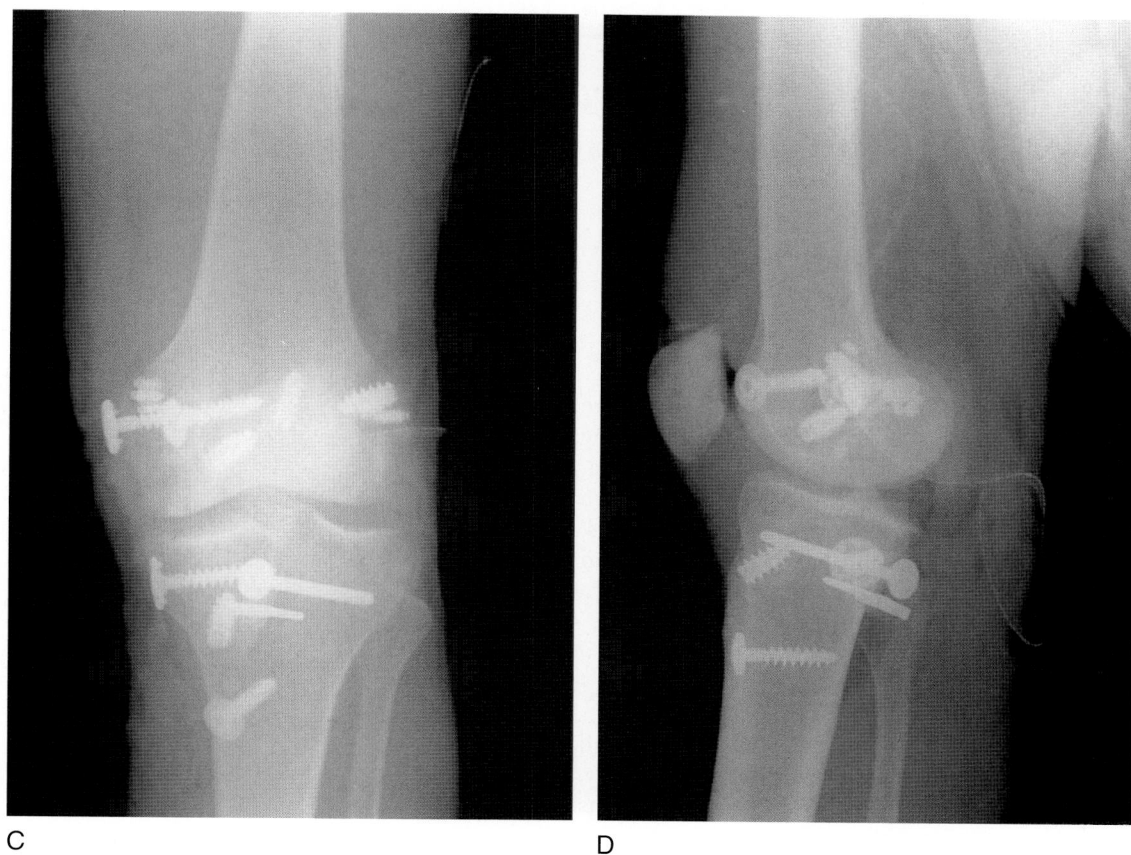

FIGURE 13–5 *Continued. C,* Anteroposterior radiograph. *D,* Lateral radiograph shows the same patient after multiple ligament reconstruction.

POSTOPERATIVE MANAGEMENT

Management of the posterior cruciate ligament should take priority. Extended use of a hinged knee brace is required for collateral ligament repairs.

COMPLICATIONS

These procedures can be lengthy and should be performed only by experienced knee surgeons. Extreme care must be taken with patient padding and positioning, with retraction of important neurovascular structures, and with ligament passage. Wound problems are common. Extended arthroscopy, especially with a pump, is strongly discouraged because of the high risk for fluid extravasation.

RESULTS

Because knee dislocations are rare, there are no large series with long-term follow-up. The literature supports operative intervention. Fanelli reported restoration of functional stability in all knees with multiple ligament injuries that were reconstructed. Although most knees were stable, some mild residual posterior instability occurred in Fanelli's series.

REFERENCES

Fanelli GC, Feldmann DD: Management of combined anterior cruciate ligament/posterior cruciate ligament/posterolateral complex injuries of the knee. Op Tech Sports Med 7:143–149, 1999.

Good L, Johnson RJ: The dislocated knee. J Am Acad Orthop Surg 3:284–292, 1995.

Sisto JD, Warren RF: Complete knee dislocation: A follow-up study of operative treatment. Clin Orthop 198:94–101, 1985.

CHAPTER 14

Treatment of Osteochondral Injuries and Osteochondritis Dissecans

INTRODUCTION

Osteochondral damage can occur as a result of an acute injury or a poorly understood osteochondrosis caused by avascular necrosis. Endocrine disorders, ischemia, genetic factors, abnormal ossification, and trauma have been implicated in the cause of osteochondritis dissecans. Osteochondritis dissecans usually occurs in the teens and can occur in skeletally immature and skeletally mature individuals.

HISTORY AND PHYSICAL EXAMINATION

Acute osteochondral injuries may be caused by a fall directly onto the knee or a twisting/shearing injury. Patients who present with osteochondritis dissecans often do not relate a specific injury but complain of insidious onset of pain and swelling. Mechanical symptoms, such as locking, can occur in both patient groups. Examination should include palpation (patients are often tender over the involved area and may have an effusion), range of motion, and stability assessment.

DIAGNOSTIC IMAGING

Plain radiographs, including a tunnel or Rosenberg view, should be obtained. Osteochondritis dissecans classically involves the lateral aspect of the medial femoral condyle (Fig. 14–1). Typically a well-circumscribed area of radiolucency can be seen above an area of subchondral bone. The presence and width of the physis should be evaluated on radiographs because this may affect the prognosis. Acute osteochondral injuries are more likely to have smaller bony fragments and may appear on plain films as a wisp of bone. MRI can be useful in the evaluation of both lesions and may help in determining whether the fragment is loose or complete.

NONOPERATIVE MANAGEMENT

Nonoperative treatment of osteochondritis dissecans is preferred in patients who have not reached skeletal maturity and in patients with minimal symptoms. A brief period of non–weight bearing and range-of-motion exercises is appropriate initially. Acute osteochondral injuries with suspected (or confirmed) loose bodies should be evaluated and treated arthroscopically.

RELEVANT ANATOMY

Epiphyseal bone is quite vascular but relies on a fragile network of small vessels. Disruption of this tenuous blood supply can lead to avascular necrosis and localized osteochondral damage. Careful evaluation of the lesion helps determine appropriate management.

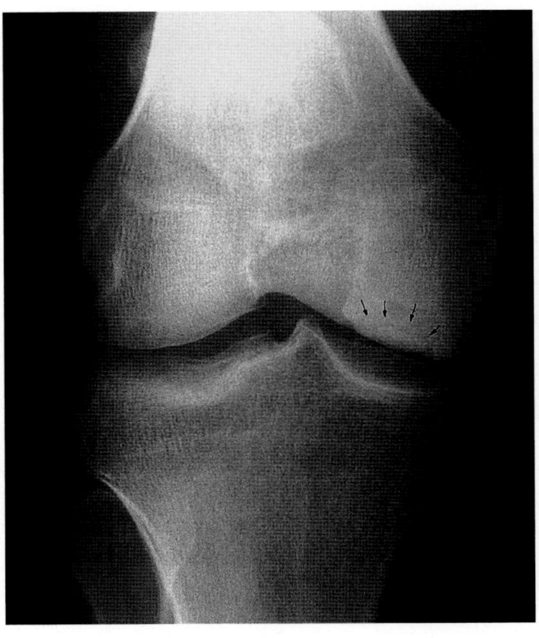

FIGURE 14–1. Plain radiograph shows OCD of the lateral aspect of the medial femoral condyle *(arrows)*.

SURGICAL *TECHNIQUE*

Indications

Indications for surgical treatment are acute osteochondral injuries with loose or detached osteochondral fragments and loose and symptomatic osteochondritis dissecans lesions, particularly in skeletally mature individuals or individuals nearing skeletal maturity.

Technique

Lesions are evaluated arthroscopically, and one of the following techniques is used.

1. Direct repair and fixation: This involves exploration and débridement of the base of the lesion and direct repair and fixation of its base (Figs. 14–2 and 14–3). In acute injuries, direct repair and fixation sometimes can be accomplished even with loose fragments. Fixation can be accomplished with absorbable pins, K-wires, various screws, and other devices.
2. Removal of loose bodies and débridement: This is necessary when there is little bone attached to the loose fragment or when the loose body is fragmented, degenerated, or otherwise unsuitable for repair. Drilling or microfracture of the base of the lesion is done to encourage fibrocartilage ingrowth.

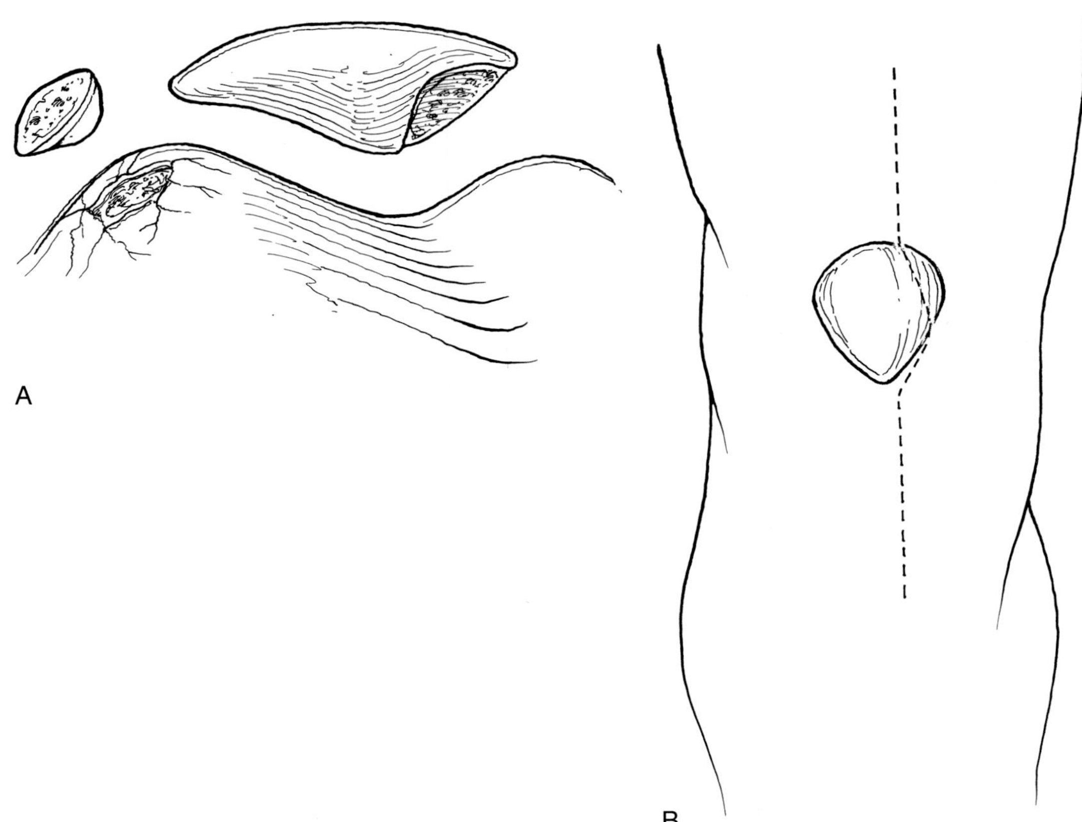

FIGURE 14–2. Treatment of osteochondral injuries to the patella. *A*, Osteochondral injury from patellar dislocation. *B*, Incision.

Illustration continued on following page

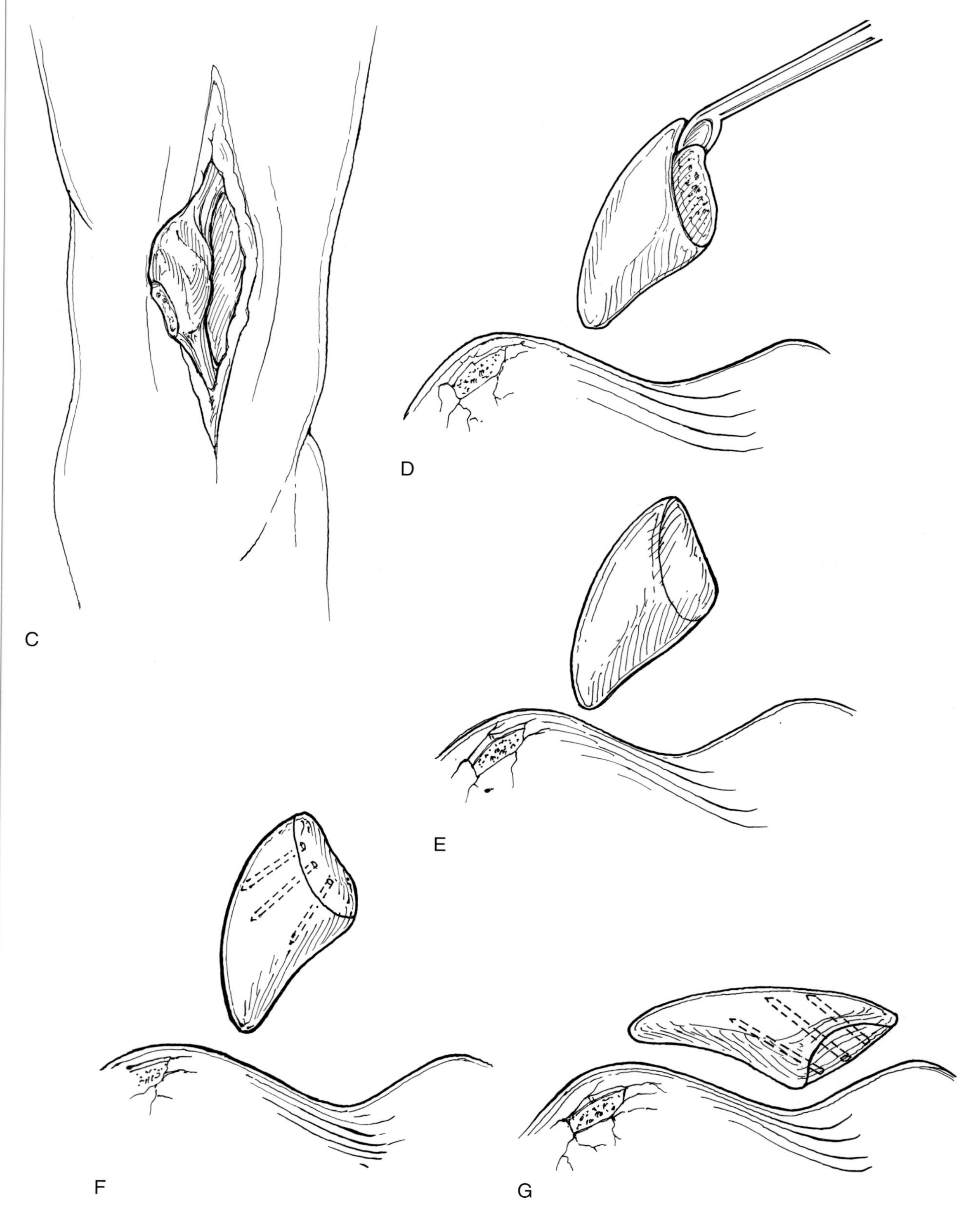

FIGURE 14–2 *Continued.* *C*, Medial parapatellar incision is made, and the patella is everted. *D*, Base of lesion is freshened. *E* and *F*, Osteochondral fragment is reduced *(E)* and fixed *(F)*. *G*, Final repair.

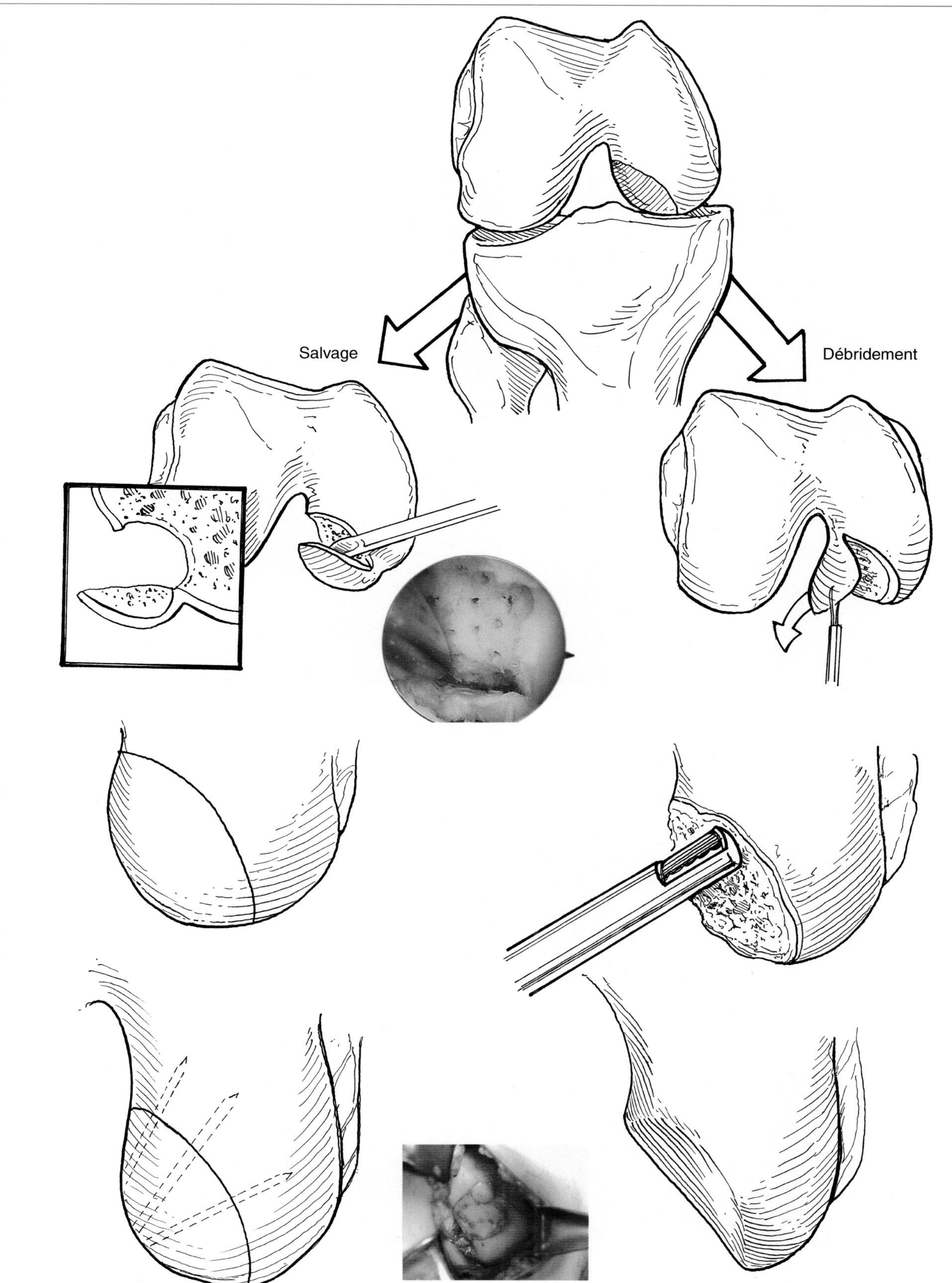

FIGURE 14–3. Salvage: The loose osteochondral lesion is probed, its base débrided, and then secured with absorbable PDS pins. Two pins and an OATS plug are inserted. Débridement: The loose fragment is removed, and the base of the lesion is débrided.

3. Chondral transfer or autologous chondrocyte implantation: These techniques, discussed in Chapter 15, have been attempted in the management of these lesions, with some early clinical success. It is unclear how chondrocyte implantation can allow differentiation of cartilage and bone, but proponents of this technique indicate that it is successful. Occasionally, bone grafting of the defect may be necessary before considering these techniques (Fig. 14–4).

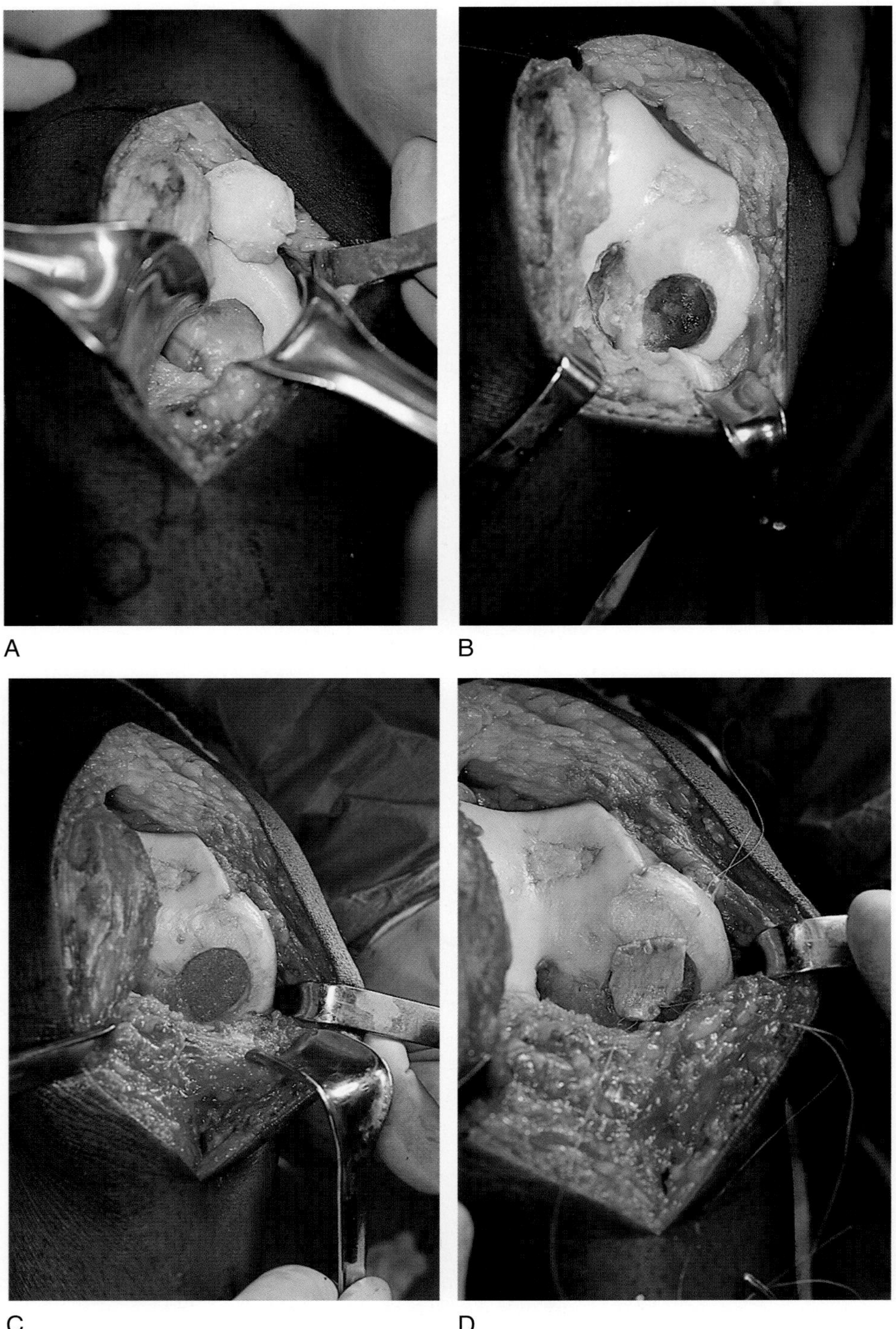

FIGURE 14–4. Bone graft and periosteal patch of large osteochondral lesion. *A*, Exposure and removal of large osteochondral fragment. The piece did not have any osteochondral bone, and the base of the lesion was fibrous. *B*, Débridement of the base of the lesion to normal bone left a large defect. *C*, Bone graft from the tibial metaphysis was packed into the defect. *D* and *E*, A periosteal patch (cambium layer out) was sewn into place.

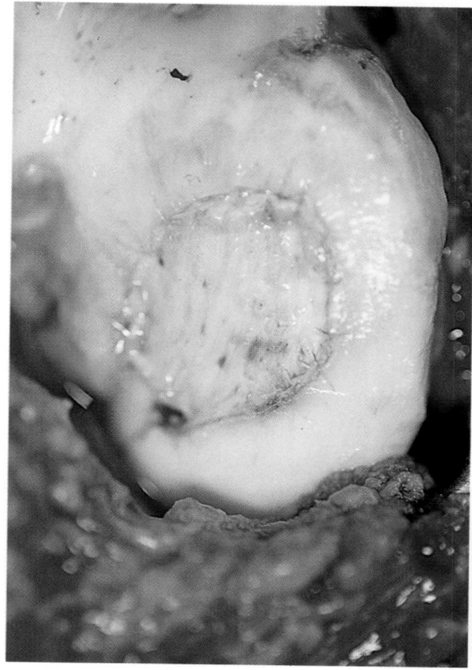

E

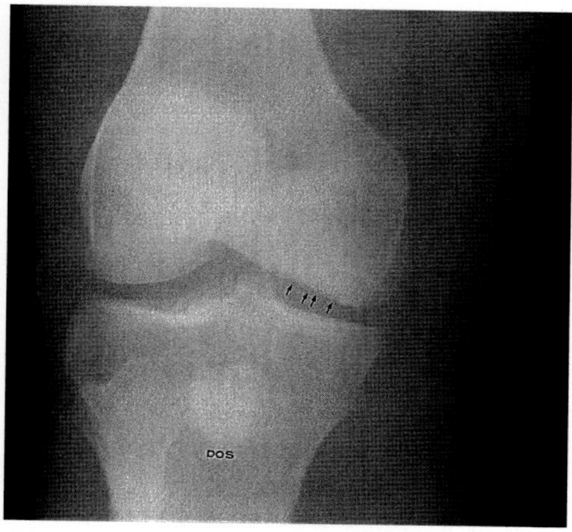

F

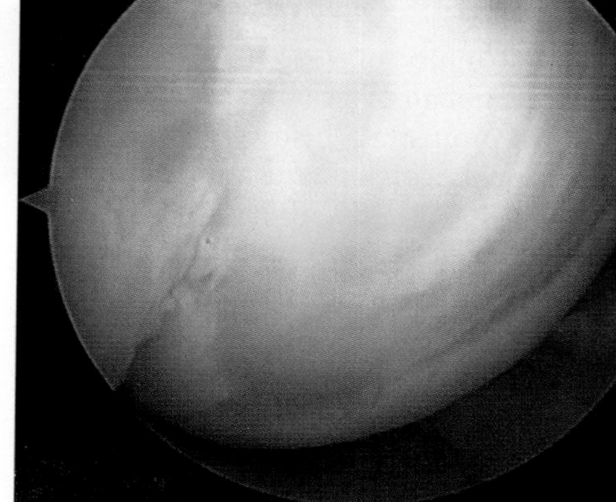

G

FIGURE 14–4 *Continued. F,* Postoperative radiograph shows final graft. This is the same patient shown in Figure 14–1. *G,* Arthroscopic view 3 months after the procedure shows articular softening but good bone incorporation.

POSTOPERATIVE MANAGEMENT

Non–weight bearing is recommended for 6 weeks. Early motion is encouraged, and continuous passive motion is preferred. Quadriceps rehabilitation and return to sports are similar to that for anterior cruciate ligament reconstruction.

COMPLICATIONS

Complications are related to the treatment chosen. Hardware can loosen or migrate, late arthrosis can develop, and a variety of other complications can occur.

RESULTS

Results are mixed. A better prognosis is associated with skeletally immature individuals, regardless of treatment.

REFERENCES

Bradley J, Dandy DJ: Osteochondritis dissecans and other lesions of the femoral condyles. J Bone Joint Surg [Br] 71:518–522, 1989.

Cahill BR: Osteochondritis dissecans of the knee: Treatment of juvenile and adult forms. J Am Acad Orthop Surg 3:237–247, 1995.

Noyes FR, Stabler CL: A system for grading articular cartilage lesions at arthroscopy. Am J Sports Med 17:505–513, 1989.

Pappas A: Osteochondritis dissecans. Clin Orthop 158:59–69, 1981.

Schenck RC, Goodnight JM: Osteochondritis dissecans: Current concepts review. J Bone Joint Surg [Am] 78:439–456, 1996.

CHAPTER 15

Treatment of Chondral Injuries and Defects

INTRODUCTION

New techniques have been introduced for the treatment of chondral injuries and defects. Although these various techniques have generated a lot of excitement, the long-term results of these procedures are not known.

HISTORY AND PHYSICAL EXAMINATION

Patients with chondral injury may or may not recall a specific injury. They complain of swelling and sometimes have mechanical symptoms. A history of recurrent swelling and the presence of an effusion on physical examination are highly associated with chondral injuries.

DIAGNOSTIC IMAGING

Plain radiographs are usually normal. A standing flexion weight-bearing posteroanterior radiograph should be obtained to ensure that there is no significant narrowing in the affected portion of the joint. MRI of chondral injuries has improved; however, consultation with a musculoskeletal radiologist can be helpful in these cases because special images can be obtained (Fig. 15–1).

NONOPERATIVE TREATMENT

Nonoperative treatment of these lesions was favored until recently. Earlier techniques that rely on fibrocartilage to fill these defects (so-called abrasion chondroplasty) did not seem to significantly alter the natural history of knees with cartilage loss. Newer techniques have shown some promise, but long-term results are unknown.

RELEVANT ANATOMY

Cartilage loss occurs most commonly on the medial femoral condyle. It is important to understand the normal curve of the condyle and to attempt to reproduce this. Cartilage transfer procedures use cartilage from areas of the knee that have minimal requirements for normal articulation. Although there is no ideal site for this harvest, contact pressure studies have shown that the superior aspect of the lateral femoral condyle is least affected.

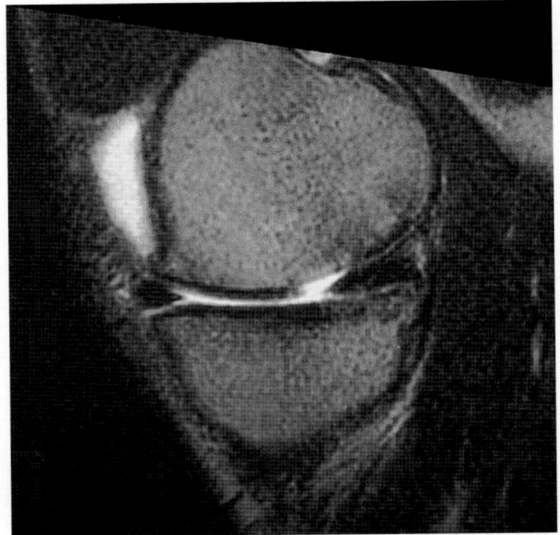

FIGURE 15–1. Gadolinium-enhanced T2-weighted sagittal MRI of chondral injury.

SURGICAL TECHNIQUE

Indications

Although many of these procedures are investigational, all of them are recommended only for symptomatic focal, discrete, full-thickness cartilage lesions without any significant accompanying arthritis in physiologically young patients. These lesions sometimes are not appreciated preoperatively, and the surgeon and patient need to be prepared with a plan ahead of time. Some of these techniques that require cartilage culture or allograft harvesting can be expensive, and some insurance plans may not cover their costs.

Technique

Four techniques are described: (1) microfracture, (2) osteochondral plugs (MosaicPlasty, Smith & Nephew, Andover, MA; OATS, Arthrex, Naples, FL; COR, Mitek, Westwood, MA), (3) autologous chondrocyte implantation (ACI), and (4) osteochondral allografts. All of these techniques begin with diagnostic arthroscopy and débridement of the edges of the lesion (Fig. 15–2).

Microfracture

This technique, developed by Steadman, begins with débridement of the lesion, including the calcified cartilage layer. A special awl is used to make multiple holes in the exposed subchondral bone plate (Fig. 15–3). Holes are placed approximately 3 to 4 mm apart (or three or four holes per square centimeter). The awl is inserted about 4 mm, and fat droplets and blood can be seen after removal of the awl. These droplets of blood are believed to create a *superclot,* which results in a *hybrid* of hyaline cartilage and fibrocartilage.

Osteochondral Plugs

This technique, developed in Hungary, uses cylindric harvesting tools to transfer plugs of cartilage and subchondral bones into specially prepared recipient defects (Fig. 15–4). The key to this technique is perpendicular harvesting and placement of the plugs. Typically the superior lateral condyle is used for plug harvest. Although some surgeons do this procedure

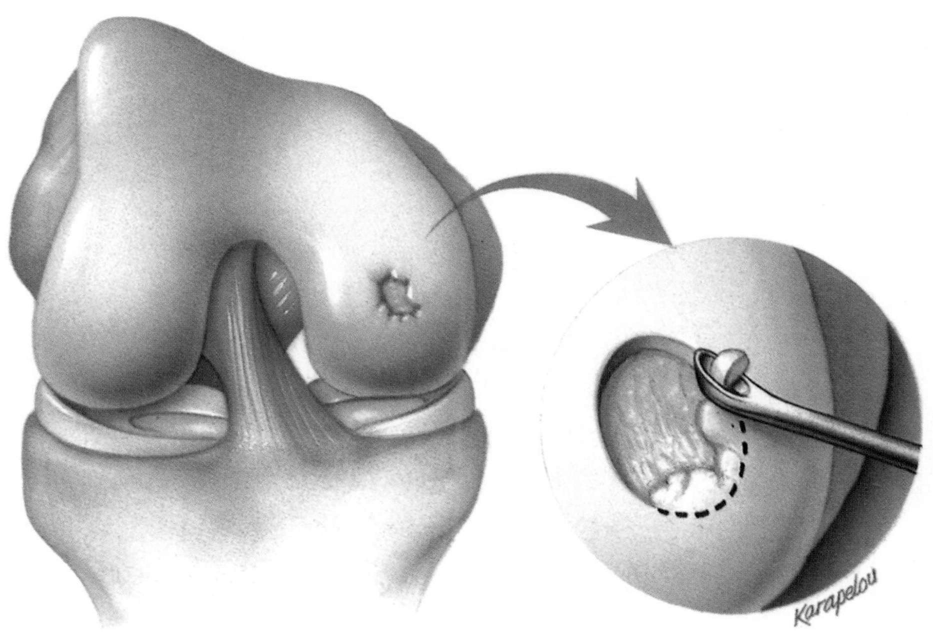

FIGURE 15–2. Débridement of full-thickness chondral injury. (From Miller MD: Atlas of chondral injury treatment. Op Tech Orthop 7:289–293, 1997.)

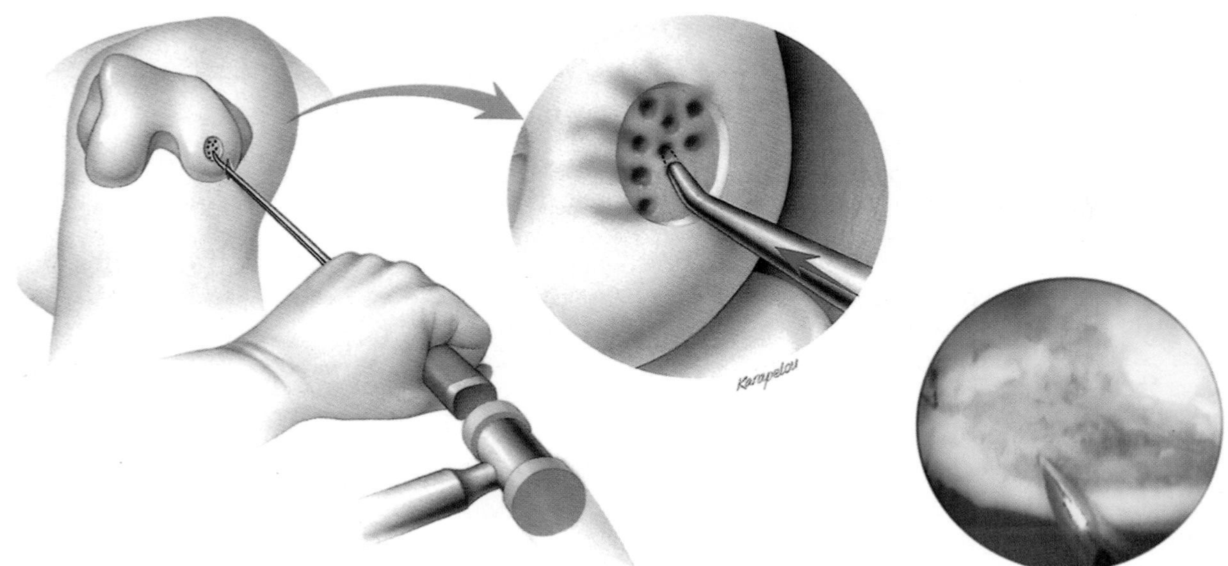

FIGURE 15–3. Microfracture. Special awls are inserted through the ipsilateral portal and penetrate the subchondral bone approximately 4 mm. (From Miller MD: Atlas of chondral injury treatment. Op Tech Orthop 7:289–293, 1997.)

A

B

C D E

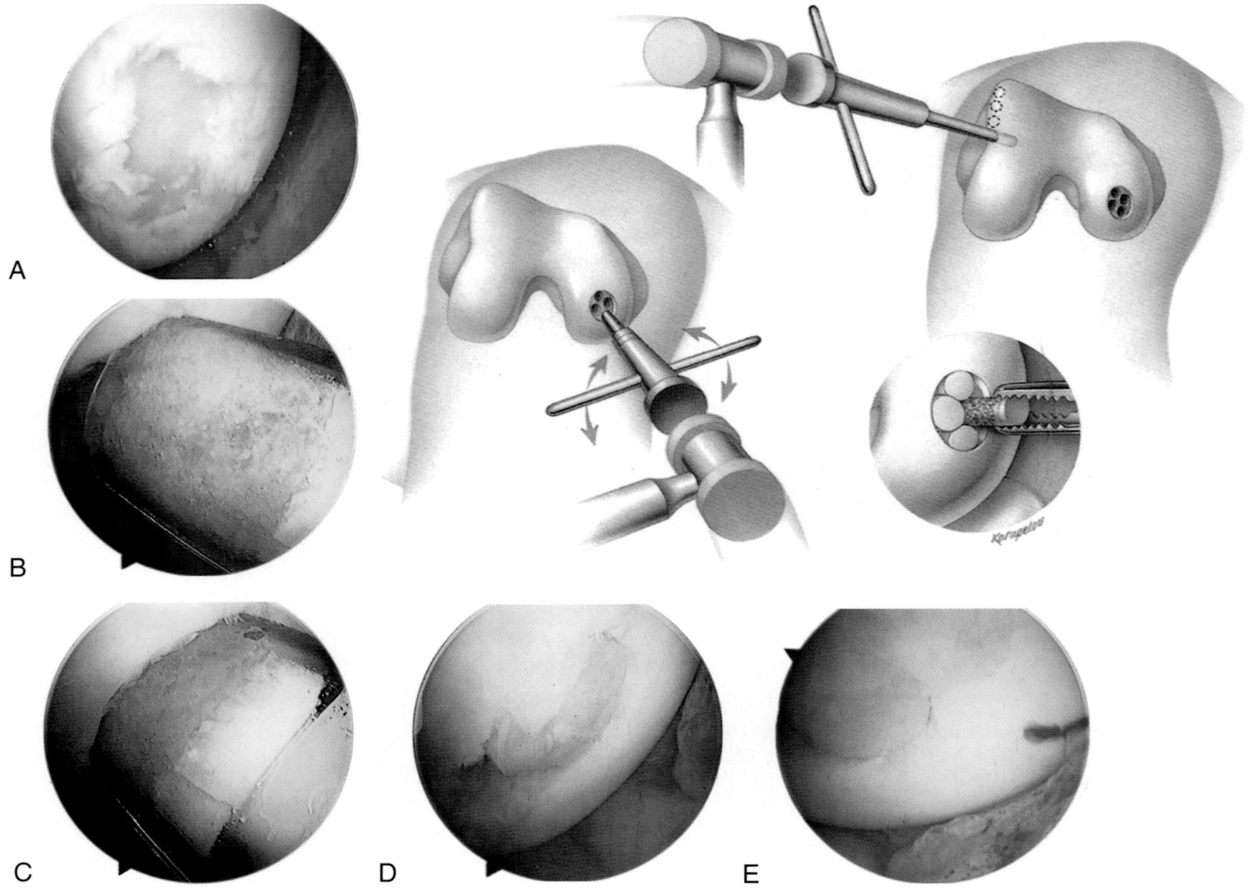

FIGURE 15–4. Osteochondral plugs. Plugs are harvested from the superolateral knee and transferred into prepared defects. *A*, Initial débridement and planning. *B*, Drilling. All steps must be done perpendicular to the joint surface. *C*, Plug delivery. *D*, Drilling for second plug. *E*, Two plugs in place. (From Miller MD: Atlas of chondral injury treatment. Op Tech Orthop 7:289–293, 1997.)

arthroscopically, we have found that a small superolateral arthrotomy facilitates plug harvesting. A surgical sponge can be placed in this incision, and the remainder of the procedure can be done arthroscopically. Some lesions, such as trochlear defects, must be repaired open (Fig. 15–5).

Autologous Chondrocyte Implantation

This procedure, pioneered in Sweden, is a two-stage technique for implanting the patient's own cultured chondrocytes. In the initial procedure, the lesion is sized, and a small amount of nonaffected cartilage is harvested. This cartilage is sent to a laboratory, where it is enzymatically digested and chondrocytes are cultured. The second stage, done several weeks later, consists of preparing a recipient site for these cells (Fig. 15–6). The defect is débrided, preserving the subchondral plate; a periosteal patch is harvested from the proximal tibia and sewn over the defect using 6–0 suture. A watertight seal is necessary, and fibrin glue is used to help achieve this.

Osteochondral Allografts

This procedure, currently done at only a few centers in North America, uses fresh, matched osteochondral allografts to replace large defects. Restoring normal mechanical alignment is a major focus of this procedure. Large osteochondral grafts (Fig. 15–7) or patch grafts (Fig. 15–8) can be used.

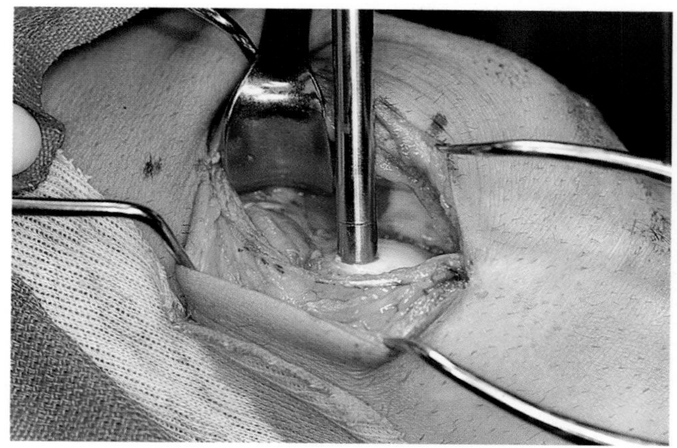

A

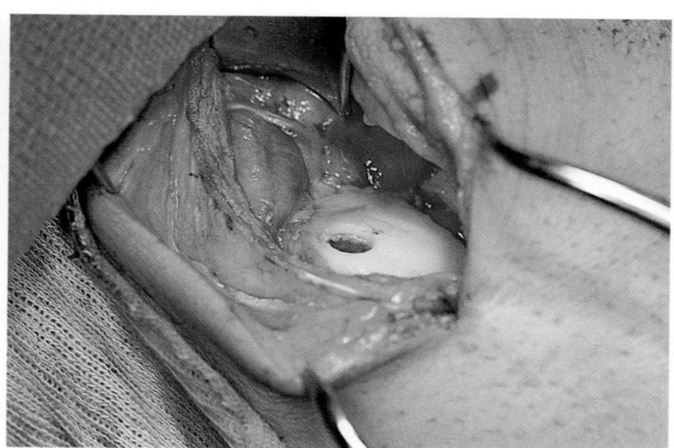

B

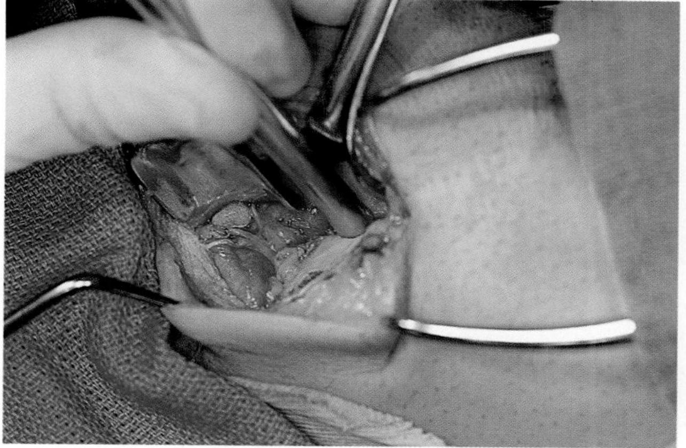

C

D

FIGURE 15–5. Osteochondral plug insertion in some areas, such as the trochlea shown here, must be done open. *A*, Plug harvesting. *B*, Defect after plug harvesting. *C*, Plug delivery. *D*, After plug delivery showing donor and recipient sites.

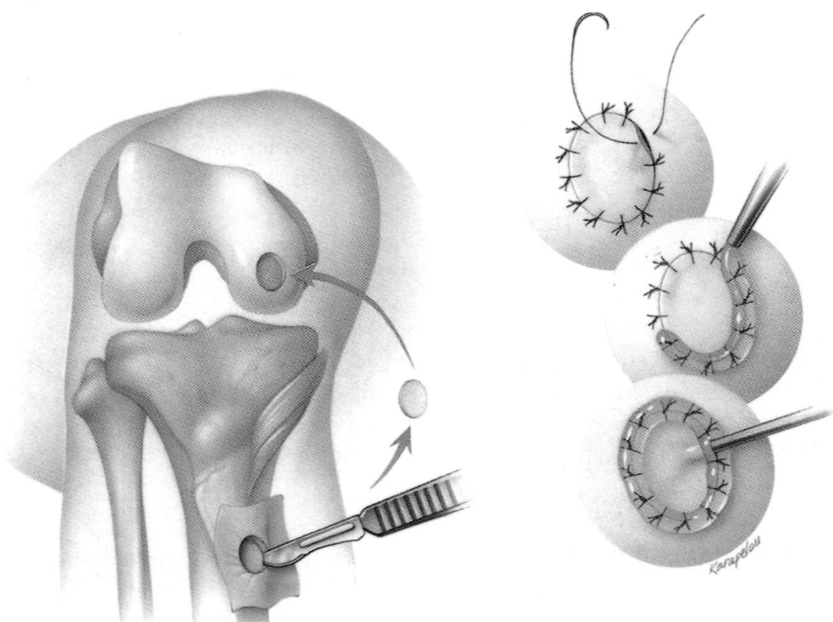

FIGURE 15–6. Autologous chondrocyte implantation. Chondrocytes, obtained from an earlier harvest, are cultured and injected into the defect. The subchondral plate is left intact, and periosteum is sewn carefully in place and sealed with fibrin glue. Cells are injected into this bed. (From Miller MD: Atlas of chondral injury treatment. Op Tech Orthop 7:289–293, 1997.)

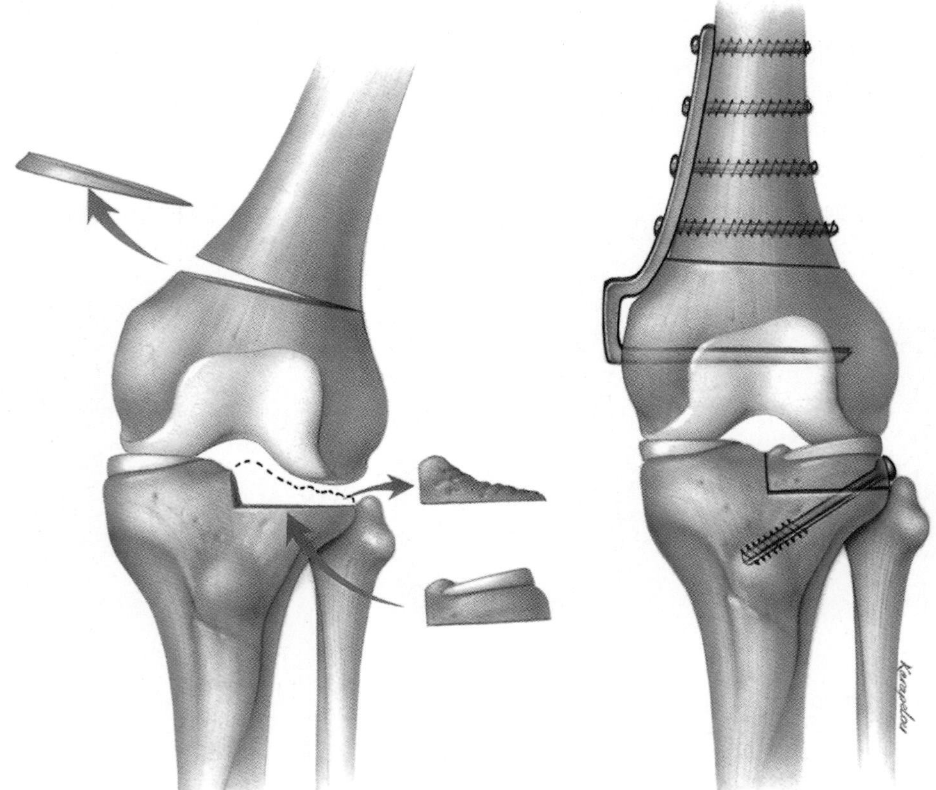

FIGURE 15–7. Osteochondral allograft. Fresh osteochondral allograft is transferred into an excised area of bone and cartilage. Mechanical alignment is restored with a concomitant osteotomy. (From Miller MD: Atlas of chondral injury treatment. Op Tech Orthop 7:289–293, 1997.)

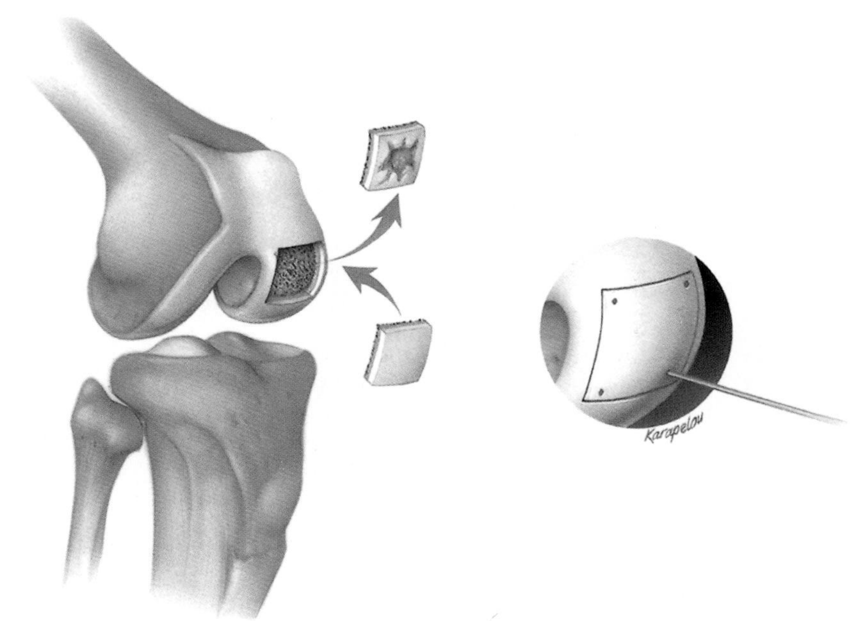

FIGURE 15–8. Patch, or shell allograft. A matched osteochondral graft is inserted into a prepared defect similar to replacing a damaged patch of lawn with fresh sod. (From Miller MD: Atlas of chondral injury treatment. Op Tech Orthop 7:289–293, 1997.)

POSTOPERATIVE MANAGEMENT

Most authors recommend a prolonged period (6 to weeks) of non–weight bearing or partial weight bearing and continuous passive motion after cartilage procedures. Closed-chain quadriceps strengthening is initiated after this period.

COMPLICATIONS

Perhaps the biggest complication is that the procedures may not hold up over time or that they do not work. Additional chondral injury, loss of motion, bleeding, infections, and a host of other complications are possible.

RESULTS

Results of all of these procedures are encouraging but preliminary. Independent evaluation of these techniques with long-term follow-up is necessary to determine the best technique.

REFERENCES

Buckwalter JA, Mankin HJ: Articular cartilage (parts I and II). J Bone Joint Surg [Am] 79:600–632, 1997.

Mandelbaum BR, Browne JE, Fu FH, et al: Articular cartilage lesions of the knee: Current concepts. Am J Sports Med 26:853–861, 1998.

Menche DS, Vangsness CT, Pitman M, et al: The treatment of isolated articular cartilage lesions in the young individual. Instr Course Lect 47:505–515, 1998.

Miller MD: Treatment of chondral injuries. Op Tech Orthop 7:261–354, 1997.

Newman AP: Articular cartilage repair: Current concepts. Am J Sports Med 26:309–324, 1998.

O'Driscoll SW: The healing and regeneration of articular cartilage: Current concepts review. J Bone Joint Surg [Am] 80:1795–1812, 1998.

CHAPTER 16

Patellar Realignment Procedures

INTRODUCTION

Patellar realignment procedures, including lateral release, proximal realignment, and tibial tubercle transfers (distal realignment), have limited indications and inconsistent results. Extended rehabilitation should be the mainstay of treatment for these often difficult patients.

HISTORY AND PHYSICAL EXAMINATION

Patients may complain of slipping of the kneecap and often never had a frank dislocation. Swelling and catching in full extension is a common complaint. Examination for tenderness, effusion, mobility, and apprehension should be completed (Fig. 16–1). Measurement of the Q angle (anterior superior iliac

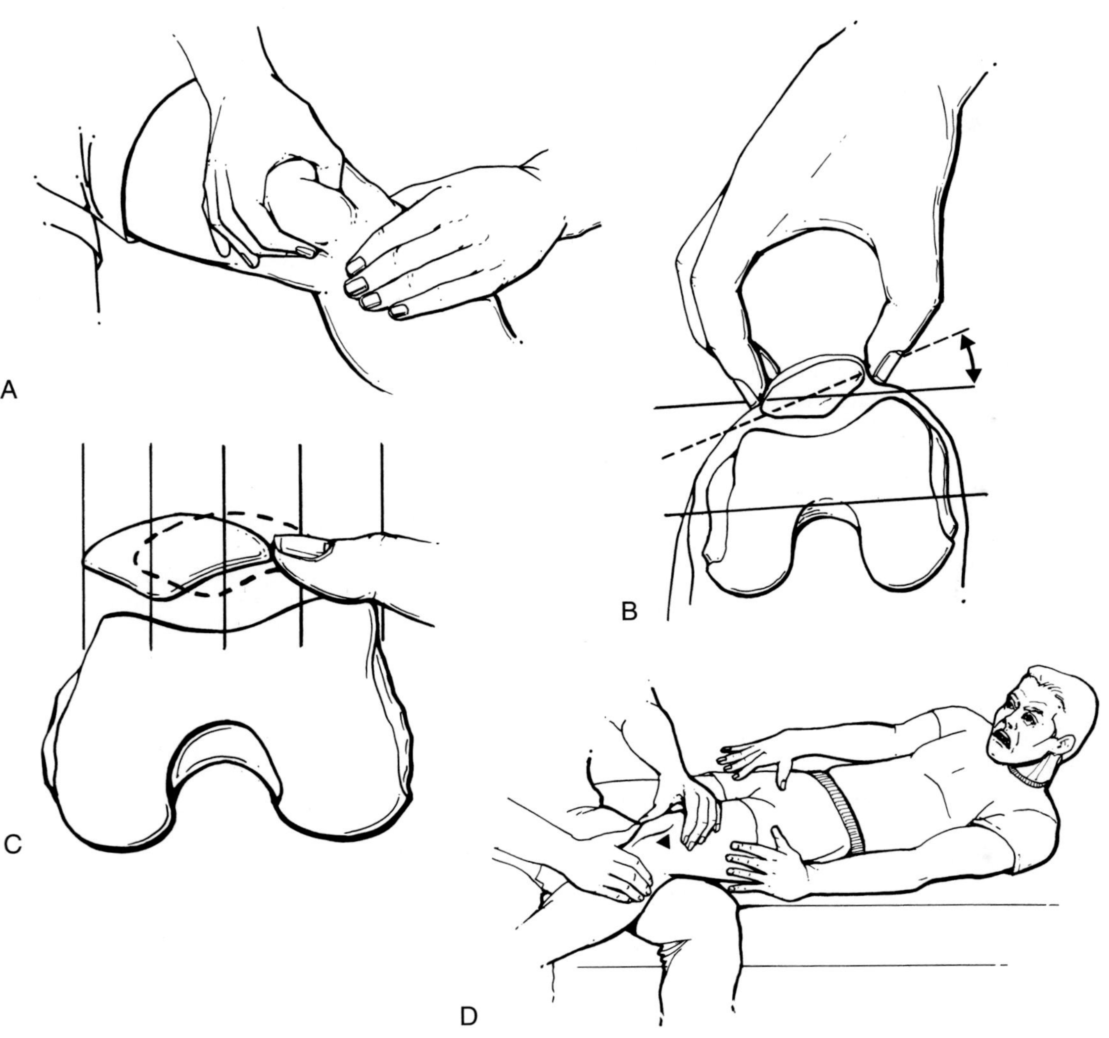

FIGURE 16–1. Patellar examination. *A*, Palpation for medial facet tenderness. *B*, Patellar tilt test. *C*, Mobility testing. *D*, Apprehension testing. (From Walsh WM: Patellofemoral joint. In DeLee JC, Drez D Jr [eds]: Orthopaedic Sports Medicine Principles and Practice. Philadelphia, WB Saunders, 1994, pp 1163–1248.)

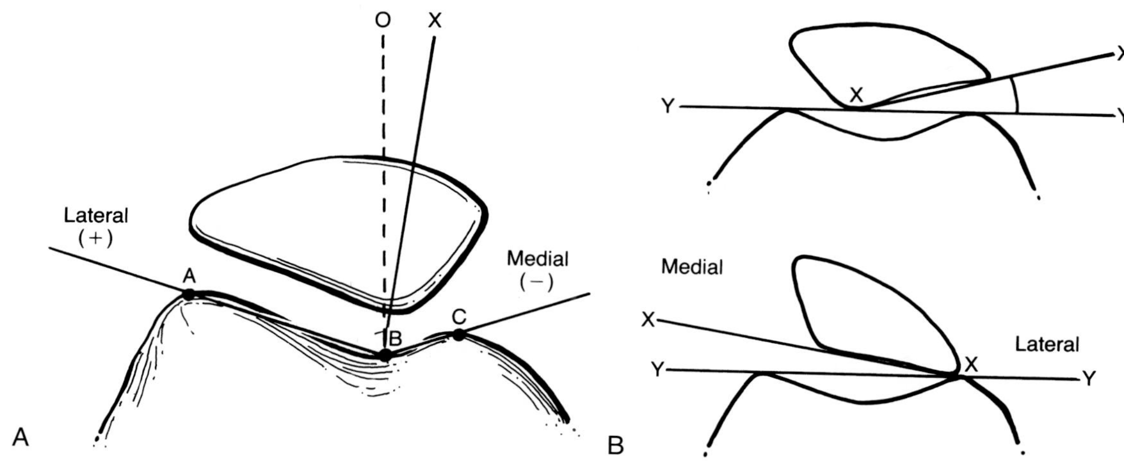

FIGURE 16–2. *A*, Merchant's congruence angle. BO bisects angle ABC (angle ABO = angle OBC). Line BX passes through the lowest point on the median ridge of the patella. Angle OBX is the congruence angle (normally −6° ± 8°). *B*, Laurin's lateral patellofemoral angle. Line YY connects the anterior aspects of the femoral trochlea. Line XX follows the slope of the lateral patellar facet. Lateral opening *(top)* is normal; medial opening *(bottom)* is abnormal. (From Walsh WM: Patellofemoral joint. In DeLee JC, Drez D Jr [eds]: Orthopaedic Sports Medicine Principles and Practice. Philadelphia, WB Saunders, 1994, pp 1163–1248.)

spine to midpatella to tibial tubercle; normally ≤15°) and the sitting Q angle (normally ≤8°) also can be helpful.

DIAGNOSTIC IMAGING

Several methods for imaging to the patellofemoral joint have been described, including the congruence angle of Merchant (normal, −6° ± 8°), Laurin's lateral patellofemoral angle (normally opens laterally), and others (Fig. 16–2). Stress views and CT evaluation also have been proposed. MRI may be helpful occasionally, especially in the evaluation of articular cartilage.

NONOPERATIVE TREATMENT

Because operative management of these disorders is poorly understood, nonoperative treatment is the first choice. Closed-chain quadriceps exercise, flexibility exercises, bracing, and taping all have a role. Correction of other problems such as foot deformities, activity modification, and nonsteroidal anti-inflammatory drugs also can be helpful.

RELEVANT ANATOMY

An appreciation of the normal extensor mechanism anatomy, including the vastus medialis obliqus (VMO), the lateral retinaculum, and the tibial tubercle (and the cross-sectional anatomy of this area), is helpful. The vascular anatomy of the patellofemoral joint also should be appreciated (Fig. 16–3).

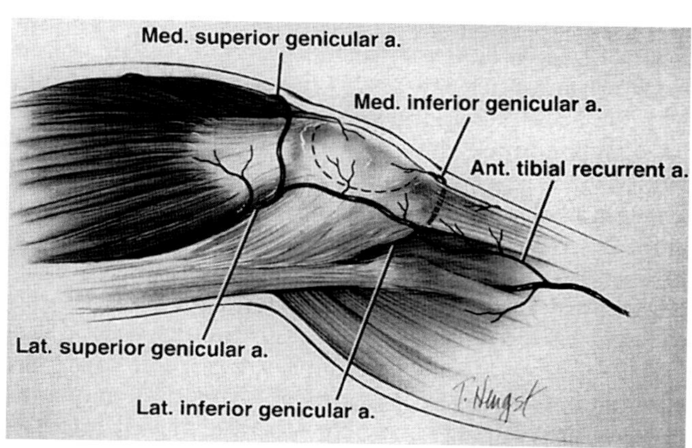

FIGURE 16–3. Arterial blood supply to the patellofemoral joint. (From Banas MP, Ferkel RD, Friedman MJ: Arthroscopic lateral retinacular release of the patellofemoral joint. Op Tech Sports Med 2:291–296, 1994.)

SURGICAL *TECHNIQUE*

Indications

1. Lateral release: Indications include pain, tight lateral retinaculum, lateral tenderness, and lateral tracking without patellar subluxation in a patient who has failed extended nonoperative management. Contraindications include advanced arthrosis, small patella, reflex sympathetic dystrophy (RSD), patella alta.
2. Proximal realignment: The indication is painful lateral subluxation with a normal Q angle (controversial) in patients who otherwise meet parameters described for lateral release procedures. It sometimes is advocated for skeletally immature patients who are not candidates for distal procedures.
3. Distal realignment: Indications are symptomatic lateral subluxation, recurrent dislocation, abnormal Q angle (and abnormal flexion Q angle), and elevated congruence angle, with or without arthrosis (oblique tibial tubercle osteotomy allows medial and anterior displacement). This represents the last step in the treatment of patellar malalignment; all other treatment methods must have failed before this procedure is considered.

Techniques

Arthroscopic Lateral Release

1. After routine arthroscopy, the scope is placed in the superomedial portal, and patellar tracking is observed (Fig. 16–4). The medial patellar facet normally contacts the medial femoral trochlea by 45° of flexion. Excessive tilt and overhang of the lateral patella also can be seen from this portal.

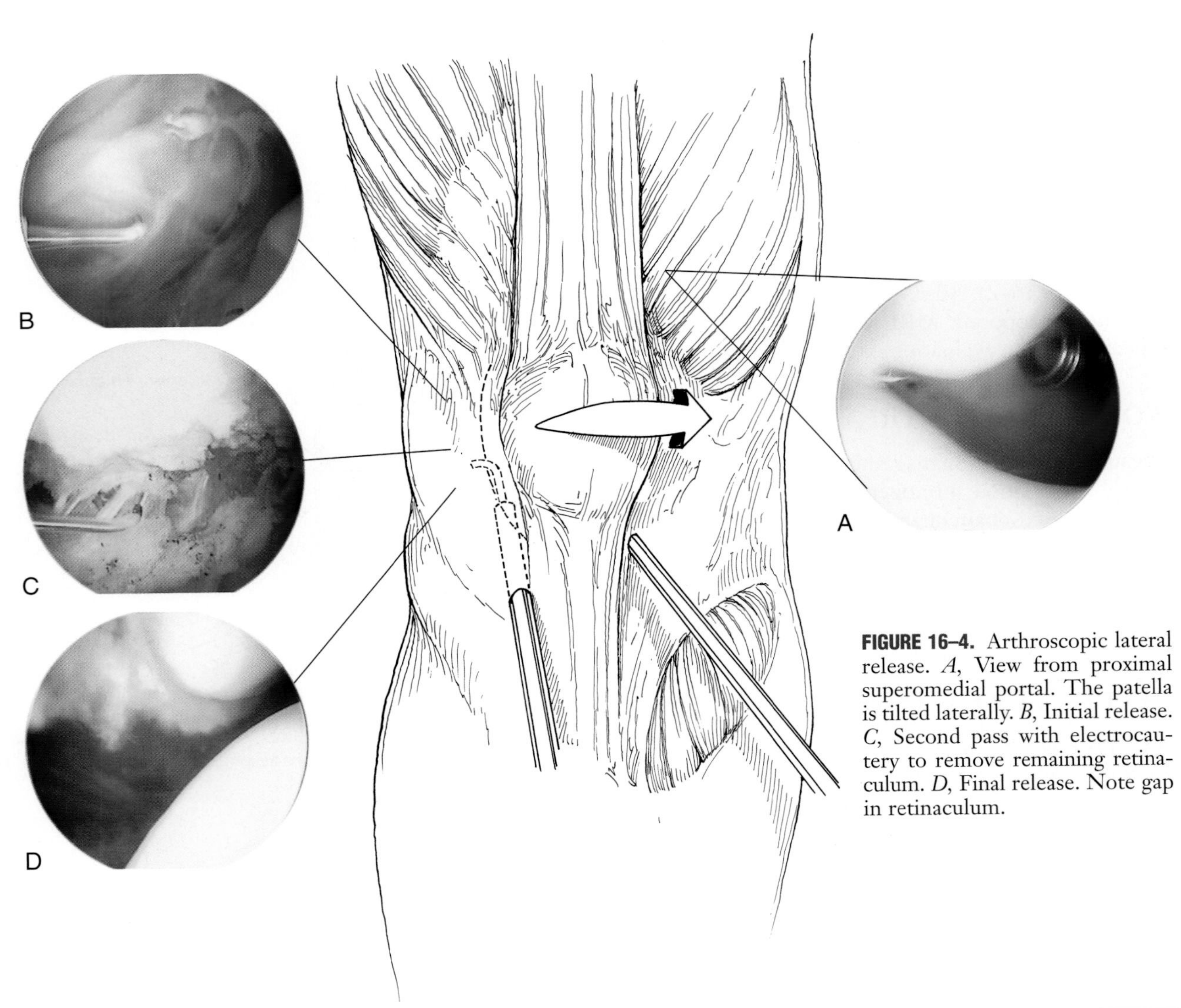

FIGURE 16–4. Arthroscopic lateral release. *A*, View from proximal superomedial portal. The patella is tilted laterally. *B*, Initial release. *C*, Second pass with electrocautery to remove remaining retinaculum. *D*, Final release. Note gap in retinaculum.

2. The electrocautery tip is inserted in the inferolateral portal, and the superomedial portal (and inferomedial portal) are used for visualization. The release is done approximately 5 mm lateral to the patella, in a straight line from proximal to distal. The release is carried out from the superior to the inferior border of the patella. After the procedure, the patella should tilt 60° to 90°, or additional release may be required (Fig. 16–5).

Open Lateral Release

Basically the same procedure is done through a small arthrotomy. The patella tilt is checked before closure.

Proximal Realignment

This technique typically includes a lateral release plus medial imbrication of the VMO (Fig. 16–6). The VMO insertion is sharply incised, and the muscle is advanced laterally and distally onto the patella. This procedure has fallen out of favor.

Anteromedialization of the Tibial Tubercle (Fulkerson)

This procedure uses an oblique osteotomy to *slide* the tibial tubercle anteriorly and medially.

1. A skin incision is made from the lateral aspect of the midpatella to a point 5 cm distal to the tibial tuberosity (Fig. 16–7). A lateral release is accomplished.
2. The patella tendon is exposed, and the anterior compartment musculature is subperiosteally dissected.
3. A parallel drill guide is used to drill a series of parallel drill bits along the planned osteotomy plane.
4. A small osteotome is used to complete the osteotomy

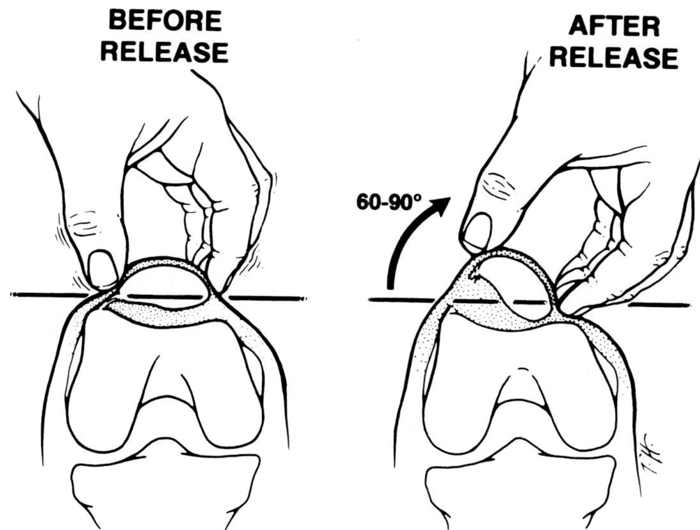

FIGURE 16–5. After lateral release, the patella should be able to be tilted 60° to 90°. (From Banas MP, Ferkel RD, Friedman MJ: Arthroscopic lateral retinacular release of the patellofemoral joint. Op Tech Sports Med 2:291–296, 1994.)

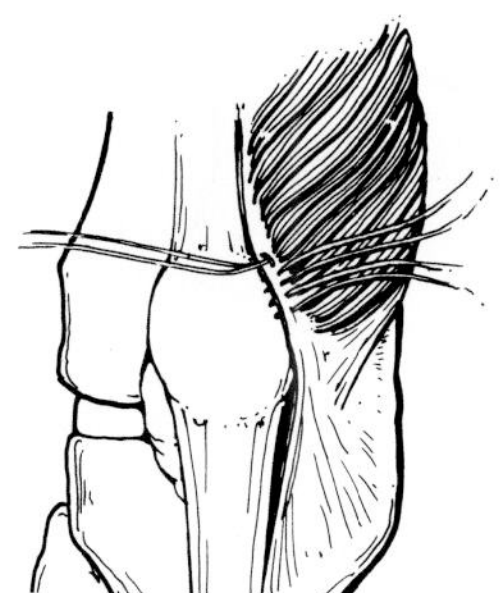

FIGURE 16–6. Proximal realignment. (From Walsh WM: Patellofemoral joint. In DeLee JC, Drez D Jr [eds]: Orthopaedic Sports Medicine Principles and Practice. Philadelphia, WB Saunders, 1994, pp 1163–1248.)

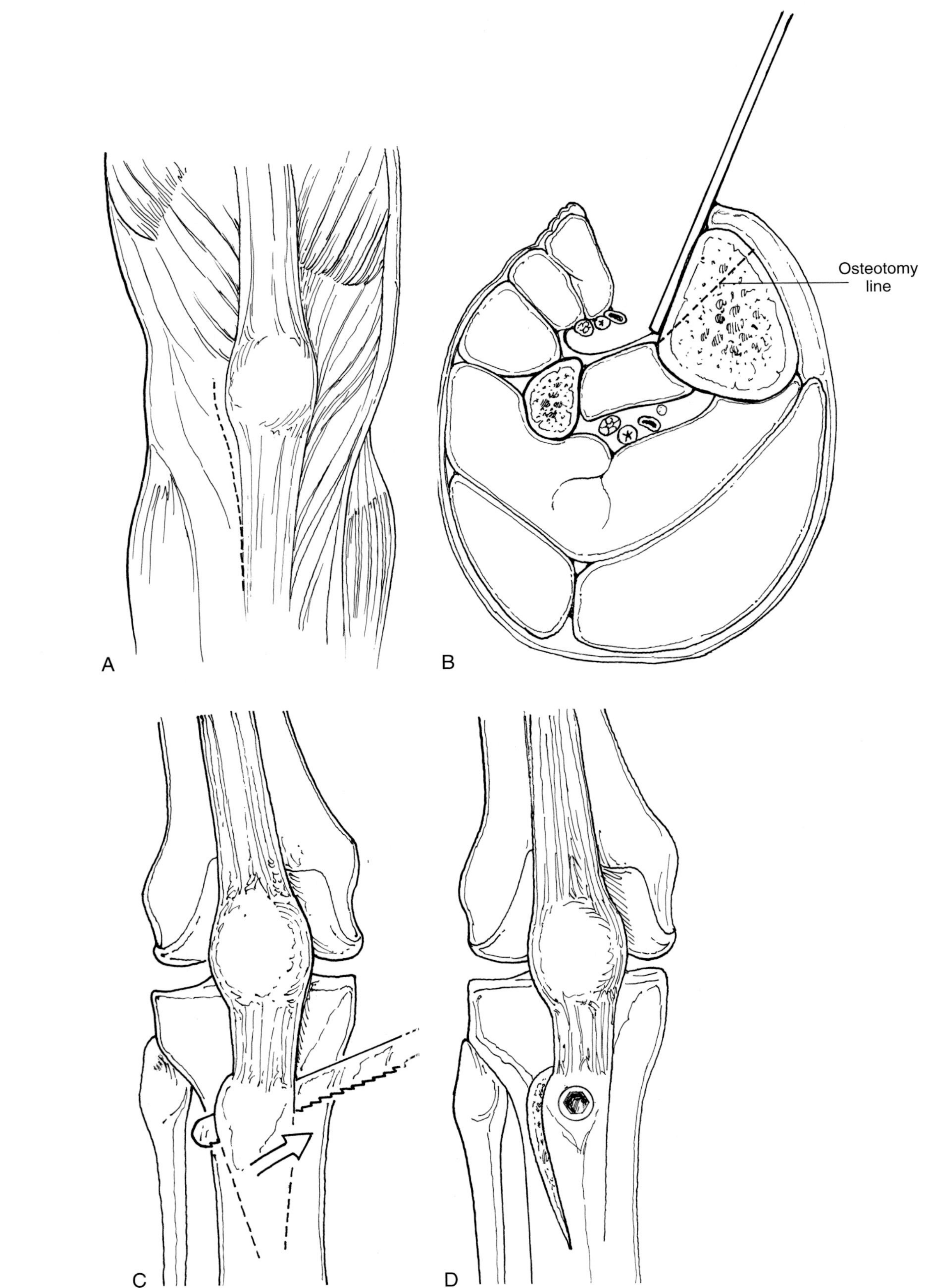

FIGURE 16–7. Anteromedialization (Fulkerson). *A*, Incision. *B*, Exposure of cross section. *C*, Osteotomy. *D*, Displacement and fixation.

proximally to a point proximal to the patellar tendon insertion.

5. The primary osteotomy is completed with a broad osteotome in the desired plane. For smaller degrees of correction, the distal aspect of the tibial tubercle can be left in place, and the proximal portion can be rotated (Elmslie-Trillat technique) (Fig. 16–8).
6. The surgeon slides the freed tibial tubercle anteriorly and medially, provisionally fixes it, and assesses patellar tracking.
7. The location of the osteotomy is adjusted as necessary, and the osteotomy is fixed with two bicortical screws, being careful not to *plunge* with the drill or depth gauge when engaging the posterior cortex.
8. Routine closure is accomplished over a drain with meticulous homeostasis.

Anteriorization of the Tibial Tubercle (Modified Maquet)

This technique is essentially a salvage procedure for advanced patellofemoral arthrosis. It has been much maligned because of the associated risk of skin breakdown; however, if the tubercle is raised only 1 cm, this is not a problem. The technique involves a proximal straight (flat) osteotomy of the tibial tubercle, leaving the distal tubercle intact. The osteotomy is opened gradually with osteotomies used as wedges until a contoured tricortical iliac crest graft can be inserted in the proximal extent of the osteotomy. Cancellous graft is packed into the remaining space (Fig. 16–9).

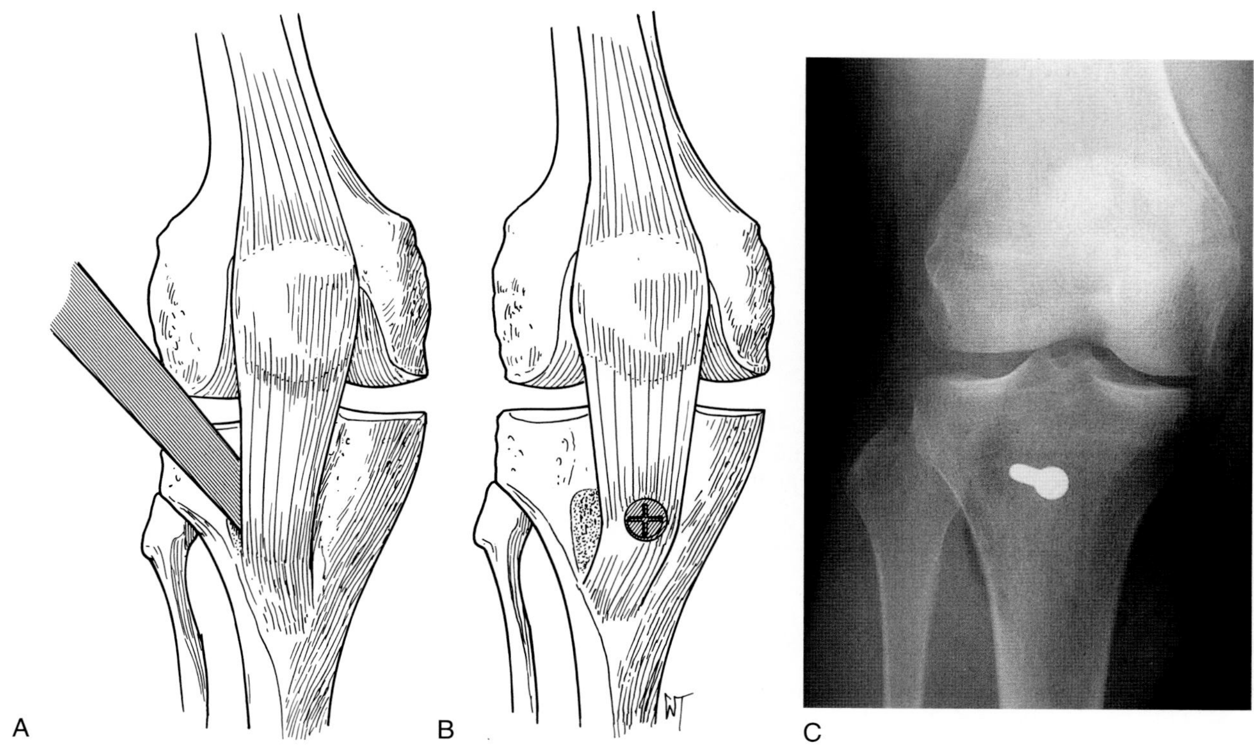

FIGURE 16–8. Elmslie-Trillat procedure leaving the distal tubercle intact. *A* and *B*, Artist's depiction. *C*, Radiograph showing screw placement after this procedure. (*A* and *B* from Insall JN: Disorders of the patella. In Insall JN [ed]: Surgery of the Knee. New York, Churchill Livingstone, 1984, pp 191–260.)

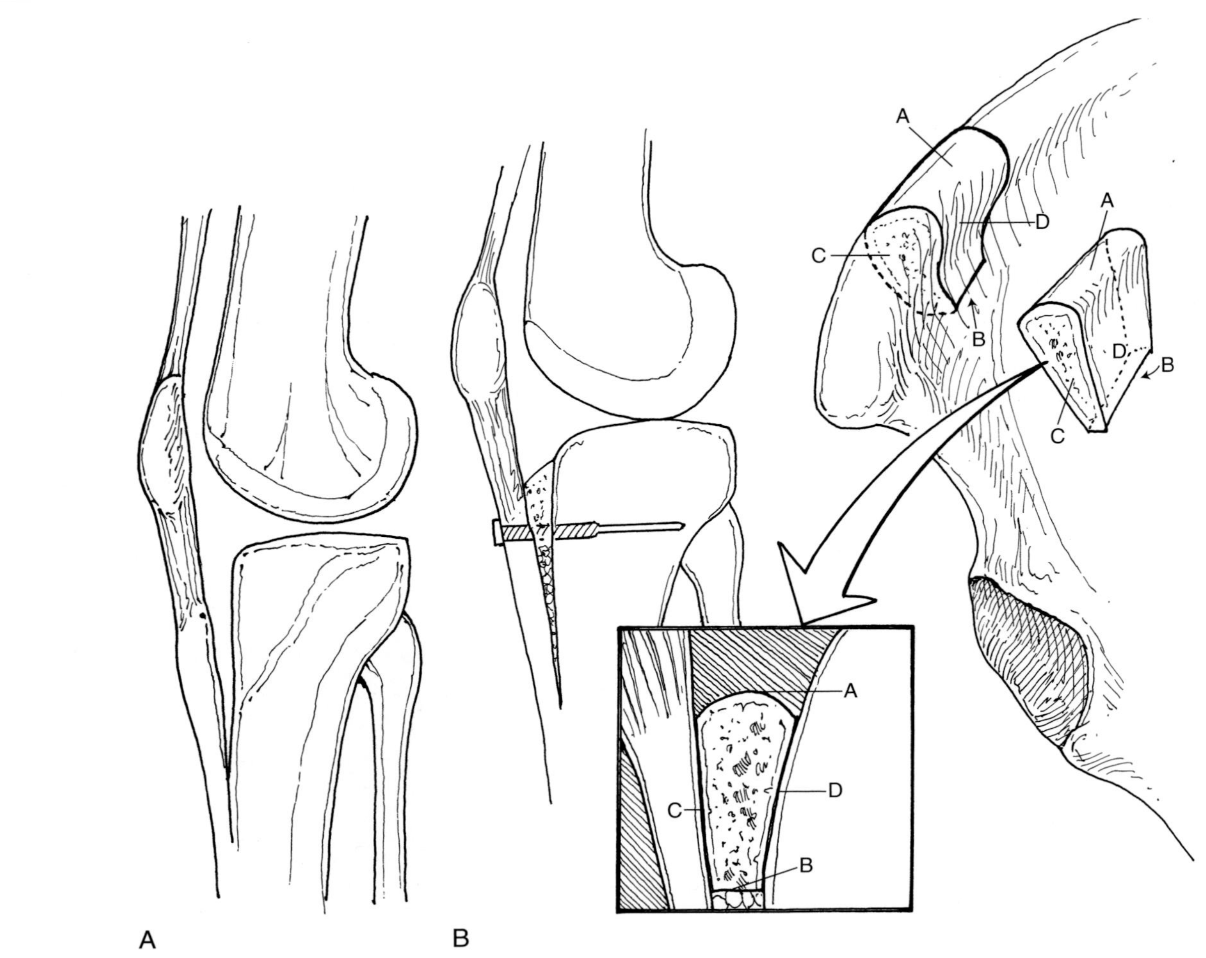

FIGURE 16–9. Anterior displacement of the tibial tubercle (Maquet procedure). *A*, A hinged osteotomy is made in the tibial tubercle. *B*, A tricortical bone graft is used to elevate the tubercle. Cancellous graft is placed distal to this graft.

POSTOPERATIVE MANAGEMENT

Early motion is encouraged for patients undergoing lateral release alone. Protected weight bearing is recommended for patients undergoing distal procedures for approximately 6 weeks. A knee immobilizer is used initially for ambulation, and range-of-motion exercises are initiated early.

COMPLICATIONS

Lateral release procedures have the highest complication rate of any arthroscopic procedure. The most common complication is hemarthrosis. Careful intraoperative control of homeostasis may reduce but not eliminate this complication. Recurrence, deep venous thrombosis, RSD, and other complications also can occur. Distal procedures have the added risk of inadvertent fractures, arterial injury (plunging drill bits), compartment syndrome, infection, deep venous thrombosis, and other problems.

RESULTS

Perhaps more than any other area in sports medicine, results of these procedures depend on proper patient selection. With select indications and good technique, good-to-excellent results can be expected in most patients.

REFERENCES

Boden BP, Pearsall AW, Garrett WE, et al: Patellofemoral instability: Evaluation and management. J Am Acad Orthop Surg 5:47–57, 1997.

Fulkerson JP: Patellofemoral pain disorders: Evaluation and management. J Am Acad Orthop Surg 2:124–132, 1994.

Kelly MA: Algorithm for anterior knee pain. Instr Course Lect 47:339–343, 1998.

Walsh WM: Patellofemoral joint. In DeLee JC, Drez D Jr (eds): Orthopedic Sports Medicine Principles and Practice. Philadelphia, WB Saunders, 1994, pp 1163–1248.

CHAPTER 17

Acute Patellar Dislocation—Medial Patellofemoral Ligament Repair

INTRODUCTION

Anatomic, biomechanical, and clinical studies have shown the importance of the medial patellofemoral ligament (MPFL) in stability of the patella. Acute patellar dislocations can result in disruption of this ligament, especially from its insertion in the medial femoral epicondyle, and may be the cause of chronic patellar instability.

HISTORY AND PHYSICAL EXAMINATION

Patellar dislocations occur as a result of a twisting injury with strong contraction of the quadriceps. An acute effusion may develop, and this diagnosis may be mistaken for the more common anterior cruciate ligament injury. The patella usually is reduced easily with extension of the knee, and the patient may never have appreciated that the patella was dislocated. If patients do note the injury, they sometimes mistakenly report that their patella dislocated medially because the uncovered medial femoral condyle is noted. Acute injuries often are accompanied by a large effusion, medial patellar and medial epicondyle tenderness, and a positive apprehension sign. Occasionally the patella may be so unstable that simple range of motion may displace it. Patellar mobility, tilt, and the Q angle also should be assessed.

DIAGNOSTIC IMAGING

Unless the patella is still dislocated, plain radiographs may be normal. Subtle osteochondral fragments sometimes can be seen and, to many, represent a surgical indication (Fig. 17–1). Patellar views should be examined, and the sulcus angle and patellar position should be assessed. MRI can be particularly helpful in the evaluation of acute patellar dislocations. Chondral injuries, not seen on plain radiographs, can be appreciated better. Rupture of the MPFL also can be seen on MRI (Fig. 17–2). Retraction of the vastus medialis obliquus (VMO), a secondary sign of MPFL injury, also can be appreciated with MRI.

NONOPERATIVE TREATMENT

Nonsurgical management of acute patellar dislocations has been the mainstay of treatment for this injury for centuries. Immobilization in a cylinder cast was recommended until more recently. So-called functional treatment has been recommended, with a reduction in recurrence and morbidity. All nonoperative management options are associated with a high recurrence rate.

RELEVANT ANATOMY

The MPFL, which contributes greater than 50% of the resistance to lateral displacement of the patella in biomechanical testing, connects the medial border of the patella to the medial femoral epicondyle (Fig. 17–3). It is located deep to the sartorius and is covered partially by fibers of the VMO.

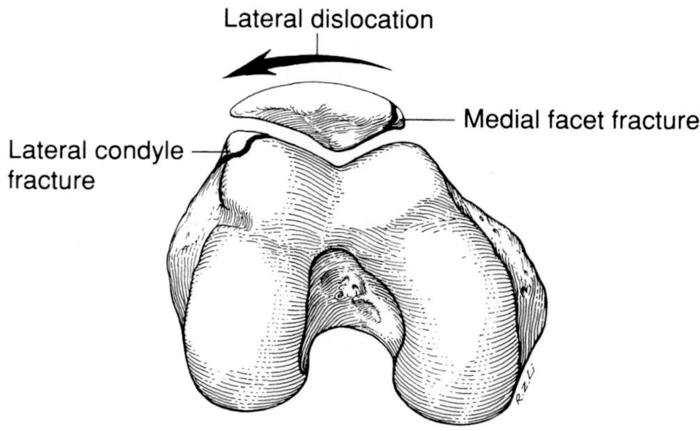

FIGURE 17–1. Patellar dislocation can be associated with osteochondral fractures of the lateral femoral condyle or the medial patellar facet. (From Tria AJ, Klein KS: An Illustrated Guide to the Knee. New York, Churchill Livingstone, 1992.)

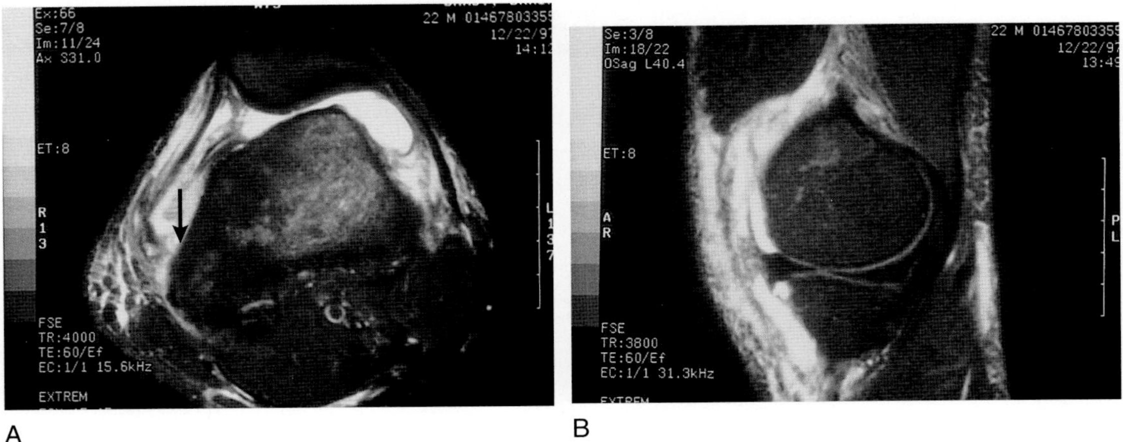

FIGURE 17–2. MRI of MPFL injury. *A*, Coronal view shows avulsion of the MPFL *(arrow)*. *B*, Sagittal view shows concavity of the VMO, which is a secondary finding.

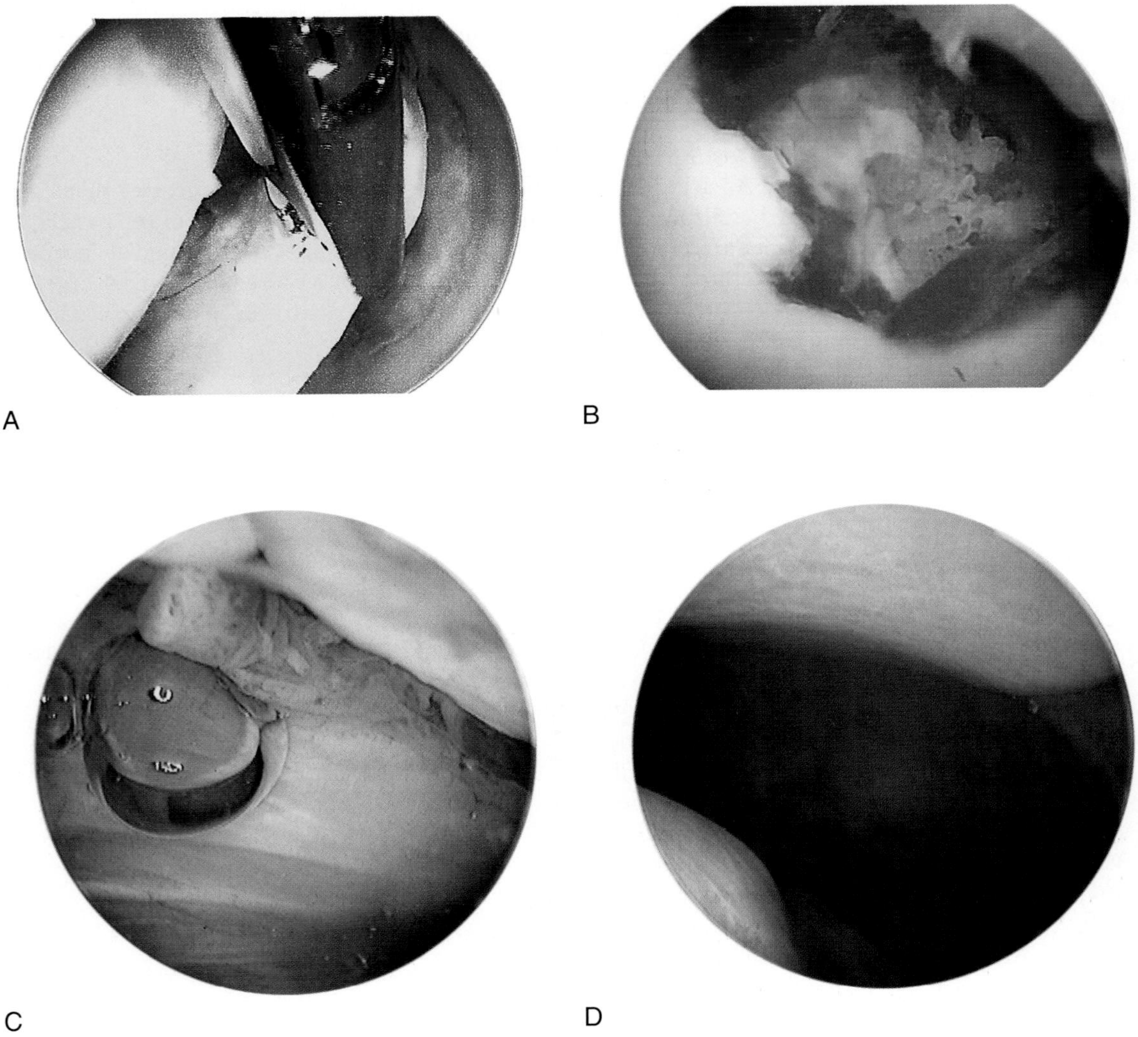

A B

C D

FIGURE 17–3. Arthroscopic view of osteochondral injuries associated with acute patellar dislocation. *A*, Loose body is removed from lateral gutter. *B*, Defect in lateral femoral condyle. *C*, MPFL avulsion off patella. *D*, Lateral displacement of patella in relation to lateral condyle.

SURGICAL TECHNIQUE

Indications

Although it is controversial, we recommend arthroscopy and MPFL repair for young athletes with first-time patellar dislocations. MRI has been helpful in identifying chondral injuries and the location of MPFL injury. In cases without an avulsion of the ligament, we have imbricated the MPFL. The presence of chondral injuries and loose bodies is greater than 50%.

Technique

1. Diagnostic arthroscopy is done in standard fashion. Large osteochondral injuries to the patella are repaired if possible. Smaller pieces with no bony components must be removed (Fig. 17–4). The bed of these defects is débrided and microfractured. Patellar tracking is observed carefully from a proximal medial portal (Fig. 17–5).
2. If the patient is tender over the medial femoral epicondyle and MRI suggests that the MPFL is avulsed from its insertion, an incision is made slightly anterior to this point. If it is not clear where the MPFL is injured or if it is merely attenuated, an incision is made midway between the medial border of the patella and the epicondyle.
3. The sartorius is incised in line with its fibers and

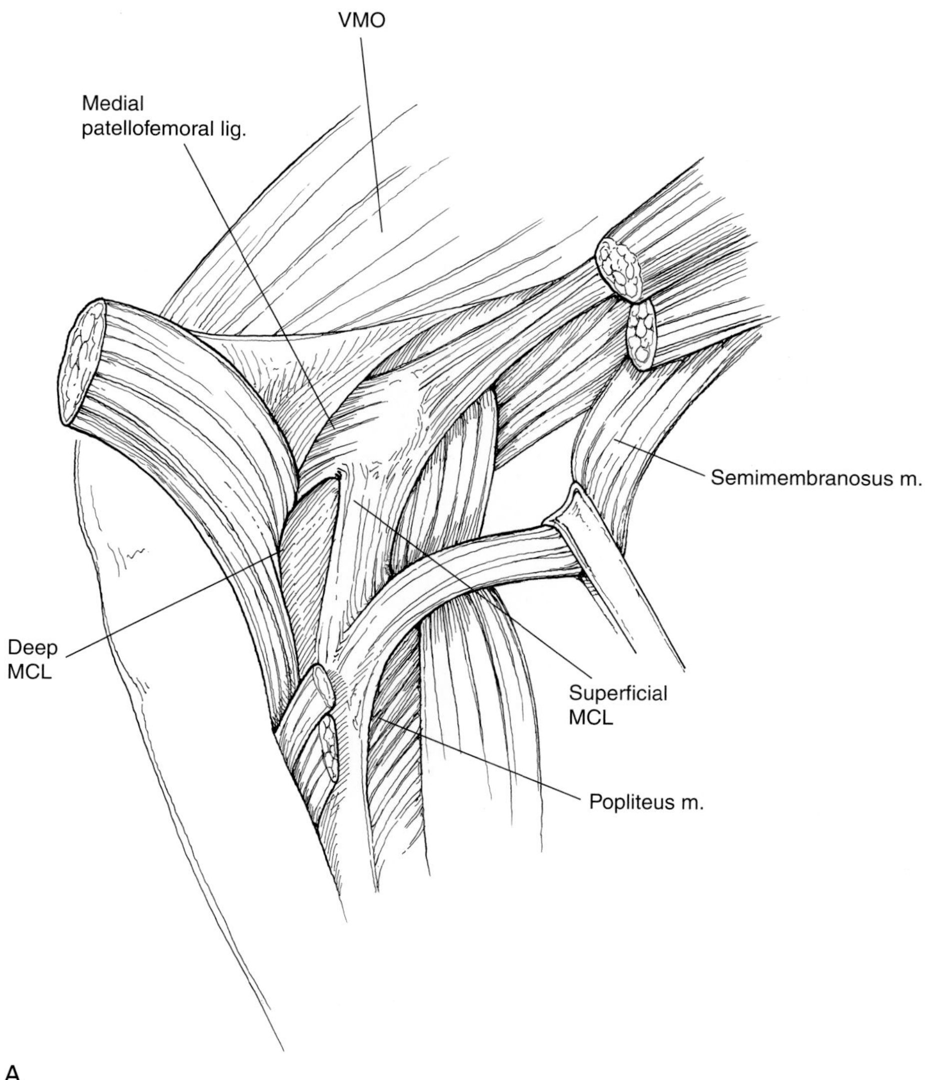

FIGURE 17–4. The medial patellofemoral ligament lies deep to the sartorius, partially covered on its superior aspect by the VMO. *A*, It attaches to the medial femoral epicondyle, perpendicular to the superficial medial collateral ligament fibers.

Illustration continued on following page

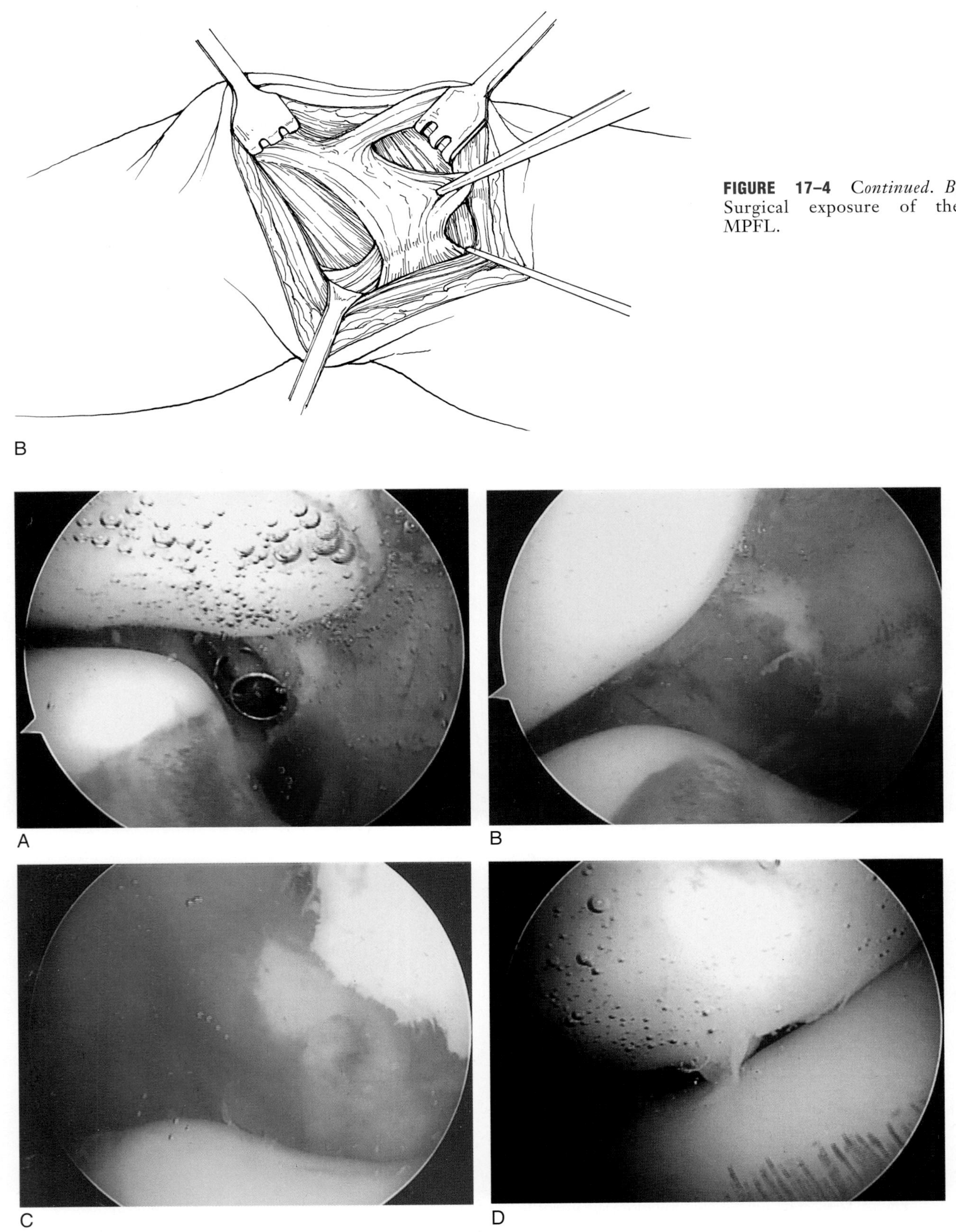

FIGURE 17–4 *Continued*. *B*, Surgical exposure of the MPFL.

FIGURE 17–5. View of patellar tracking from a proximal medial portal. Note lateral displacement of patella. *A*, Excessive lateral overhang of the patella before MPFL repair. *B*, Same view after repair. *C*, View of the patella in relation to the trochlea before MPFL repair. *D*, Same view after repair. The patella now engages the trochlea.

retracted. The inferior border of the VMO is identified, and the MPFL is reflected off its inferior surface. The MPFL is explored with particular attention to its medial insertion. Often there may be hemorrhage in the area of injury.

4. The torn end is freed, débrided, and reinserted into its attachment using suture anchors (Fig. 17–6). If the MPFL is not torn but is lax, it can be imbricated in a pants-over-vest fashion (Fig. 17–7).
5. Before final fixation, arthroscopy is done to reassess patellar tracking.
6. Wounds are closed in standard fashion.

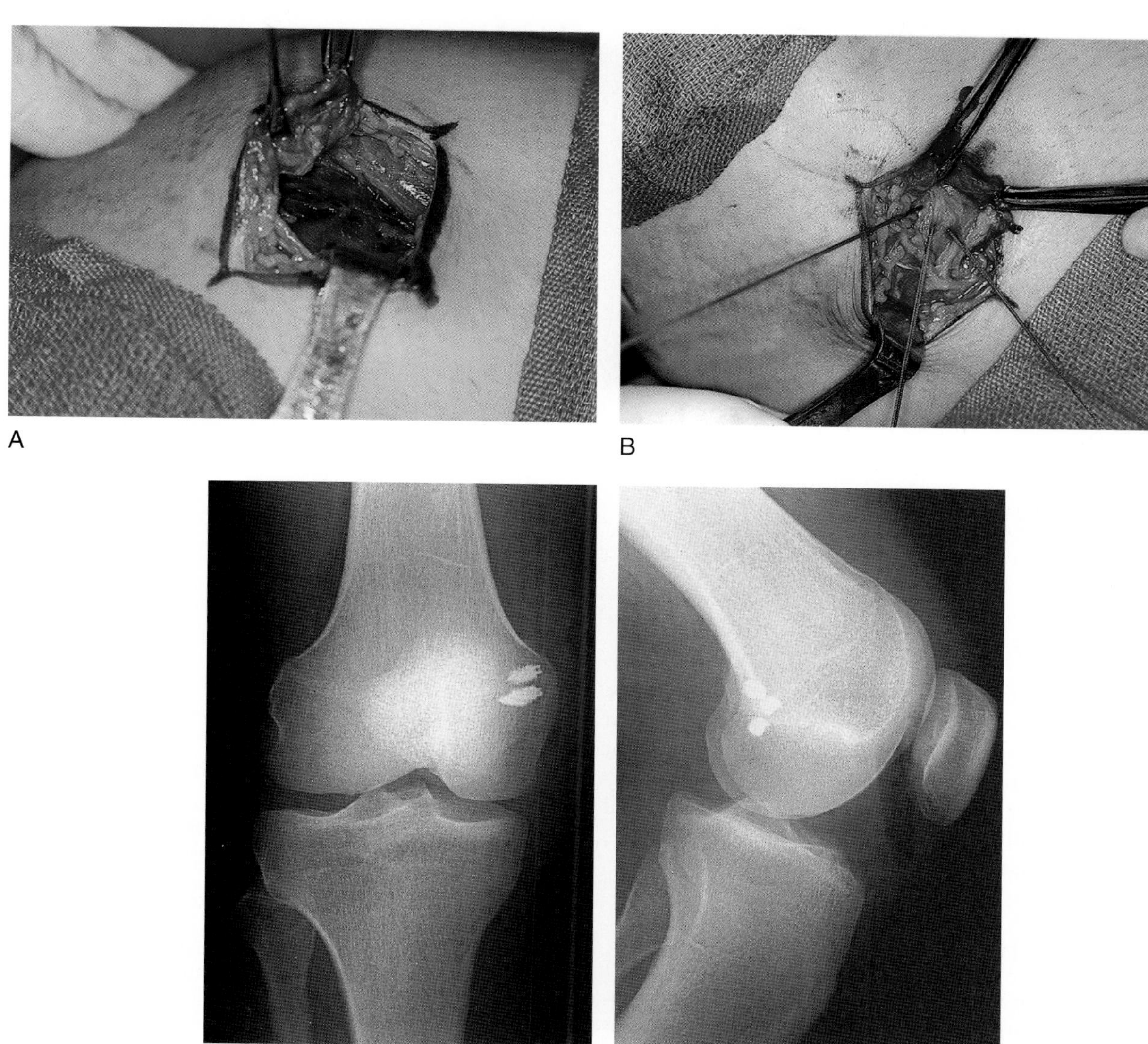

FIGURE 17–6. Operative repair of MPFL injury. *A*, The MPFL (clamps) is dissected free from its torn bed. *B*, Repair using suture anchors. *C* and *D*, Anteroposterior and lateral views of suture anchor placement.

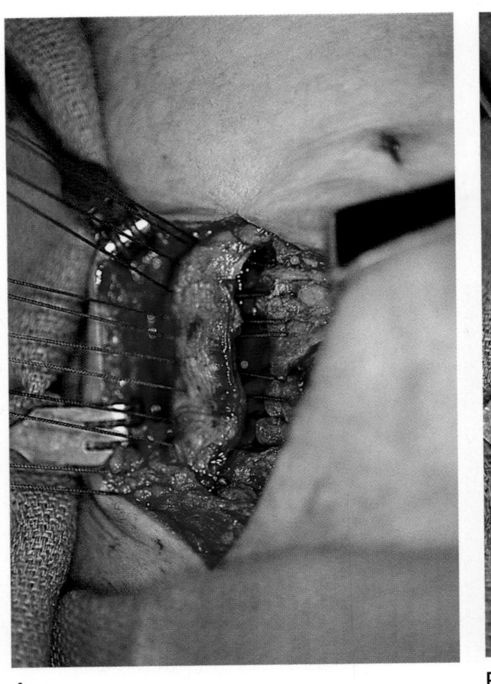

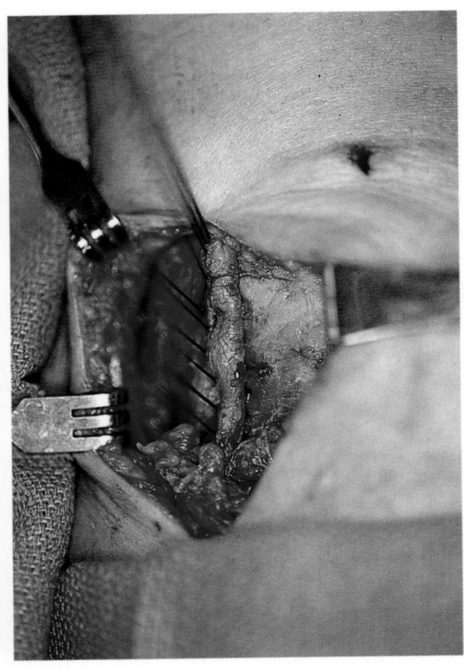

A B

FIGURE 17–7. MPFL imbrication. *A*, The MPFL is dissected and incised vertically in its midsubstance. Sutures are placed in a pants-over-vest fashion. *B*, Tension is placed on these sutures; patellar tracking is assessed arthroscopically; and if it is adequate, the sutures are tied.

POSTOPERATIVE MANAGEMENT

Although a brief period of immobilization may be beneficial to wound healing, early motion is important in these patients. Similar to acute anterior cruciate ligament surgery, arthrofibrosis can be devastating. We routinely place patients in a dynamic patellar brace (with medial support) and begin range of motion and quadriceps rehabilitation immediately.

COMPLICATIONS

As mentioned earlier, loss of motion in the early postoperative period is a problem. Redislocation after this procedure is a small risk, although much less than with other forms of treatment. Wound problems, neurovascular injuries, and other complications that occur with any open procedure are possible.

RESULTS

Acute repair of the MPFL has been suggested only more recently, and there are no long-term studies of this technique. Early results are encouraging, and the risk for redislocation can be improved greatly.

REFERENCES

Burks RT, Luker MG: Medial patellofemoral ligament reconstruction. Techniques Orthop 12:185–191, 1997.

Conlan T, Garth WP, Lemos JD: Evaluation of the medial soft-tissue restraints of the extensor mechanism of the knee J Bone Joint Surg Am 75:682–693, 1993.

Garth WP, Pomphrey M, Merrill K: Functional treatment of patellar dislocation in an athletic population. Am J Sports Med 24:785–791, 1996.

Sallay PI, Poggi J, Speer KP, Garrett WE: Acute dislocation of the patella: A correlative pathoanatomic study. Am J Sports Med 24:52–60, 1996.

CHAPTER 18

Knee Osteotomies

INTRODUCTION

Although knee realignment procedures are not classically considered sports medicine, many older recreational athletes develop osteoarthritis of one compartment of the knee. Knee realignment procedures, most commonly valgus upper or *high* tibial osteotomies, are believed to delay the need for a total knee arthroplasty (not covered in this book).

HISTORY AND PHYSICAL EXAMINATION

Patients typically complain of activity-related knee pain localized primarily in either the medial or the lateral compartment. Significant swelling is uncommon. Mechanical symptoms may or may not be present. Osteotomies are recommended more commonly for young, active patients with unicompartmental arthritis, often from a prior meniscectomy. Physical examination should include an evaluation of range of motion, ligamentous stability, and gait. Patients who have significant lateral compartment opening (>10 mm) and a lateral thrust during the stance phase of gait may have advanced degrees of instability that may not do well with conventional osteotomies.

DIAGNOSTIC IMAGING

Standard radiographic views, including a patellar view, should be evaluated carefully to ensure that the patient has primarily single-compartment involvement. The flexion posteroanterior weight-bearing radiograph is also important. A full-length (hip-ankle) anteroposterior radiograph is necessary to measure the mechanical axis of the knee (Fig. 18–1). Typically the mechanical axis falls in the affected compartment, and the goal of the osteotomy is to shift this axis into the less affected compartment. Technetium bone scans sometimes are helpful in confirming that there is primarily unicompartmental disease.

NONOPERATIVE TREATMENT

Realignment procedures are elective, and other forms of management, including physical therapy, nonsteroidal anti-inflammatory drugs, and the use of a cane, should be tried first. Other operative procedures, such as arthroscopic débridement (typically provides only short-term relief) and total knee arthroplasty (for physiologically older patients with more extensive involvement), also should be considered.

RELEVANT ANATOMY

Closing wedge proximal tibial osteotomies require subperiosteal dissection of anterior compartment leg muscles and disruption of the proximal tibiofibular joint (Fig. 18–2). Care should be taken because of the location of the peroneal nerve, which crosses the neck of the fibula. Distal femoral varus osteotomies require a subvastus approach.

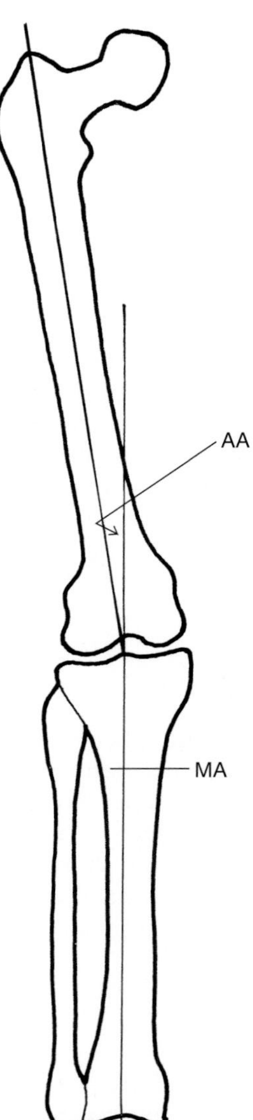

FIGURE 18–1. The mechanical axis is drawn from the center of the femoral head to the center of the ankle mortise. The anatomic axis is drawn along the diaphysis of the femur and tibia, and the angle formed at the intersection of these two lines between the tibial eminences (normally 5° to 6° of valgus) is used to determine the desired correction angle.

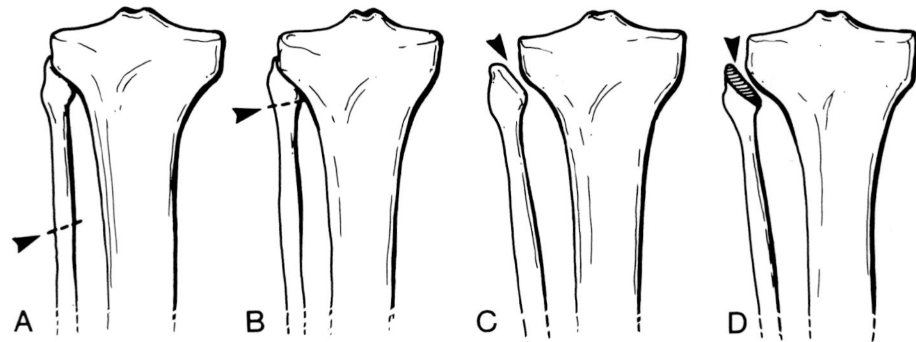

FIGURE 18–2. Methods to release the proximal tibiofibular joint. *A*, Shaft osteotomy. *B*, Head excision. *C*, Division of the proximal tibiofibular joint. *D*, Partial excision of the fibular head. (From Sisk TD: Knee realignment and replacement in the recreational athlete. In DeLee JC, Drez D Jr [eds]: Orthopaedic Sports Medicine: Principles and Practice. Philadelphia, WB Saunders, 1994, pp 1475–1501.)

SURGICAL TECHNIQUE

Indications

Knee realignment is indicated for physiologically young, active patients with moderate medial compartment osteoarthritis (tibial osteotomy) or lateral compartment osteoarthritis (femoral osteotomy). Contraindications include rheumatoid or inflammatory arthritis, deformities greater than than 10°, range of motion less than 90°, flexion contractures 15° or more, significant ligamentous instability or subluxation, and pain at rest.

Techniques

Closing Wedge Proximal Tibial Osteotomy

1. Standing long leg cassettes are used to plan the amount of correction necessary. Although there is some disagreement, most authors attempt to achieve approximately 5° to 7° or more of valgus.
2. A midline or lateral incision is made, and the proximal tibia is exposed. The anterior compartment muscles are subperiostally stripped off the tibia (Fig. 18–3), and the proximal tibiofibular joint is released with a Cobb elevator.
3. Using freehand techniques or commercially available guides, an appropriately sized wedge of bone is removed (Fig. 18–4). Ideally the medial cortex of the tibia is left intact, and the osteotomy is closed carefully with sequential pressure. Fenestrating the medial cortex with a series of drill holes can be helpful.
4. Fixation can be achieved with a variety of techniques, including offset staples, external fixation, and plates.

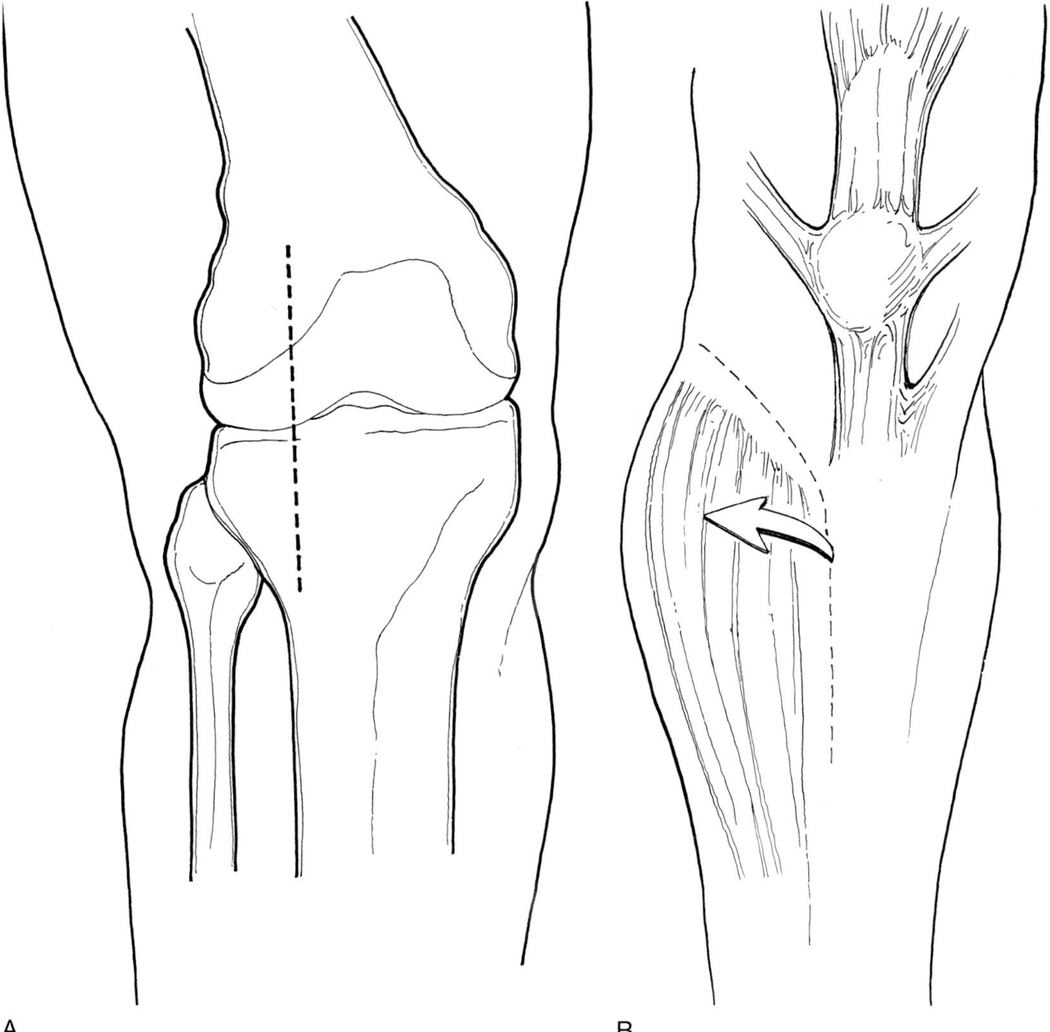

FIGURE 18–3. *A*, Incision. *B*, Subperiosteal dissection of anterior compartment muscles.

Illustration continued on following page

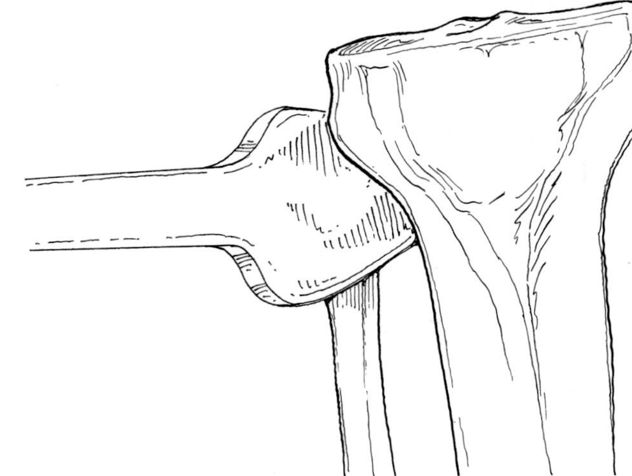

FIGURE 18–3 Continued. *C*, Tibial-fibular release.

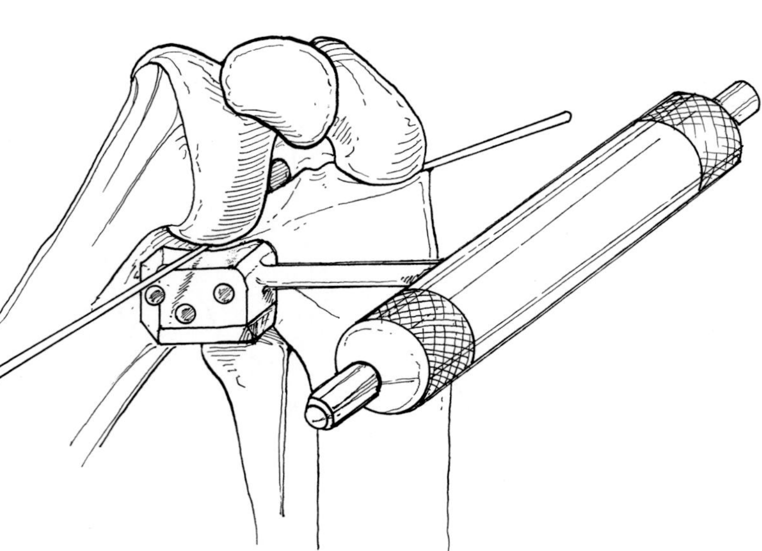

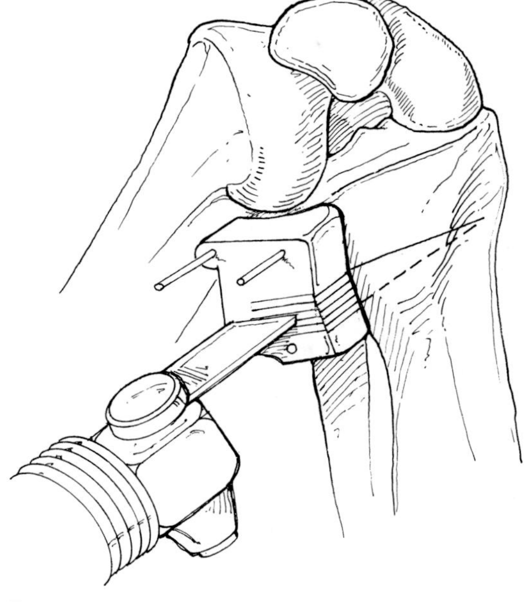

FIGURE 18–4. Osteotomy of the proximal tibia. *A*, Initial guide placement. *B*, Cutting guide.

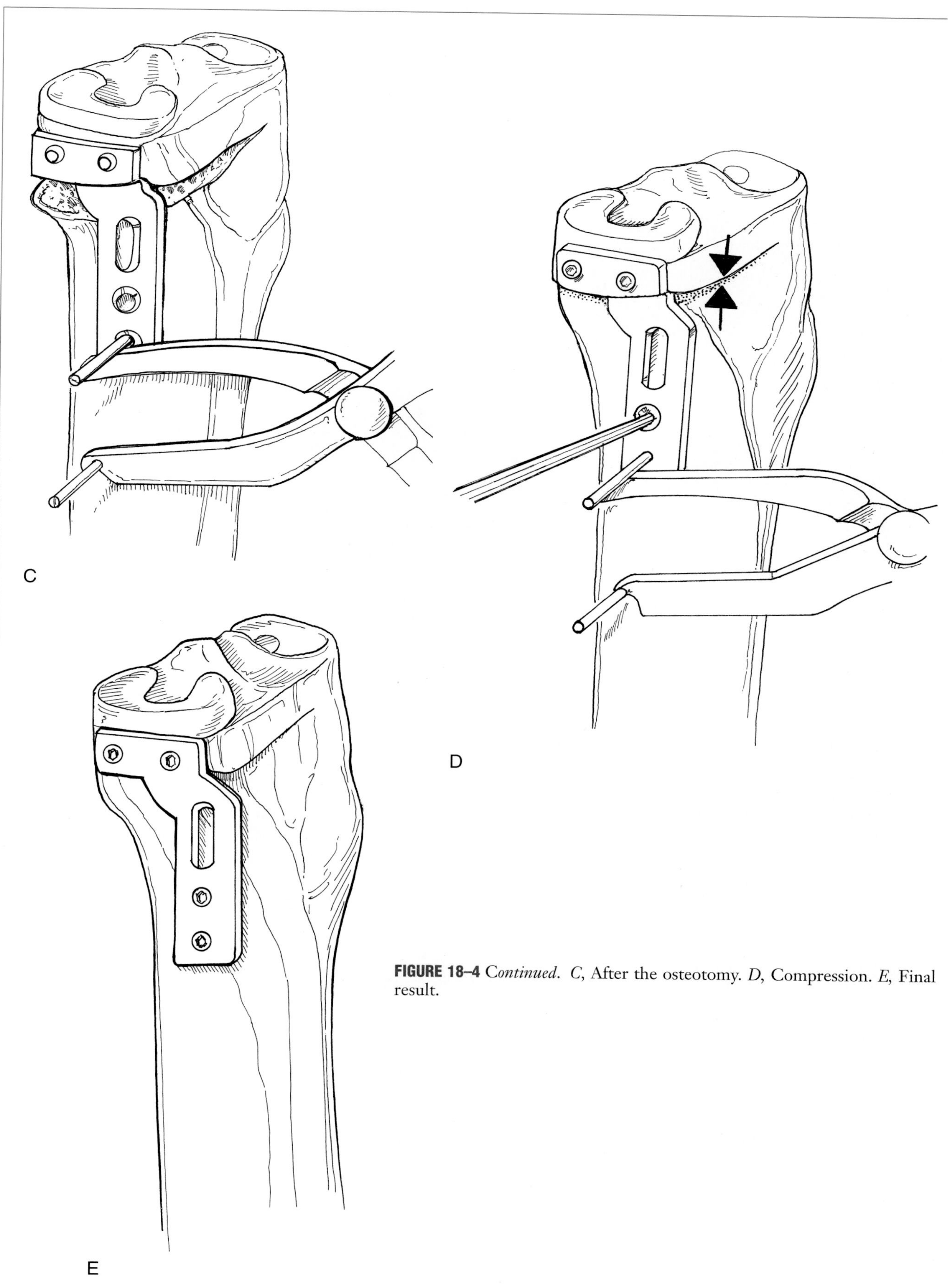

FIGURE 18–4 C*ontinued*. *C*, After the osteotomy. *D*, Compression. *E*, Final result.

Staples require additional protection, and fixators can be associated with pin tract infections and peroneal nerve palsy; we prefer plate fixation (Fig. 18–5).

5. The anterior compartment muscles are closed over a drain, and the subcutaneous tissues and skin are closed in standard fashion.

Opening Wedge Proximal Tibial Osteotomy

Because of the concern with delayed union or nonunion or loss of correction if the graft is absorbed, opening wedge osteotomies have not been popular in the United States. Newer techniques and fixation methods,

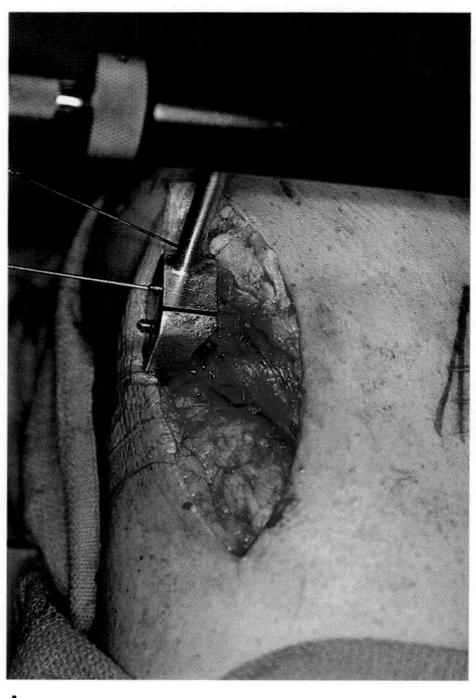

A

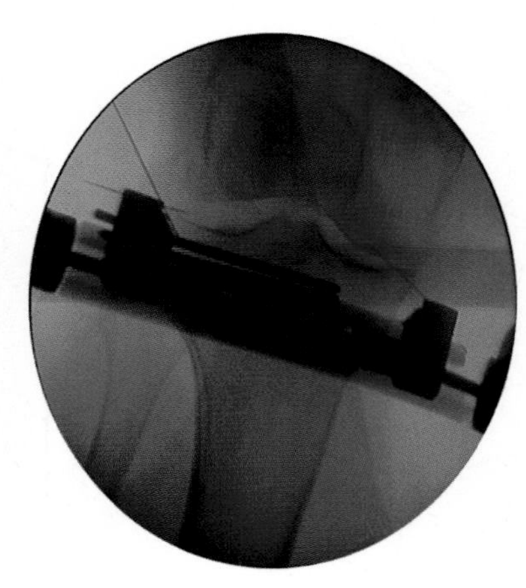

B

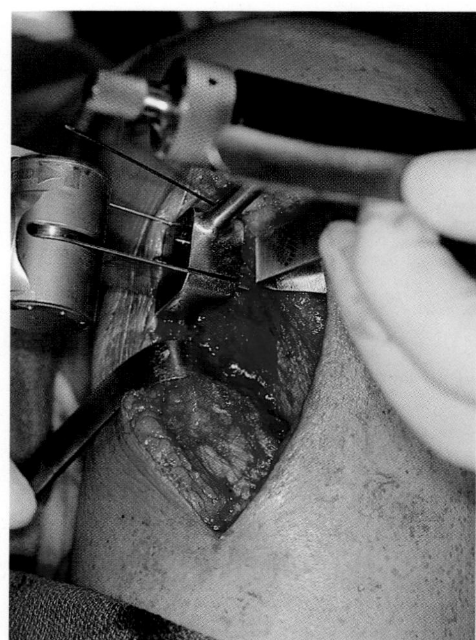

C

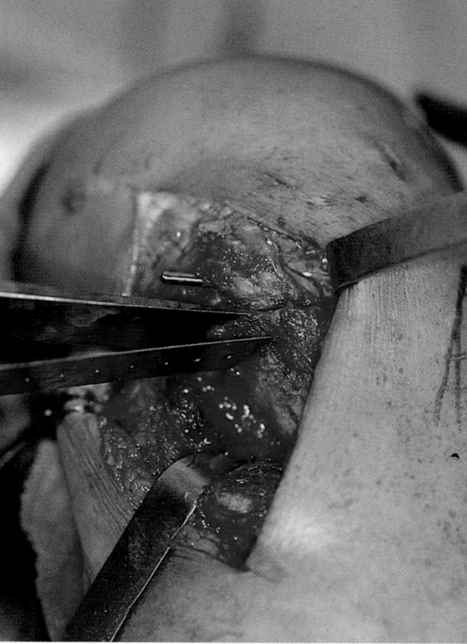

D

FIGURE 18–5. Upper tibial osteotomy with Intermedics system. *A*, After initial dissection, the joint line is identified, and the guide is placed just distal to it. *B*, The location of the guide is checked with fluoroscopy. *C*, Using a slotted guide, a saw is used to complete the osteotomy. The guide is slotted for various degrees of wedges based on preoperative planning. *D*, The wedge is outlined.

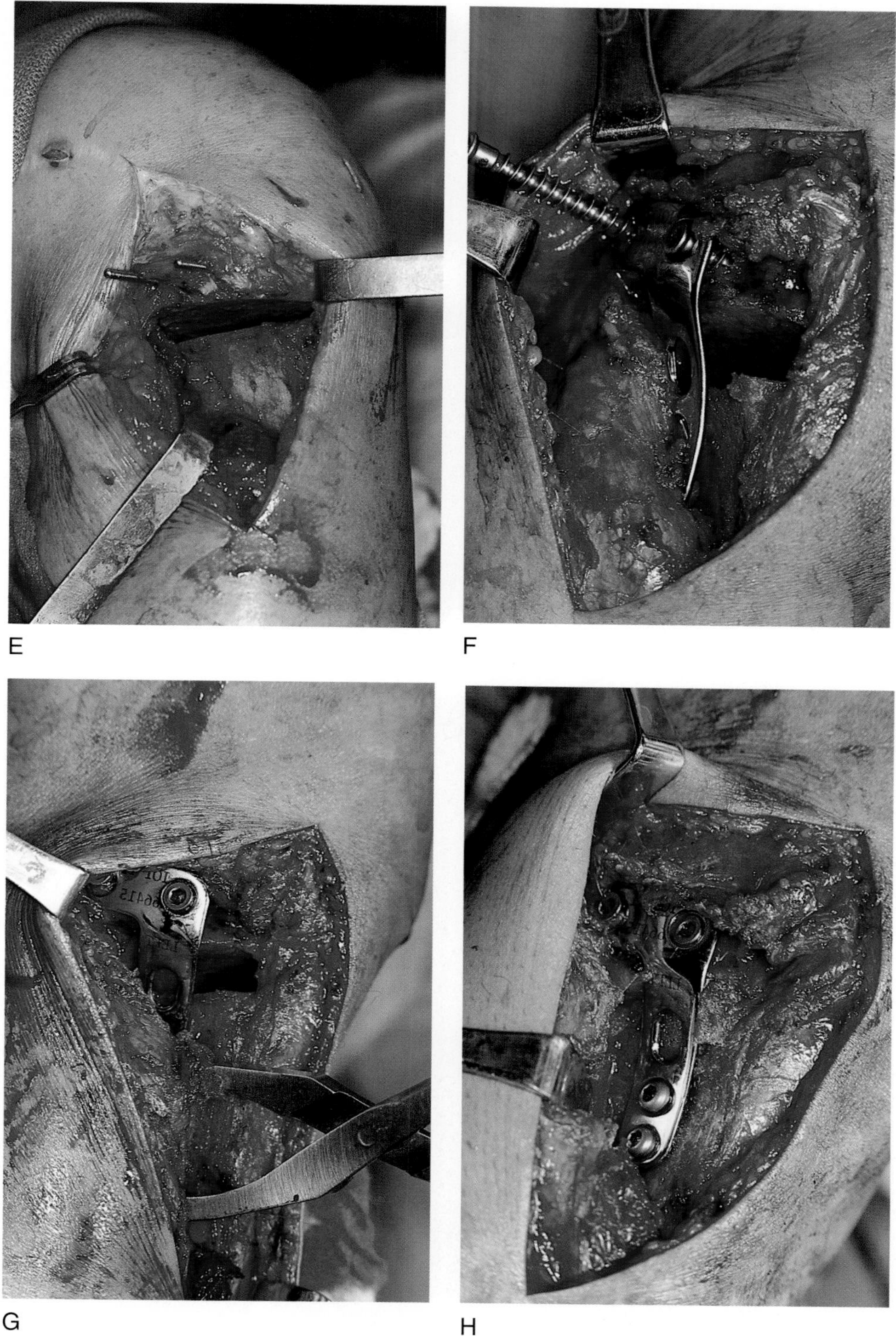

FIGURE 18–5 *Continued. E,* The wedge is removed. *F,* The plate is applied. *G,* The plate is tensioned. *H,* Final osteotomy and plate application before closure.

including the use of external fixators for distraction callistasis and wedge plates, may increase the popularity of this approach. Opening wedge osteotomies offer some advantages, including preservation of leg length and correction of posterolateral corner problems. One technique, illustrated in Figure 18–6, involves an oblique osteotomy distal to the tibial tubercle.

Closing Wedge Distal Femoral Osteotomy

This technique is recommended for patients with lateral compartment osteoarthritis and valgus deformities. Proximal tibial osteotomies (especially >10° to 12°) are not recommended because of excessive medial tilt to the joint line. The technique is as follows.

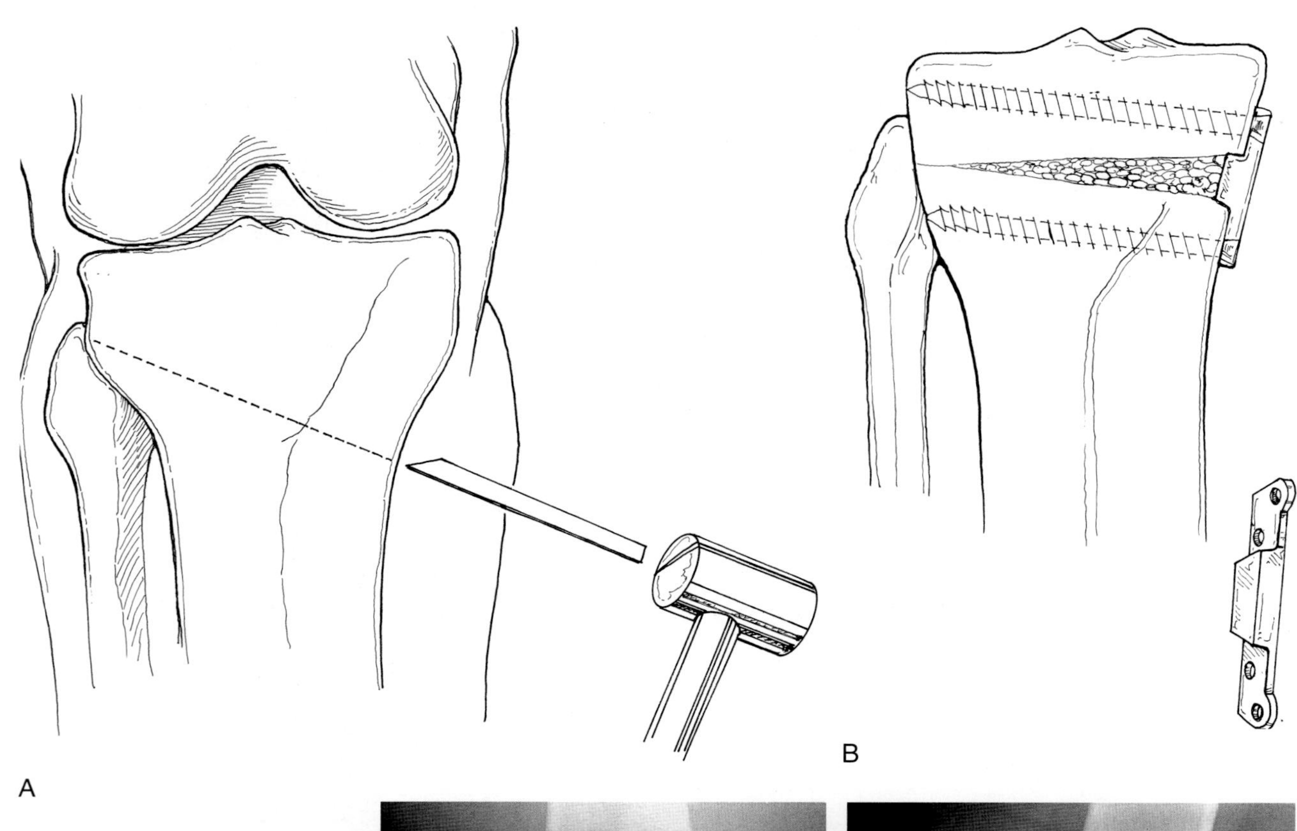

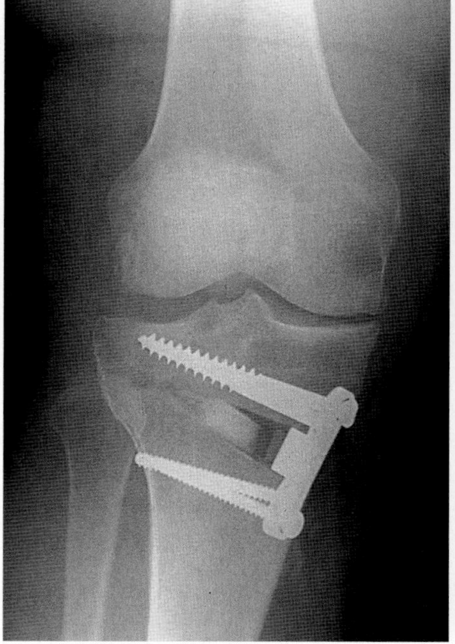

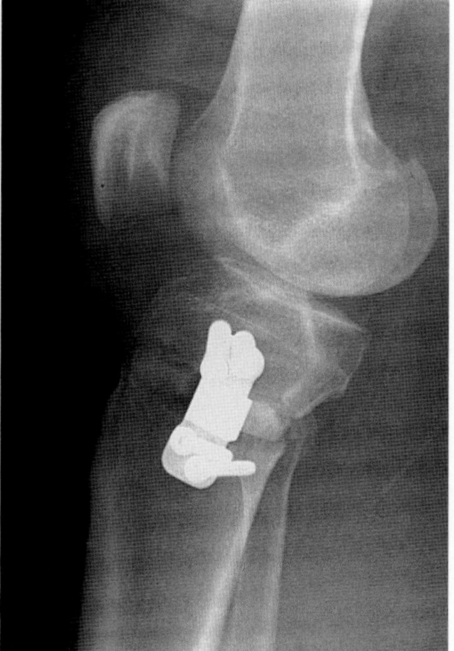

FIGURE 18–6. Opening wedge proximal tibial osteotomy. *A*, Planned osteotomy. *B*, Opening wedge and plate placement. *C* and *D*, Anteroposterior and lateral radiographs after osteotomy.

1. Standing long anteroposterior radiographs are used for preoperative planning. A resulting neutral anatomic axis is planned.
2. A midline longitudinal incision and subvastus approach are used. The vastus medialis is retracted anteriorly and laterally to expose the shaft of the femur, leaving a cuff of tissue with the medial intermuscular septum to protect the femoral vessels.
3. With the knee flexed 90° and with fluoroscopic assistance, guide wires are passed through the joint and 1 cm proximal to the joint, parallel to the articular surface (Fig. 18–7).
4. Drill holes are made in line with the anticipated chisel placement (1 cm proximal to second guide wire) to prevent comminution of the femoral cortex. The chisel is inserted to a depth of 50 to 70 mm.
5. A femoral osteotomy is made just proximal to the adductor tubercle using a saw or osteotome, and an appropriately sized wedge of bone is removed.
6. One of the three 90° variable offset blades available is inserted, and the plate is secured to the medial cortex with standard AO technique.

Opening Wedge Distal Femoral Osteotomy

A lateral opening wedge osteotomy can be used in lieu of a medial closing osteotomy for valgus deformities. Special plates with opening wedges (Arthrex, Naples, FL) are used. An oblique osteotomy is made in the metaphysis, and a wedge is inserted to the appropriate depth to accommodate the plate. The plate is secured, and bone graft is packed into the defect. Figure 18–8 shows a final radiograph.

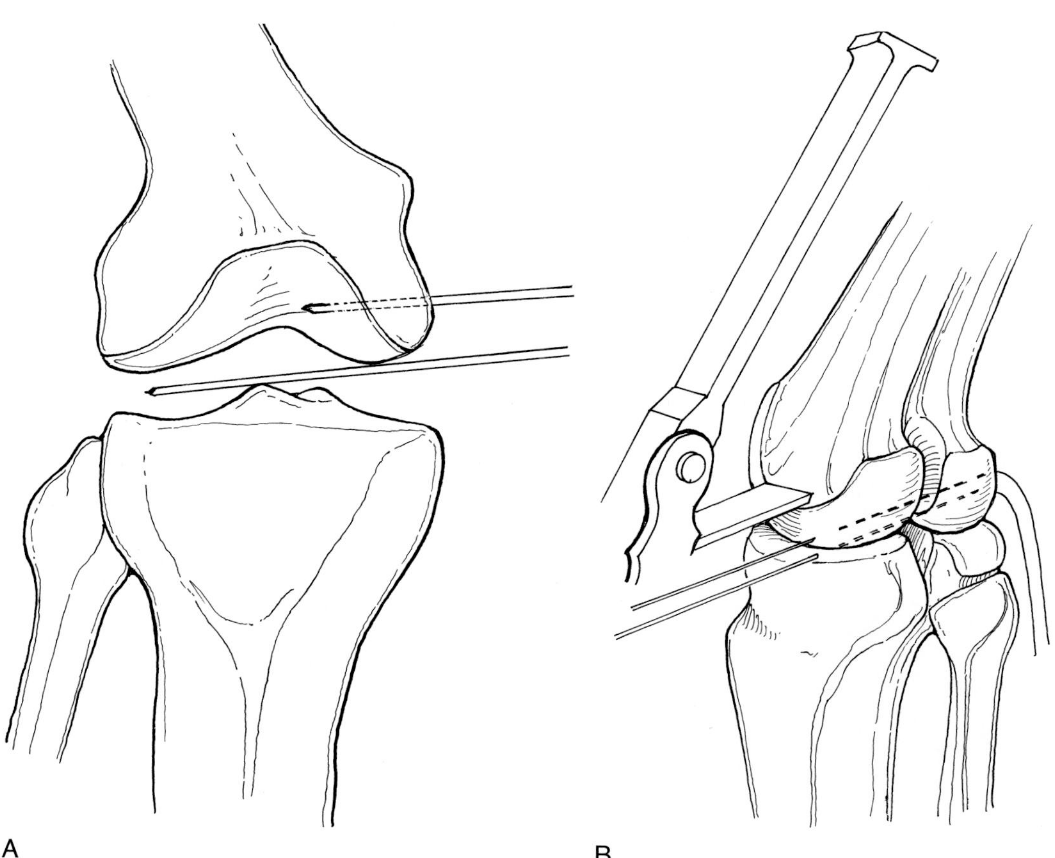

FIGURE 18–7. Closing wedge distal femoral osteotomy. *A*, Initial pin placement. *B*, Blade plate placement.

Illustration continued on following page

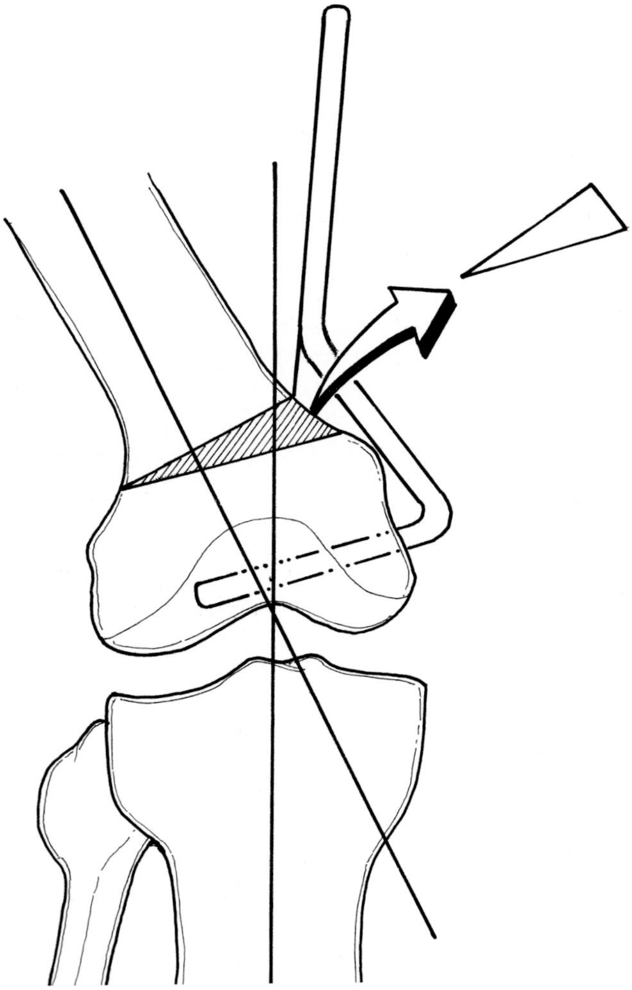

C

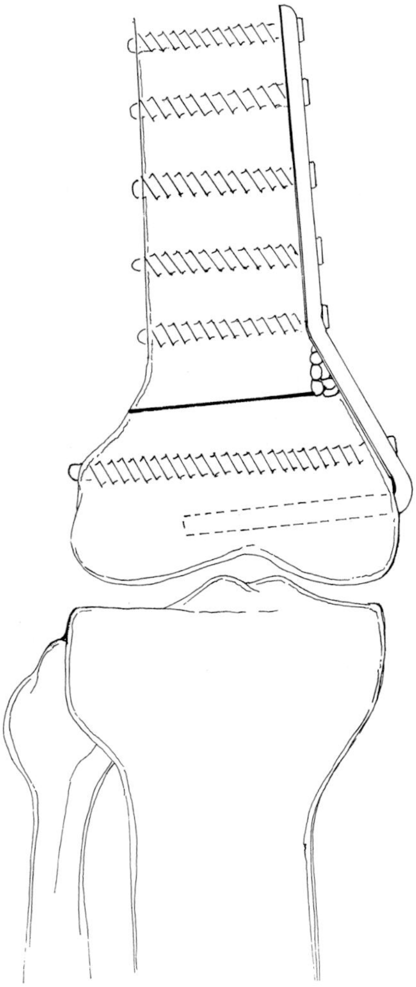

D

FIGURE 18–7 *Continued.* *C*, Wedge of bone removed. *D*, Final osteotomy.

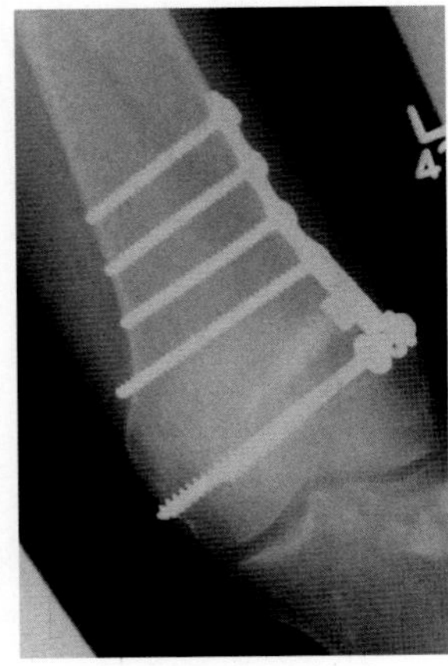

A

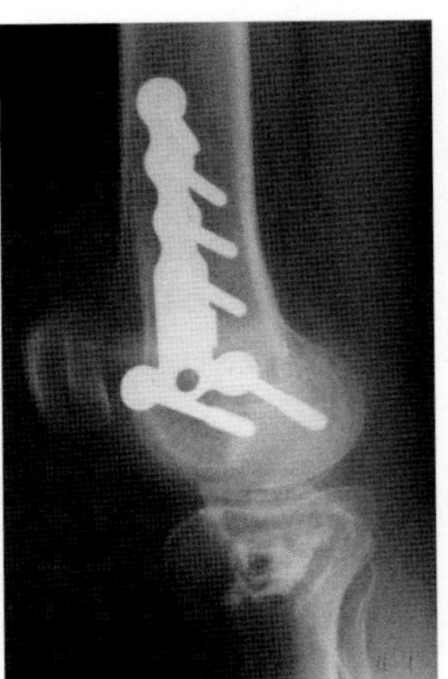

B

FIGURE 18–8. *A* and *B*, Anteroposterior and lateral radiographs show distal femoral opening wedge osteotomy.

POSTOPERATIVE MANAGEMENT

If rigid fixation is obtained, patients may begin weight bearing as tolerated immediately. Continuous passive motion use is advocated by some surgeons, but early range of motion is essential. Quadriceps rehabilitation is initiated immediately.

COMPLICATIONS

A common complication is undercorrection. Careful preoperative planning is essential for a successful result. Intraoperative complications include fracture (the osteotomy must be at least 2 cm from the joint and extend up to the opposite cortex), neurovascular injury, and hardware failure. Postoperative complications include deep venous thrombosis, compartment syndrome, infection, delayed union or nonunion, and loss of correction.

RESULTS

Although intermediate-term results are encouraging, it is unclear how successful these procedures are in meeting their established goal of delaying the need for knee replacement.

REFERENCES

Coventry MB: Upper tibial osteotomy for osteoarthritis. J Bone Joint Surg [Am] 67:1136–1140, 1985.

McDermott AG, Finkelstein JA, Farine I, et al: Distal femoral varus osteotomy for valgus deformity of the knee. J Bone Joint Surg [Am] 70:110, 1988.

Murray PB, Rand JA: Symptomatic valgus knee: The surgical options. J Am Acad Orthop Surg 1:1–9, 1993.

Sisk TD: Knee realignment and replacement in the recreational athlete. In DeLee JC, Drez D Jr (eds): Orthopaedic Sports Medicine Principles and Practice. Philadelphia, WB Saunders, 1994, pp 1475–1501.

CHAPTER 19

Treatment of Patellar and Quadriceps Tendon Ruptures

INTRODUCTION

Although patellar and quadriceps tendon ruptures typically occur in older patients, patients on prolonged steroids, and patients with systemic disease, they can occur on a regular basis in athletes.

HISTORY AND PHYSICAL EXAMINATION

Patients classically describe a sudden pop while applying stress to the extensor mechanism. They may have immediate inability to bear weight and may report significant displacement of the kneecap. On examination, there may be a displaced patella, hemarthrosis, and an inability to extend the knee. Quadriceps tendon rupture typically occurs in an older age group than does patellar dislocation.

DIAGNOSTIC IMAGING

Plain radiographs may show proximal (patellar tendon rupture) or distal (quadriceps tendon rupture) displacement of the patella (best seen on lateral radiographs) (Fig. 19–1). MRI can be helpful in questionable cases.

NONOPERATIVE MANAGEMENT

Unless there are extenuating circumstances, nonoperative management of complete injuries is not recommended.

RELEVANT ANATOMY

An appreciation of the normal tendon anatomy and insertions is helpful. Repair should be close to the articular margin to prevent *snowplowing* of the patella into the trochlea.

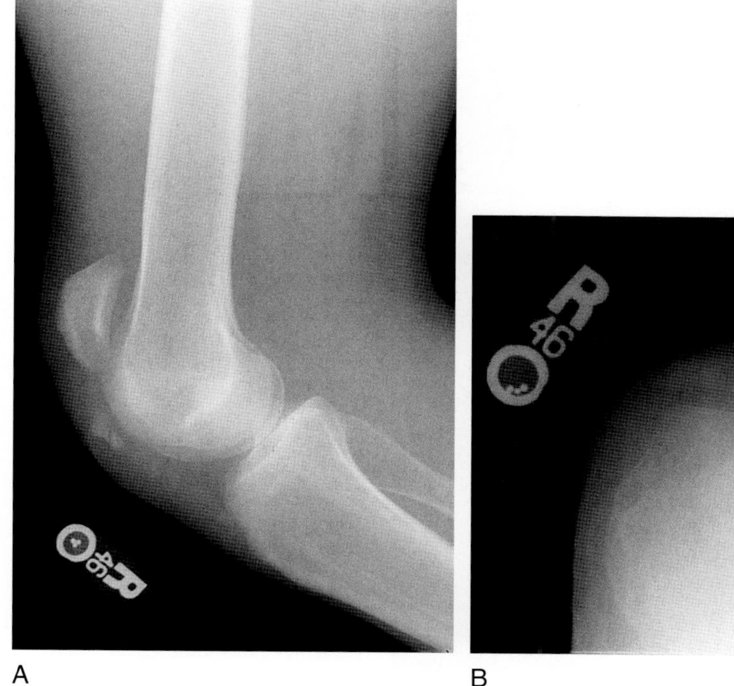

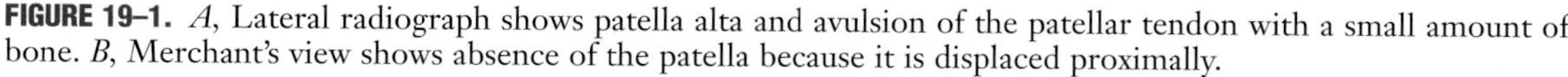

FIGURE 19–1. *A*, Lateral radiograph shows patella alta and avulsion of the patellar tendon with a small amount of bone. *B*, Merchant's view shows absence of the patella because it is displaced proximally.

SURGICAL *TECHNIQUE*

Indications

Surgery is indicated for acute tendon rupture with disruption of the extensor function.

Technique

Patellar Tendon Rupture

The tendon is exposed, the edges are trimmed, and the tendon is reapproximated through drill holes (Figs. 19–2 and 19–3). A McLaughlin wire—in this case, a PDS cable (Ethicon, Somerville, NJ)—is used to protect the repair.

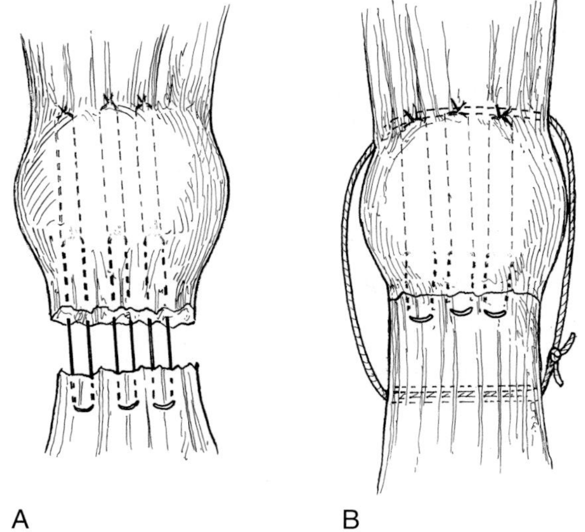

FIGURE 19–2. Technique for patellar tendon repair. *A*, Primary repair through drill holes in bone. *B*, McLaughlin reinforcement.

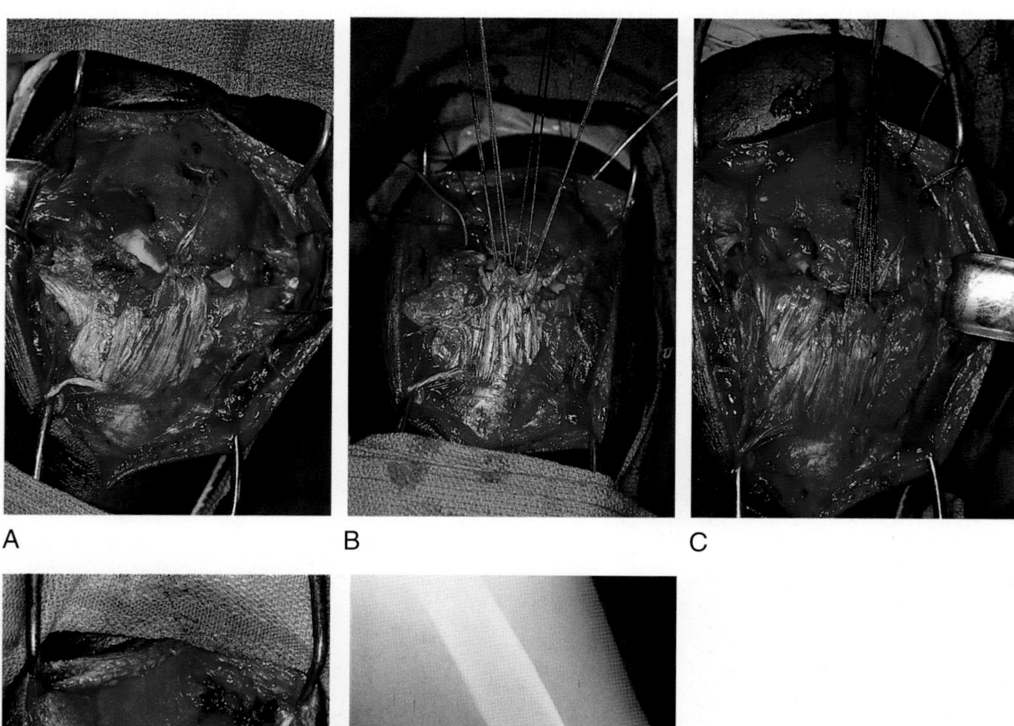

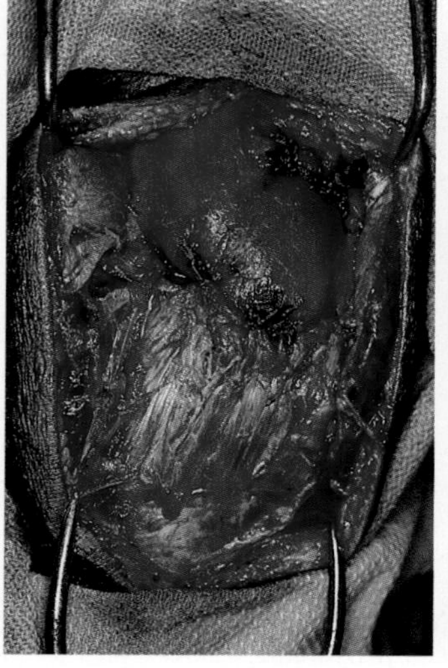

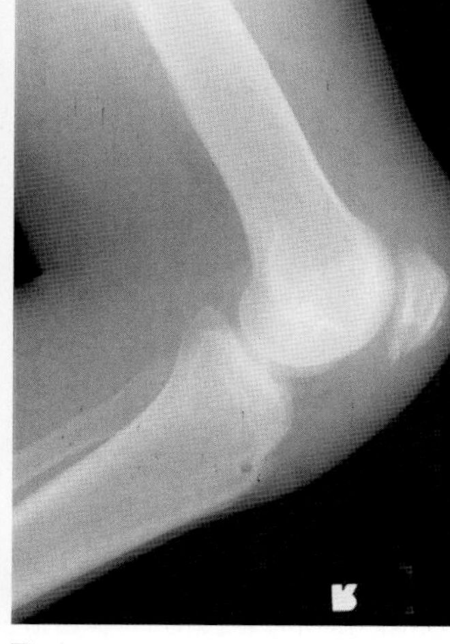

FIGURE 19–3. Patellar tendon repair. *A*, Initial exposure. Tendon is completely avulsed from the patella. *B*, Initial suture placement. *C*, Sutures are placed through drill holes from inferior to superior. Additional sutures are placed to reinforce the repair. *D*, Final repair. *E*, Lateral radiograph after patellar tendon repair. Note the presence of the McLaughlin suture at the tibial tubercle drill hole.

Quadriceps Tendon Repair

Heavy nonabsorbable Bunnell-type sutures are placed in the edge of the ruptured tendon and secured through drill holes (Fig. 19–4). For both repairs, reestablishment of the normal patellar height is recommended. A *turn-down* flap of quadriceps fascia can be used to reinforce the repair (Fig. 19–5).

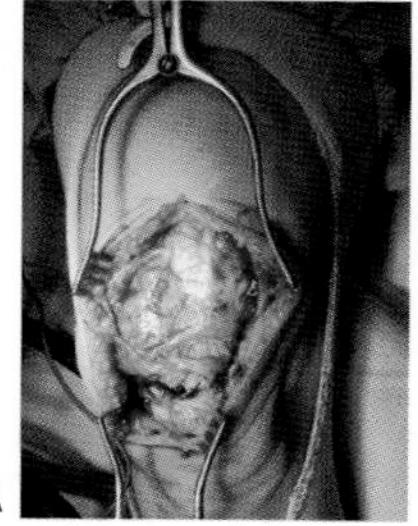

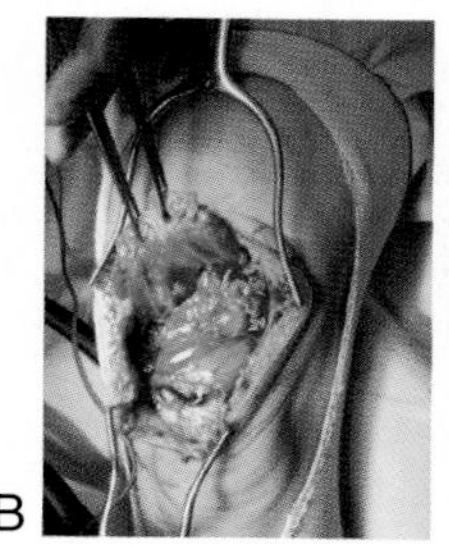

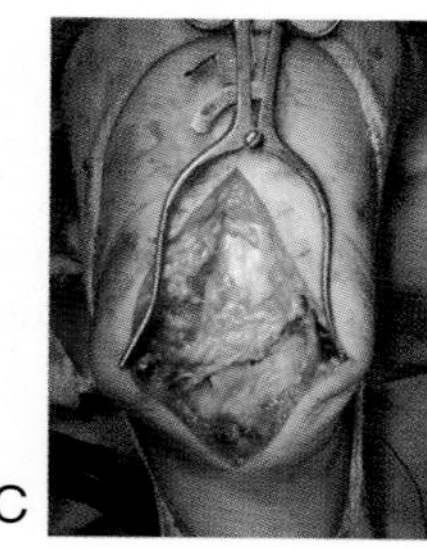

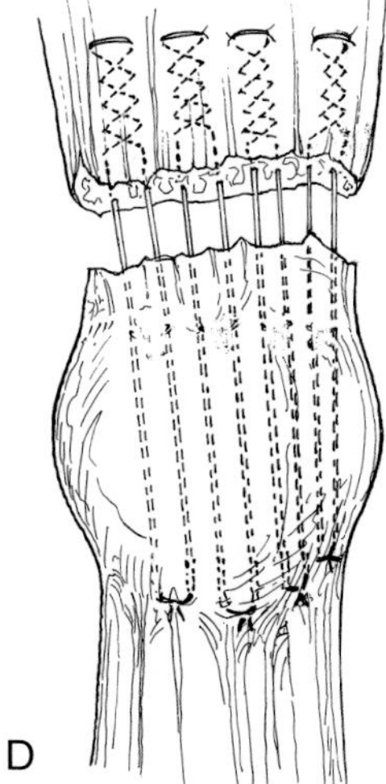

FIGURE 19–4. Quadriceps tendon repair. *A*, Clinical photo of quadriceps tendon rupture. *B*, Tendon is mobilized (Allis clamps). *C*, Final repair. *D*, Artist's depiction.

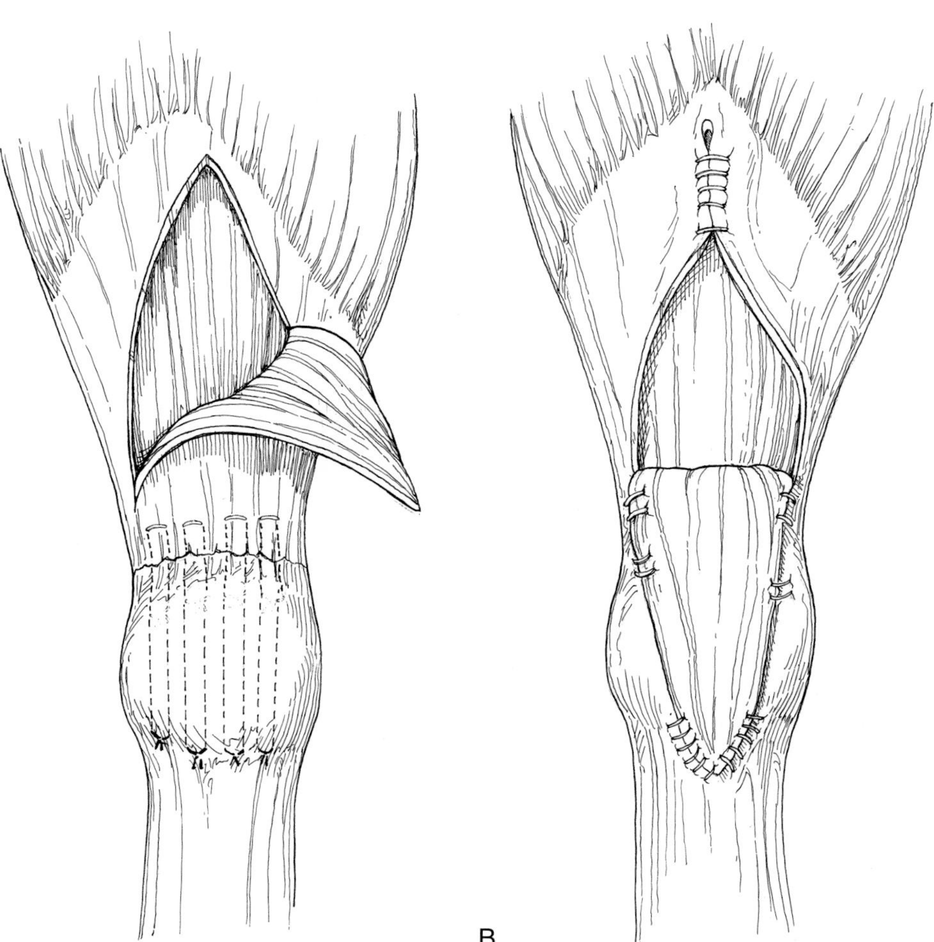

FIGURE 19–5. Turn-down flap of quadriceps fascia may be used to reinforce the repair. *A*, Triangular flap of tissue is turned down. *B*, Flap is used to reinforce repair.

POSTOPERATIVE MANAGEMENT

Protected weight bearing in extension and early range of motion are encouraged.

COMPLICATIONS

Rerupture, failure to restore normal patellar height, dysfunction, chronic pain, and other problems can occur after repair.

RESULTS

Patellar tendon repair is usually successful. Less successful results have been reported for quadriceps tendon repairs. Rasul noted excellent results, however, in 17 of 17 patients with quadriceps tendon ruptures treated acutely.

R E F E R E N C E S

Matava MJ: Patellar tendon ruptures. J Am Acad Orthop Surg 4:287–296, 1996.

Rasul AT, Fischer DA: Primary repair of quadriceps tendon ruptures: Results of treatment. Clin Orthop 289:205–207, 1993.

Sanders R, Gregory PR: Patella fractures and extensor mechanism injuries. In Browner BD, Jupiter JB, Levine AM, Trafton PG (eds): Skeletal Trauma, 2nd ed. Philadelphia, WB Saunders, 1998, pp 2081–2113.

CHAPTER 20

Treatment of Patellar Fractures

INTRODUCTION

Although not considered a sports medicine procedure per se, internal fixation of patellar fractures is an important technique for the knee surgeon. Patellar fractures can occur as a complication after patellar and quadriceps tendon graft harvest.

HISTORY AND PHYSICAL EXAMINATION

Patellar fractures typically result from direct trauma to the anterior knee. Occasionally, violent extensor mechanism contraction can result in patellar fracture. If the fracture is not displaced, tenderness may be the only examination finding. With displaced fractures, a defect may be present, and the extensor function may be compromised.

DIAGNOSTIC IMAGING

Plain radiographs usually show the extent of injury. Patellar fractures are classified based on their location and amount of comminution (Fig. 20–1).

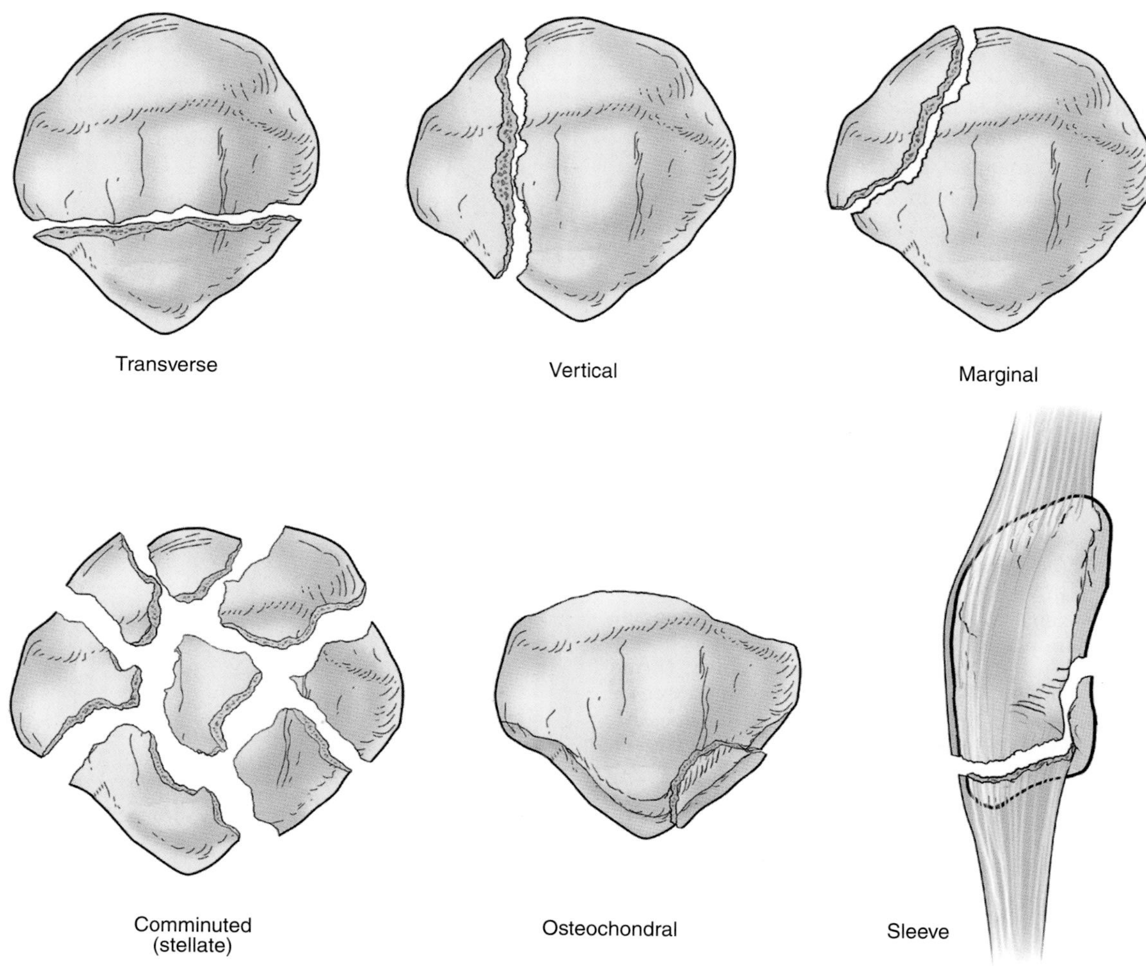

FIGURE 20–1. Classification of patellar fractures based on fracture configuration. (Redrawn from Cramer KE, Moed BR: Patellar fractures: Contemporary approach to treatment. J Am Acad Orthop Surg 5:323, 1997.)

NONOPERATIVE MANAGEMENT

Undisplaced fractures can be treated with immobilization. Motion should be initiated as soon as practical. Displaced fractures require operative stabilization.

RELEVANT ANATOMY

The key is to restore the normal articular surface. Arthroscopy can be a helpful adjunct (Fig. 20–2).

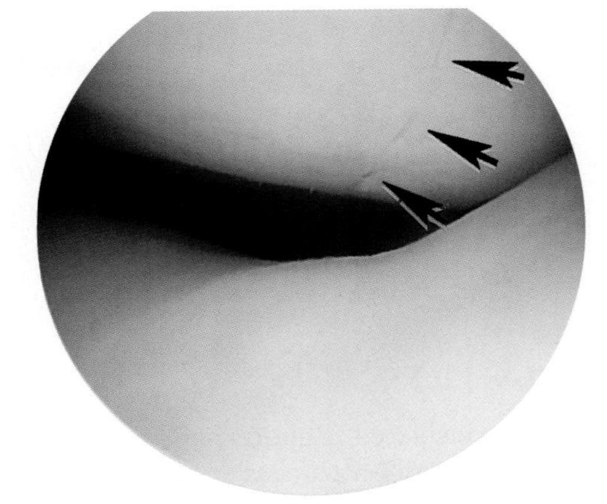

FIGURE 20–2. Arthroscopic view of patellar fracture *(arrows)* after reduction.

SURGICAL *TECHNIQUE*

Indications

Surgery is indicated for displaced patellar fracture.

Technique

A midline incision is used, clots are removed, the edges are irrigated, and the articular continuity is restored. Simple transverse fractures do well with tension band wiring. More comminuted fractures require additional techniques and fixation (Figs. 20–3 through 20–6).

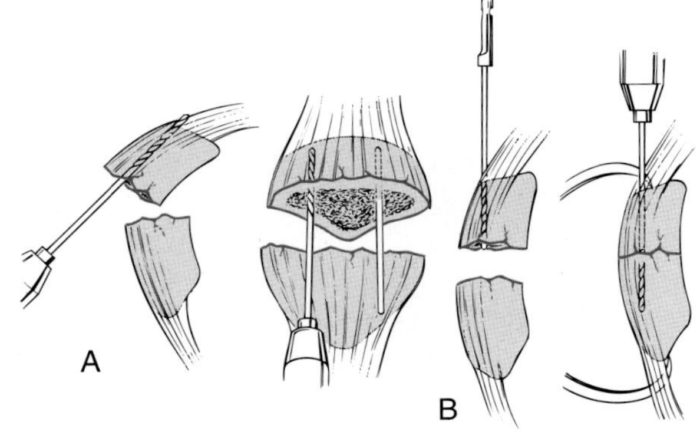

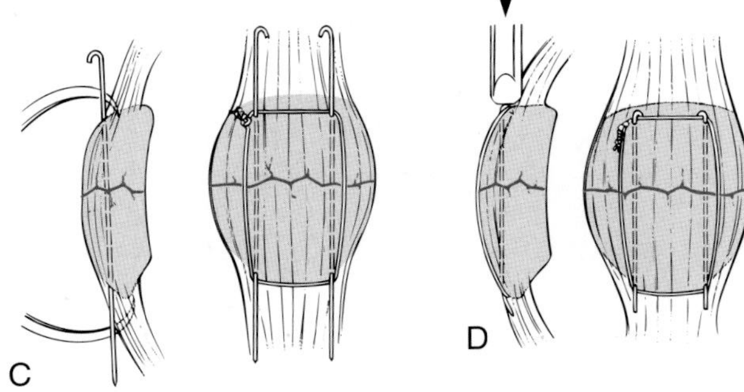

FIGURE 20–3. Technique for open reduction and internal fixation of transverse patellar fractures. *A*, Retrograde drilling of proximal fragment. *B*, Reduction and antegrade drilling. *C*, Wire placed deep to the wires and immediately adjacent to the patella. *D*, Tensioning and fixation. (From Sanders R, Gregory PR: Patella fractures and extensor mechanism injuries. In Browner BD, Jupiter JB, Levine AM, Trafton PG [eds]: Skeletal Trauma, 2nd ed. Philadelphia, WB Saunders, 1998, pp 2081–2113.)

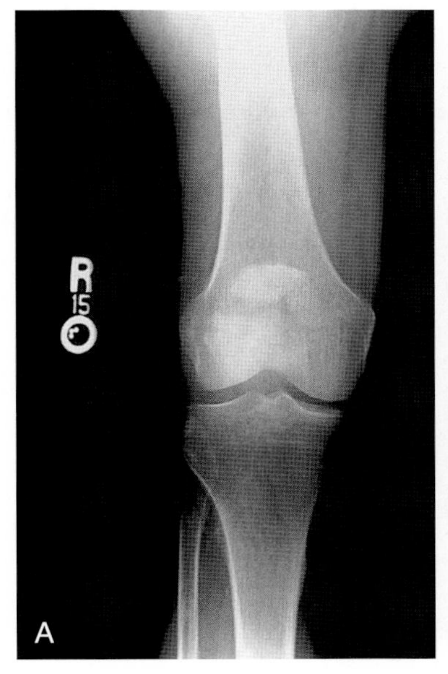

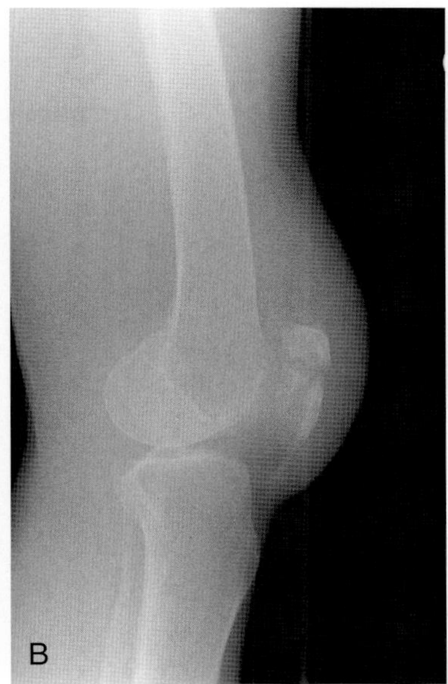

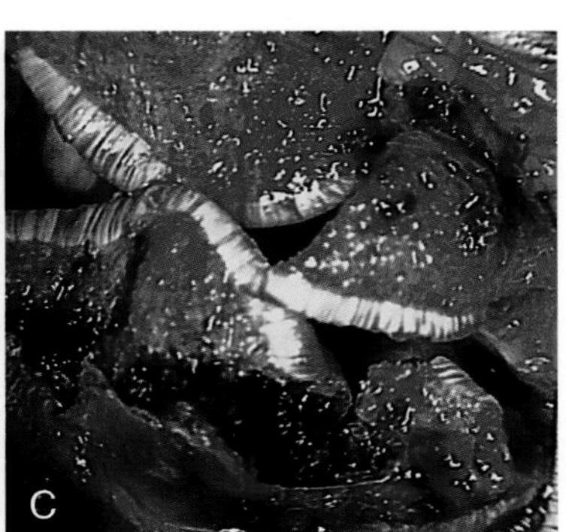

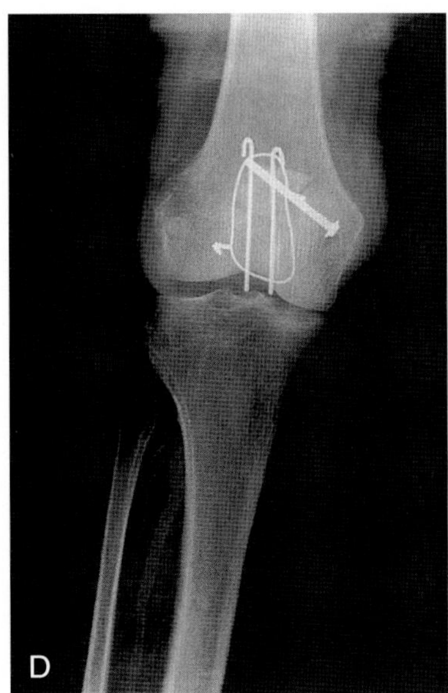

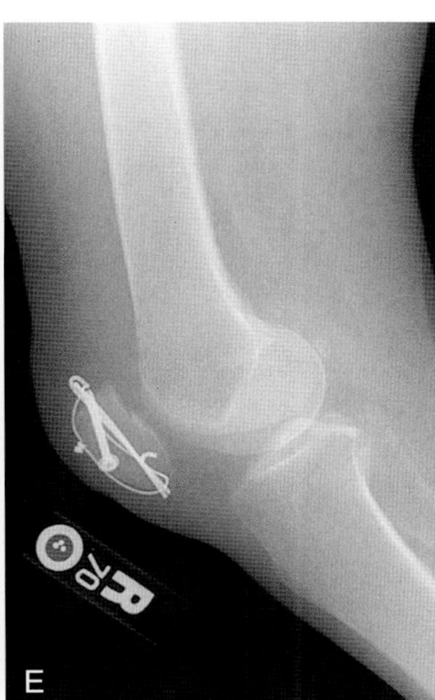

FIGURE 20–4. Open reduction and internal fixation of a transverse patellar fracture with proximal comminution. *A* and *B*, Anteroposterior and lateral radiographs show patellar fracture. *C*, Fracture after exposure. *D* and *E*, Anteroposterior and lateral radiographs show fracture after open reduction and internal fixation.

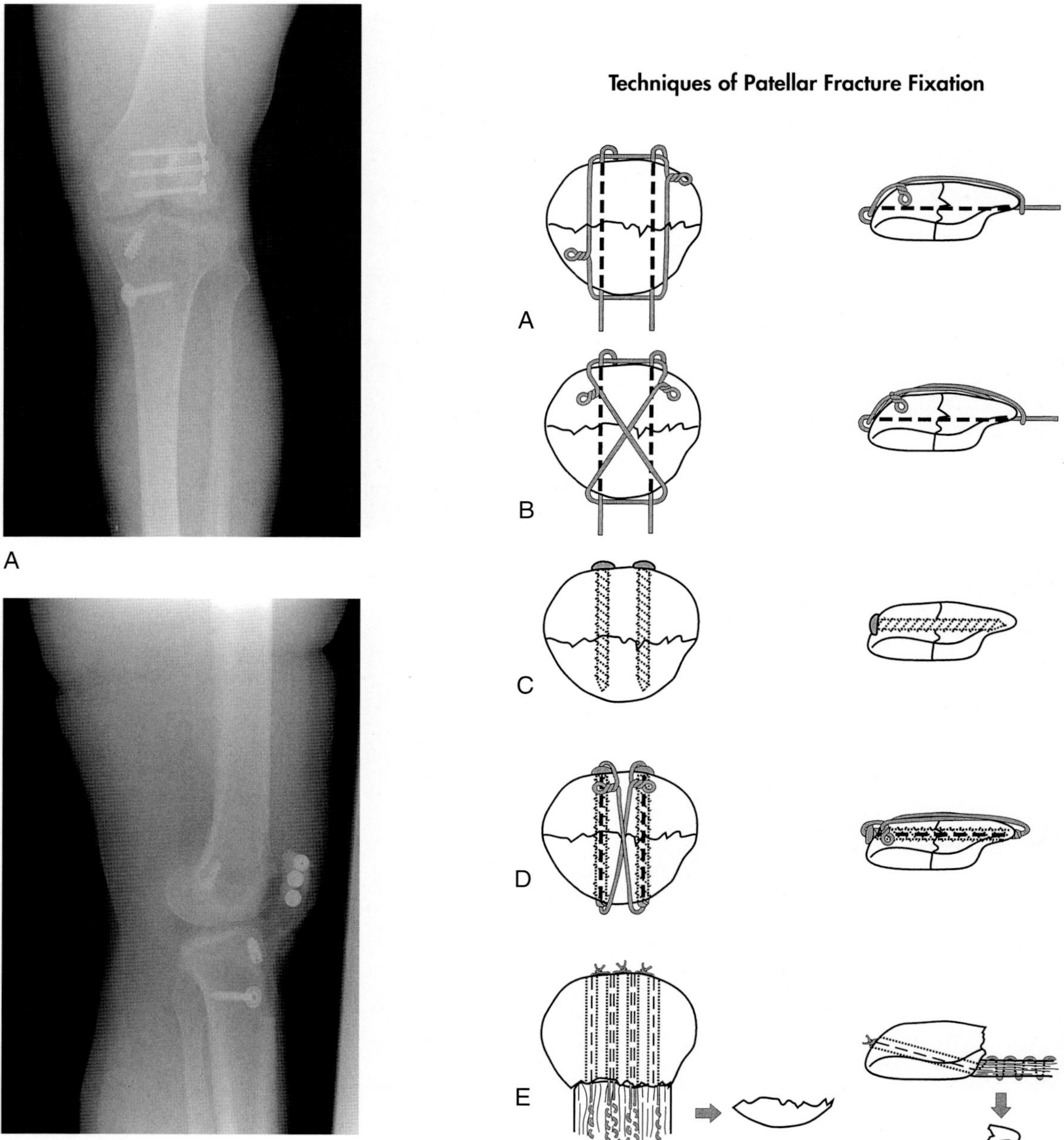

FIGURE 20–5. *A* and *B*, Anteroposterior and lateral radiographs show open reduction and internal fixation of a patellar fracture that occurred during anterior cruciate ligament reconstruction with bone patellar tendon–bone graft harvesting.

FIGURE 20–6. Various methods of fixation for patellar fractures. *A*, Modified tension band wiring using a circular configuration. *B*, Modified tension band wiring using a figure-eight configuration. *C*, Lag-screw fixation. *D*, Combination cannulated lag screw and tension band wiring. *E*, Partial patellectomy. (From Ross PW, Miller MD: Extensor mechanism injuries. In Brinker MR [ed]: Review of Orthopaedic Trauma. Philadelphia, WB Saunders, 2001, pp 101–117.)

POSTOPERATIVE MANAGEMENT

Protected weight bearing in extension and early range-of-motion exercises are encouraged.

COMPLICATIONS

Refracture, nonunion, infection, chronic pain, and other problems can occur.

RESULTS

With careful technique, most fractures heal uneventfully.

REFERENCES

Carpenter JE, Kasman R, Matthews LS: Fractures of the patella. Instr Course Lect 43:97–108, 1994.

Cramer KE, Moed BR: Patellar fractures: Contemporary approach to treatment. J Am Acad Orthop Surg 5:323–331, 1997.

Rispolli D, Miller MD: Extensor mechanism injuries. In Brinker MR (ed): Review of Orthopaedic Trauma. Philadelphia, WB Saunders, 2000, pp 101–117.

Sanders R, Gregory PR: Patella fractures and extensor mechanism injuries. In Browner BD, Jupiter JB, Levine AM, Trafton PG (eds): Skeletal Trauma, 2nd ed. Philadelphia, WB Saunders, 1998, pp 2081–2113.

SECTION II

LEG, ANKLE, AND FOOT

CHAPTER 21

Ankle Arthroscopy

INTRODUCTION

Ankle arthroscopy is now a well-established diagnostic and therapeutic tool. Improvements in noninvasive distraction techniques have expanded the use of the arthroscope.

POSITIONING

Most surgeons perform ankle arthroscopy with the patient supine. Several commercially available ankle distractors are available and allow improved visualization (Fig. 21–1). Alternatively a looped gauze bandage can be fashioned and used. Standard 4.0-mm scopes or smaller 2.7-mm scopes can be used.

PORTALS

Although a variety of portals have been described, three portals commonly are used: the anterolateral, anteromedial, and posterolateral (Fig. 21–2). The anterolateral portal is just lateral to the peroneus tertius tendon at the joint line. The *nick and spread* technique is used to avoid damage to superficial peroneal nerve branches. The anteromedial portal is just medial to the tibialis anterior tendon (avoid the saphenous vein). Other portals were largely abandoned because of neurovascular risks, including the anterocentral portal (dorsalis pedis and deep peroneal nerve) and the posteromedial portal (posterior tibial artery and tibial nerve). It is important to understand that in contrast to knee arthroscopy, ankle arthroscopy and instrumentation is performed at an angle almost

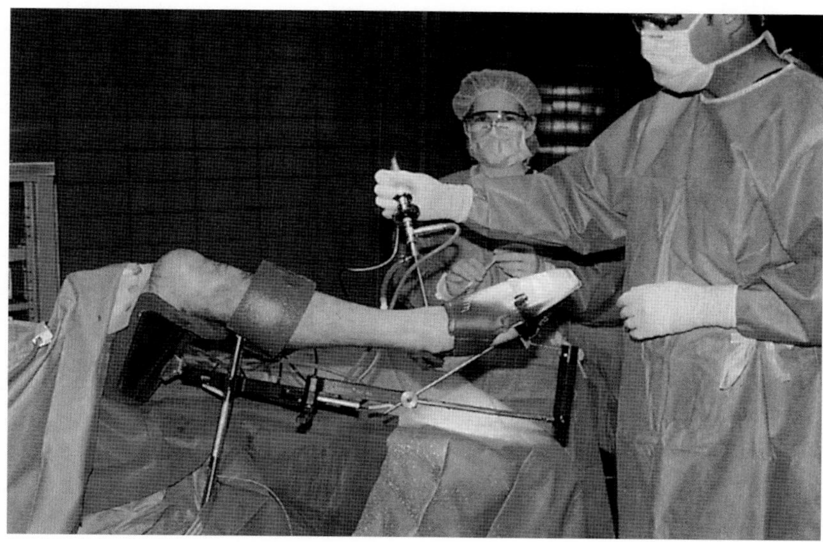

FIGURE 21–1. Positioning for ankle arthroscopy with a commercially available distractor. (From Miller MD, Osborne JR, Warner JJP, Fu FH: MRI-Arthroscopy Correlative Atlas. Philadelphia, WB Saunders, 1997, p 133.)

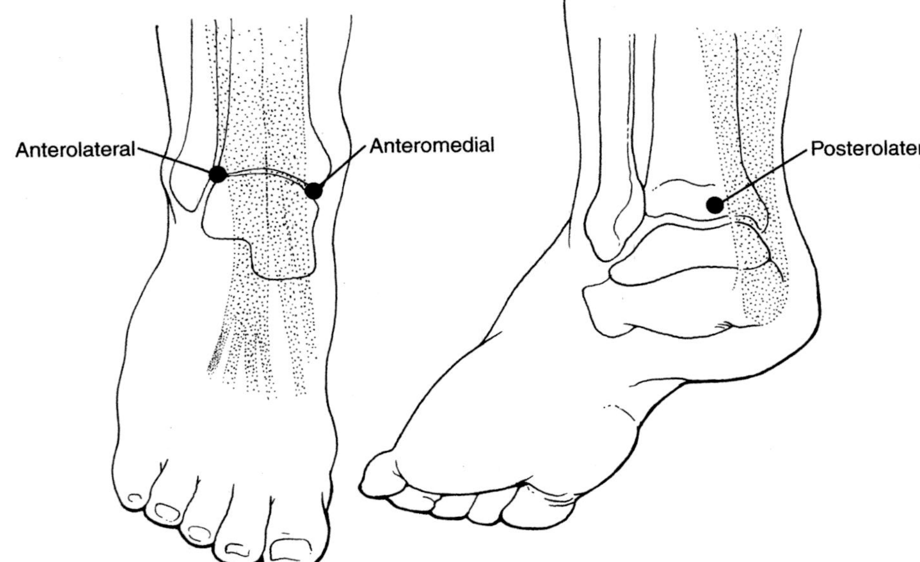

FIGURE 21–2. Portals for ankle arthroscopy. (From Miller MD, Osborne JR, Warner JJP, Fu FH: MRI-Arthroscopy Correlative Atlas. Philadelphia, WB Saunders, 1997, p 134.)

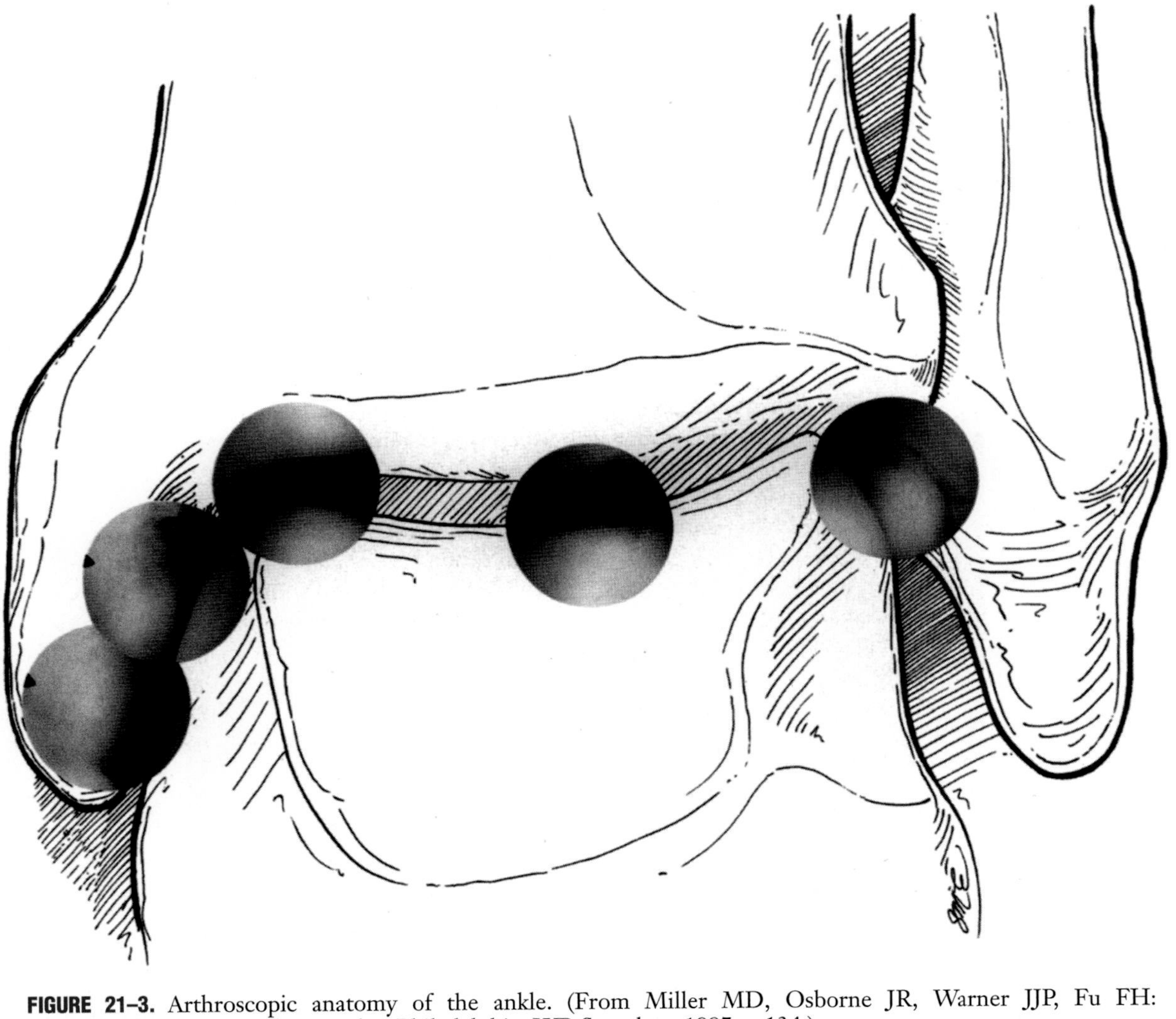

FIGURE 21–3. Arthroscopic anatomy of the ankle. (From Miller MD, Osborne JR, Warner JJP, Fu FH: MRI-Arthroscopy Correlative Atlas. Philadelphia, WB Saunders, 1997, p 134.)

perpendicular to the tibia and does not usually require deep penetration. Subtalar arthroscopy can be done through anterolateral and posterolateral portals. Two accessory portals (accessory anterolateral and accessory posterolateral) can be used for instrumentation.

ARTHROSCOPIC ANATOMY

The anterolateral portal is used most commonly for visualization of the tibiotalar joint. The entire dome of the talus and both gutters can be visualized easily (Fig. 21–3).

REFERENCES

Drez D, Guhl JF, Gollehon DL: Ankle arthroscopy: Technique and indications. Foot Ankle 2:138–142, 1981.

Ewing JW, Tasto JA, Tippett JW: Arthroscopic surgery of the ankle. Inst Course Lect 44:325–340, 1995.

Ferkel RD, Karzel RP, Del Pizzo W, et al: Arthroscopic treatment of anterolateral impingement of the ankle. Am J Sports Med 19:440–446, 1991.

Stetson WB, Ferkel RD: Ankle arthroscopy. J Am Acad Orthop Surg 4:17–34, 1996.

CHAPTER 22

Arthroscopic Débridement of Anterior Impingement

INTRODUCTION

Anterior soft tissue impingement of the ankle is relatively common after ankle sprains and other injuries. Thickened *meniscoid* connective tissue, which often is located between the talus and fibula, can occur in the superior portion of the anterior talofibular ligament, in the distal portion of the anteroinferior tibiofibular ligament, and within the anterior synovium of the ankle joint. Bony impingement is typically a result of tibiotalar osteophytes that occur secondary to trauma and degenerative changes.

HISTORY AND PHYSICAL EXAMINATION

Patients with anterior soft tissue impingement have persistent anterolateral pain despite prolonged conservative treatment, including rest, immobilization, nonsteroidal anti-inflammatory drugs (NSAIDs), local steroid injections, and physical therapy. Patients with bony impingement complain of anterior pain and may have decreased range of motion, catching, and swelling. Typically the pain is worse with walking upstairs, squatting, or running. Dorsiflexion is limited, and localized tenderness is common.

DIAGNOSTIC IMAGING

Soft tissue impingement is often not appreciated on standard imaging modalities. Even MRI is not sensitive. Bony impingement can be shown on lateral radiographs. Reduction of the tibiotalar angle to less than 60° is diagnostic (Fig. 22–1). Bony impingement has been classified radiographically by Scranton and McDermott (Fig. 22–2). A bone scan sometimes can be helpful in the identification of symptomatic pathology.

NONOPERATIVE MANAGEMENT

Rest, NSAIDs, a heel lift, and intra-articular steroid injections sometimes can effect a definitive cure. Conservative management should be attempted for at least 3 months.

RELEVANT ANATOMY

It is important to understand the location of the anterior inferior tibiofibular ligament and the anterior talofibular ligament (Fig. 22–3) because thickening of these ligaments is often responsible for soft tissue impingement. It also is crucial to appreciate that tendons and neurovascular structures are immediately adjacent to the ankle joint capsule.

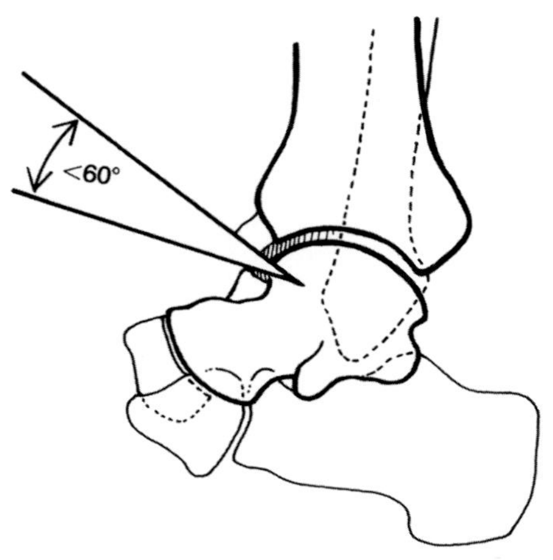

FIGURE 22–1. Osteophytes from the distal tibia and talar neck can result in reduction of the tibiotalar angle to less than 60°. (From Miller MD, Cooper DE, Warner JJP: Review of Sports Medicine and Arthroscopy, 2nd ed. Philadelphia, WB Saunders, 1995.)

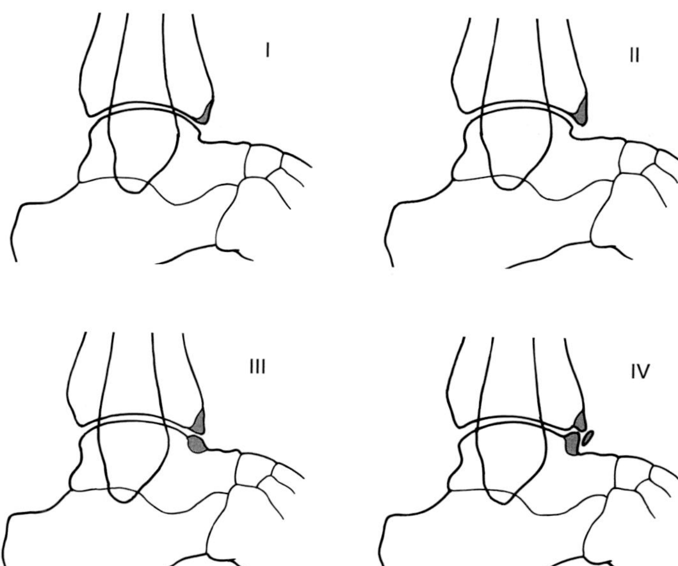

FIGURE 22–2. Scranton and McDermott's radiologic classification of anterior ankle bony impingement (I through IV). (From Scranton PE, McDermott JE: Anterior tibiotalar spurs: A comparison of open versus arthroscopic debridement. Foot Ankle 13:125–129, 1992.)

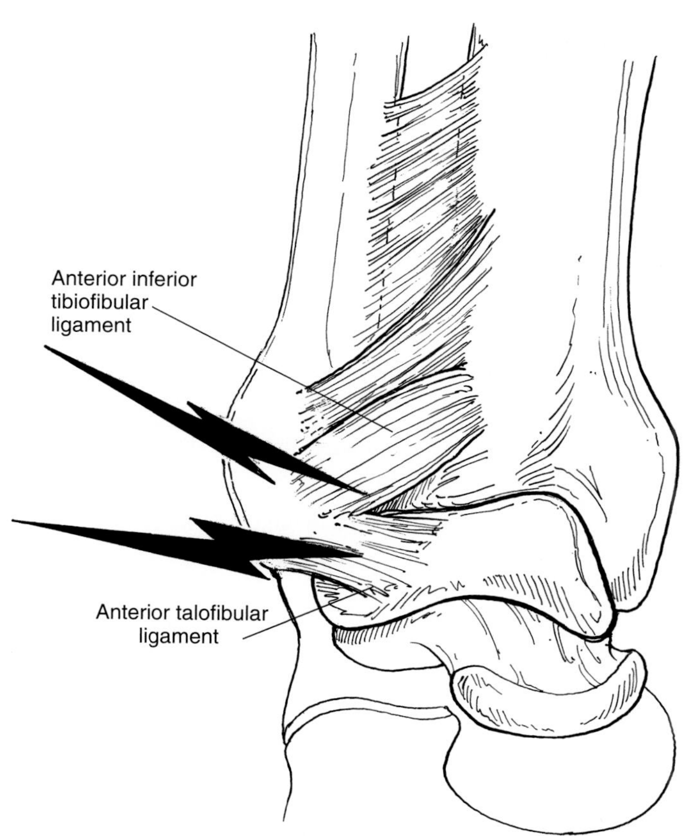

FIGURE 22–3. The inferior portion of the anterior inferior tibiofibular ligament and the superior portion of the anterior talofibular ligament can impinge on the lateral talar dome.

SURGICAL *TECHNIQUE*

Indications

The procedure is indicated for persistent symptoms refractory to nonoperative management.

Technique

1. Positioning: The patient is positioned supine, and a commercially available ankle distractor is placed on the foot.
2. Diagnostic arthroscopy: Diagnostic arthroscopy is done, and the extent of impingement is appreciated. A full radius shaver is used to débride hypertrophic synovium (Fig. 22–4).
3. The location and extent of bony impingement is appreciated (Fig. 22–5). A shaver and a burr are used through alternate portals to débride this area. An intraoperative lateral radiograph is often helpful to ensure that adequate bony resection is obtained.

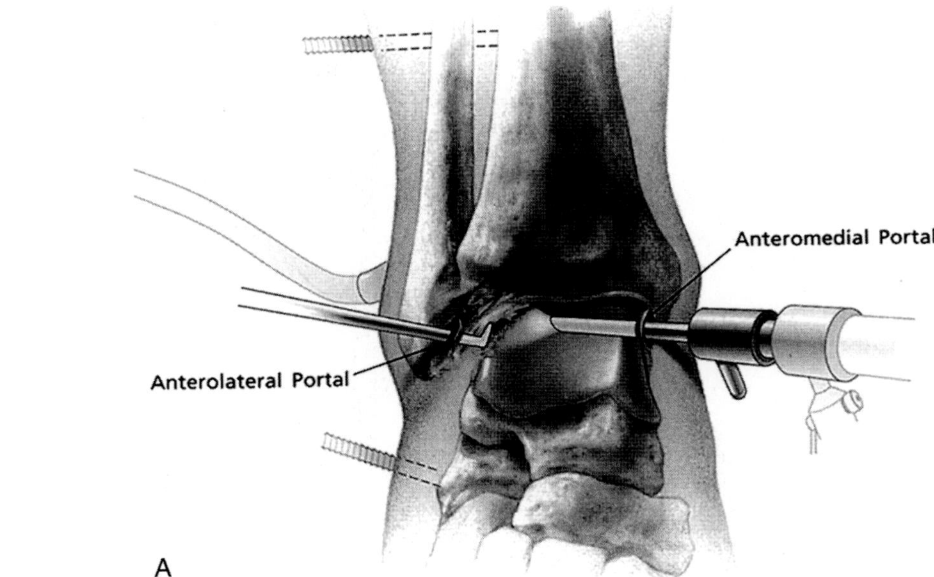

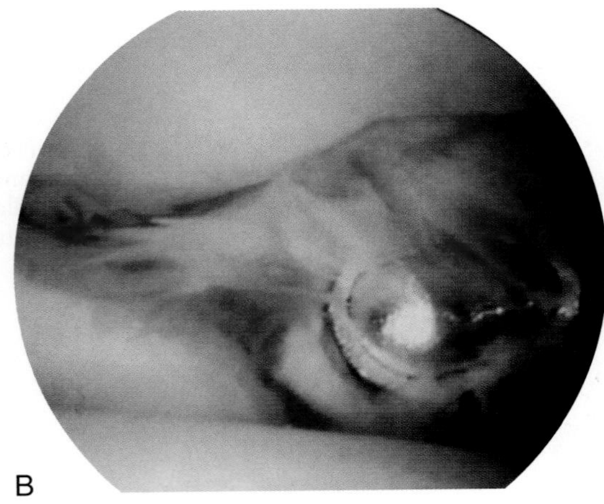

FIGURE 22–4. *A*, With the arthroscope in the anteromedial portal, the impinging lesion is seen and palpated through the anterolateral portal. *B*, Full radius shaver, placed through the anterolateral portal. (From Ferkel RD, Ruland CM: Operative arthroscopy of the ankle. In Andrews JR, Timmerman LA [eds]: Diagnostic and Operative Arthroscopy. Philadelphia, WB Saunders, 1997, p 439.)

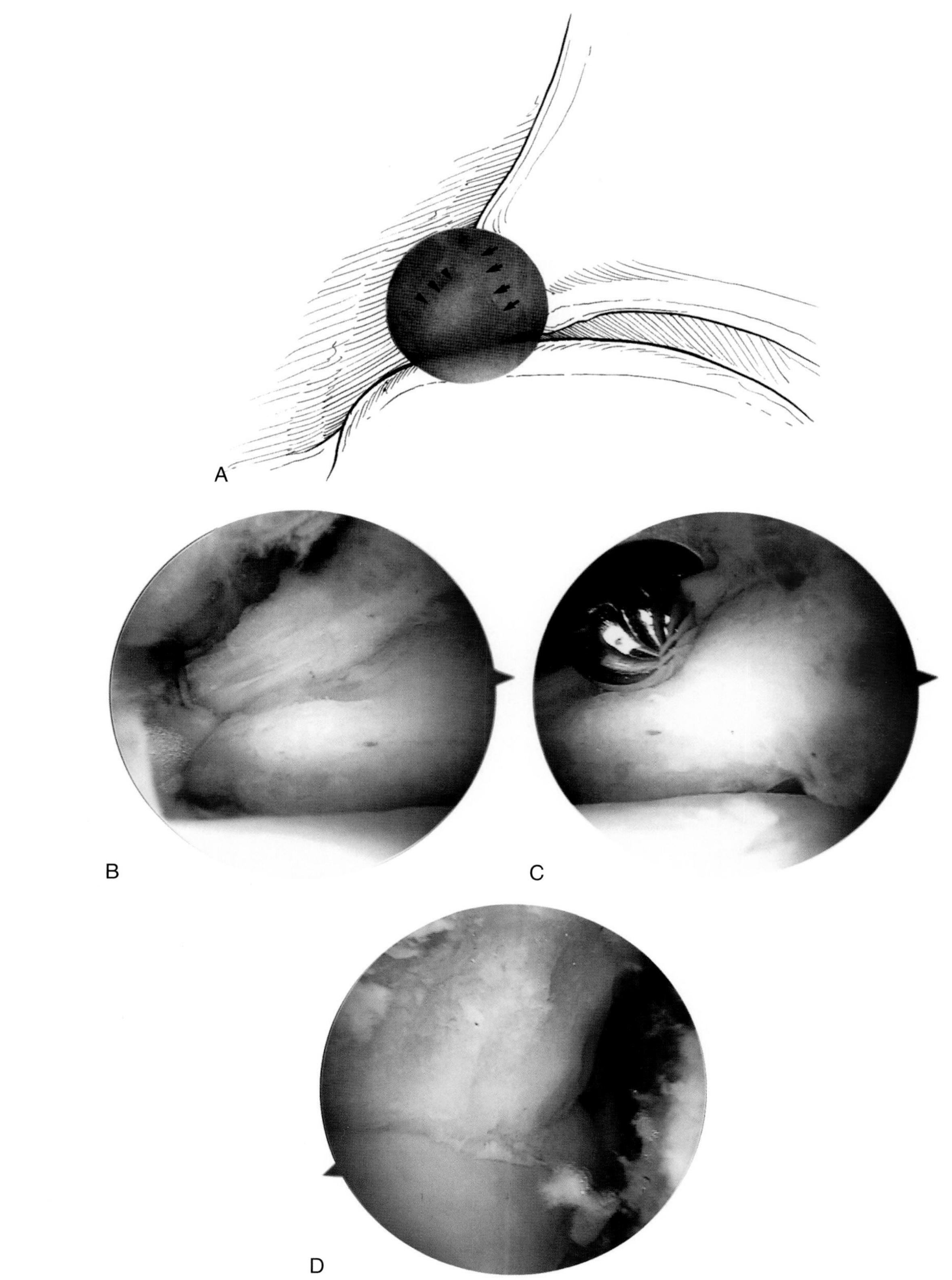

FIGURE 22–5. Tibiotalar spur resection. *A*, Artist's depiction of tibiotalar spur *(arrowheads)*. *B*, Note a large spur with overlying soft tissue. *C*, A burr is introduced through the contralateral portal, and the spur is resected. *D*, Final spur resection. (From Miller MD, Osborne JR, Warner JJP, Fu FH: MRI-Arthroscopy Correlative Atlas. Philadelphia, WB Saunders, 1997, p 140.)

POSTOPERATIVE MANAGEMENT

Because of the risk of fistula development after ankle arthroscopy, a bulky splint is applied for the initial 5 to 7 days postoperatively. Gradual weight bearing is allowed after this period, and range-of-motion exercises and strengthening are initiated about 2 weeks postoperatively.

COMPLICATIONS

Neurovascular injury can occur during portal placement. Fistulas can occur if the ankle is not immobilized postoperatively. Articular cartilage injury also can occur unless extreme care is taken during ankle arthroscopy.

RESULTS

Long-term results of arthroscopic synovectomy and débridement for anterolateral impingement are good to excellent in 75% to 90% of patients. Arthroscopic removal of bony spurs has decreased morbidity and greater success than open methods.

REFERENCES

Ferkel RD, Karzel RP, Del Pizzo W, et al: Arthroscopic treatment of anterolateral impingement of the ankle. Am J Sports Med 19:440–446, 1991.

Ferkel RD, Ruland CM: Operative arthroscopy of the ankle. In Andrews JR, Timmerman LA (eds): Diagnostic and Operative Arthroscopy. Philadelphia, WB Saunders, 1997.

Ogilvie-Harris DJ, Mahomed N, Demaziere A: Anterior impingement of the ankle treated by arthroscopic removal of bony spurs. J Bone Joint Surg [Br] 75:437, 1993.

Scranton PE Jr, McDermott JE: Anterior or tibiotalar spurs: A comparison of open versus arthroscopic debridement. Foot Ankle 13:125, 1992.

Slater GL, O'Malley MJ: Anterior bony ankle impingement. Foot Ankle Clin 4:303–317, 1995.

CHAPTER 23

Treatment of Osteochondral Injuries of the Talus

INTRODUCTION

Osteochondral lesions of the talus represent a complete spectrum of pathology, ranging from fibrous defects to large osteochondral fractures. They may or may not be associated with trauma. These lesions typically are located on either the medial or the lateral side of the talus with the following characteristics:

Lesion	*Location*	*Depth*	*Characteristics*	*Cause*
Medial	Posterior	Deep	Nondisplaced	Often unknown
Lateral	Anterior	Shallow	Displaced	Traumatic

HISTORY AND PHYSICAL EXAMINATION

Patients typically complain of chronic ankle pain and may relate a history of trauma (e.g., a severe ankle sprain). Other symptoms include swelling, stiffness, weakness or giving way, and occasional locking or catching. The examination is most often nonspecific.

DIAGNOSTIC IMAGING

Plain radiographs often show the lesion. CT and MRI also have been recommended, especially for subtle lesions (Fig. 23–1). Several classification schemes have been developed based on the appearance of these lesions. The Berndt and Harty classification is perhaps most universally accepted. Loomer and colleagues added a fifth category based on MRI of subtle fibrous lesions (type V), which they found to be the most common in their series (Fig. 23–2).

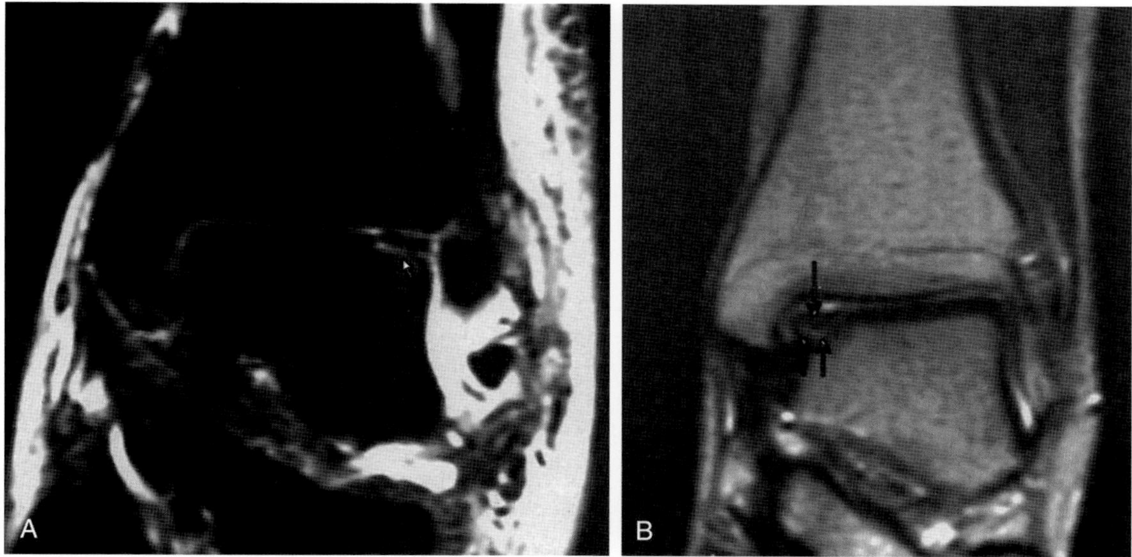

FIGURE 23–1. *A*, Coronal short tau inversion recovery (STIR) image shows shallow lateral talar lesion *(arrow)*. *B*, Coronal fat-suppressed echo T2-weighted image shows a deep medial talar lesion *(arrows)*. (From Miller MD, Osborne JR, Warner JJP, Fu FH: MRI-Arthroscopy Correlative Atlas. Philadelphia, WB Saunders, 1997, pp 136–137.)

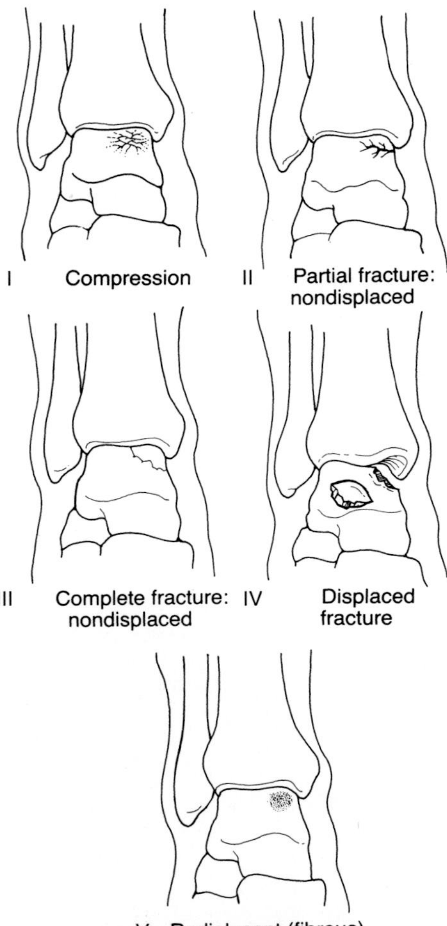

FIGURE 23–2. Loomer and colleagues' modification of the Berndt and Harty classification of osteochondral lesions of the talus. (From Miller MD, Cooper DE, Warner JJP: Review of Sports Medicine and Arthroscopy, 2nd ed. Philadelphia, WB Saunders, 2002, p 105.)

NONOPERATIVE MANAGEMENT

Nonoperative treatment usually is recommended first, especially for early, nondisplaced lesions. Treatment consists of 6 to 12 weeks of casting with partial weight bearing.

RELEVANT ANATOMY

Access to these lesions, especially the medial talar lesions, which are more posterior, can be difficult. The surgeon should be familiar with open approaches to the ankle, including transmalleolar osteotomies (Fig. 23–3) and the posteromedial approach (Fig. 23–4).

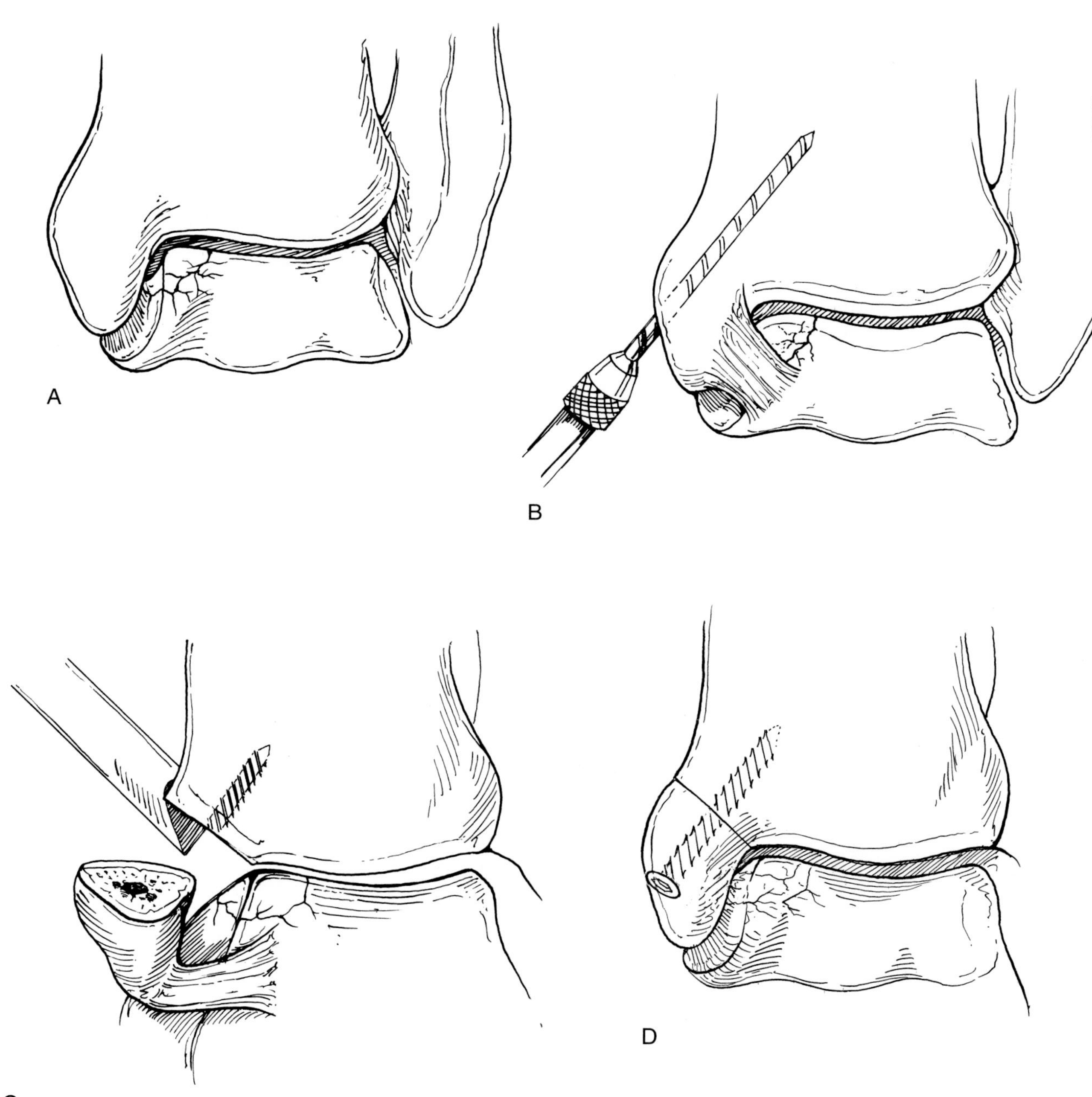

FIGURE 23–3. Medial malleolar osteotomy for access to medial osteochondral lesion of the talus. *A*, Medial talar lesions are typically more posterior and deeper than lateral lesions. *B*, The medial malleolus is predrilled. *C*, An osteotomy is made, and the medial malleolus is reflected. Note that the deltoid attachment is preserved. *D*, Reduction and fixation of the osteotomy.

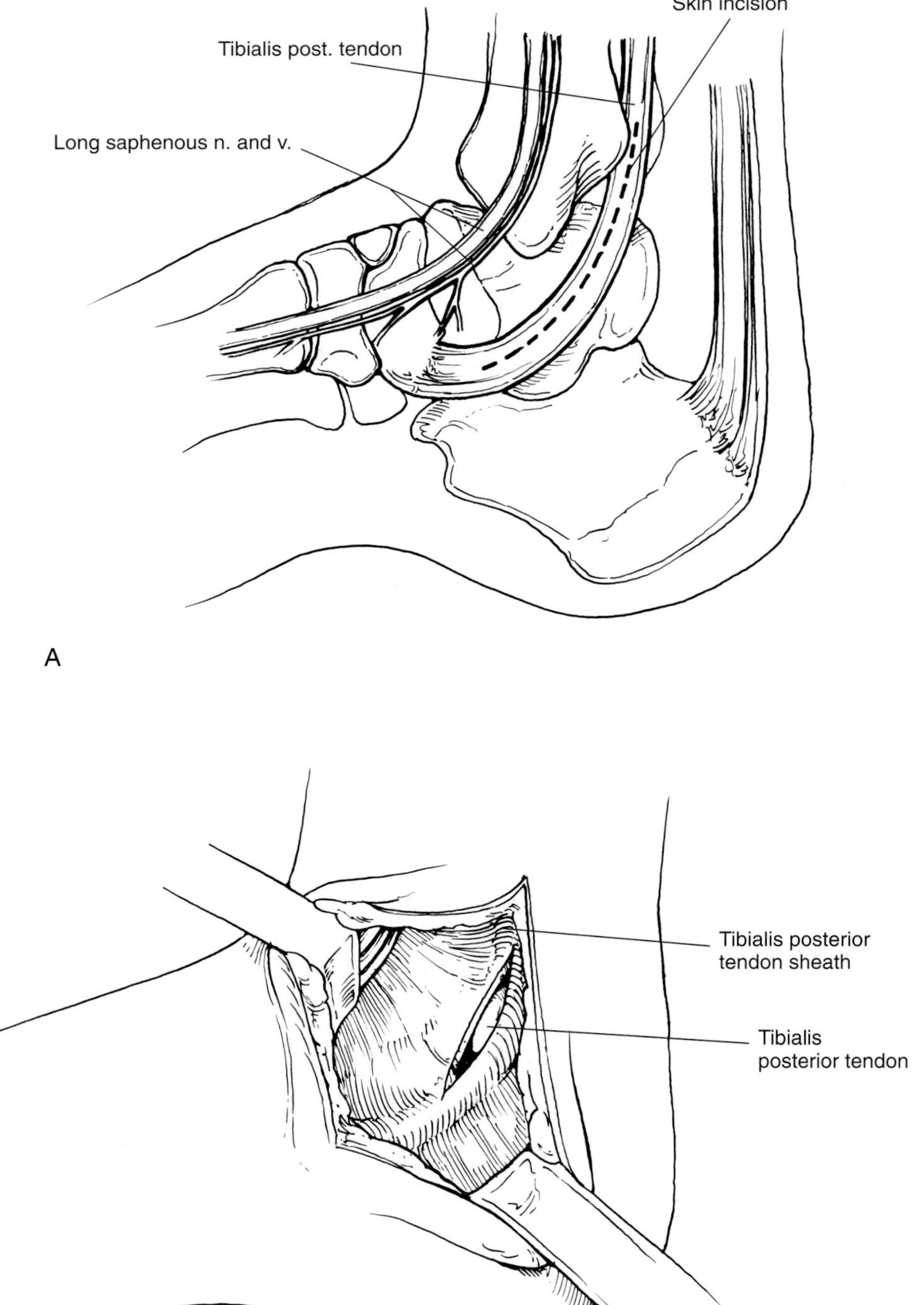

FIGURE 23–4. Posteromedial approach to the medial malleolus. *A*, The approach is through the posterior tibial tendon sheath. A skin incision is planned over the tendon. *B*, The tendon sheath is sharply incised.

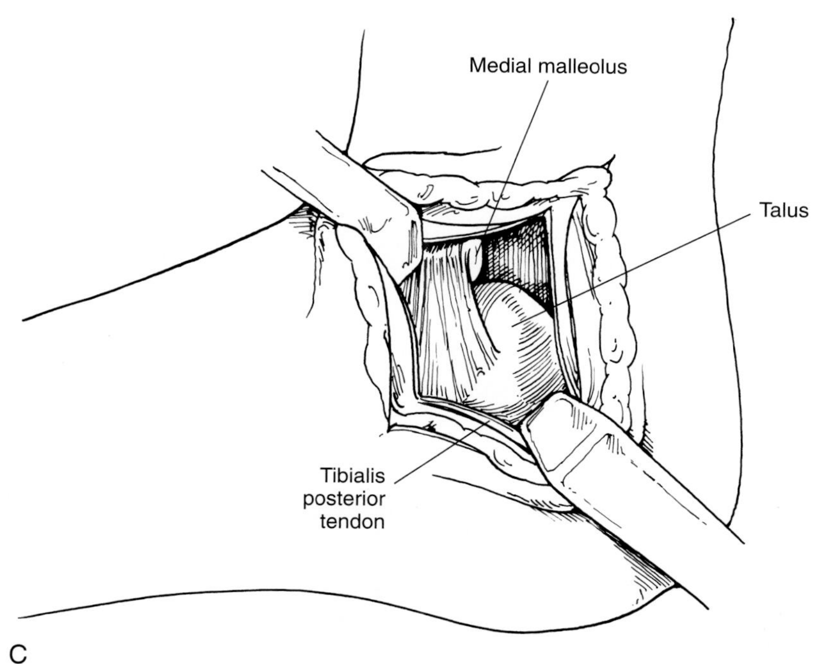

FIGURE 23–4 *Continued. C,* The talus is exposed.

SURGICAL *TECHNIQUE*

Indications

Indications for this procedure are persistent symptoms that have failed nonoperative management including immobilization. Surgery is indicated for some acute, displaced lesions.

Technique

1. Positioning: Positioning is similar to ankle arthroscopy.
2. Diagnostic arthroscopy: Visualization and probing of the lesion from both anterior portals are carried out. Loose bodies are identified and removed.
3. Débridement: The lesion is identified, and a curette and shaver are used to smooth the edges and remove any loose flaps. Exposed bone is drilled using a transmalleolar technique (usually using an anterior cruciate ligament drill guide placed in the ipsilateral anterior portal) (Fig. 23–5), or a microfracture awl is used to penetrate the subchondral bone (Fig. 23–6).

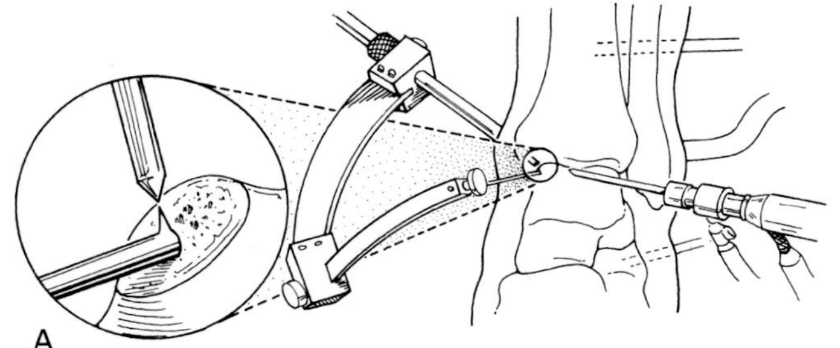

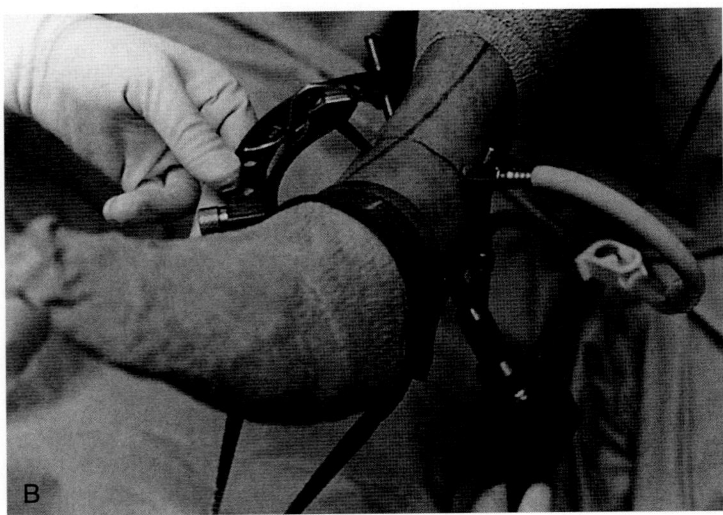

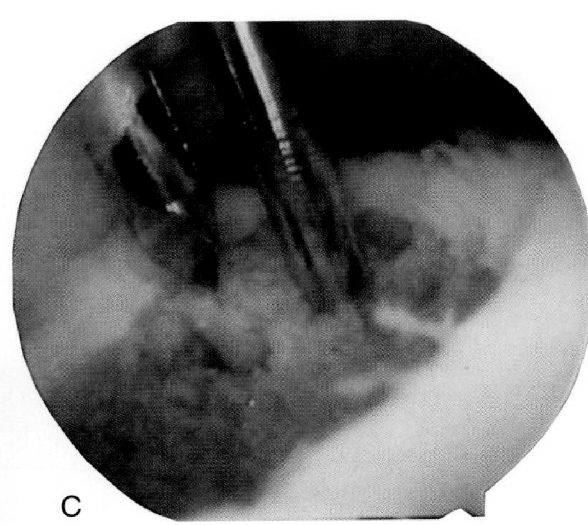

FIGURE 23–5. Transmalleolar drilling. *A*, Artist's depiction. *B*, Operative photo showing technique, external view. *C*, Arthroscopic view from posterolateral portal. (*A* from Miller MD, Cooper DE, Warner JJP: Review of Sports Medicine and Arthroscopy, 2nd ed. Philadelphia, WB Saunders, 2002, p 105. *B* and *C* from Ferkel RD, Ruland CM: Operative arthroscopy of the ankle. In Andrews JR, Timmerman LA [eds]: Diagnostic and Operative Arthroscopy. Philadelphia, WB Saunders, 1997, p 442.)

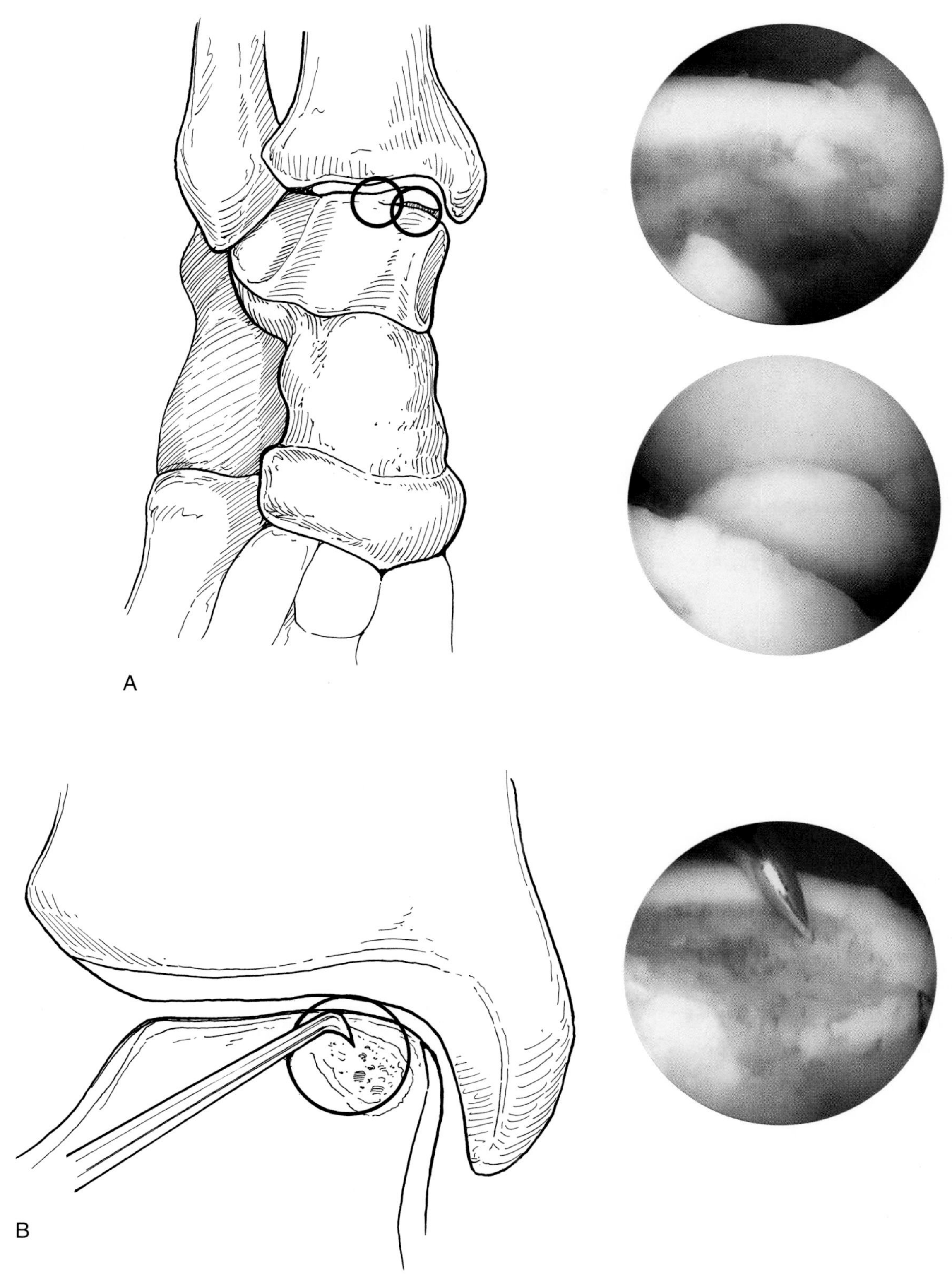

FIGURE 23–6. Microfracture of medial talar lesion. *A*, Lesion includes a defect and a loose body that is removed. *B*, A microfracture awl is introduced through the contralateral portal and used to create subchondral holes in the bone.

Illustration continued on following page

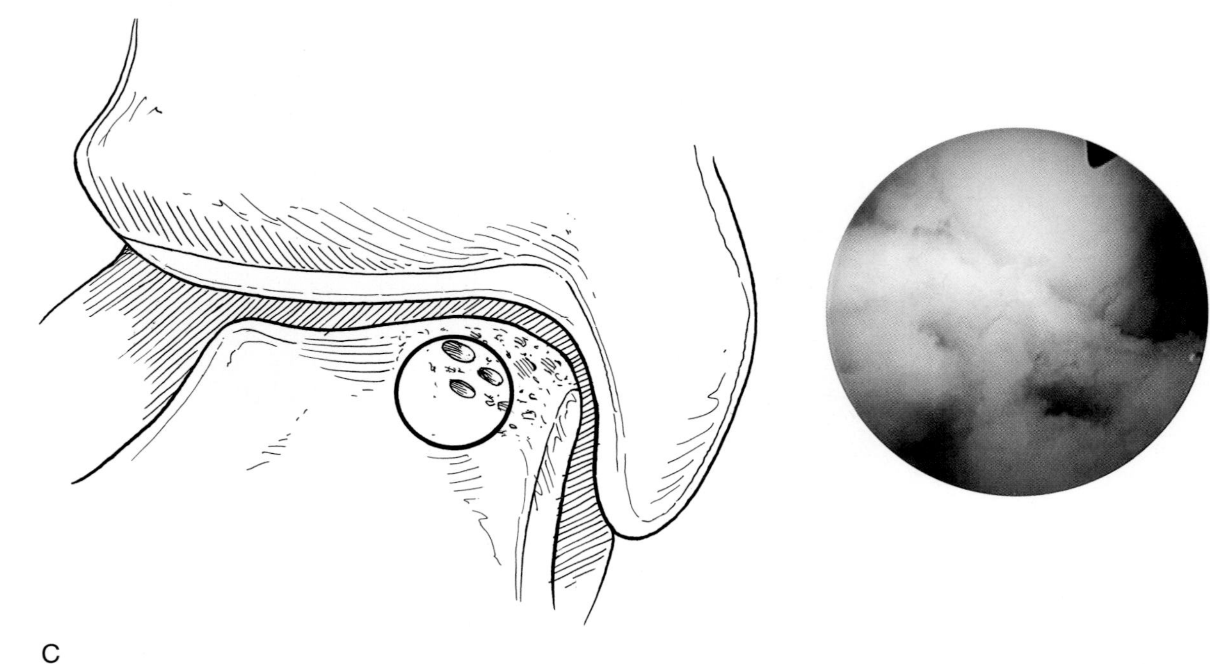

FIGURE 23–6 *Continued. C,* Talar lesion after microfracture.

4. Osteochondral plug technique: Although it is still investigational, Hungody and associates described a technique for osteochondral transfer, similar to that in the knee. The lesion is identified and exposed, and the edges are tapered. Small (4-mm-diameter) osteochondral plugs are harvested from the knee and placed into drill holes in the defect. This technique creates a *mosaic* or cobblestone-like articular surface with the transferred articular cartilage (Fig. 23–7).

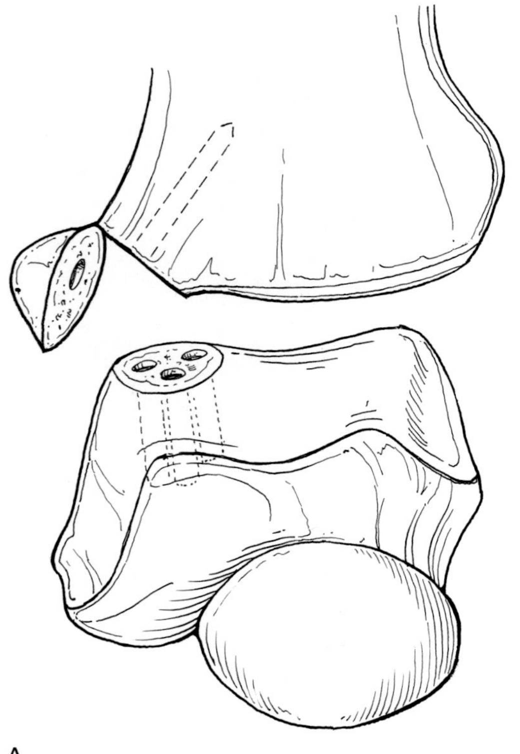

FIGURE 23–7. Treatment of medial osteochondral lesion with osteochondral plugs. *A,* Recipient holes are created in the talus in a geometric pattern allowing the most coverage of the defect.

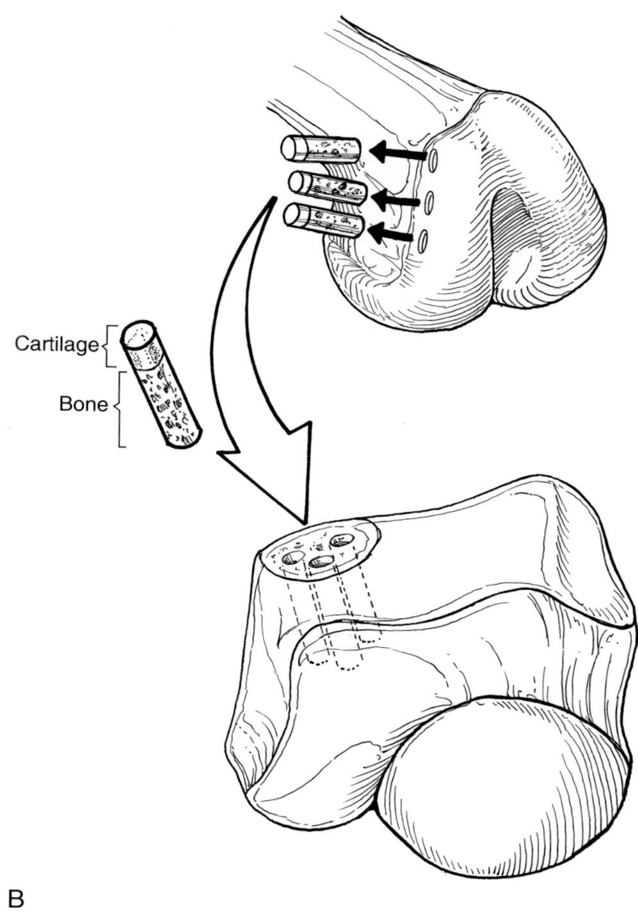

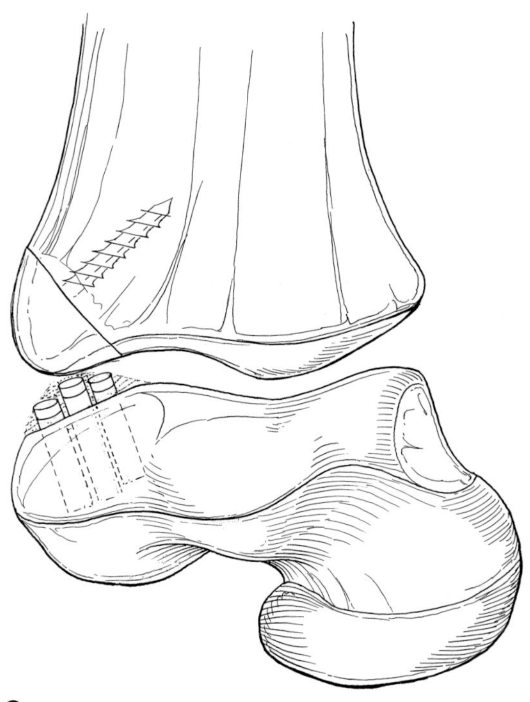

FIGURE 23–7 *Continued. B,* Osteochondral plugs are harvested from the knee and placed into the defect. *C,* Final plug placement.

POSTOPERATIVE MANAGEMENT

Depending on the technique, the ankle usually is immobilized in a bulky splint for 1 week. This is followed by range-of-motion exercises. Weight bearing usually is avoided for approximately 6 weeks.

RESULTS

The results of arthroscopic treatment of these lesions are as good as or better than with open treatment. Arthroscopic treatment also is associated with lower morbidity and a shorter recovery time.

REFERENCES

Bassett FH, Billys JB, Gates HS: A simple surgical approach to the posteromedial ankle. Am J Sports Med 21:144–146, 1993.

Ferkel RD, Ruland CM: Operative arthroscopy of the ankle. In Andrews JR, Timmerman LA (eds): Diagnostic and Operative Arthroscopy. Philadelphia, WB Saunders, 1997.

Kish G, Modis L, Hungody L: Osteochondral mosaicplasty for the treatment of focal chondral and osteochondral lesions of the knee and talus. Clin Sports Med 18:45–66, 1999.

Loomer R, Fisher C, Lloyd-Smith R, et al: Osteochondral injuries of the talus. Am J Sports Med 21:13–19, 1993.

Parisien JS: Arthroscopic treatment of osteochondral lesions of the talus. Am J Sports Med 14:211, 1986.

Stone JW: Osteochondral lesions of the talar dome. J Am Acad Orthop Surg 4:63–73, 1996.

CHAPTER 24

Ligamentous Reconstruction for Recurrent Ankle Instability

INTRODUCTION

Ankle sprains are common injuries in sports. The anterior talofibular ligament (ATFL) is the most commonly injured ligament. The calcaneofibular ligament (CFL) is the second most commonly injured ligament. Most often, ligamentous injuries can be managed successfully nonoperatively. Recurrent ankle sprains may require operative stabilization.

HISTORY AND PHYSICAL EXAMINATION

Patients who present with acute ankle sprains typically describe an inversion injury, pain, and swelling. Examination consists of the anterior drawer test (to test the ATFL) and the tilt test (to test the CFL) (Fig. 24–1). It is important to palpate the proximal fibula to rule out a fracture with a syndesmosis injury (Maisonneuve's fracture). The squeeze test and external rotation test should be done to rule out a syndesmotic injury (Fig. 24–2). Subtalar instability can be tested by locking the talus in the mortise, then testing for excessive tilt in this joint.

DIAGNOSTIC IMAGING

Plain radiographs are usually normal after ankle sprains. Radiographs may not be required if the patient does not have any bony tenderness over the medial malleolus and distal fibula, the navicular, or the fifth metatarsal base and can walk without support. Stress radiographs may be helpful in the evaluation of chronic ankle instability. Greater than 5 mm of anterior displacement of the talus with drawer stress testing is consistent with an ATFL

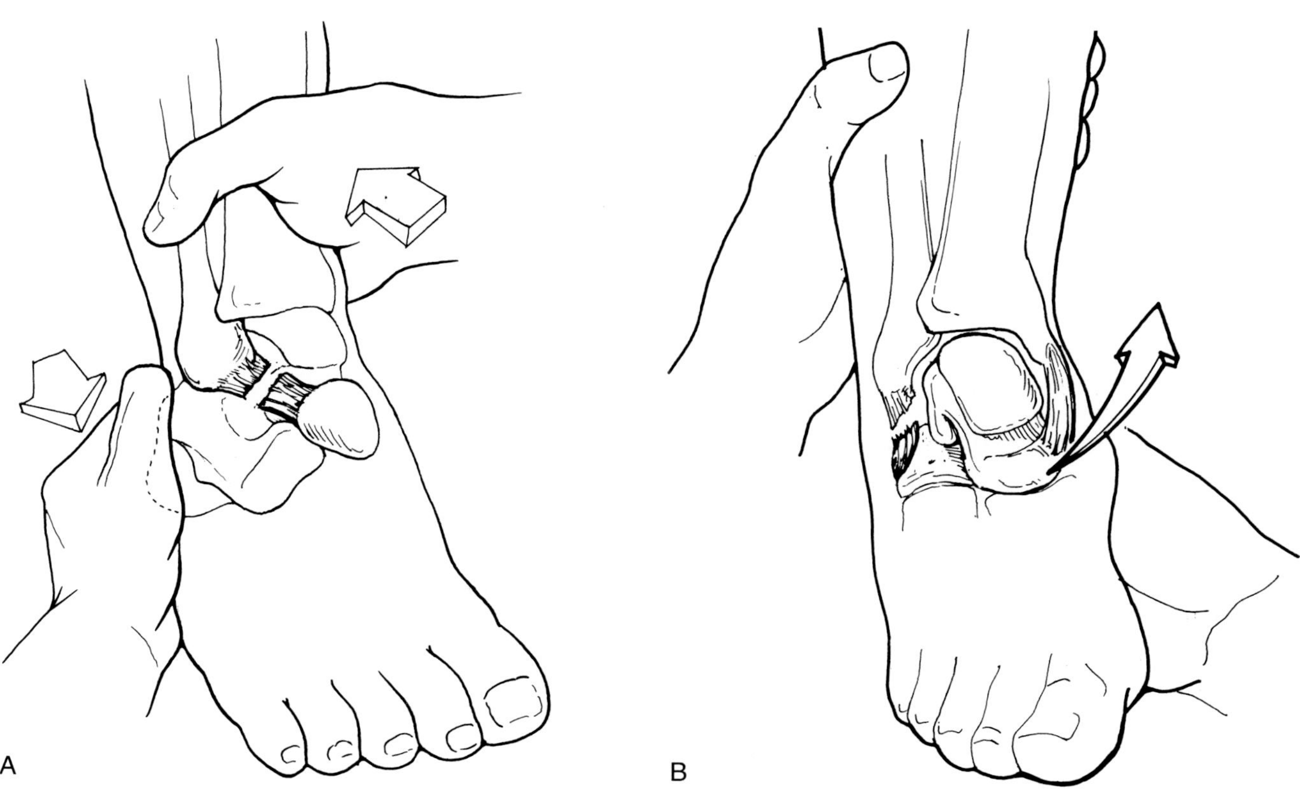

FIGURE 24–1. *A*, Anterior drawer test. *B*, Talar tilt test.

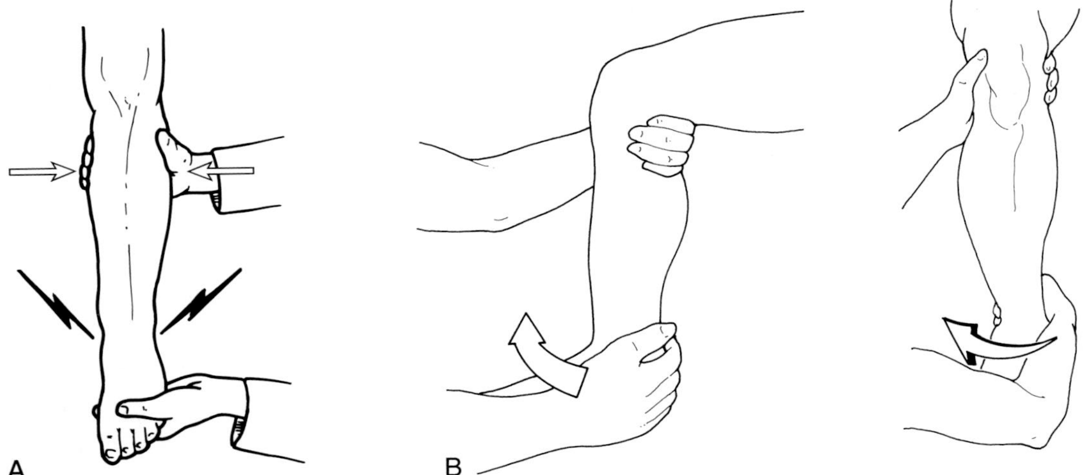

FIGURE 24–2. Squeeze test *(A)* and abduction-external rotation stress test *(B)* are used to rule out a syndesmotic injury. (From Miller MD, Cooper DE, Warner JJP: Review of Sports Medicine and Arthroscopy, 2nd ed. Philadelphia, WB Saunders, 2002, p 103.)

injury. Greater than 15 mm of tibiotalar tilt or greater than 5° of asymmetry with tilt testing suggests CFL instability. CT and MRI are usually not helpful in the evaluation of ankle instability.

NONOPERATIVE MANAGEMENT

Conservative treatment is the mainstay of ankle sprain treatment. RICE—*r*est, *i*ce, *c*ompression, and *e*levation—is initiated in the early phase. RICE is followed by supervised therapy, including peroneal strengthening and proprioceptive training. The use of an orthotic device is often helpful.

RELEVANT ANATOMY

An appreciation of the anatomy of the lateral aspect of the ankle is important before operating in this area (Fig. 24–3). The ATFL, which is a thickening in the joint capsule, is located deep to the inferior extensor retinaculum. The CFL lies deep to the peroneal tendons. The sural and superficial peroneal nerve branches should be avoided.

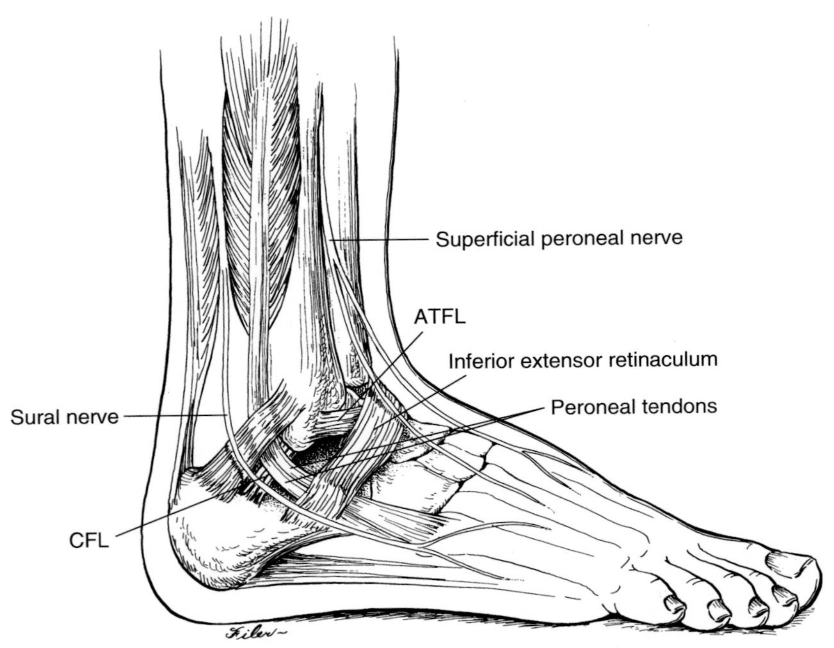

FIGURE 24–3. Anatomy of the lateral ankle. ATFL, anterior talofibular ligament; CFL, calcaneofibular ligament. (Modified from Taranow WS, Conti SF: Surgical treatment of lateral ankle instability. Op Tech Orthop 5:284–289, 1995.)

SURGICAL TECHNIQUE

Indications

Objective evidence of recurrent instability that has failed extended nonoperative management as outlined earlier is an indication for surgical treatment.

Technique

Modified Brostrom Procedure

1. Positioning: The patient is placed in the supine position, and a tourniquet is applied to the ipsilateral thigh.
2. Incision: A J-shaped incision is made from the anterior aspect of the distal fibula and curved inferiorly and posteriorly (Fig. 24–4).
3. The inferior extensor retinaculum is retracted inferiorly.
4. The ATFL is isolated and sharply incised in its midsubstance. Sutures are placed in the inferior flap from deep to superficial. These same sutures are placed in the superior flap from deep to superficial. In this manner, a pants-over-vest imbrication is accomplished. The foot is held in an inverted position for the remainder of the case.
5. The CFL is isolated, trimmed, and repaired in a similar fashion.
6. The inferior extensor retinaculum can be used to reinforce the repair as described by Gould.
7. The wound is closed in standard fashion, and a cast is applied with the foot in an inverted position.

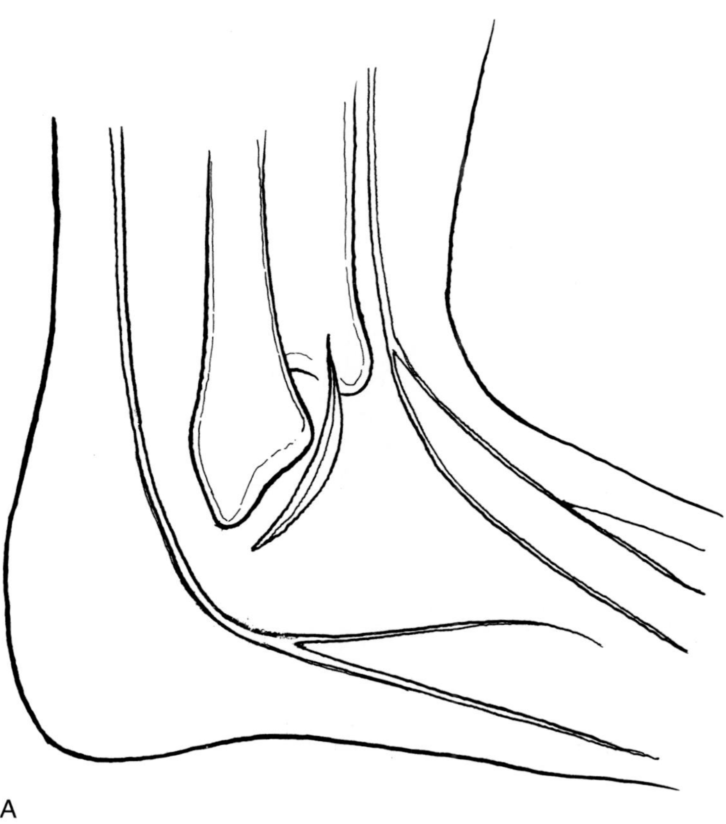

FIGURE 24–4. Brostrom technique. *A*, Incision.

Illustration continued on following page

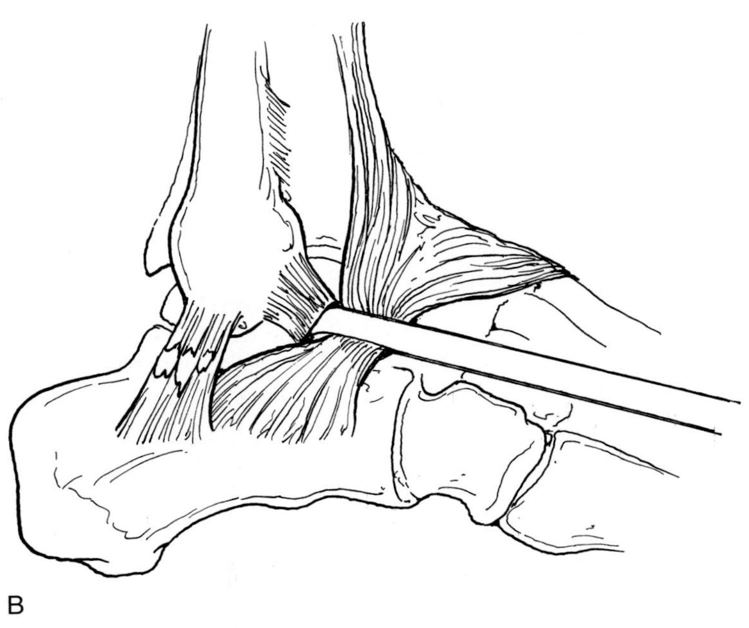

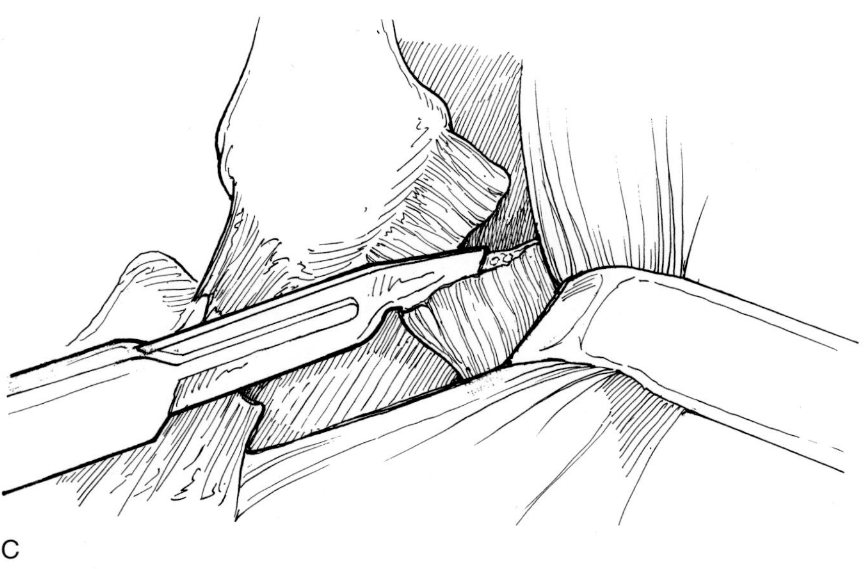

FIGURE 24–4 *Continued. B*, Retraction of extensor retinaculum. *C*, Longitudinal incision in ATFL.

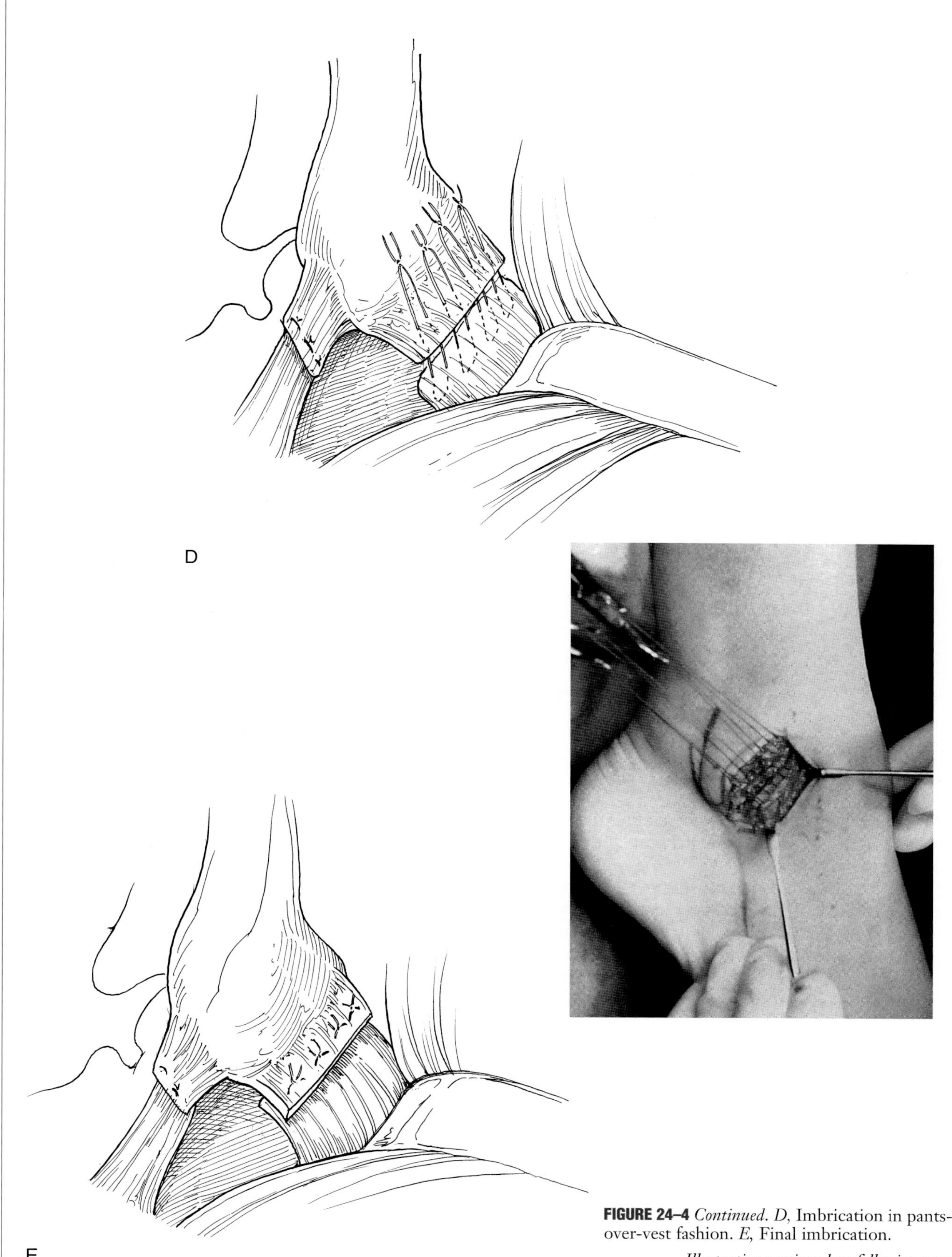

FIGURE 24–4 *Continued. D,* Imbrication in pants-over-vest fashion. *E,* Final imbrication.

Illustration continued on following page

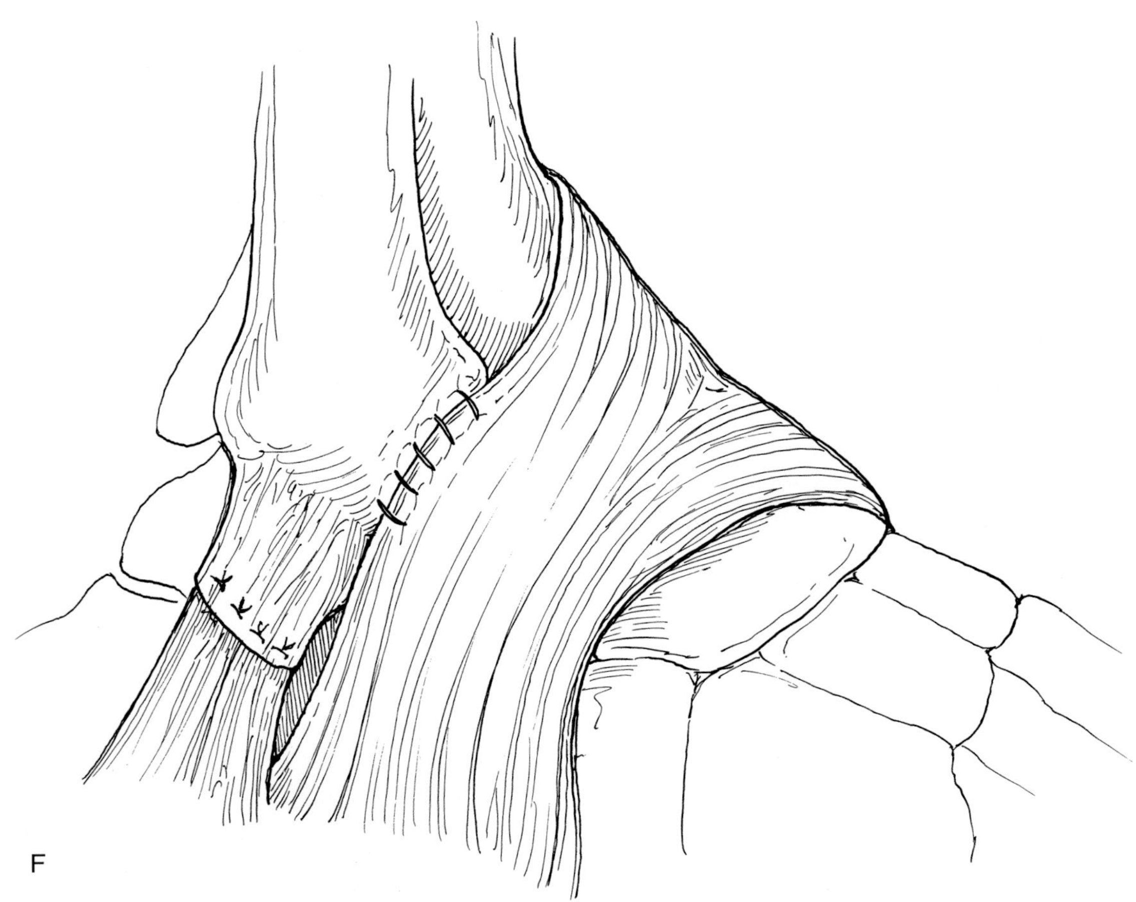

FIGURE 24–4 *Continued. F,* Extensor retinaculum is used to reinforce repair.

Tendon Augmentation Procedures

Although the Brostrom procedure is adequate for most cases of ankle instability, some surgeons prefer tendon augmentation procedures. Most of these procedures provide additional stability (especially to the subtalar joint). Many techniques have been described, including those of Evans, Chrisman-Snook, Watson-Jones, and Elmslie. Colville and Grondel described an anatomic augmentation that also is biomechanically superior to other techniques and is described (Fig. 24–5).

1. Positioning: The patient is placed in the supine position with a large bump under the affected leg or is placed in a decubitus position. A tourniquet is applied to the thigh and usually is insufflated for the procedure.
2. Incision: A 10-cm longitudinal incision is made from the base of the fifth metatarsal proximally over the lateral malleolus and along the posterior border of the fibula. The sural nerve is identified and protected.
3. The peroneal tendon sheath is opened, and the tendons are identified. The peroneus brevis tendon is located immediately behind the malleolus and frequently has distal muscle fibers that can be seen. The ATFL and CFL are identified and, if possible, repaired.
4. The anterior half of the peroneus brevis tendon is harvested, leaving the distal attachment intact. A whip stitch is placed in the proximal free end to facilitate passage.
5. Bone tunnels 4.5 mm in diameter are drilled in the calcaneus, fibula, and talus in the anatomic location of the ligaments. The calcaneal tunnel is drilled transversely, the fibular tunnel is oriented obliquely, and the talar tunnel is oriented vertically.
6. The graft is passed from the calcaneus (distal to proximal), the fibula (posterior to anterior), and the talus (superior to inferior) and sutured back to itself with the foot in eversion and neutral dorsiflexion.
7. The peroneal tendon sheath is repaired, and the wound is closed in layers.

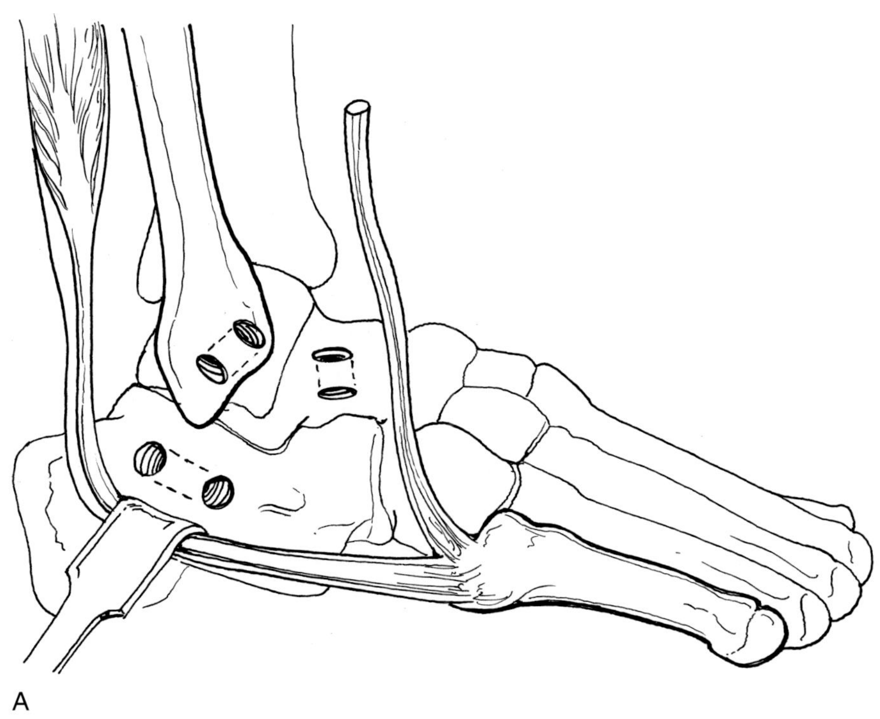

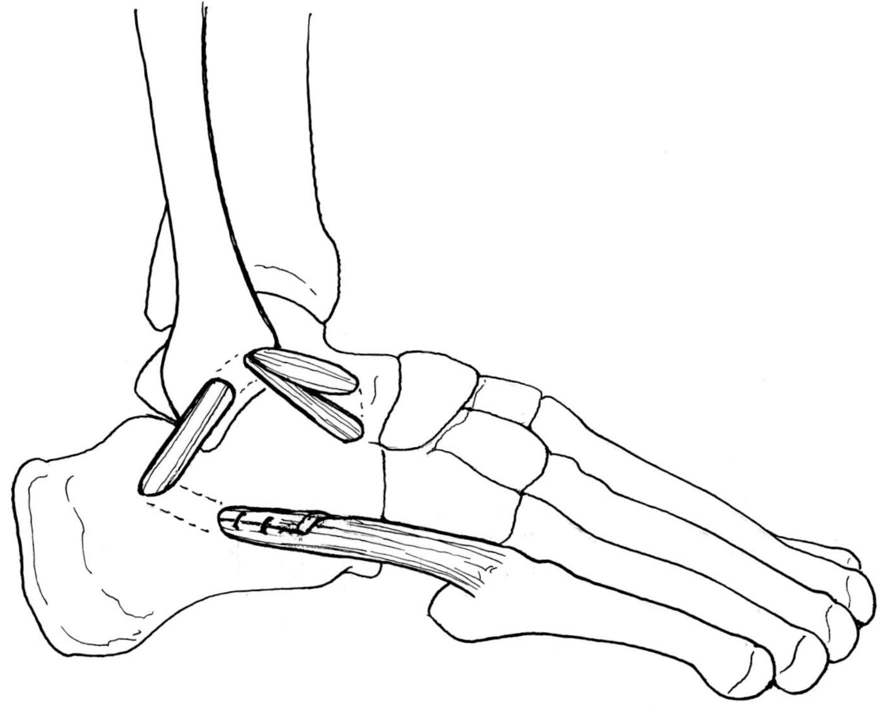

FIGURE 24–5. Colville technique using a strip of the peroneus brevis. *A*, Drill hole locations. *B*, Final reconstruction.

POSTOPERATIVE MANAGEMENT

Patients are immobilized in a below-knee cast for 6 weeks. Therapy is instituted, emphasizing range of motion and progressive resistive and proprioception exercises. Use of an ankle brace is encouraged for 6 months.

COMPLICATIONS

Complications include recurrence (<5%), overtightening, fracture, bleeding, infection, skin breakdown, and other problems.

RESULTS

The Brostrom procedure has proved to be an effective technique for most cases of ankle instability. Tendon augmentation procedures also are successful. Colville reported 10 of 12 patients with no functional limitations and an average strength of 90% of the opposite side with his technique.

REFERENCES

Brostrom L: Sprained ankles: VI. Surgical treatment of "chronic" ligament ruptures. Acta Chir Scand 132:551–565, 1966.

Colville MR: Surgical treatment of the unstable ankle. J Am Acad Orthop Surg 6:368–377, 1998.

Colville MR, Grondel RJ: Anatomic reconstruction of the lateral ankle ligaments using a split peroneus brevis tendon graft. Am J Sports Med 23:210—213, 1995.

Renstrom PAHF, Kannus P: Management of ankle sprains. Op Tech Sports Med 2:58–70, 1994.

Taranow WS, Conti SF: Surgical treatment of lateral ankle instability. Op Tech Orthop 5:284–289, 1995.

CHAPTER 25

Treatment of Posterior Tibial Tendon Dysfunction

INTRODUCTION

Posterior tibial tendon dysfunction is analogous to impingement syndrome and rotator cuff tears in the shoulder. Posterior tibial tendinitis, like impingement, is an overuse/attritional injury. Posterior tibial tendon rupture, similar to a rotator cuff tear, represents the other end of the spectrum.

HISTORY AND PHYSICAL EXAMINATION

Patients with posterior tibial tendinitis may relate a history of recent excessive training. Examination of their shoewear may suggest that they run with a pronated foot. Ruptures of the tendon typically occur in older women with no apparent trauma, although ruptures can occur in athletes. Pain and localized swelling may be present. A planovalgus deformity may be present in chronic cases. Tenderness, localized swelling, inability to heel walk, and decreased inversion strength are common. Additionally, the "too many toes sign," or an apparent asymmetry of the feet when viewed from behind, may be seen.

DIAGNOSTIC IMAGING

Plain radiographs are often normal. Long-standing disorders may have associated arthritis or a displacement of the calcaneus in relation to the tibia. MRI can be helpful in the diagnosis as well.

NONOPERATIVE MANAGEMENT

Early treatment includes modification of training and a medial heel wedge. Occasionally, cast or orthotic management may be necessary.

RELEVANT ANATOMY

Anatomy of the posteromedial aspect of the ankle should be well understood before embarking on surgical treatment (Fig. 25–1). The posterior tibial tendon lies in a groove immediately behind the medial malleolus. The flexor digitorum longus tendon and neurovascular structures lie immediately behind the tendon. The flexor retinaculum covers these structures.

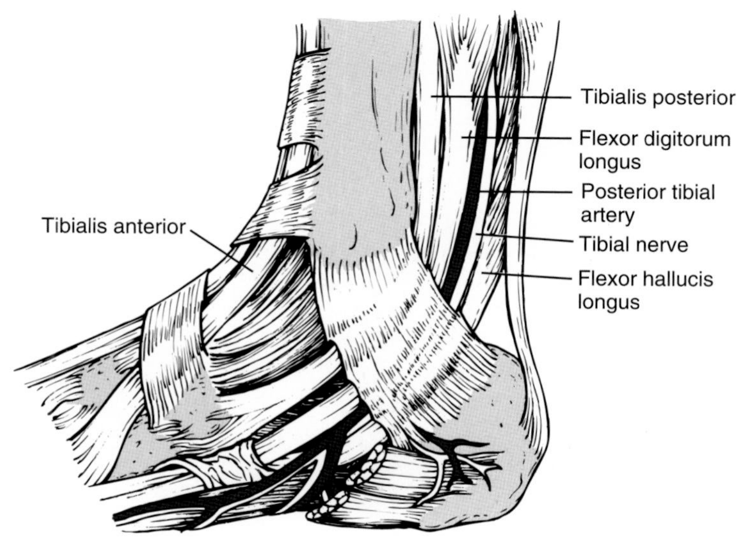

FIGURE 25–1. Anatomy of the posteromedial ankle. (From Carr JB, Trafton PG: Malleolar fractures and soft tissue injuries of the ankle. In Browner BD, Jupiter JB, Levine AM, Trafton PG [eds]: Skeletal Trauma, 2nd ed. Philadelphia, WB Saunders, 1998, pp 2327–2404.)

SURGICAL *TECHNIQUE*

Indications

Refractory tendinitis that has failed several months of nonoperative treatment is an indication for surgery. Complete ruptures with a flexible hindfoot (fixed hindfoot procedures may require fusions that are beyond the scope of this text) are another indication.

Technique

Débridement and Repair

1. Incision: A 10-cm incision is made from 3 cm proximal to the medial malleolus to the insertion of the posterior tibialis tendon at the navicular (Fig. 25–2).
2. Tenosynovectomy: The flexor retinaculum is released, and the tendon is inspected. Hypertrophic synovium is débrided.
3. Tendon débridement and repair: The tendon is débrided carefully, and torn portions are repaired with running 4–0 absorbable sutures and buried knots.
4. Groove deepening: The groove behind the posterior malleolus is deepened with a 0.25 gouge up to 2 cm proximal to the medial malleolus. The area is rasped, and bone wax is applied.
5. Pulley reconstruction: Two or three rectangular flaps are elevated off the flexor retinaculum and sutured on the opposite side of the tendon to prevent subluxation.

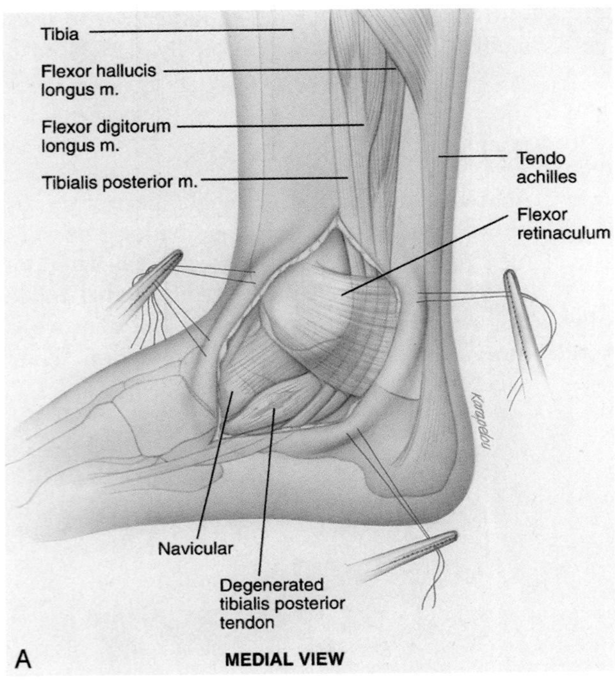

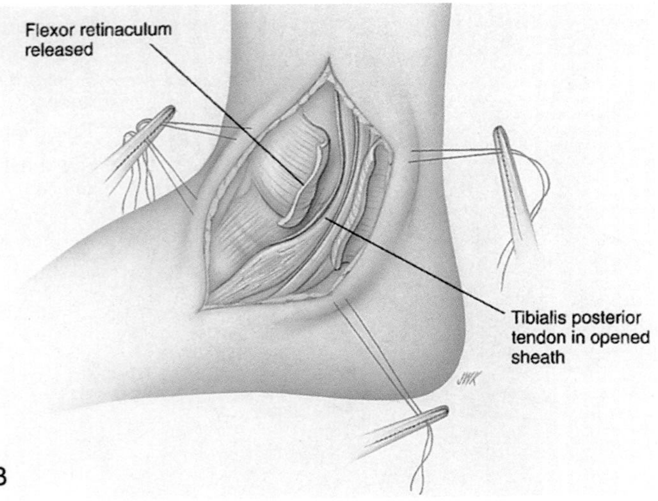

FIGURE 25–2. Débridement and repair of the posterior tibial tendon. *A*, Incision. *B*, Release of flexor retinaculum. *C*, Groove deepening. *D*, Tendon débridement and repair and development of pulleys from flexor retinaculum. *E*, Final pulley reconstruction and closure. (From Trevino SG: Alternative treatment of posterior tibial tendon dysfunction. Op Tech Orthop 6:197–202, 1996.)

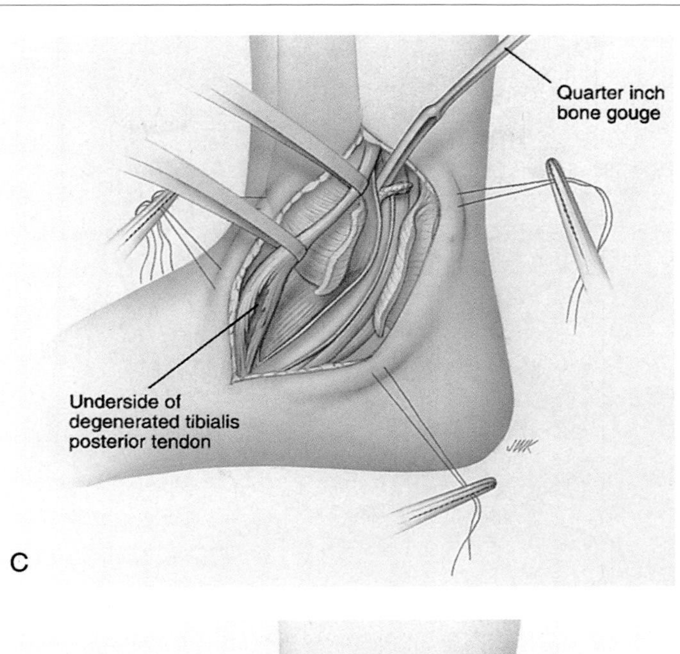

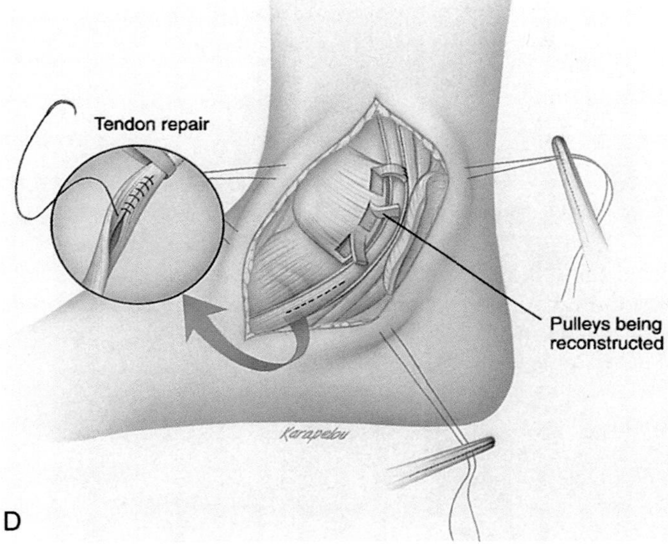

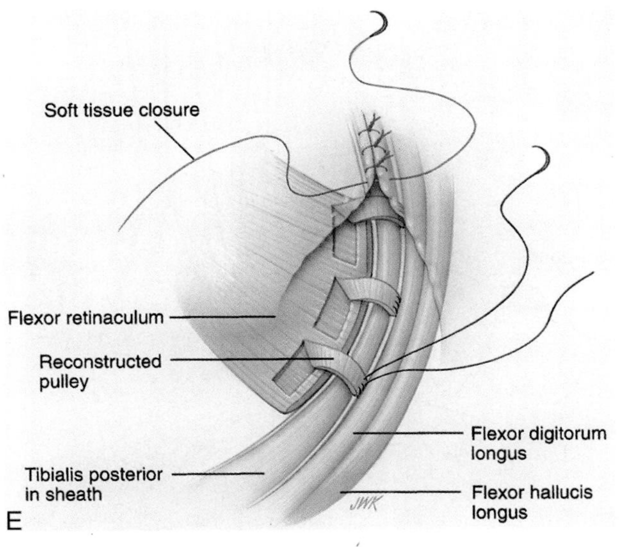

FIGURE 25–2 *Continued*

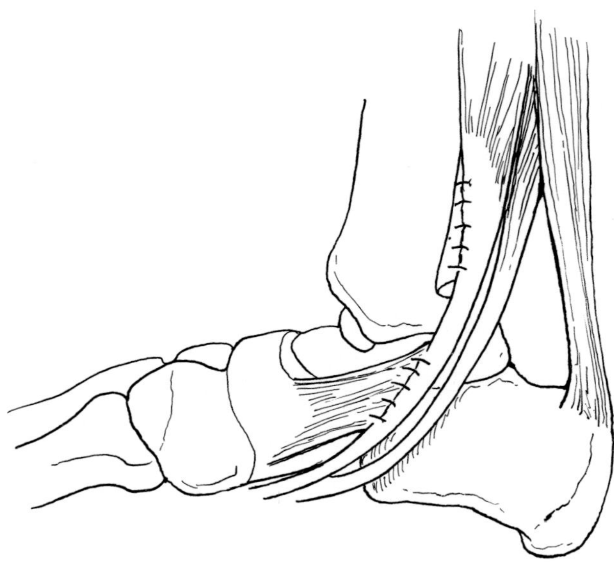

FIGURE 25–3. After release of the tendon sheath of the flexor digitorum longus, the proximal and distal portions of the posterior tibialis tendon are sutured to the intact flexor tendon.

Transfer

1. Incision and débridement are similar to that described previously.
2. If primary repair is not possible and the posterior tibial tendon is scarred and retracted within the tendon sheath, transfer of the flexor digitorum is recommended. The proximal and distal portions of the posterior tibial tendon are sutured to the intact flexor digitorum longus tendon (Fig. 25–3).
3. Alternatively, the tendinous portion of the flexor digitorum longus is transferred over to the posterior tibialis tendon, drilled through the navicular (the posterior tibialis insertion), and sutured back to itself (Fig. 25–4).

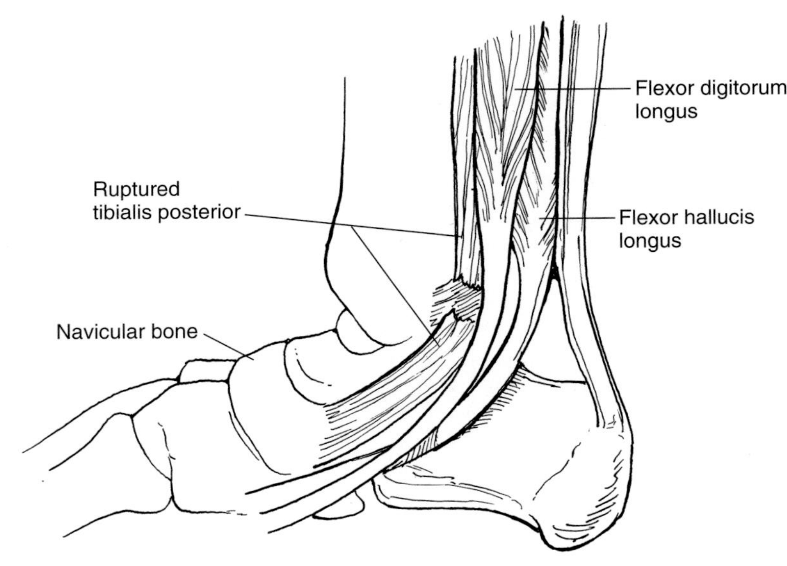

FIGURE 25–4. Reconstruction of the posterior tibialis tendon with flexor digitorum longus tendon. *A*, Posterior tibialis rupture.

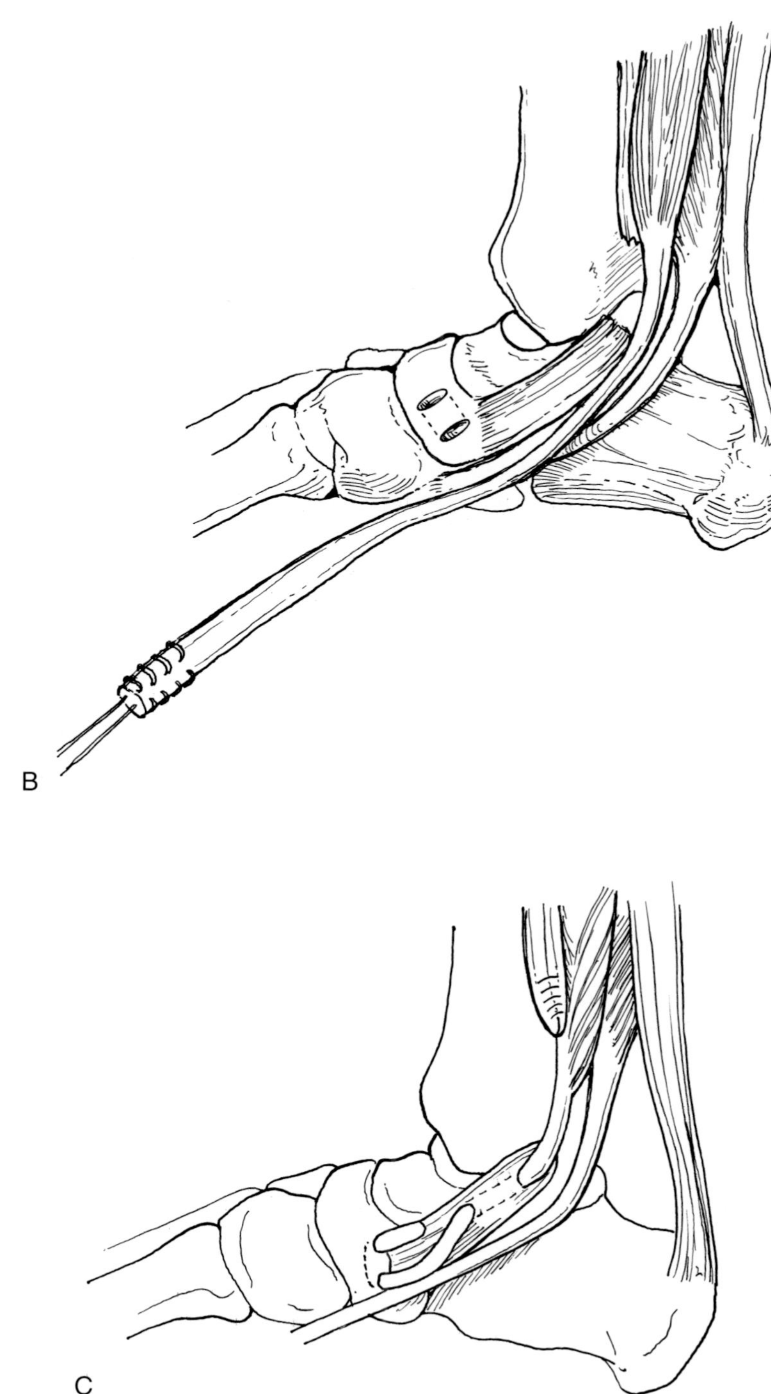

FIGURE 25–4 *Continued. B* and *C*, Reconstruction. The flexor tendon is detached from its insertion and reinserted through a drill hole in the navicular at the posterior tibialis insertion before it is sewn back to itself and the distal stump of the posterior tibialis.

POSTOPERATIVE MANAGEMENT

Postoperative management of tendon débridement and repair requires early motion. Transfers should be immobilized, however, for 4 to 6 weeks before motion is initiated. Strengthening is allowed after motion returns. Postoperative orthotic management for the residual flatfoot deformity and forefoot varus should be implemented to prevent recurrence.

COMPLICATIONS

Complications include loss of motion, rerupture, and skin problems.

RESULTS

Early results with débridement and repair are encouraging. Transfer procedures have a long history of moderate success; however, transfer does require sacrifice of a normal tendon.

REFERENCES

Conti SF: Posterior tibial tendon problems in athletes. Orthop Clin North Am 25:109–121, 1994.

Greenfield G, Stanish WD: Tendinitis and tendon ruptures. Op Tech Sports Med 2:9–17, 1994.

Jones DC: Tendon disorders of the foot and ankle. J Am Acad Orthop Surg 1:87–94, 1993.

Trevino SG: Alternative treatment of posterior tibial tendon dysfunction. Op Tech Orthop 6:197–202, 1996.

CHAPTER 26

Achilles Tendon Repair

INTRODUCTION

Achilles tendon ruptures typically occur in 30- to 50-year-old men and may be related to lack of vascularity in the tendon (2 to 3 cm proximal to its insertion in the calcaneus).

HISTORY AND PHYSICAL EXAMINATION

Achilles tendon injuries usually occur in jumping sports when an eccentric force is placed on the tendon with the foot dorsiflexed. It can follow Achilles tendinitis. Most patients report feeling a sudden snap, with warmth and swelling. A gap often can be palpated. The Thompson test (squeezing the calf normally plantar flexes the foot if the Achilles tendon is intact) is a very helpful test for diagnosing Achilles tendon rupture (Fig. 26–1).

DIAGNOSTIC IMAGING

Plain radiographs are typically normal. MRI identifies the rupture, but it usually is not required because the diagnosis usually is made based on the history and physical examination.

NONOPERATIVE MANAGEMENT

Cast immobilization (in progressively less plantar flexion) is still a reasonable treatment option. This treatment avoids anesthesia risks, hospitalization, and potential wound complications; however, the re-rupture rate after casting is more than twice the rate following surgical repair, and the strength and endurance are 20% to 30% less with cast treatment.

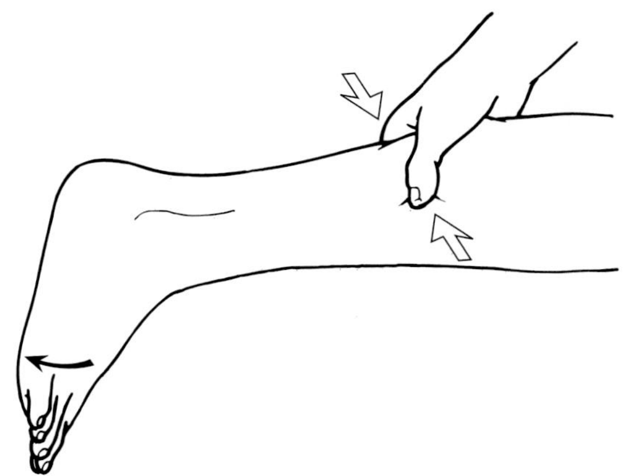

FIGURE 26–1. Thompson test for Achilles tendon injury consists of squeezing the injured calf and seeing if the foot plantar flexes. (Redrawn from Gould JA III, Davis GJ: Orthopedic Sports Physical Therapy. St. Louis, CV Mosby, 1985.)

RELEVANT ANATOMY

The Achilles tendon lies in its own sheath. The sural nerve is lateral to the tendon, and the plantaris tendon (sometimes used to supplement repairs) is medial to the tendon. The posterior tibial artery and tibial nerve are further medial (Fig. 26–2).

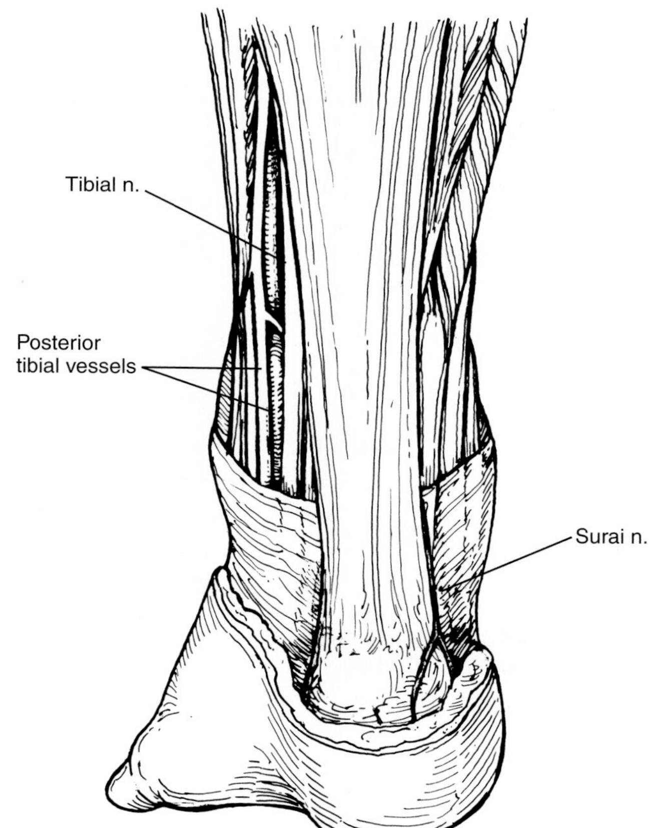

FIGURE 26–2. Achilles tendon anatomy.

SURGICAL TECHNIQUE

Indications

A physiologically young individual with an Achilles tendon rupture who does not wish to accept increased chances of re-rupture is a candidate for this procedure.

Technique

1. Incision: A 10-cm incision is made on the medial side of the tendon. Flaps are not created because this can disrupt the already tenuous skin.
2. Tendon exploration: The tendon sheath is identified and sharply incised longitudinally. The tendon is explored and débrided. Typically, the tendon does not tear cleanly but has a "mop end" appearance.
3. Tendon repair: Typically, a Bunnell suture with a heavy (No. 5) nonabsorbable suture is used for a core stitch to bring the tendon ends into close approximation. This approximation can be reinforced with multiple absorbable sutures (Fig. 26–3).
4. Alternatively, if the ends do not reapproximate well, a *three-bundle* technique can be used (Fig. 26–4).
5. If desired, the repair can be reinforced with the plantaris tendon (Fig. 26–5). The plantaris tendon also can be avulsed from its musculotendinous origin with an abrupt tug, and the tendon itself can be used with a free needle to reinforce the repair.
6. Chronic ruptures can be repaired with a V-Y flap, a strip of triceps surae fascia, or allograft.

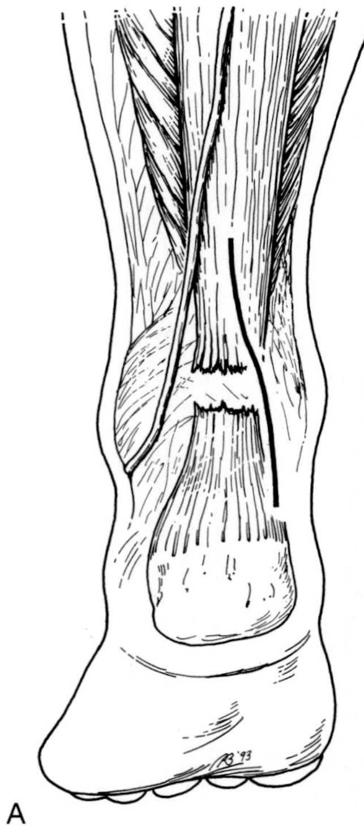

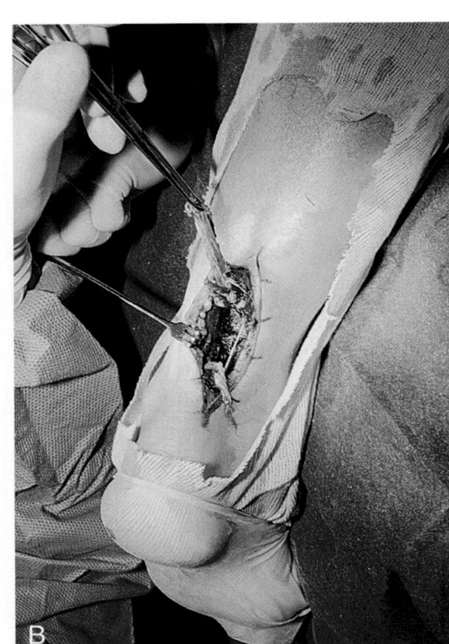

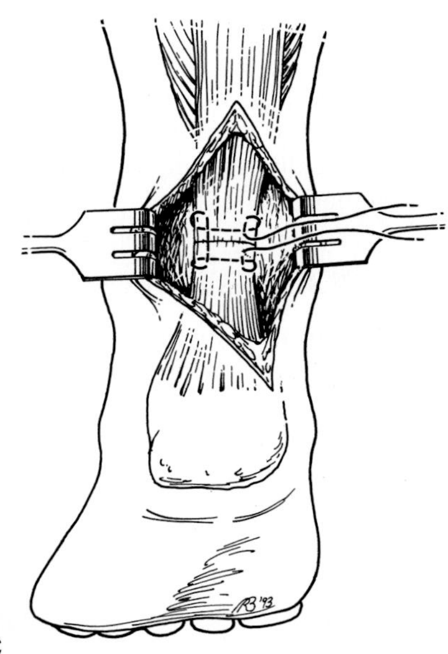

FIGURE 26–3. Primary repair using a Bunnell stitch. *A*, Incision. *B*, Exposure and mobilization. *C*, Repair. (*A* and *C* from Greenfield G, Stanish WD: Tendinitis and tendon ruptures. Op Tech Sports Med 2:9–17, 1994.)

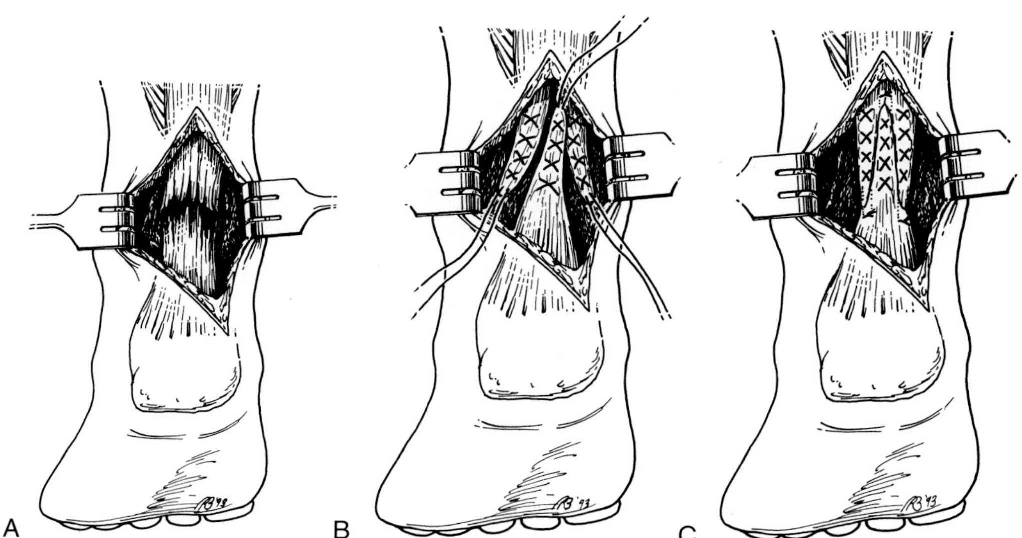

FIGURE 26–4. Three-bundle technique for Achilles tendon repair. *A*, Achilles tendon rupture. *B*, Fibers gathered into three bundles. *C*, Approximation of the fibers. (From Greenfield G, Stanish WD: Tendinitis and tendon ruptures. Op Tech Sports Med 2:9–17, 1994.)

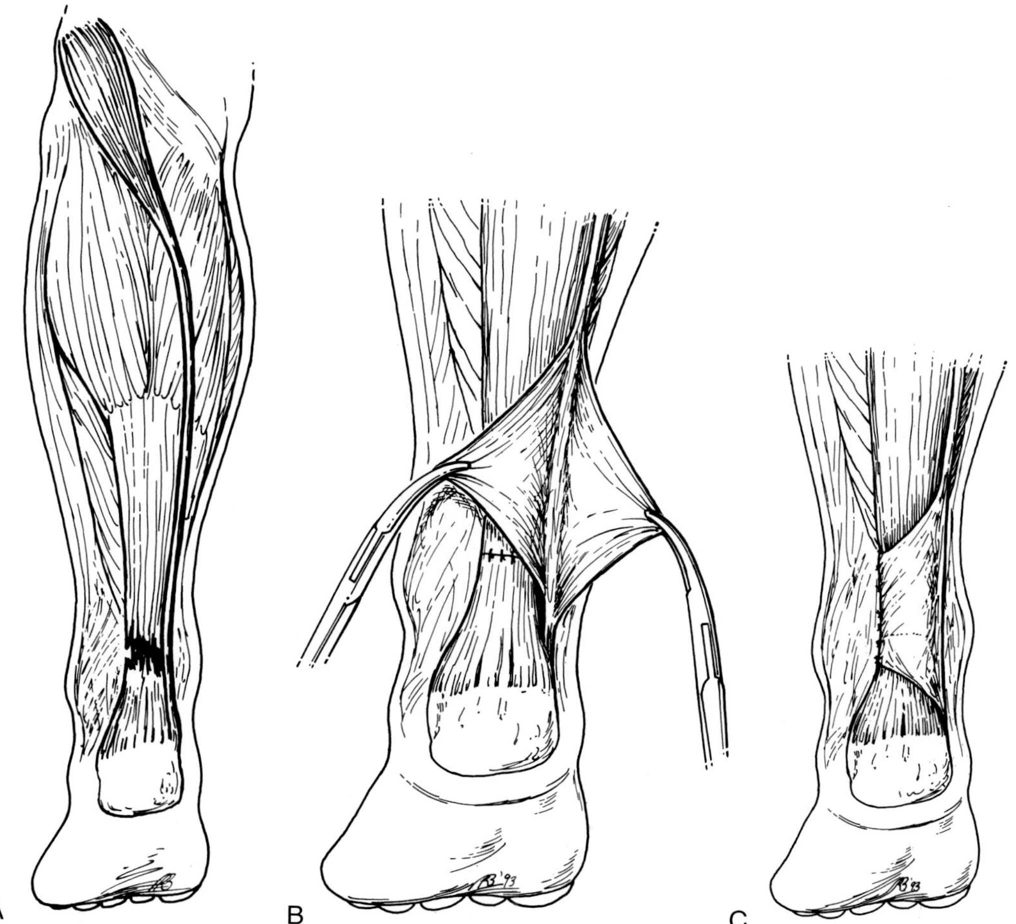

FIGURE 26–5. Reinforcement with plantaris tendon. *A*, Rupture. *B*, Achilles tendon is repaired, and plantaris tendon is divided and fanned. *C*, Plantaris tendon is used to reinforce repair. (From Greenfield G, Stanish WD: Tendinitis and tendon ruptures. Op Tech Sports Med 2:9–17, 1994.)

POSTOPERATIVE MANAGEMENT

The patient is placed in a cast or brace in approximately 15° of plantar flexion for about 1 month. This is followed by a heel lift and gentle, progressive, active-assisted exercises. Eccentric muscle strengthening is initiated 2 to 3 months postoperatively.

COMPLICATIONS

Infection and skin slough are risks with operative treatment of Achilles tendon ruptures, especially with a history of steroid use or steroid injections, peripheral vascular disease, or diabetes. Re-rupture, although less than half as common as with cast treatment, can occur in 10% of cases.

RESULTS

As indicated earlier, results are generally good. Most re-ruptures occur within a couple of weeks after cast removal, so extra care should be taken during this period.

REFERENCES

Greenfield G, Stanish WD: Tendinitis and tendon ruptures. Op Tech Sports Med 2:9–17, 1994.

Myerson MS, McGarvey W: Disorders of the insertion of the Achilles tendon and Achilles tendinitis. J Bone Joint Surg [Am] 80:1814–1824, 1998.

Saltzman CL, Tearse DJ: Achilles tendon injuries. J Am Acad Orthop Surg 6:316–325, 1998.

CHAPTER 27

Treatment of Peroneal Tendon Subluxation and Dislocation

INTRODUCTION

Displacement of the peroneal tendons from the back of the distal fibula can occur as a result of violent dorsiflexion of an inverted foot coupled with reflex contraction of these tendons. Excessive stress on the tendons causes them to tear the superior peroneal retinaculum.

HISTORY AND PHYSICAL EXAMINATION

Peroneal tendon displacement occurs most commonly in football or skiing injuries. In skiing injuries, skiers fall forward after the ski tip is caught in the snow. Patients may complain of pain and popping. Examination may confirm recurrent subluxation with provocative maneuvers.

DIAGNOSTIC IMAGING

Plain radiographs are usually normal; however, a rim fracture of the lateral aspect of the distal fibula may confirm the diagnosis (Fig. 27–1).

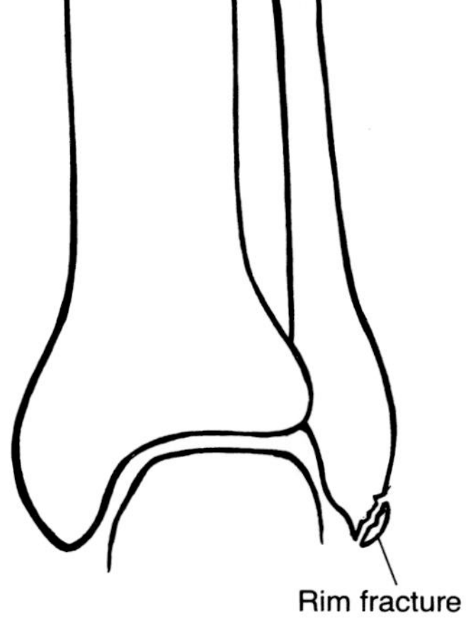

FIGURE 27–1. Rim fracture of the lateral aspect of the distal fibula associated with recurrent displacement of the peroneal tendons. (From Miller MD, Cooper DE, Warner JJP: Review of Sports Medicine and Arthroscopy, 2nd ed. Philadelphia, WB Saunders, 2002, p 85.)

NONOPERATIVE MANAGEMENT

An initial trial of casting in equinus sometimes can be successful, but it is unpredictable.

RELEVANT ANATOMY

Injury to the superior peroneal retinaculum disrupts the cartilaginous ridge and adjacent periosteum that usually keeps the peroneal tendons in their groove (Fig. 27–2).

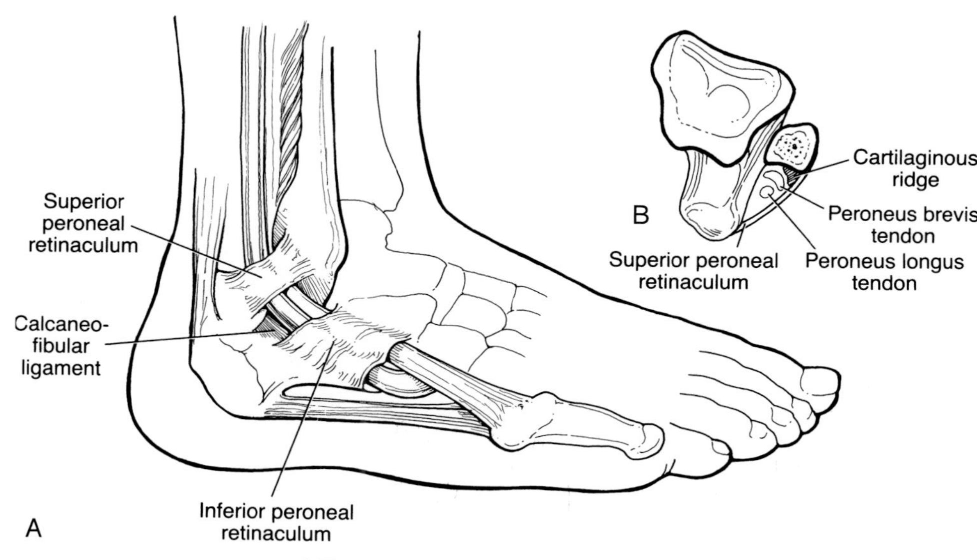

FIGURE 27–2. Normal relationship of peroneal tendons and the distal fibula. The superior peroneal retinaculum and a cartilaginous ridge hold the tendons in their groove behind the fibula. *A*, Lateral view. *B*, Superior view. (From Miller MD, Cooper DE, Warner JJP: Review of Sports Medicine and Arthroscopy, 2nd ed. Philadelphia, WB Saunders, 2002, p 85.)

SURGICAL *TECHNIQUE*

Indications

Surgery is indicated for recurrent displacement of the peroneal tendons in patients who have failed or are unwilling to attempt nonoperative management.

Technique

1. Positioning: The patient is positioned in a supine position with a bump under the ipsilateral side or in a lateral decubitus position with the injured leg up.
2. Approach: A reverse J incision is made along the posterior and inferior aspect of the distal fibula. The peroneal tendons are identified, and the overlying superior peroneal retinaculum is sharply incised (Fig. 27–3).
3. The tendons are replaced into their groove, and the periosteal flap and normal cartilaginous ridge are restored (Fig. 27–4).
4. If additional reinforcement is needed, a tendon slip from the Achilles tendon can be passed through drill holes in the fibula and sutured back to itself (Fig. 27–5). Other techniques (not shown) include groove deepening and bone block procedures.
5. Tendinitis of the peroneal tendons is unusual in athletes but can be addressed with primary débridement and repair or transfer (similar to posterior tibial tendinitis).

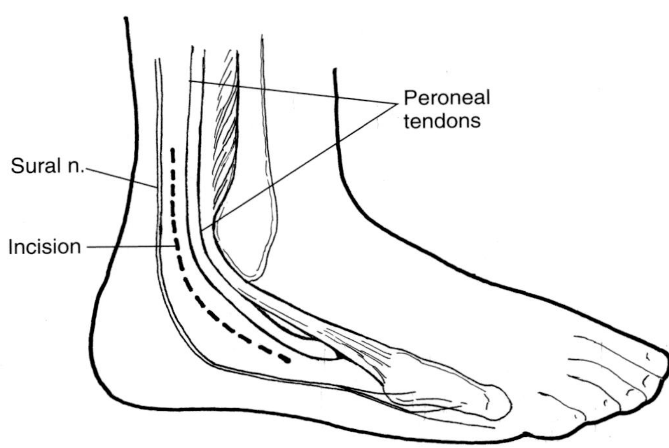

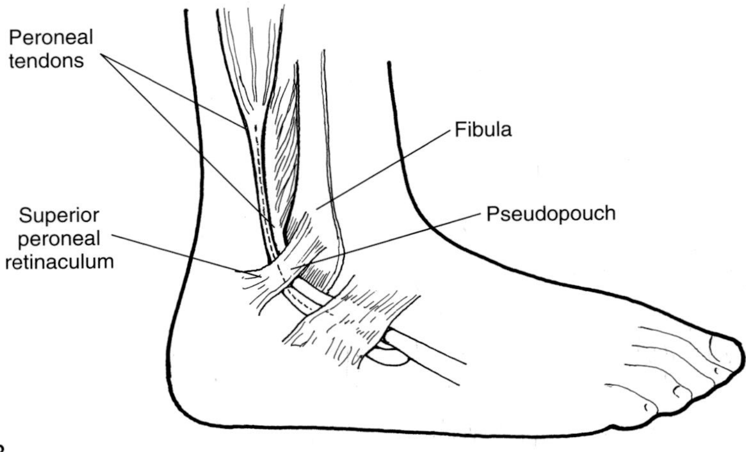

FIGURE 27–3. Initial dissection and exposure of the peroneal tendons. *A*, Incision. *B*, Initial dissection.

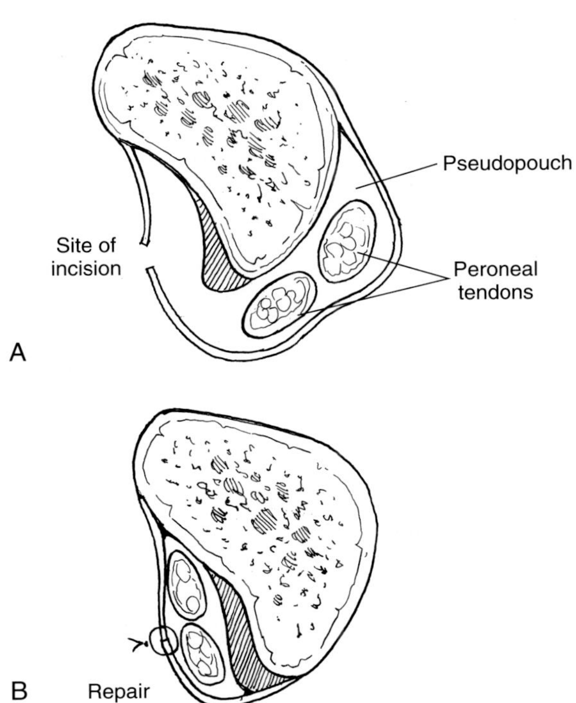

FIGURE 27–4. Open reduction of displaced tendons. *A*, Retinacular incision. *B*, Reduction. If the osteocartilaginous rim is injured, it also must be repaired (usually with suture anchors).

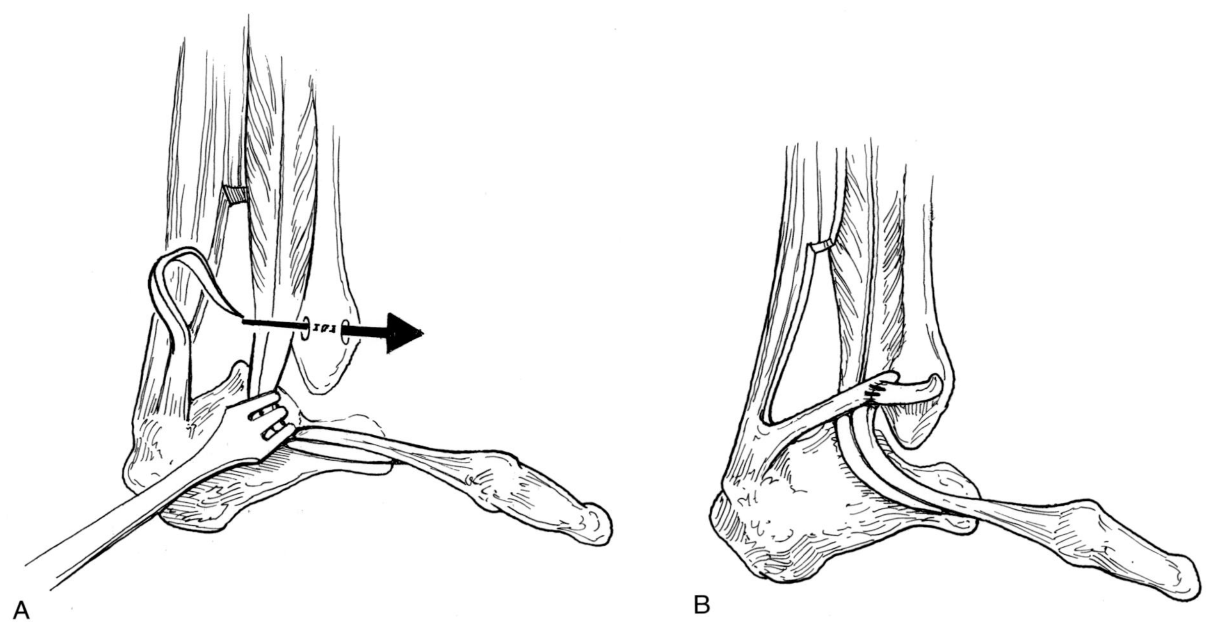

FIGURE 27–5. Reinforcement of the retinaculum with a strip of Achilles tendon. *A*, A strip of Achilles tendon is harvested and pulled through a transverse drill hole in the fibula. *B*, Final reinforcement.

POSTOPERATIVE MANAGEMENT

Patients are placed in a cast or a brace for approximately 1 month. Range-of-motion and strengthening exercises follow.

COMPLICATIONS

The sural nerve must be identified and protected throughout the case. Redisplacement risk can be reduced with careful attention to technique.

RESULTS

In general, results with these techniques are good, but it is difficult to return a professional athlete to the same level of performance after this surgery.

REFERENCES

Arrowsmith SR, Flemming LL, Allman FL: Traumatic dislocations of the peroneal tendons. Am J Sports Med 11:142, 1983.

Brage ME, Hansen ST: Traumatic subluxation/dislocation of the peroneal tendons. Foot Ankle 13:423–430, 1992.

Greenfield G, Stanish WD: Tendinitis and tendon ruptures. Op Tech Sports Med 2:9–17, 1994.

Renstrom PAHF: Mechanism, diagnosis, and treatment of running injuries. Instr Course Lect 42:225–234, 1993.

Sammarco J: Peroneal tendon injuries. Orthop Clin North Am 25:135–145, 1994.

CHAPTER 28

Treatment of Os Trigonum

INTRODUCTION

The unfused or fractured os trigonum can cause impingement in certain athletes, especially in dancers. Although this condition is frequently asymptomatic, it can cause significant problems in dancers because full plantar flexion of the foot and ankle is necessary to dance en pointe.

HISTORY AND PHYSICAL EXAMINATION

Dancers may complain of posterolateral pain that is exacerbated when their foot in placed in the demi-pointe and full-pointe positions (Fig. 28–1). Patients must be examined carefully to determine that the location of the tenderness is behind the peroneal tendons. Forced passive flexion of the ankle mimics the symptoms of which the patient complains. Injection of local anesthetic into the area relieves these symptoms.

DIAGNOSTIC IMAGING

Lateral radiographs typically reveal the os trigonum. Stress radiographs taken with the foot maximally plantar flexed may show impingement (Fig. 28–2*A*). Positive radiographs must be correlated carefully with patient symptoms. Bone scans can be helpful, if positive. The role of CT and MRI is controversial. MRI may be helpful, however, in the evaluation of associated flexor hallicus longus tendinitis (Fig. 28–2*B* and *C*).

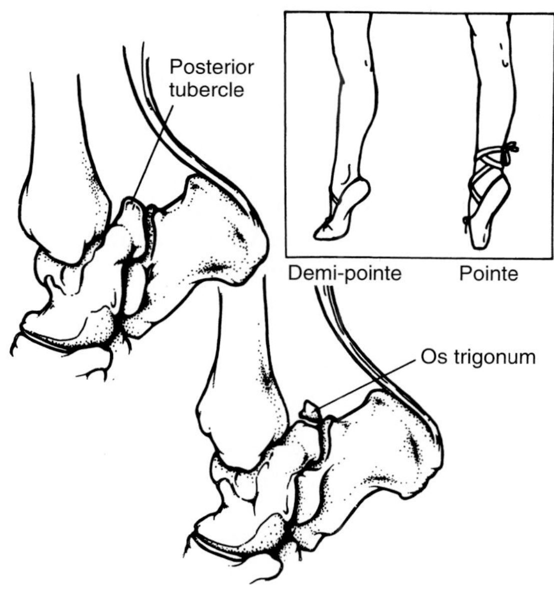

FIGURE 28–1. Positioning of the foot in demi-pointe and full-pointe can result in impingement in patients with an unfused os trigonum *(below)*. (From Hardaker WT Jr: Foot and ankle injuries in classical ballet dancers. Orthop Clin North Am 20:621–627, 1989.)

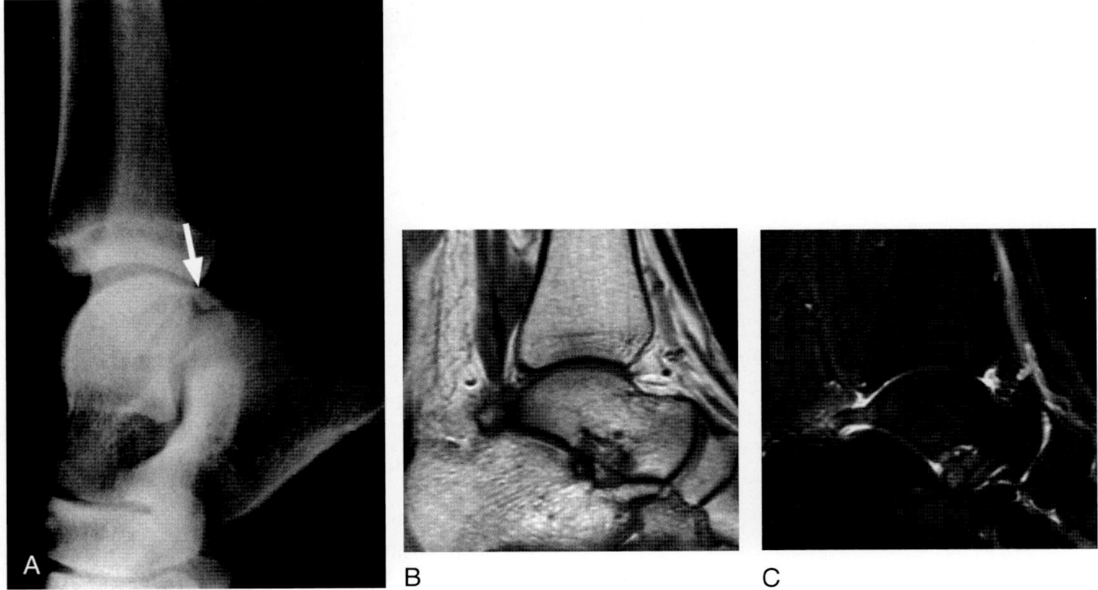

FIGURE 28–2. *A*, Radiograph of ankle in full plantar flexion with os trigonum *(arrow)*. T1-weighted *(B)* and T2-weighted *(C)* MRI shows os trigonum and associated flexor hallucis longus tendinitis. (*A* from Quirk R: Common foot and ankle injuries in dance. Orthop Clin North Am 25:123–133, 1994.)

NONOPERATIVE MANAGEMENT

Initial treatment attempts to disrupt the chronic cycle of pain and swelling caused by impingement. Activity modification (avoiding pointe work), nonsteroidal anti-inflammatory drugs, ice, and physical therapy should be attempted. Low-heeled shoes, strapping, taping, and orthotic devices may help, particularly if they restrict extreme plantar flexion. Limited steroid injections may be considered.

RELEVANT ANATOMY

The unfused os trigonum represents an ununited posterior tubercle of the talus. There is some variability in this process (Fig. 28–3). The posterior aspect of the talus can be approached from either the medial or the lateral side. Because of the location of the neurovascular structures behind the medial malleolus, excision of a symptomatic os trigonum usually is done through a lateral incision.

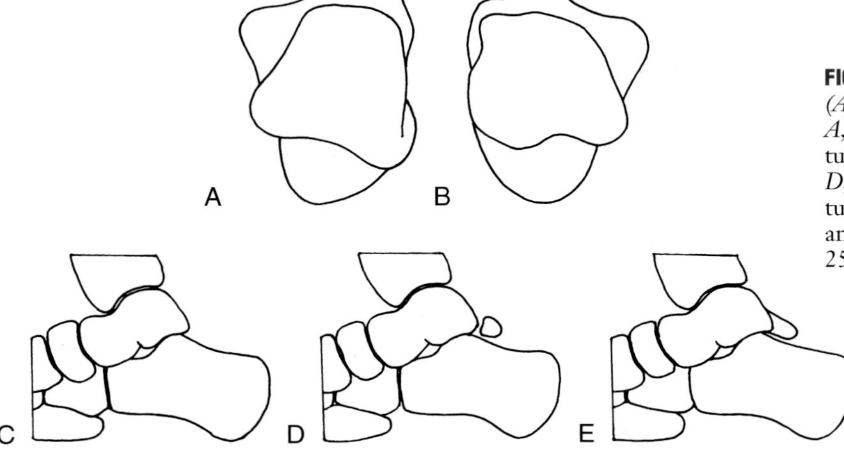

FIGURE 28–3. Posterior talus as seen from above (*A* and *B*) and in lateral view (*C*, *D*, and *E*). *A*, Unfused os trigonum. *B*, Normal posterior tubercle. *C*, Absence of posterior protuberance. *D*, Unfused os trigonum. *E*, Large posterior tubercle. (From Quirk R: Common foot and ankle injuries in dance. Orthop Clin North Am 25:123–133, 1994.)

SURGICAL *TECHNIQUE*

Indications

Indications for surgery are recurrent or refractory symptoms after extended nonoperative treatment.

Technique

A 5-cm incision is made behind the lateral malleolus (Fig. 28–4). The sural nerve is identified and protected. The peroneal tendons are retracted anteriorly, and the retrocalcaneal space is exposed. The os trigonum is denuded of all attachments, and the remaining surface is smoothed with a rasp. Standard closure is accomplished.

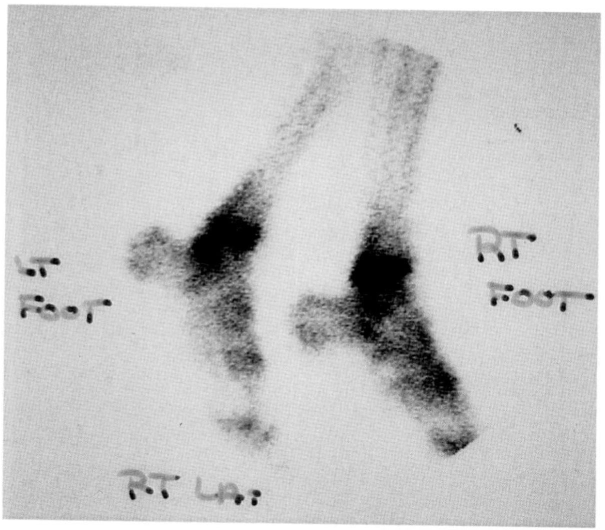

A

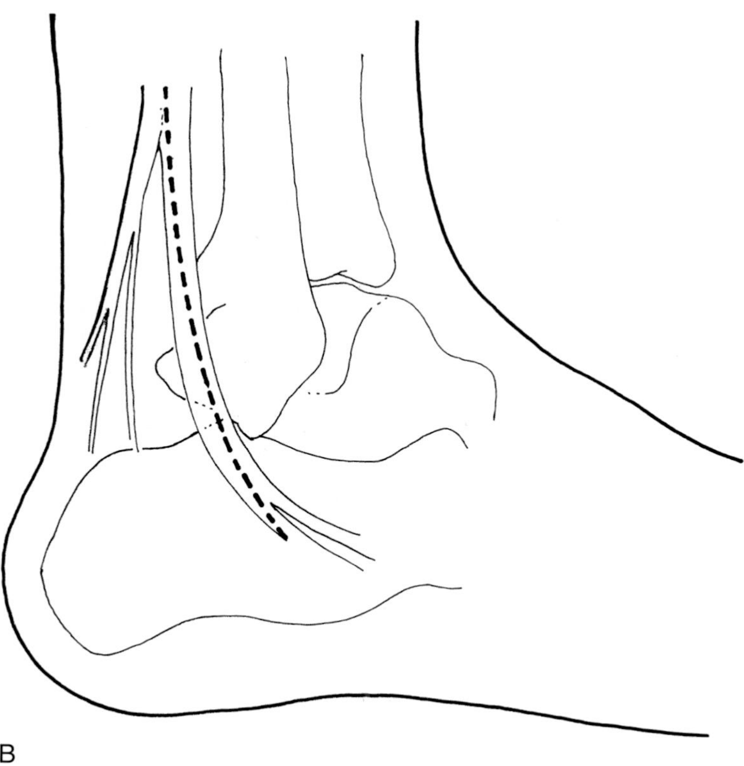
B

FIGURE 28–4. Surgical technique for excision of os trigonum. *A*, Preoperative bone scan shows focal uptake in the area of the os. *B*, Planned incision

Illustration continued on following page

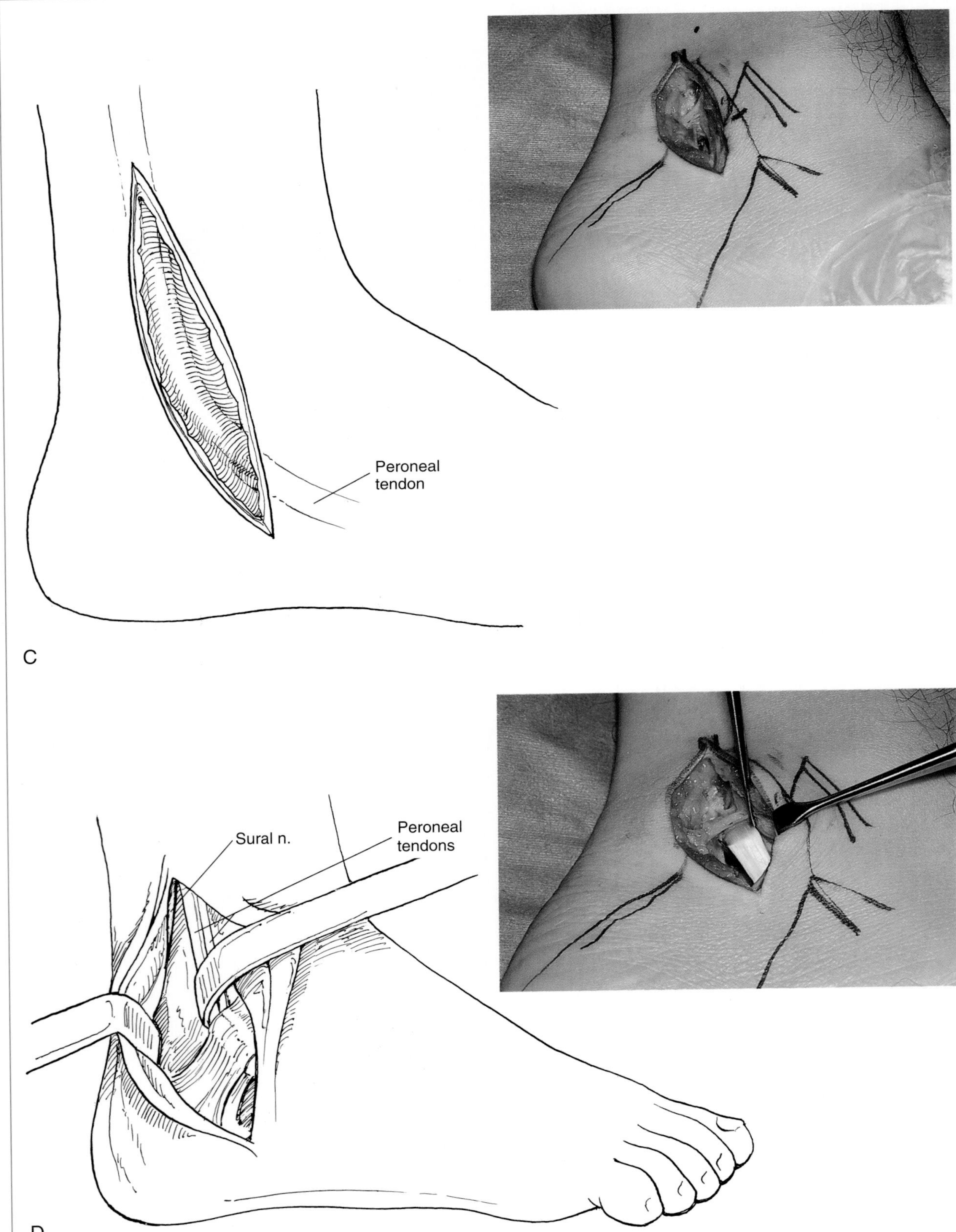

FIGURE 28–4 *Continued. C,* Subcutaneous dissection exposing peroneal tendon sheath. *D,* Retraction of the peroneal tendons and the sural nerve.

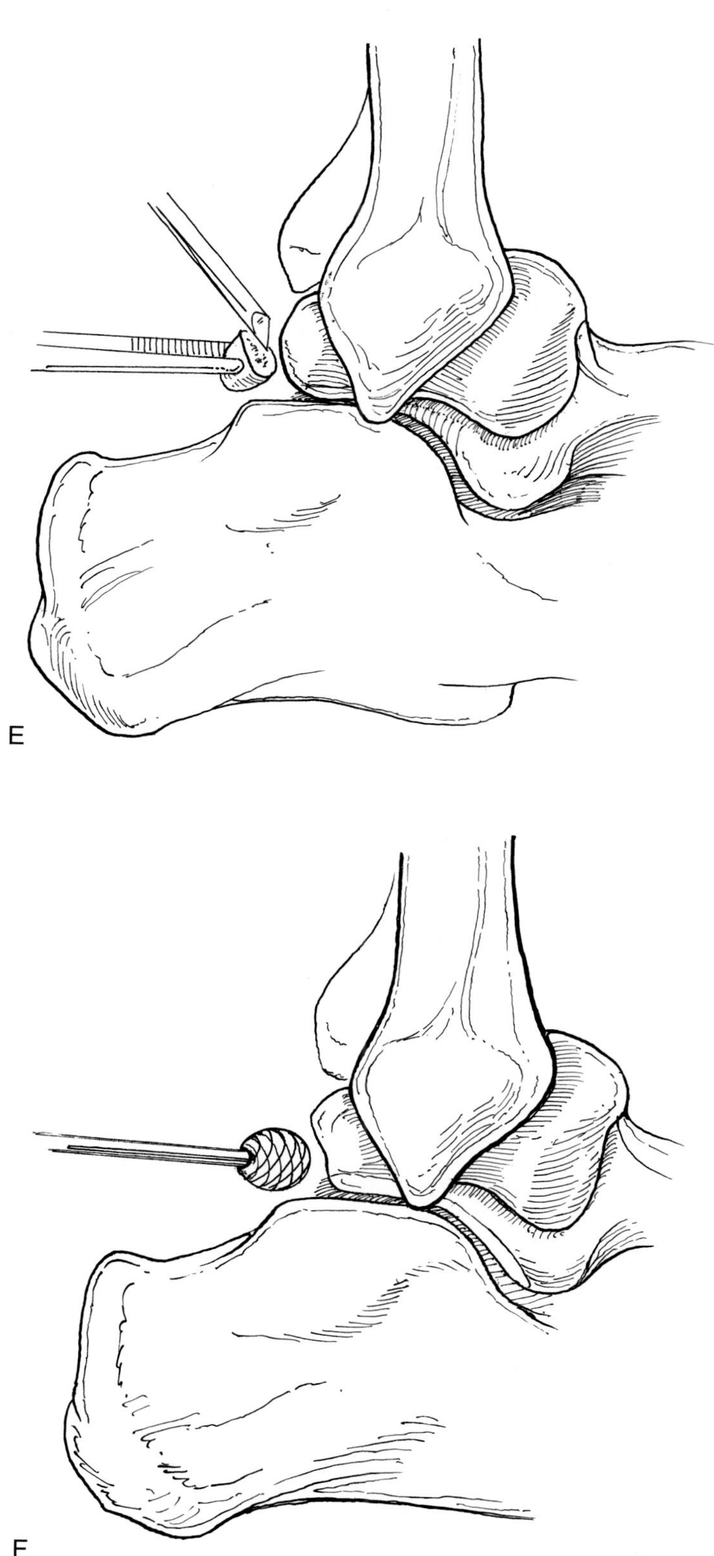

FIGURE 28–4 *Continued. E,* Excision of the os. *F,* Smoothing of the bed.

Illustration continued on following page

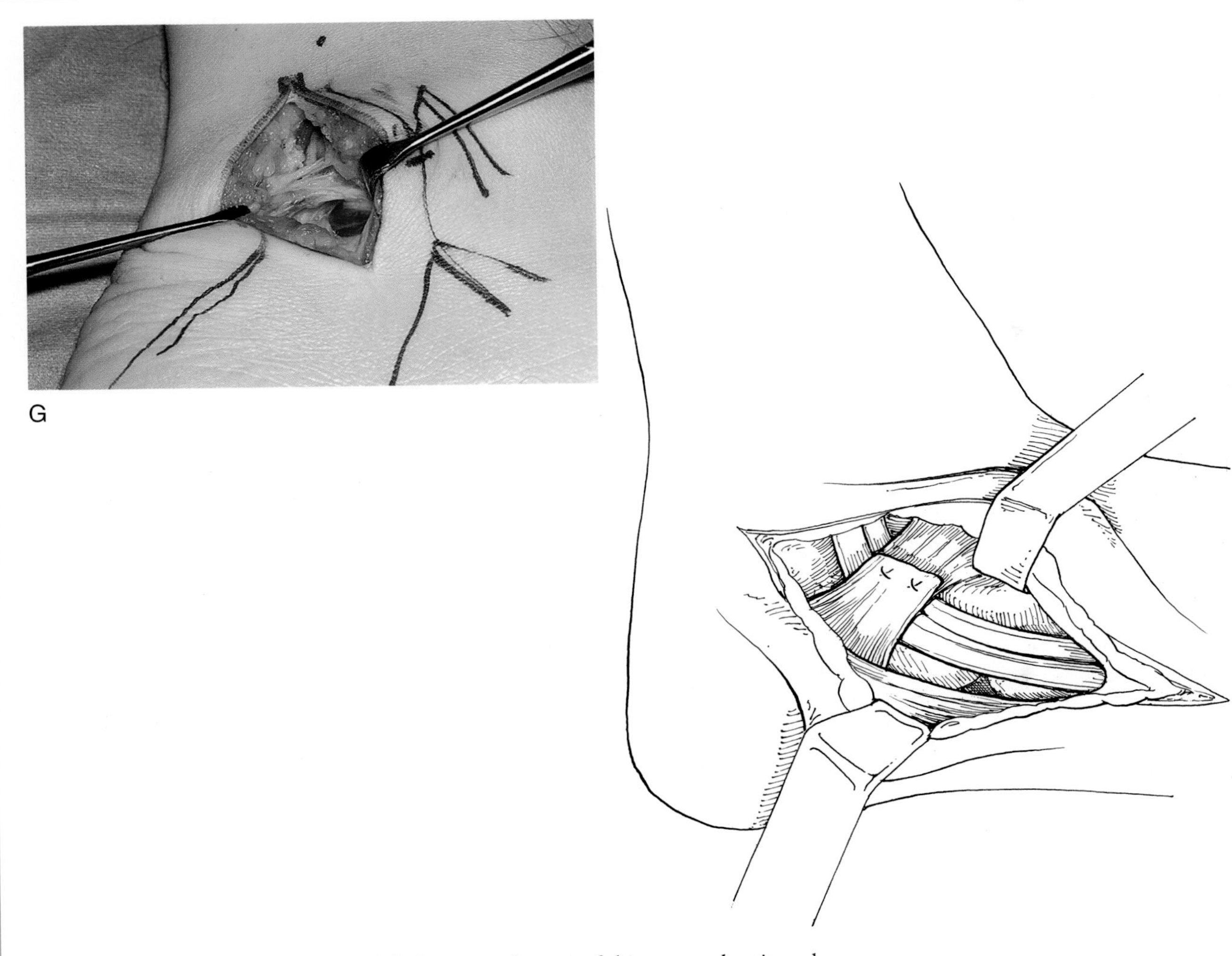

FIGURE 28–4 *Continued. G,* Closure includes reattachment of the peroneal retinaculum.

POSTOPERATIVE MANAGEMENT

A compressive dressing is applied, and the ankle is immobilized 10 to 14 days. Immobilization is followed by range-of-motion exercises and progressive weight bearing. Full return to dancing may take 6 months.

COMPLICATIONS

Perhaps the most common complication is failure to relieve symptoms, related to a failure to identify whether the os is responsible for the patient's pain. Other problems, such as bleeding and infection, also can occur.

RESULTS

Although it may take some time to return to sports or dancing, good results can be expected. In a series reported by Hamilton, 15 of 17 patients had a good result with this procedure.

REFERENCES

Hamilton WG: Stenosing tenosynovitis of the flexor hallucis longus tendon and posterior impingement upon the os trigonum in ballet dancers. Foot Ankle 3:74–80, 1982.

Hardaker WT Jr: Foot and ankle injuries in classical ballet dancers. Orthop Clin North Am 20:621–627, 1989.

Marotta JJ, Micheli LJ: Os trigonum impingement in dancers. Am J Sports Med 20:533–536, 1992.

Quirk R: Common foot and ankle injuries in dance. Orthop Clin North Am 25:123–133, 1994.

Renstrom PAHF, Kannus P: Injuries of the foot and ankle. In DeLee JC, Drez D Jr (eds): Orthopaedic Sports Medicine: Principles and Practice. Philadelphia, WB Saunders, 1994, pp 1705–1767.

CHAPTER 29

Treatment of Sports-Related Lower Extremity Fractures

INTRODUCTION

Although it is difficult to generalize, several fractures occur commonly in sports and may require surgical management by the sports medicine physician.

HISTORY AND PHYSICAL EXAMINATION

Several key features of sports-related lower extremity fractures are as follows:

Fracture	*Mode of Injury*	*Physical Examination*
Hallux sesamoids (medial < lateral)	Overuse injuries	Pain, tenderness
	Direct trauma	Pain with passive dorsiflexion
	Forced dorsiflexion	Pain relief with lidocaine injection
Fifth metatarsal base (Jones)	Inversion ankle injury Chronic (lateral overuse)	Point tenderness pain with inversion stress; may be insidious
Tarsometatarsal (Lisfranc) (lateral > medial)	Motor vehicle accident, sports (force to plantar flexed foot)	Pain, swelling, inability to bear weight
Tarsal navicular	Jumping sports/ overuse	Vague, diffuse foot pain; pain during activity
Ankle	Inversion injury	Pain, deformity
Tibial stress	Overuse	Pain with activity

DIAGNOSTIC IMAGING

Radiographic views and findings are as follows:

Fracture	*Radiographic Views*	*Findings*
Hallux sesamoids	Anteroposterior, lateral, lateral oblique	Lateral oblique shows lateral sesamoid
	Tibial sesamoid, axial sesamoid	Tibial sesamoid view taken perpendicular
Fifth metarsal base (Jones)	Anteroposterior, lateral, oblique	Fracture line, intramedullary sclerosis
Lisfranc	Anteroposterior, lateral, oblique	Medial edge of second metatarsal base aligns with medial edge of middle cuneiform on anteroposterior and oblique
Tarsal navicular	Anteroposterior, lateral, oblique Bone scan, computed tomography	Most in sagittal plane, in central one third
Ankle	Anteroposterior, lateral, mortise	Fracture line, displacement of mortise
Tibial stress	Anteroposterior, lateral	"Dreaded black line" on lateral

NONOPERATIVE MANAGEMENT

Nonoperative management can be attempted for nondisplaced acute sesamoid fractures, acute nondisplaced Jones and tarsal navicular fractures (non–weight bearing), minor Lisfranc injuries with stable reductions, and initial management of tibial stress fractures.

RELEVANT ANATOMY

Each of these difficult-to-treat sports-related fractures occurs in areas that have a tenuous blood supply.

SURGICAL *TECHNIQUE*

Hallux Sesamoid Fractures

Indications

Indications are symptoms occurring for at least 6 months and stress fractures that do not respond to 12 weeks of casting.

Technique

A 3-cm medial straight incision is made, and the retinacular hood overlying the medial capsule and abductor hallucis is incised. The capsule is incised, exposing the sesamoids. The medial sesamoid is removed by incision of the intersesamoid ligament. A small blade is used to incise along the plantar and articular surface of the sesamoid, protecting the flexor hallucis longus, and the sesamoid is removed. The medial capsule and skin are closed, and a bulky dressing and short-leg cast are applied (Fig. 29–1).

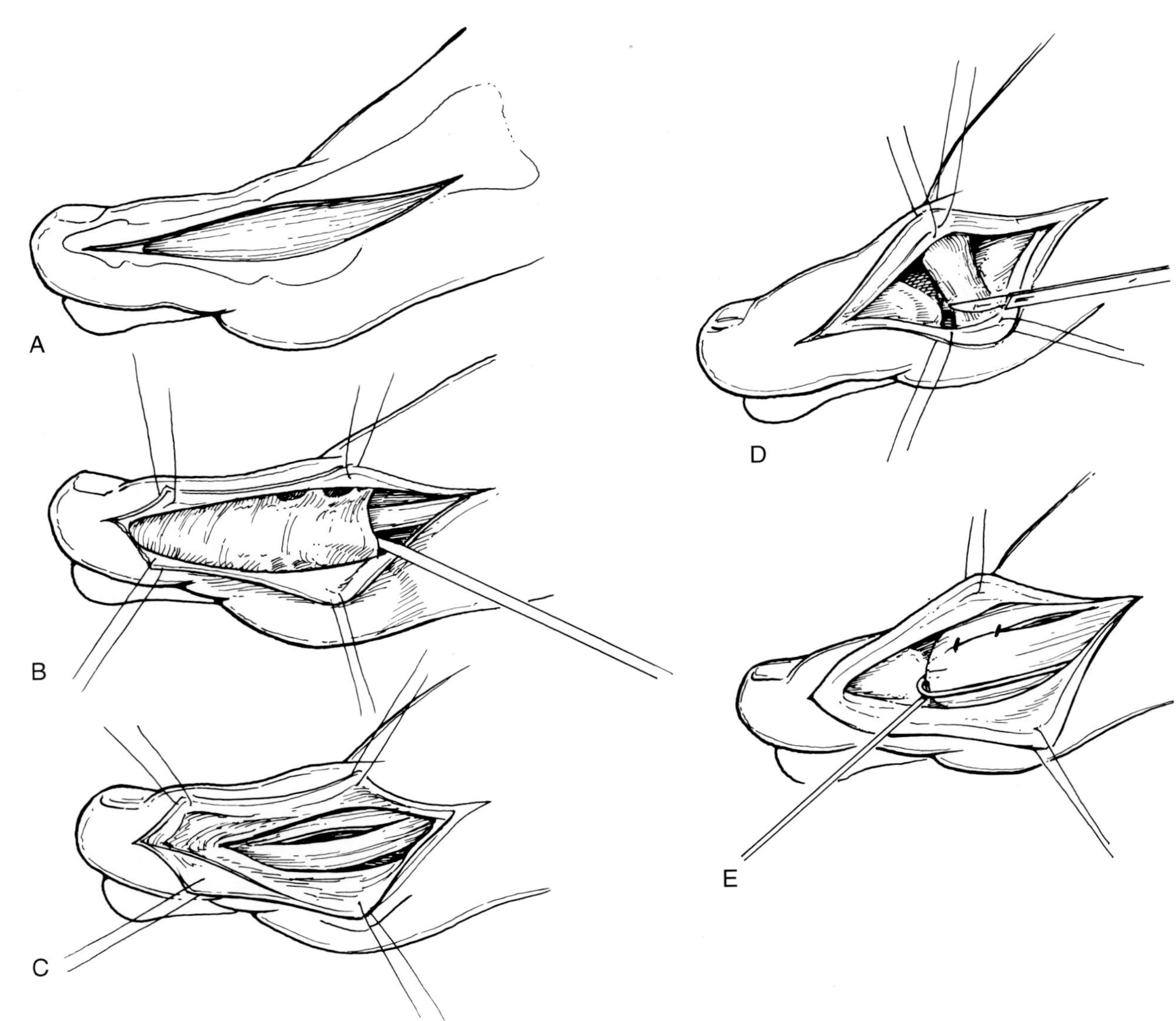

FIGURE 29–1. Excision of tibial sesamoid. *A*, Skin incision. *B*, Incision of tendon sheath. *C*, Exposure of flexor tendons. *D*, Sesamoid excision. *E*, Closure.

Fifth Metatarsal Base Fractures

Indications

Indications include failure of conservative management, especially in high-performance athletes with evidence of chronic (preexisting stress) fractures.

Technique

A 2- to 3-cm horizontal incision is made over the base of the fifth metatarsal, and the two branches of the sural nerve are identified and protected. A cannulated guide wire is placed down the shaft of the fifth metatarsal under fluoroscopic guidance. The wire is measured, left in place, and overdrilled with a cannulated drill. A 4.5-mm partially threaded cancellous screw is placed over the wire after tapping. Bone graft may be placed in the fracture site if desired, but it is usually not required. A bulky dressing and short-leg cast are applied (Fig. 29–2).

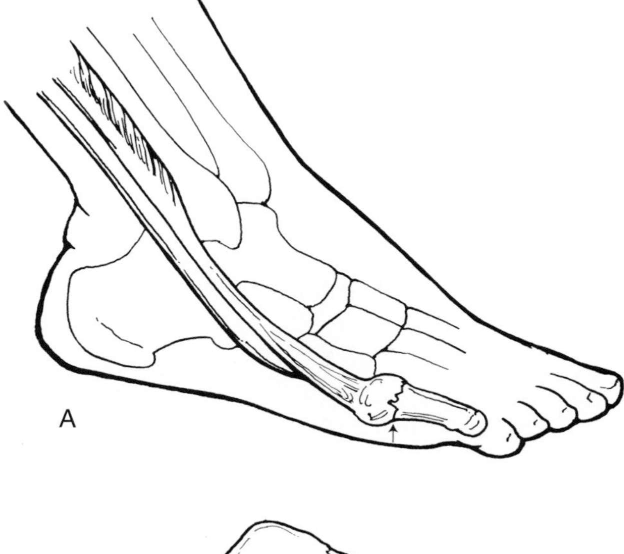

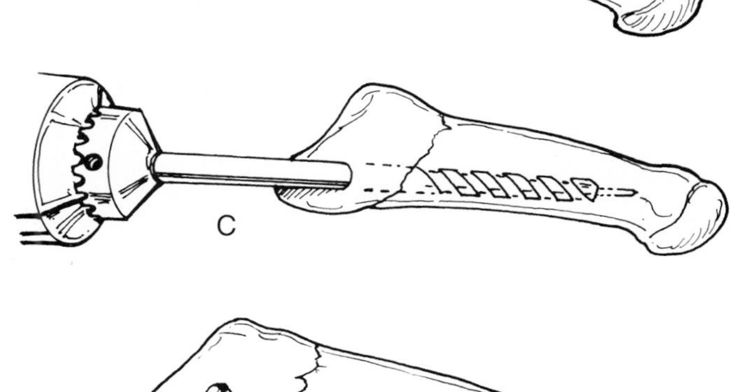

FIGURE 29–2. Open reduction and internal fixation of a Jones fracture. *A*, Fracture is typically at the metaphyseal/diaphyseal junction *(arrow)*. *B*, Guide wire insertion. *C*, Drilling. *D*, Screw insertion. *E*, Clinical AP radiograph of an acute Jones fracture. *F*, AP radiograph after lateral medullary fixation and fracture healing.

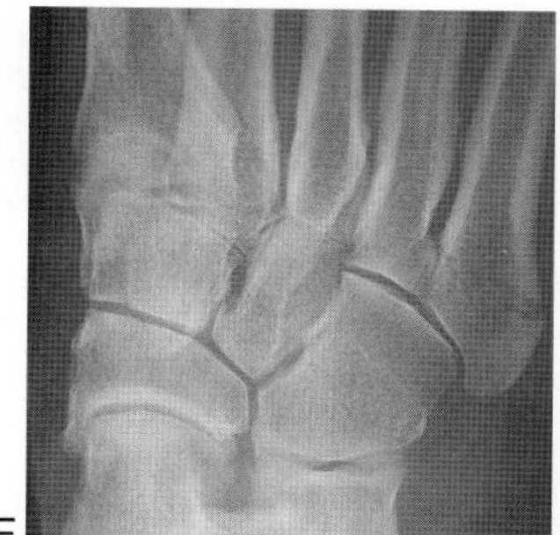

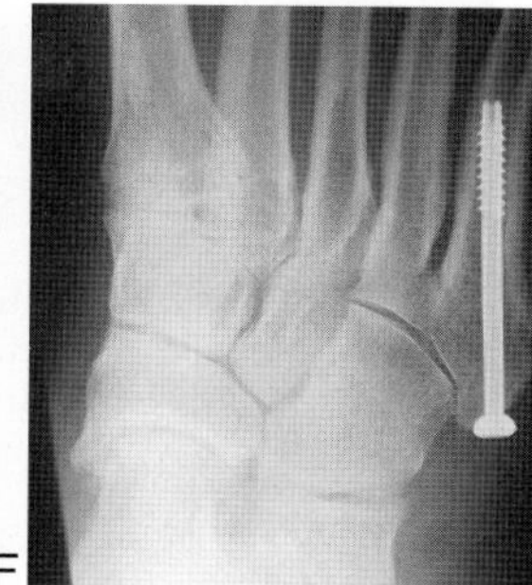

Lisfranc Fractures

Indications

Failure to obtain a stable anatomic reduction with closed methods is an indication for surgery.

Technique

A 4- to 5-cm longitudinal incision is made in the first intermetatarsal space. The extensor hallucis longus, dorsalis pedis artery, and deep peroneal nerve are identified and protected. The second metatarsal base is identified, and the second metatarsal phalangeal joint is opened and débrided. If the medial cuneiform is displaced, it is reduced and pinned to the middle cuneiform. The second metatarsal is then reduced and fixed to the middle cuneiform. If the first metatarsal is involved, it also is reduced and stabilized to the middle cuneiform. If the lateral three metatarsals remain unreduced, a second incision is made in the third intermetatarsal space, the joints are débrided and reduced, and the fifth metatarsal is stabilized to the cuboid. A bulky dressing and splint are applied (Fig. 29–3).

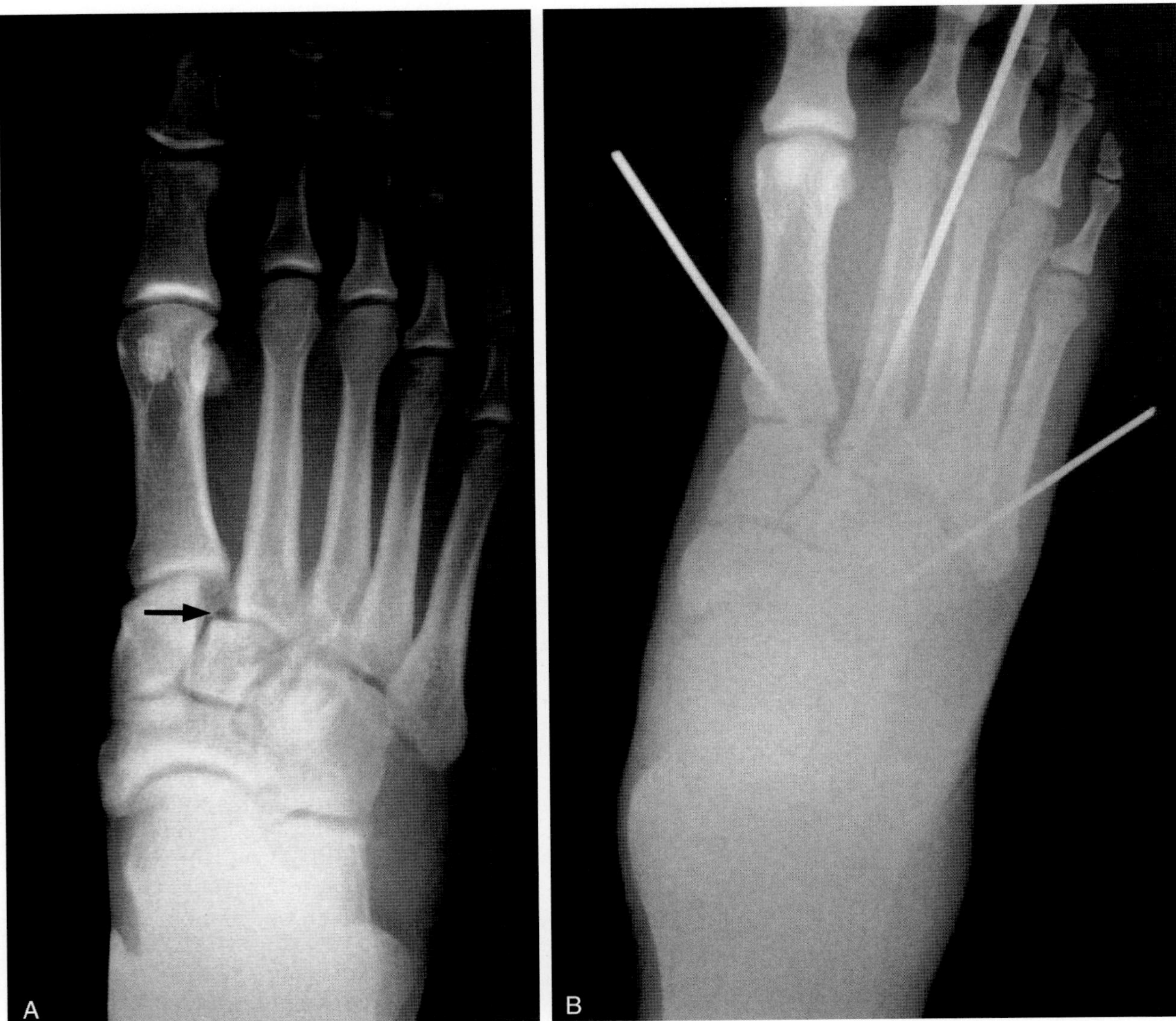

FIGURE 29–3. *A*, Anteroposterior radiograph shows a displaced Lisfranc injury. Note disruption of the alignment of the second metatarsal base with the medial edge of the middle cuneiform *(arrow)*. *B*, Fixation with K-wires. (*A* and *B* from Whittle AP: Fractures of the foot in athletes. Op Tech Sports Med 2:43–57, 1994.)

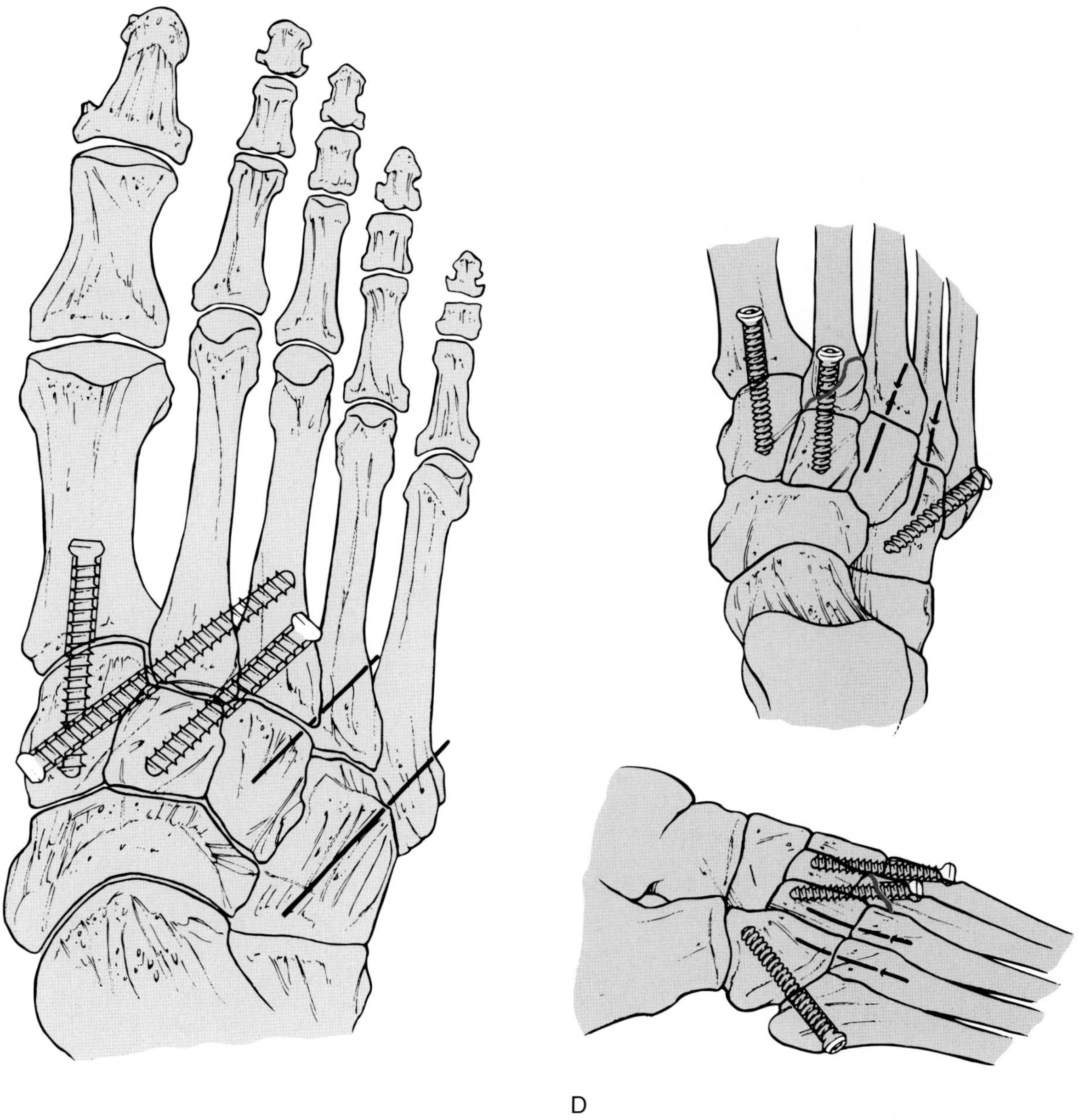

FIGURE 29–3 *Continued. C* and *D*, Alternative fixation options using screws. (*C* and *D* from Hansen ST Jr: Foot injuries. In Browner BD, Jupiter JB, Levine AM, Trafton PG [eds]: Skeletal Trauma, 2nd ed. Philadelphia, WB Saunders, 1998, pp 2405–2438.)

Illustration continued on following page

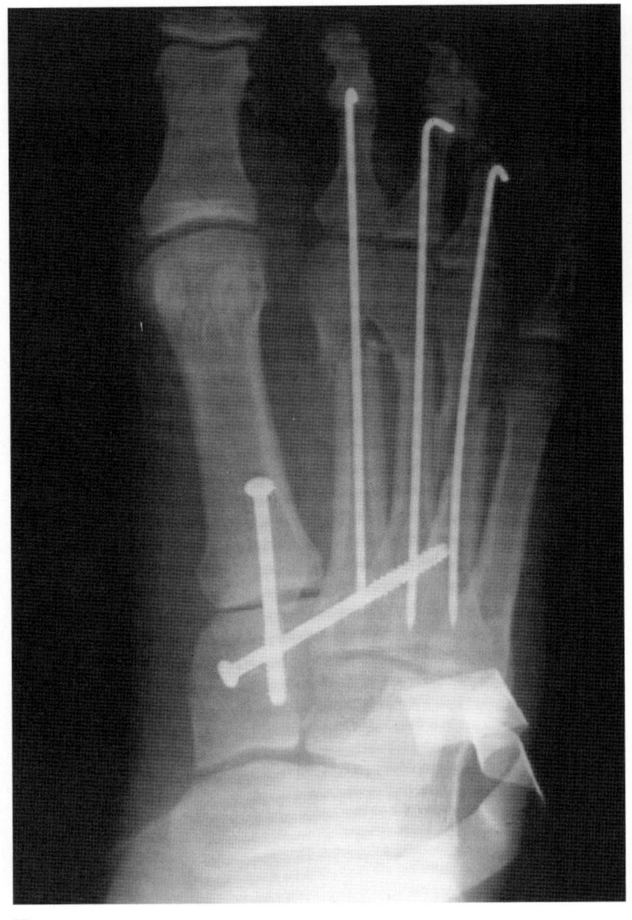

E

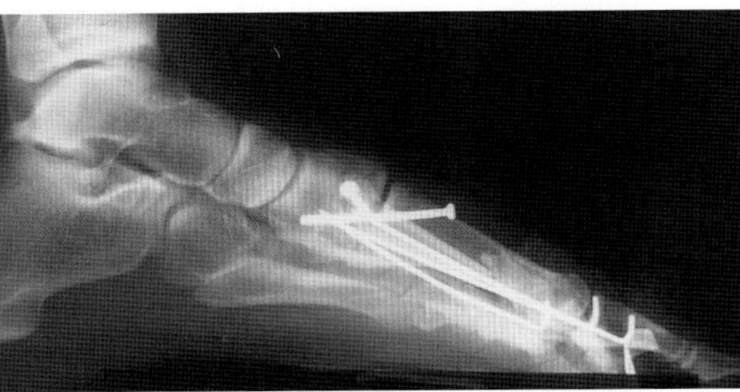

F

FIGURE 29–3 *Continued. E* and *F*, Clinical example of Lisfranc and metacarpal fractures, open reduction and internal fixation.

Tarsal Navicular Fractures

Indications

Failure of nonoperative management (short-leg non–weight-bearing cast) for 6 to 8 weeks is an indication for surgery.

Technique

A 3-cm dorsal vertical incision is made just distal to the tibialis tendon insertion. The neurovascular structures are retracted laterally. The navicular is exposed, and the fracture is débrided with a curette. Bone graft can be inserted into the defect, or an osteotome can be used to create a gutter in the cortex for bone graft. Two 3.5-mm lag screws are inserted perpendicular to the fracture from the lateral to the medial direction through a small separate incision (Fig. 29–4).

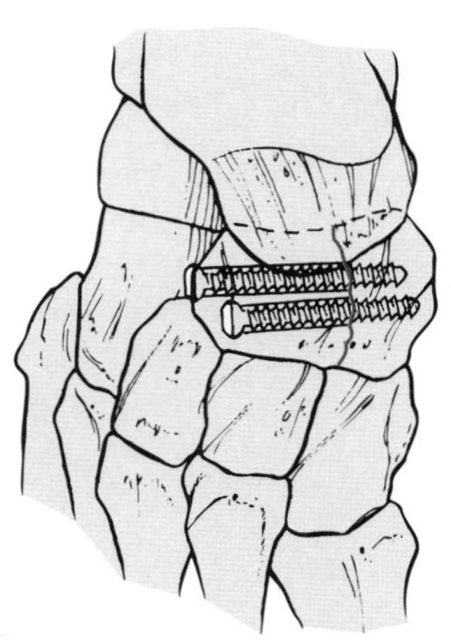

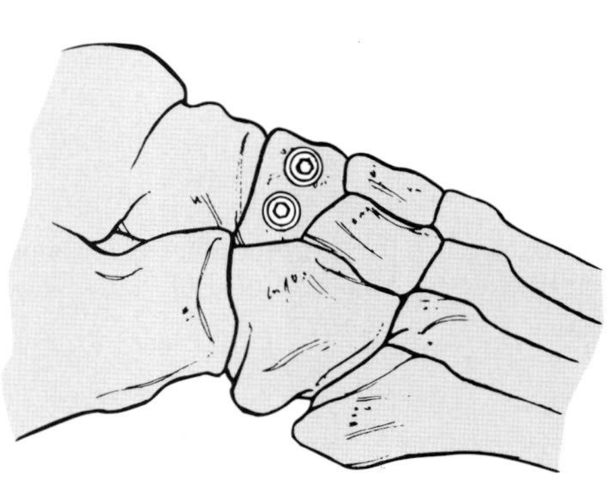

FIGURE 29–4. Fixation of tarsal navicular fractures using two screws (with or without bone graft). The screws are inserted from lateral to medial because the lateral side is smaller than the medial side. (From Hansen ST Jr: Foot injuries. In Browner BD, Jupiter JB, Levine AM, Trafton PG [eds]: Skeletal Trauma, 2nd ed. Philadelphia, WB Saunders, 1998, pp 2405–2438.)

Ankle Fractures

Indications

Indications include significant displacement and failure of closed reduction.

Technique

A posterolateral incision is made, and the posterolateral aspect of the distal fibula is exposed. A one-third tubular antiglide plate is placed posteriorly, and lag screws can be placed through the plate or from anterior to posterior (Fig. 29–5). The medial malleolus can be fixed with a variety of methods through a separate medial incision (Fig. 29–6). The integrity of the syndesmosis can be tested using fluoroscopy and the *hook test*. The stabilized fibula is hooked, and distraction is attempted away from the tibia. The anterolateral corner of the joint is assessed for excessive movement of the fibula and talus during this maneuver. If there is instability of the mortise, one of the screws in the plate (preferably one approximately 3 cm above the plafond) is exchanged for a longer 4.5-mm malleolar screw that is inserted from lateral to medial up to or through the medial cortex of the tibia, oriented 30° anteriorly with the foot held in full dorsiflexion.

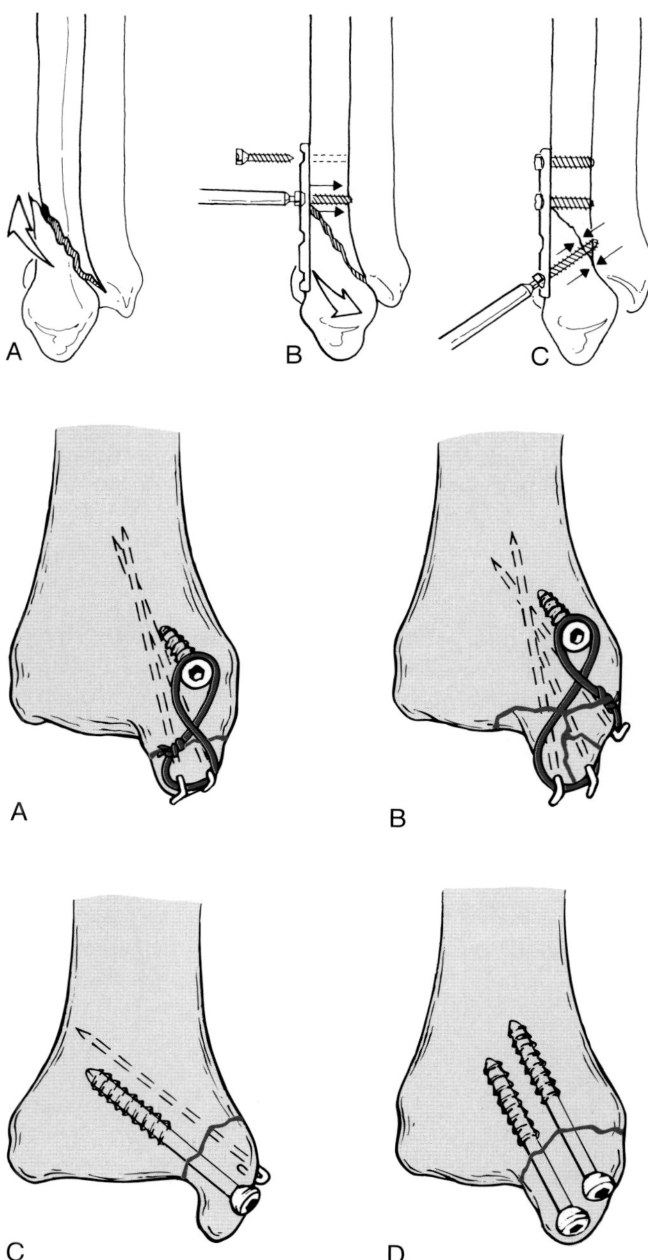

FIGURE 29–5. Fixation of a lateral malleolus fracture using a posterior antiglide plate. *A*, Fracture pattern and displacement *(arrow)*. *B*, Indirect reduction. *C*, Interfragmentary fixation can be accomplished through the plate. (From Miller MD, Cooper DE, Warner JJP: Review of Sports Medicine and Arthroscopy, 2nd ed. Philadelphia, WB Saunders, 2002, p 109.)

FIGURE 29–6. Fixation of medial malleolus fractures. Smaller fractures *(A)* and comminuted fractures *(B)* are best treated with K-wires and a tension band wire. Larger fractures *(C* and *D)* can be treated with K-wires or K-wires and a screw. (From Carr JB, Trafton PG: Malleolar fractures and soft tissue injuries of the ankle. In Browner BD, Jupiter JB, Levine AM, Trafton PG [eds]: Skeletal Trauma, 2nd ed. Philadelphia, WB Saunders, 1998, pp 2327–2404.)

Tibial Stress Fractures

Indications

Indications for surgical treatment are activity-related pain and the presence of a "dreaded black line" (Fig. 29–7) for more than 6 months (especially with a positive bone scan).

Technique

There is some disagreement as to whether local bone grafting, a reamed intramedullary rod, or both should be used for treatment of this difficult problem. Because of the concern that the dreaded black line can progress to a complete fracture, we recommend rigid fixation with a rod, but this alone sometimes is inadequate. The rod is inserted in the standard fashion. The starting point for the rod is behind the patellar tendon, and the tendon must be retracted throughout the case. A flexible reamer is used, and the rod is inserted and locked. The nonunion site is exposed and freshened, and bone graft (preferably iliac crest autograft) is inserted into the fracture site (Fig. 29–8).

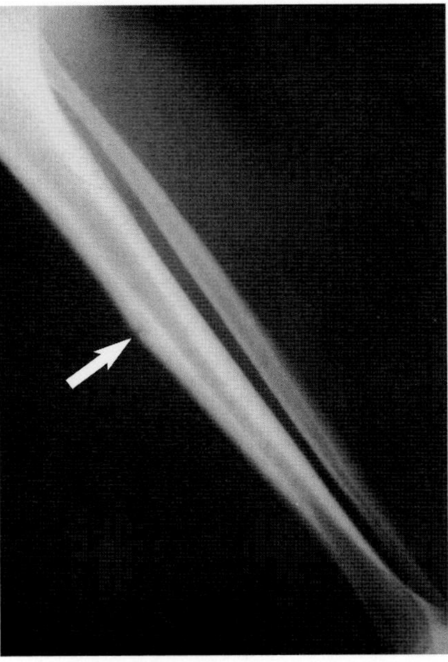

FIGURE 29–7. Radiograph shows the "dreaded black line" *(arrow)* associated with an impending complete fracture from an anterior tibial stress fracture. (From Miller MD, Cooper DE, Warner JJP: Review of Sports Medicine and Arthroscopy, 2nd ed. Philadelphia, WB Saunders, 2002, p 83.)

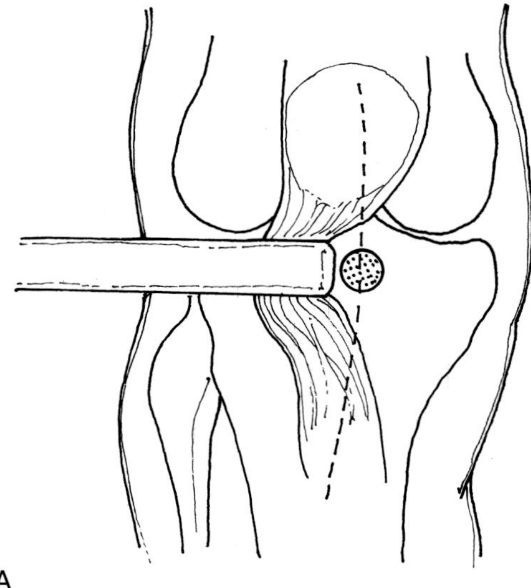

FIGURE 29–8. Technique for intramedullary rodding and bone grafting for an anterior tibial stress fracture. *A*, Retraction of patellar tendon to access starting point. *B*, Guide wire placement and initial reaming. In some cases, the fracture must be exposed, necrotic bone is removed, and the area is freshened. *C*, Intramedullary nail insertion. *D*, The nail is rigidly fixed with proximal and distal locking screws. Bone graft is packed into the defect if it was exposed.

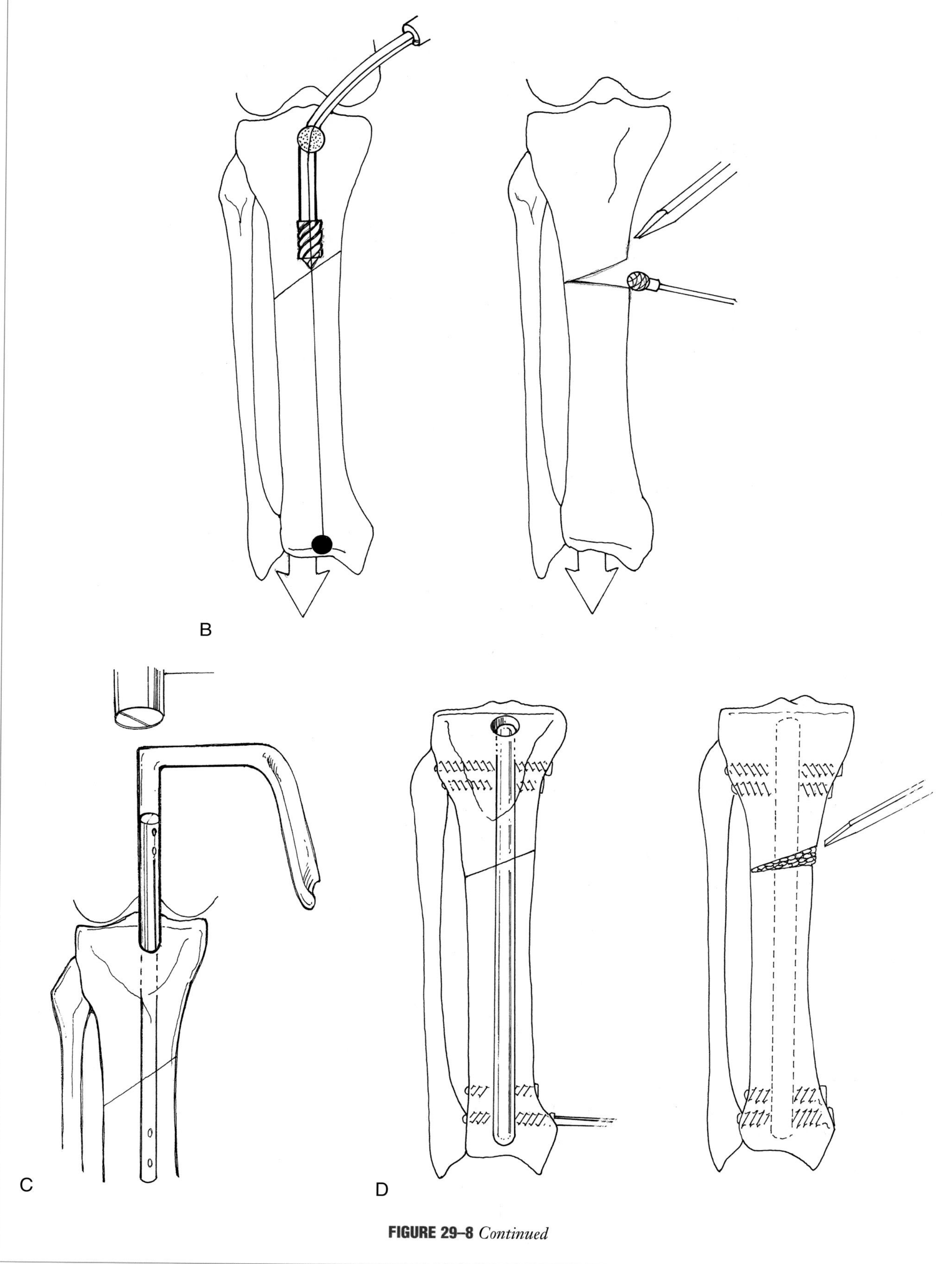

FIGURE 29–8 *Continued*

POSTOPERATIVE MANAGEMENT

Hallux Sesamoid Fractures

The cast is removed after 1 week, but the patient remains non–weight bearing for 3 weeks. Sports may begin 6 weeks postoperatively

Fifth Metatarsal Base Fractures

The patient is kept non–weight bearing for the initial 2 to 4 weeks. Sports may resume when clinical and radiographic healing has occurred (6 to 10 weeks).

Lisfranc Fractures

The patient is placed in a non–weight-bearing cast for the initial 6 to 8 weeks. If K-wires are used, they are removed at 6 to 8 weeks. If screws are used, they should remain in place for 12 to 16 weeks. A longitudinal arch support should be used for 6 to 12 months. Return to sports may take several months.

Tarsal Navicular Fractures

The patient is placed in a short-leg cast and kept non–weight bearing for 6 weeks. Gradual return to activities is based on symptoms.

Ankle Fractures

Typically a short-leg cast is applied, and minimal weight bearing is allowed for 6 to 8 weeks. Progressive range-of-motion and strengthening exercises are allowed after cast removal.

Tibial Stress Fractures

Partial weight-bearing and the use of a long AirCast (Ethicon, Summit, NJ) brace is recommended until callus formation is seen.

COMPLICATIONS

Complications are similar for all procedures and include nonunion, infection, and neurovascular injuries.

RESULTS

Although the fractures described in this chapter can be difficult to manage, results on the whole are encouraging.

REFERENCES

Hansen ST Jr: Foot injuries. In Browner BD, Jupiter JB, Levine AM, et al (eds): Skeletal Trauma. Philadelphia, WB Saunders, 1992, pp 1959–1991.

Whittle AP: Fractures of the foot in athletes. Op Tech Sports Med 2:43–57, 1994.

CHAPTER 30

Treatment of Exertional Compartment Syndrome

INTRODUCTION

Exertional compartment syndrome (ECS) is a result of increased tissue pressure within a noncompliant compartment space. Resultant pain, only partially caused by muscle ischemia, persists until the pressure diminishes.

HISTORY AND PHYSICAL EXAMINATION

Patients classically report pain that gradually increases during exercise, ultimately restricting their performance. This pain often occurs bilaterally in patients younger than age 30 and is common in runners. Individuals have no pain at rest, and their examination at rest is normal. The diagnosis is made primarily by intracompartment pressure measurements taken before and after exercise. A value of greater than or equal to 15 mm Hg 15 minutes after exercise is diagnostic of ECS. Other criteria sometimes used include absolute values of greater than or equal to 15 mm Hg at rest, greater than or equal to 30 mm Hg immediately after exercise, and greater than or equal to 20 mm Hg 5 minutes after exercise.

DIAGNOSTIC IMAGING

Plain radiographs are normal in patients with ECS. Although some investigators suggested there may be subtle changes in MRI immediately after exercise in patients with ECS, this does not seem to be a practical tool for routine evaluation of these patients. A new evaluation method that currently is being studied is near-infrared spectroscopy.

NONOPERATIVE MANAGEMENT

Nonoperative treatments, such as physical therapy, anti-inflammatory drugs, and orthotic devices, play an important role in the management of many causes of exercise-induced leg pain; however, they usually are not effective in the management of ECS.

RELEVANT ANATOMY

Before embarking on operative treatment of ECS, it is crucial to understand the anatomy of the four compartments of the leg and especially where the important neurovascular structures are within these compartments (Fig. 30–1). The anterior compartment is most frequently involved in ECS. There is often a fascial defect (and muscle hernia) in the lateral compartment where the superficial peroneal nerve exits this compartment and becomes subcutaneous. The following are important features of each compartment:

Compartment	*Muscles*	*Nerve*	*Artery*
Anterior	Foot dorsiflexors	Deep peroneal	Anterior tibial
Lateral	Peroneus longus/brevis	Superficial peroneal	
Superficial posterior	Foot plantar flexors	Sural	
Deep posterior	Toe flexors, posterior tibialis	Tibial	Tibial

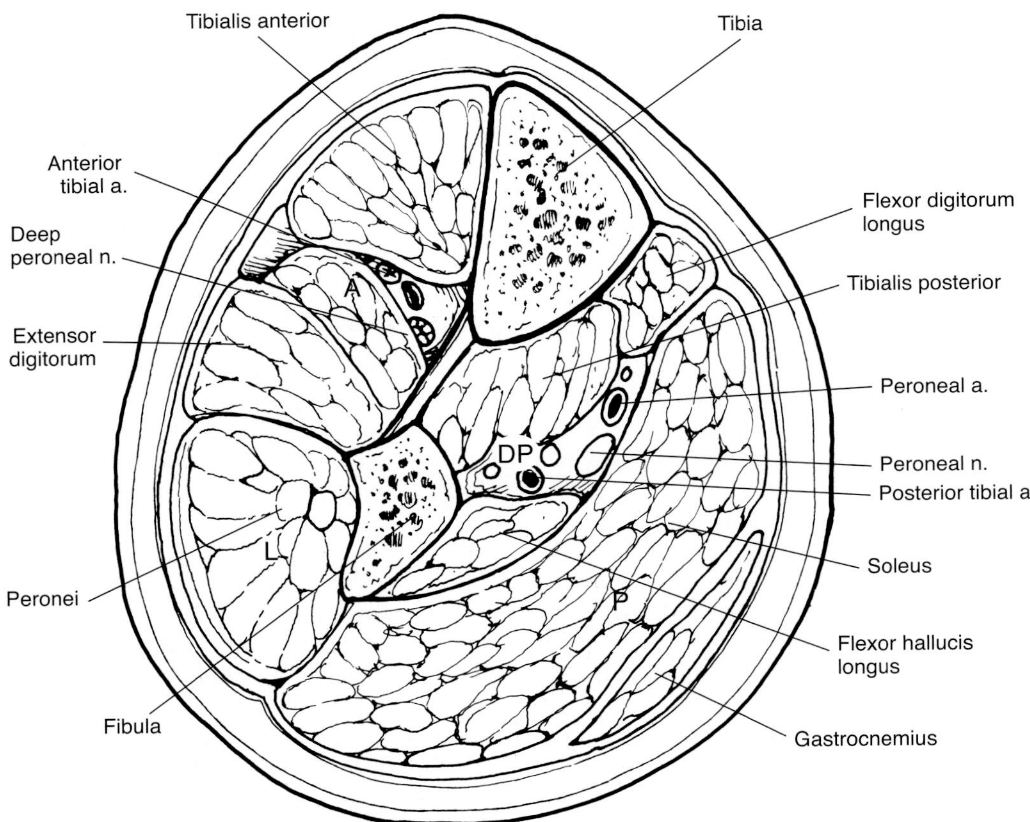

FIGURE 30–1. Cross-sectional view of the four compartments of the leg. A, anterior; DP, deep posterior; L, lateral; P, posterior.

SURGICAL *TECHNIQUE*

Indications

Surgery is indicated for chronic exertional leg pain with documented compartment pressures that exceed the values stated earlier.

Technique

1. Positioning: The patient is positioned supine on a standard operating table. A tourniquet is applied to the thigh but not routinely used.
2. Anterior and lateral compartment decompression: This is accomplished through one 3- to 4-cm incision (and sometimes a second, more proximal incision) placed in the midportion of the leg, halfway between the fibular shaft and tibial crest. If a fascial hernia is present, the incision is placed more distally, directly over the defect. It may be necessary to use a second, more proximal incision in some cases. The skin edges are undermined, and a small transverse incision is made in the fascia to identify the anterior intermuscular septum separating the anterior and lateral compartments. A 12-inch Metzenbaum scissors and a fasciotome are used to release the fascia proximal and distal to the incision in both compartments with a *pushing* action directed away from the superficial peroneal nerve (Fig. 30–2).

FIGURE 30–2. Anterior and lateral compartment release. *A*, A 5-cm incision is made beginning approximately 12 cm proximal to the distal tip of the lateral malleolus, and the fascia is exposed. The superficial peroneal nerve is identified and dissected so that it can be protected during the release. *B*, A long scissors or a fasciotome is used to release the fascia overlying the anterior compartment proximally and distally.

Illustration on opposite page

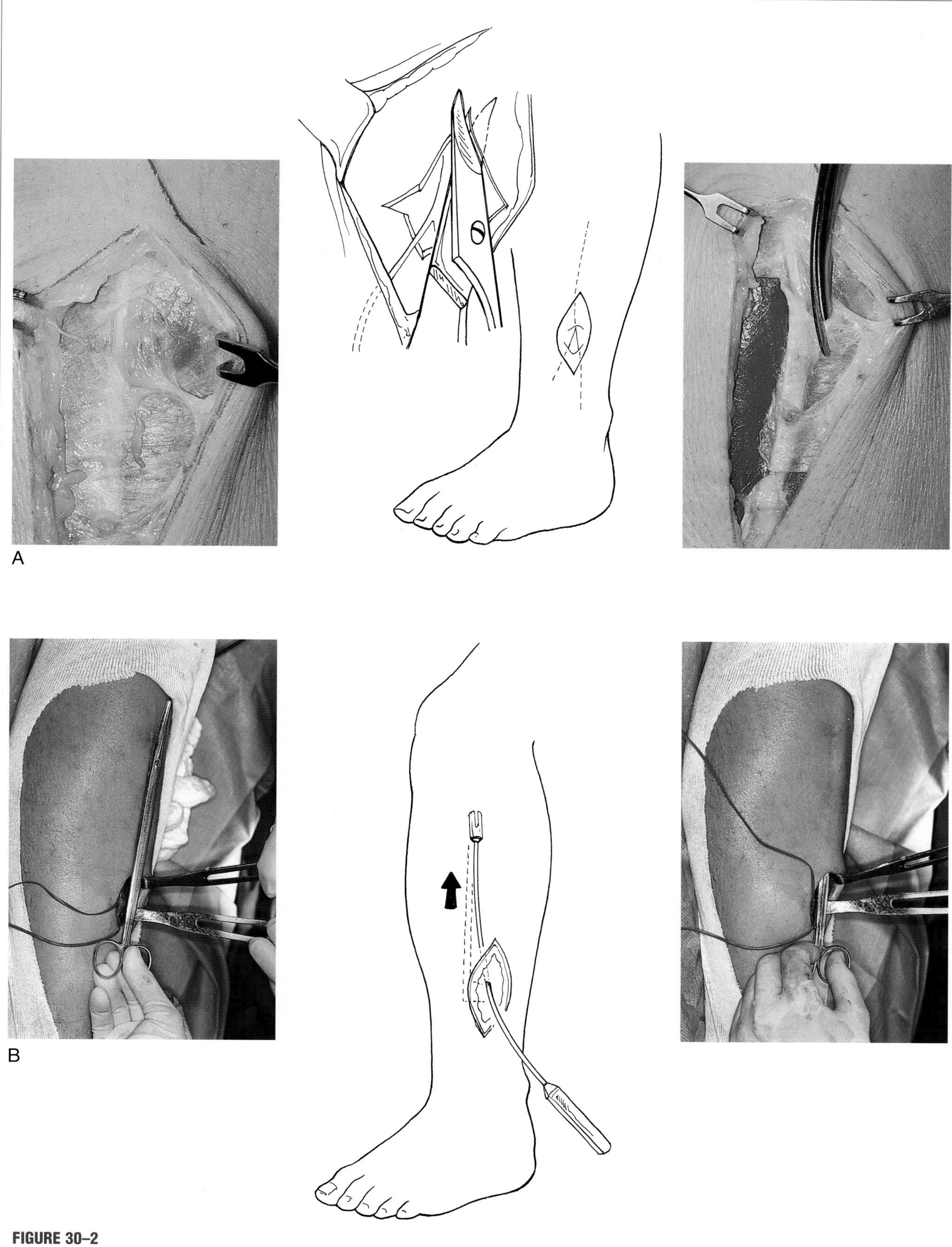

FIGURE 30–2

Illustration continued on following page

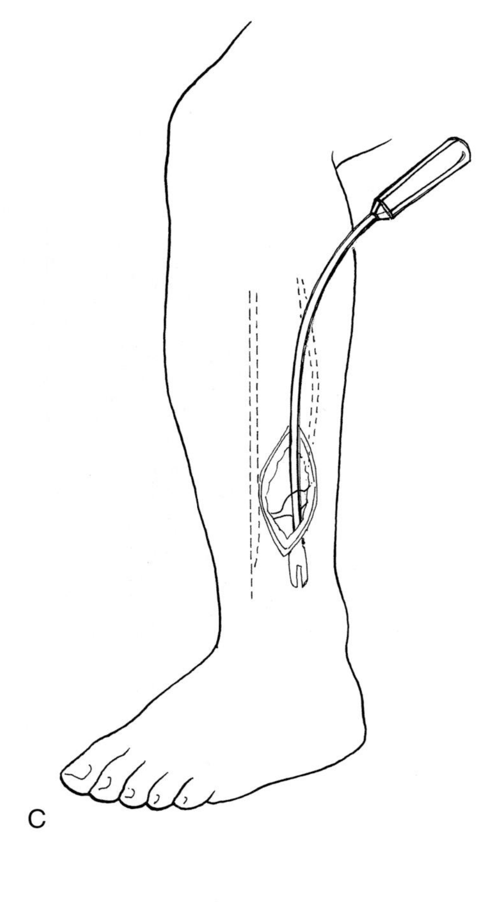

FIGURE 30–2 *Continued. C,* The lateral compartment is released in a similar fashion.

3. Posterior compartment decompression: This is completed through a 3- to 4-cm medial incision at the junction of the middle and distal third of the leg (Fig. 30–3). It is placed 2 cm posterior to the posterior tibial margin. The saphenous nerve and vein are identified and retracted anteriorly. A transverse fascial incision is made, and the septum between the deep and superficial posterior compartments is identified. The superficial compartment (overlying the Achilles tendon) is released first. The deep compartment (overlying the tendon of the flexor digitorum longus) is released distally behind the medial malleolus, then proximally under the soleus bridge.
4. Wound closure: The subcutaneous tissue and skin are closed in standard fashion. A drain is optional; if it is used, it is removed on the first postoperative day.

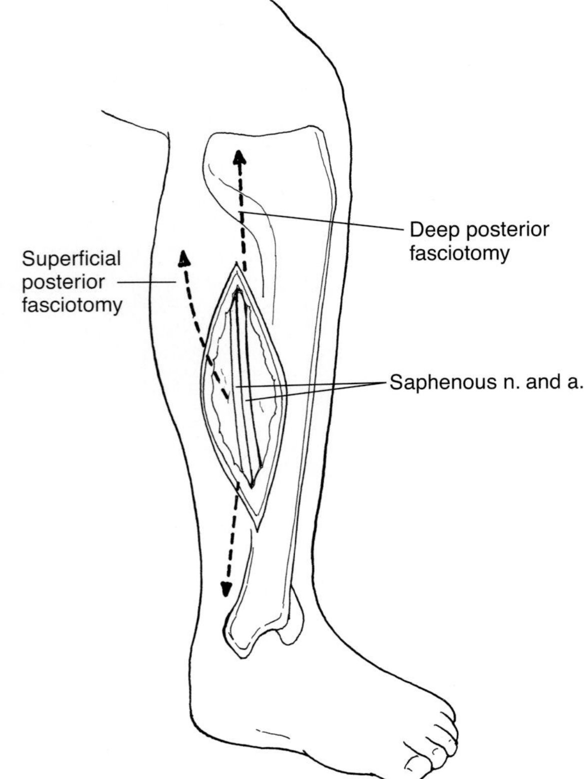

FIGURE 30–3. Superficial and deep posterior compartment release.

POSTOPERATIVE MANAGEMENT

A bulky dressing is applied, and weight bearing is allowed as tolerated. Physical therapy is initiated, and return to sports may occur at 4 to 6 weeks.

COMPLICATIONS

Neurovascular injury is a big risk with this procedure; however, with careful incisions and techniques, the risk can be minimized. Recurrence may be a result of an incomplete release.

RESULTS

The success rate of decompressive fasciotomy is high. When intramuscular pressures are remeasured, the resting and postexercise pressures are normal. Of patients in one study, 90% had complete resolution of symptoms and returned to normal activities.

REFERENCES

Mubarak SJ: Surgical management of chronic compartment syndromes of the leg. Op Tech Sports Med 3:259–266, 1995.

Pedowitz RA, Hargens AR, Mubarak SJ, et al: Modified criteria for objective diagnosis of chronic compartment syndrome of the leg. Am J Sports Med 18:35–40, 1990.

Rampersaud YR, Amendola A: The evaluation and treatment of exertional compartment syndrome. Op Tech Sports Med 3:267–273, 1995.

Rorabeck CH, Bourne RB, Fowler PJ, et al: The surgical treatment of exertional compartment syndrome in athletes. J Bone Joint Surg [Am] 65:1245–1251, 1983.

Rorabeck CH, Bourne RB, Fowler PJ, et al: The role of tissue pressure measurement in diagnosing chronic anterior compartment syndrome. Am J Sports Med 16:143–146, 1988.

CHAPTER 31

Treatment of Lower Extremity Nerve Entrapment

INTRODUCTION

Many potential sites of nerve entrapment are in the lower extremity. This chapter includes only the most common of these rare problems. Nerve entrapment can occur at many levels, and the diagnosis is often difficult. Certain diagnostic clues and tests are helpful in the management of these problems.

HISTORY AND PHYSICAL EXAMINATION

Although symptoms may be specific to the region of the entrapment, pain, numbness, paresthesias, and occasionally a palpable mass may be present. Motor involvement is variable. It is important to have a good understanding of the anatomy when considering lower extremity nerve entrapment. Physical examination should include an evaluation of range of motion, sensation, and motor function distal to the suspected entrapment.

DIAGNOSTIC IMAGING

Plain radiographs are typically normal; however, it is important to rule out the possibility of exostoses or bony abnormalities that may cause nerve entrapment. MRI can be helpful if there are any masses or space-occupying lesions impinging on the affected nerve. The key diagnostic tests, although not always reliable, are electromyography and nerve conduction studies.

NONOPERATIVE MANAGEMENT

Depending on the cause of the entrapment, an initial nonoperative approach may be warranted. Activity modification, nonsteroidal anti-inflammatory drugs, ice or heat, various modalities (electrical stimulation, transcutaneous electrical nerve stimulation, ultrasound, or iontophoresis), various orthoses, and occasionally local steroid injections may have a role in the treatment of these disorders. If impingement or injury is suspected, operative treatment may be justified early.

RELEVANT ANATOMY

Saphenous Nerve

The saphenous nerve is the terminal branch of the femoral nerve and can be entrapped at the level of the adductor canal and as it courses between the sartorius and gracilis distally in the thigh (Fig. 31–1). Infrapatellar branches of the nerve commonly are injured with medial and anterior incisions about the knee and medial meniscal repairs.

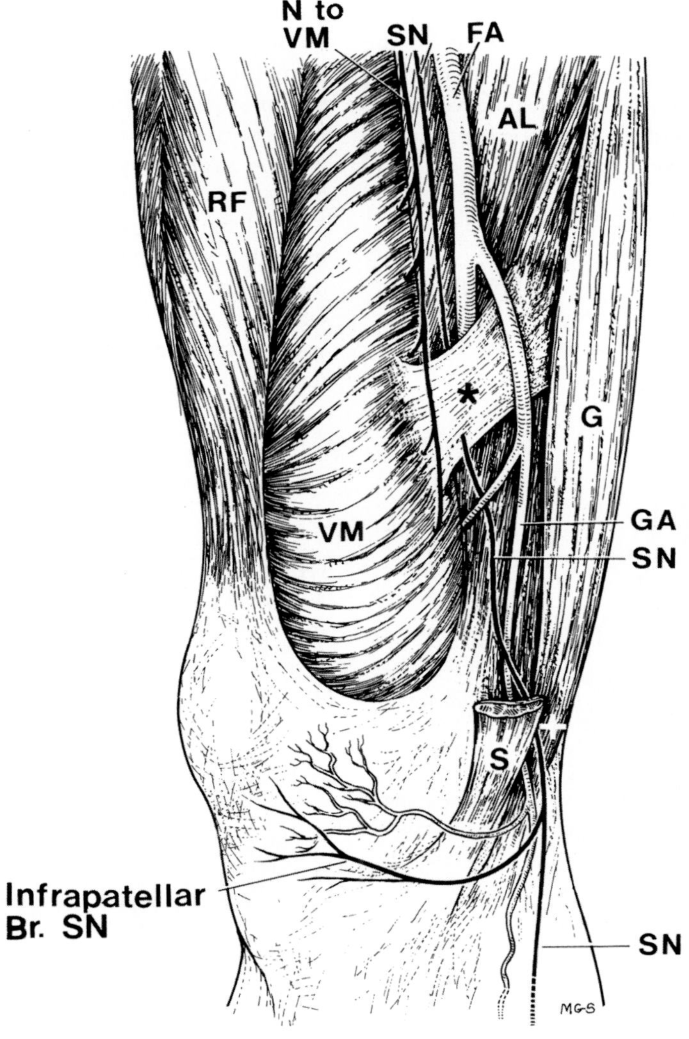

FIGURE 31–1. Saphenous nerve (SN) entrapment can occur at the level of the adductor canal (*) and more distally, as it passes between the sartorius (S) and gracilis (G) (+). RF, rectus femoris; VM, vastus medialis; N to VM, nerve to vastus medialis; FA, femoral artery; AL, adductor longus; GA, geniculate artery. (Modified from Kalenak A: Saphenous nerve entrapment. Op Tech Sports Med 4:40–45, 1996.)

Peroneal Nerve

The peroneal nerve, one of two main branches of the sciatic nerve, begins in the popliteal fossa. It crosses laterally and inferiorly and wraps around the neck of the fibula. It then passes through a fibro-osseous tunnel and bifurcates into a deep branch and a superficial branch (Fig. 31–2). Because it is superficial as it passes around the fibula, it is commonly injured at this location. The superficial peroneal nerve also can be entrapped distally as it pierces the deep fascia of the anterolateral compartment, approximately 12 cm proximal to the tip of the lateral malleolus. Fascial defects and muscle herniations are common in this area. The deep peroneal nerve can be entrapped distally at the level of the extensor retinaculum (anterior tarsal tunnel syndrome).

Posterior Tibial Nerve

The posterior tibial nerve, the continuation of the other main branch of the sciatic nerve, is entrapped most commonly as it passes under the flexor retinaculum behind the medial malleolus, at the tarsal tunnel (Fig. 31–3). The nerve bifurcates into medial and lateral plantar nerves. The medial plantar nerve can be entrapped more distally, near the knot of Henry (where the flexor hallucis longus and flexor digitorum longus tendons cross), causing a syndrome commonly referred to as *jogger's foot*. A branch of the lateral plantar nerve (the motor branch to the abductor digiti quinti) can be entrapped beneath the plantar aspect of the deep investing fascia of the abductor hallucis muscle as it courses laterally across the foot. This may be a relatively common (and treatable) form of heel pain, and release of Baxter's nerve may be beneficial. More distally, the medial and lateral plantar nerves divide into digital branches. Entrapment under the transverse metatarsal ligament (especially in the third web space where the medial and lateral branches may overlap) can lead to the development of an intradigital (Morton's) neuroma.

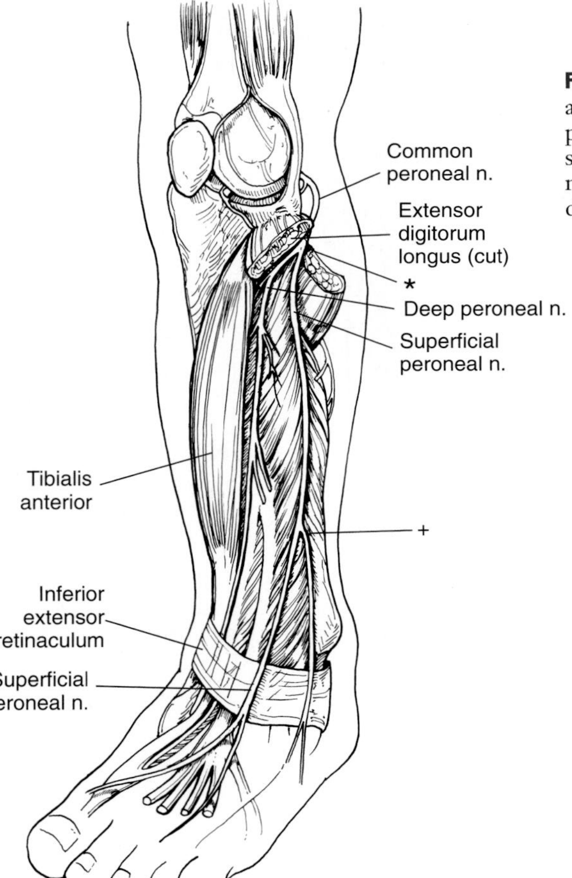

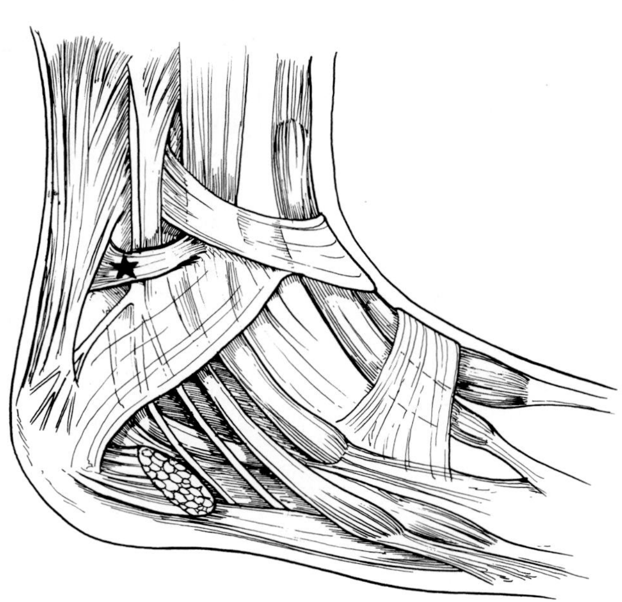

FIGURE 31–2. *A*, The peroneal nerve is injured most commonly as it passes around the neck of the fibula (*). The superficial peroneal nerve branch also commonly is entrapped as it passes superficially, approximately 12 cm proximal to the lateral malleolus (+). *B*, The deep peroneal nerve may be entrapped distally, as it passes under the extensor retinaculum (*).

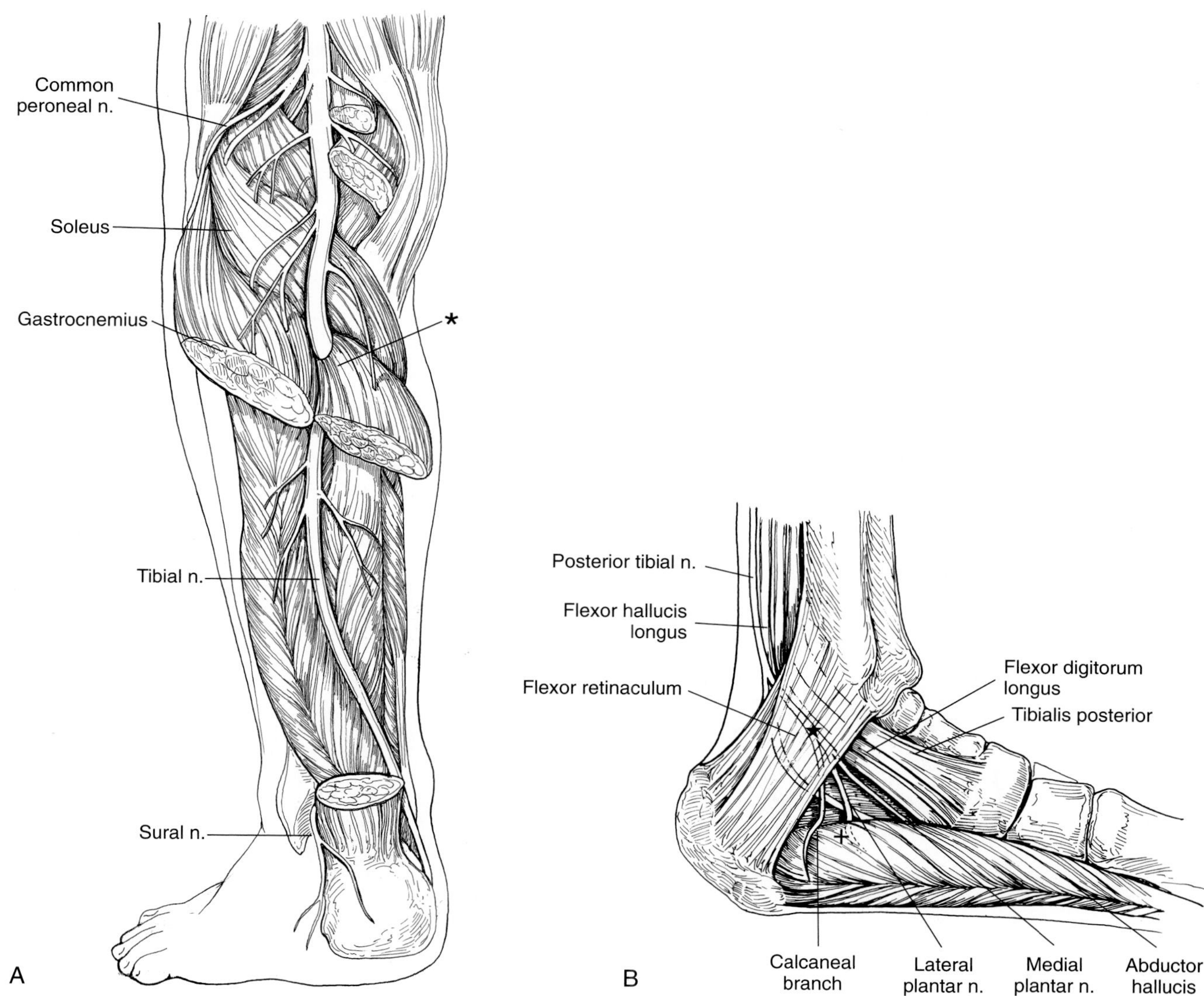

FIGURE 31–3. *A* and *B*, The tibial nerve can be entrapped at any location along its course, including between the two heads of the gastrocnemius (*) *(A)* and at the tarsal tunnel (*) or more distally (+) at the origin of the abductor hallucis muscle *(B)*.

SURGICAL *TECHNIQUE*

Indications

Pain and other symptoms that fail to respond to nonoperative methods are indications for surgery.

Technique

In general, the technique is to identify the affected nerve, trace its course, and remove any impinging structures.

Saphenous Nerve Entrapment

A 5- to 7-cm incision is made parallel to the anterior border of the sartorius, at the junction of the middle and distal thirds of the thigh, centered approximately 10 cm proximal to the superior pole of the patella (Fig. 31–4*A*). The aponeurotic sheath of the adductor canal is identified between the origin of the vastus medialis and the adductor muscles, and it is incised, freeing the nerve (Fig. 31–4*B*).

Common Peroneal Entrapment

A 10-cm incision is made just anterior to the fibular head. The peroneal nerve is identified at the posterior border of the biceps tendon (Fig. 31–5). The peroneal nerve is isolated, and any impingement is relieved.

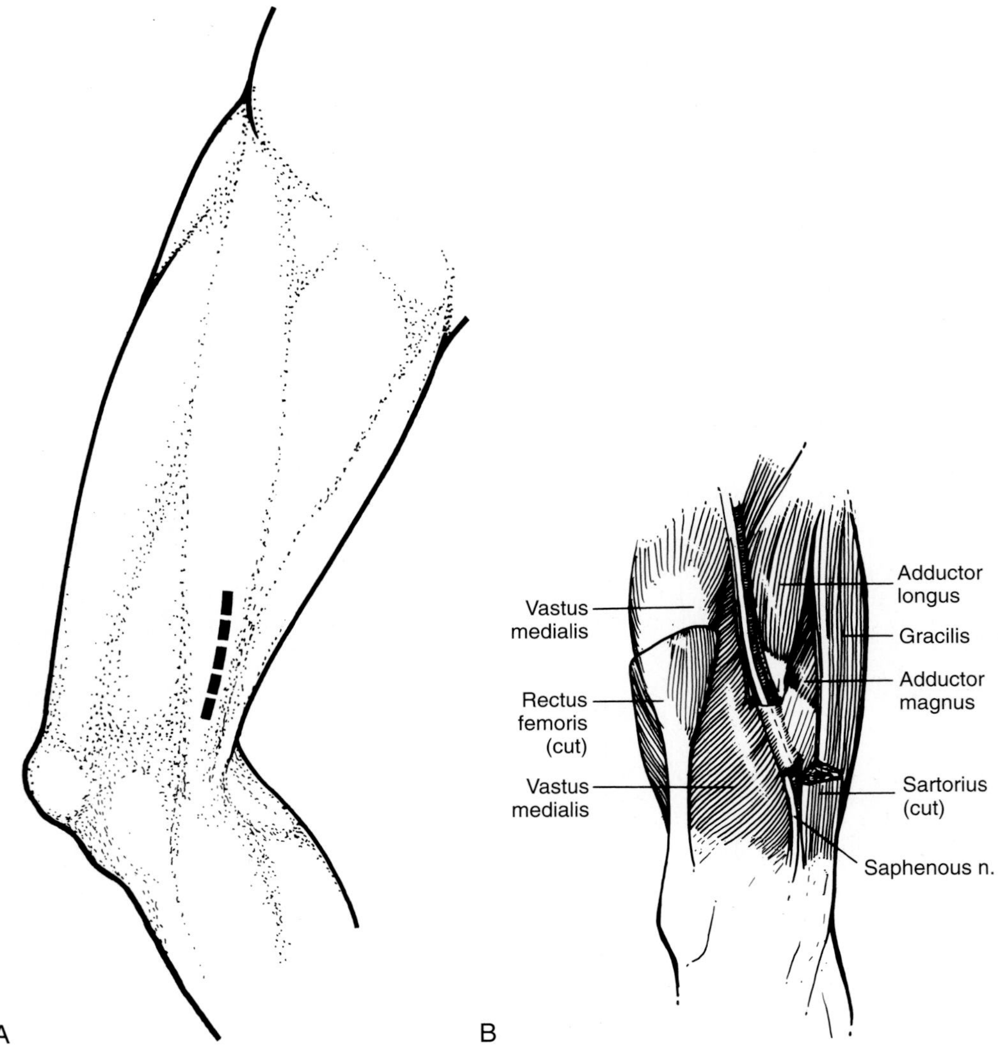

FIGURE 31–4. Release of the saphenous nerve at the level of the adductor canal. *A*, A 5- to 7-cm incision is made directly over the canal. *B*, The nerve is released from its sheath. (*A* from Kalenak A: Saphenous nerve entrapment. Op Tech Sports Med 4:40–45, 1996. *B* from Cox JS, Blanda JB: Peripatellar pathologies. In DeLee JC, Drez D Jr [eds]: Orthopaedic Sports Medicine: Principles and Practice. Philadelphia, WB Saunders, 1994, pp 1249–1260.)

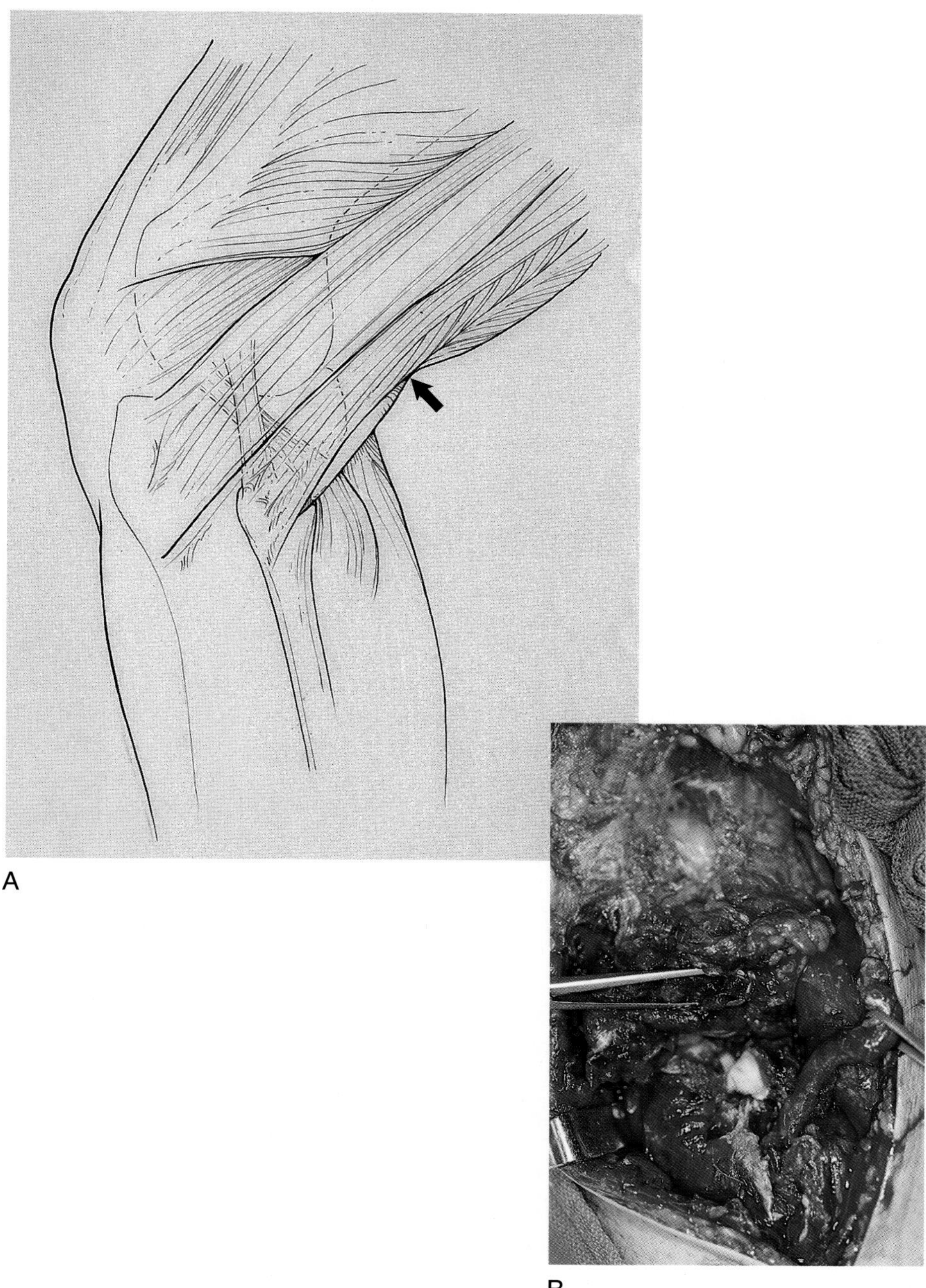

FIGURE 31–5. Common peroneal nerve entrapment typically occurs at the fibular neck. *A*, The nerve is identified at the posterior border of the biceps tendon proximally and traced distally *(arrow)*. *B*, The injured nerve shown here (blue vessel loop) has been dissected free before proceeding with posterolateral knee reconstruction.

Superficial Peroneal Nerve

A 5-cm incision is made on the anterolateral aspect of the leg centered approximately 12 cm proximal to the lateral malleolus. Often there is a hernia in this location. The nerve is identified and protected, and the fascia is released using a subcutaneous technique (Fig. 31–6).

Tarsal Tunnel Release

A 10-cm incision is made behind the medial malleolus. The investing retinaculum is opened behind the posterior tibial tendon sheath. The posterior tibial nerve lies just posterior to the flexor digitorum longus tendon, and it is dissected free from the proximal portion of the sheath distally. The medial and lateral plantar branches are

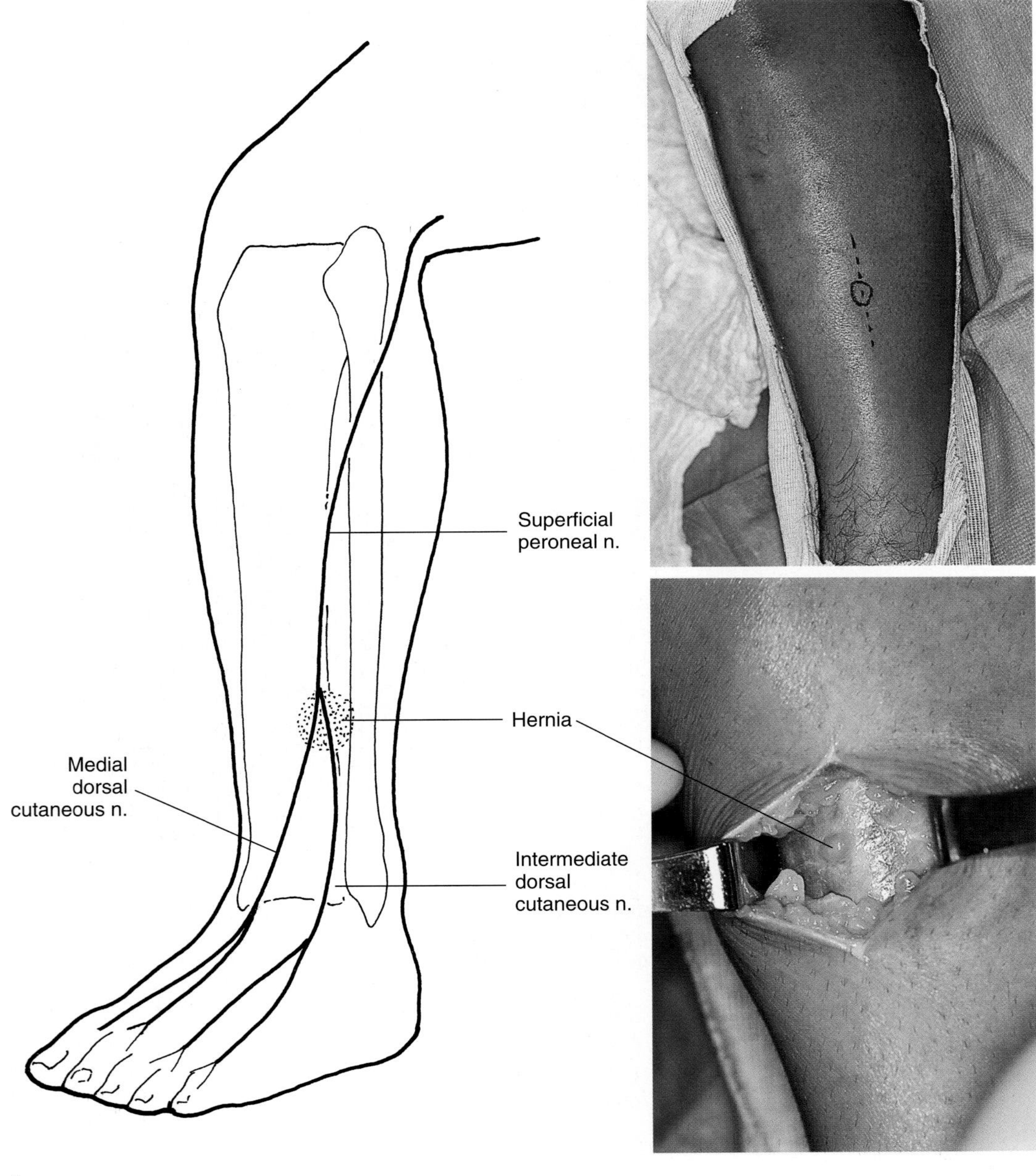

FIGURE 31–6. Superficial peroneal nerve release. *A*, Incision and exposure of fascial hernia.

traced distally, and they too are freed as necessary (Fig. 31–7). Additional releases of distal branches can be accomplished as indicated in Figure 31–8.

Excision of Interdigital Neuroma

Most authors now recommend that interdigital neuromas be excised through a dorsal approach (Fig. 31–9). The incision is made in the web space and carried down between the two metatarsals. The transverse metatarsal ligament is incised, and the common digital nerve is identified. The nerve is traced proximal to the metatarsal head and excised. The nerve is traced distally and excised just distal to its bifurcation.

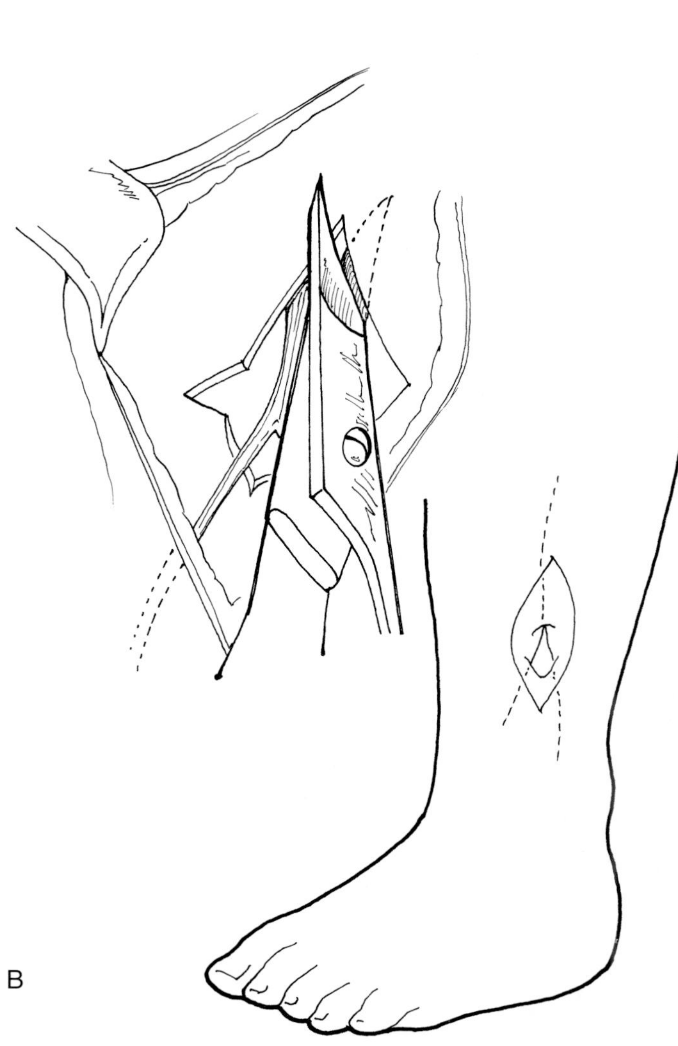

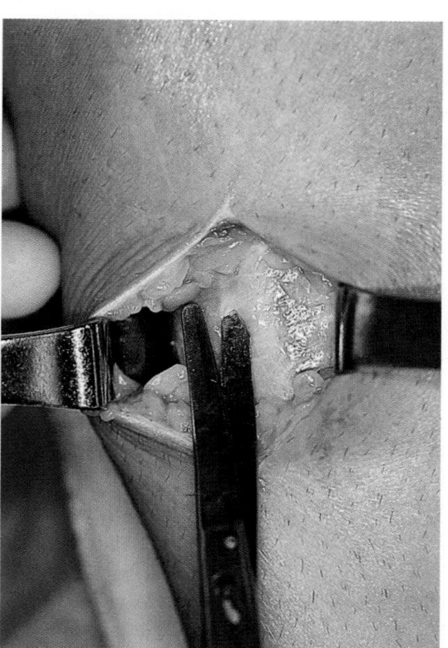

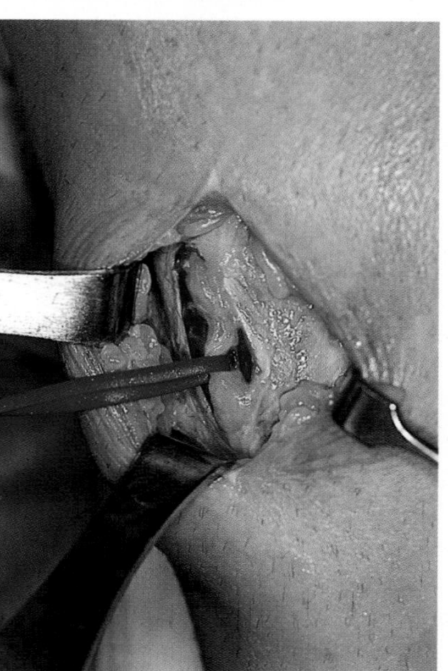

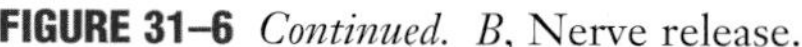

FIGURE 31–6 *Continued. B*, Nerve release.

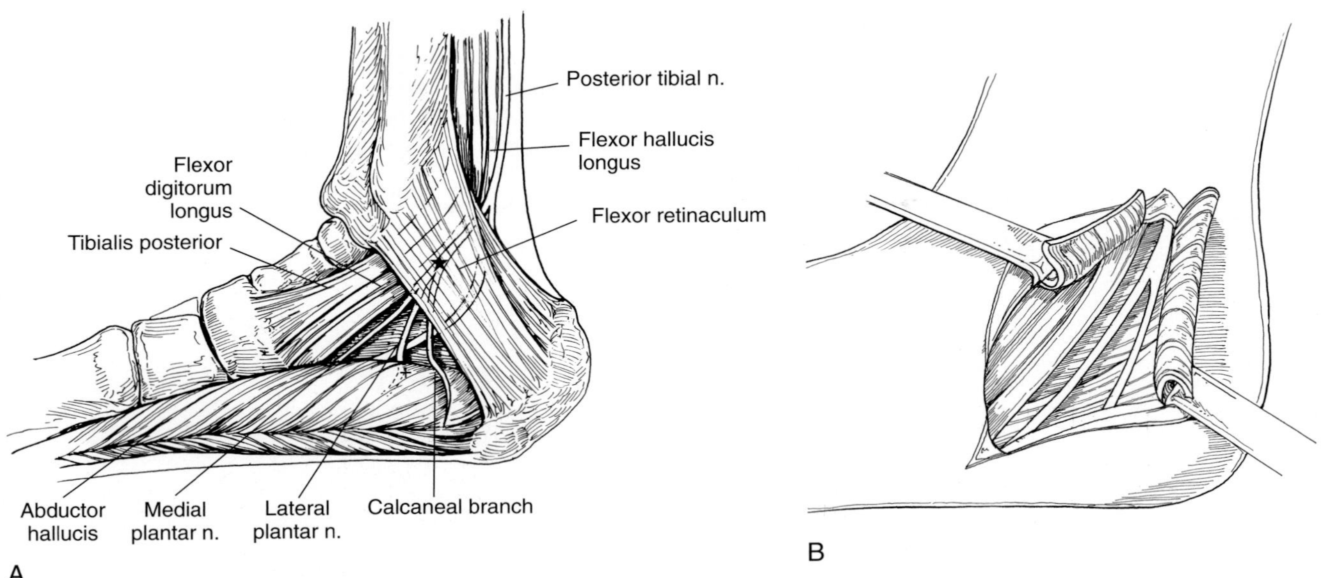

FIGURE 31–7. Tarsal tunnel release. *A*, Exposure of tarsal tunnel. *B*, After release.

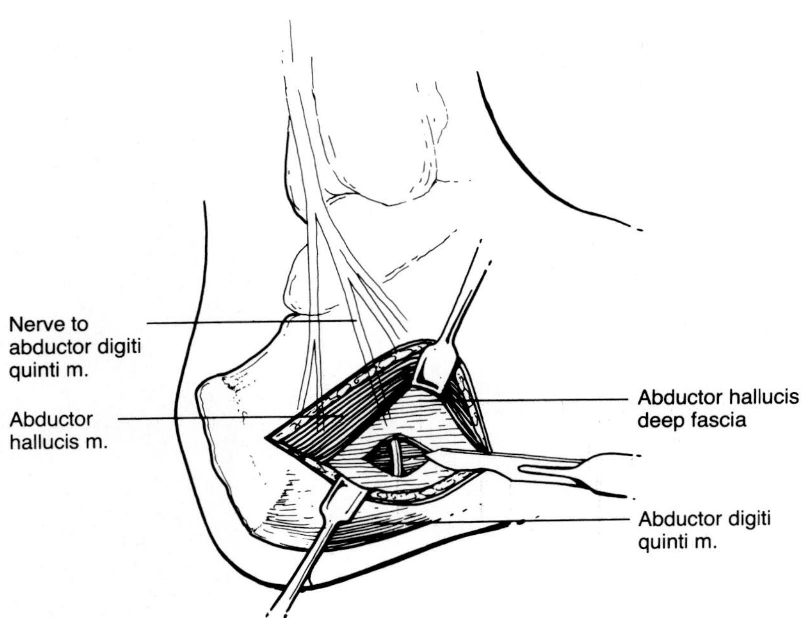

FIGURE 31–8. Release of lateral plantar nerve branch to the abductor digiti quinti muscle (Baxter's nerve). (From Mann RA: Entrapment neuropathies of the foot. In DeLee JC, Drez D Jr [eds]: Orthopaedic Sports Medicine: Principles and Practice. Philadelphia, WB Saunders, 1994, pp 1831–1841.)

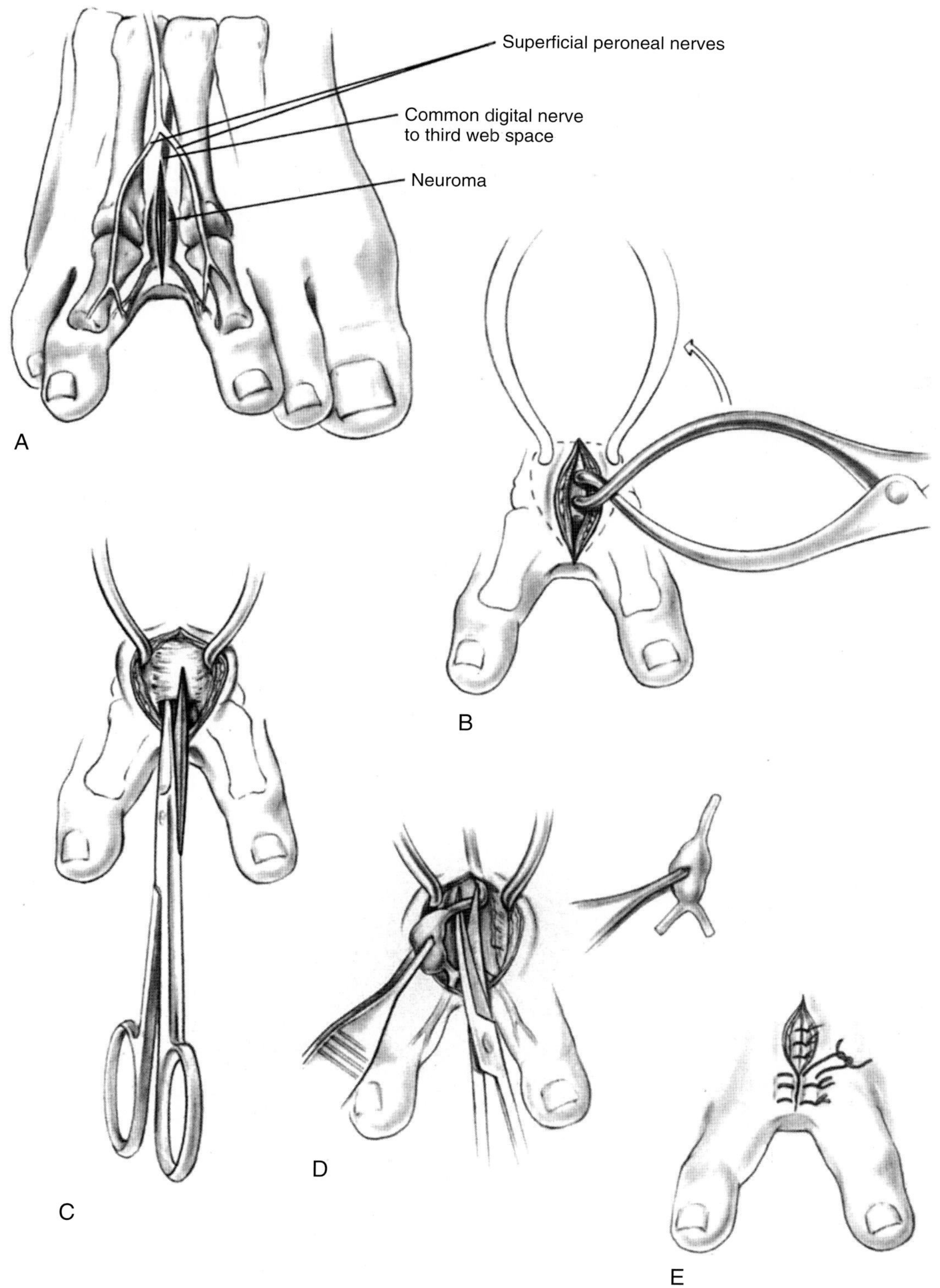

FIGURE 31–9. Excision of interdigital neuroma. *A,* A 3-cm incision is made proximal to the web space. *B,* A spreader is inserted, and tension is applied to the transverse metatarsal ligament. *C,* The ligament is divided, and the neuroma is exposed. *D,* The neuroma is excised. *E,* Skin closure. (From Berberian WS, Lin SS: Surgical treatment of interdigital neuroma. Op Tech Orthop 9:55–61, 1999.)

POSTOPERATIVE MANAGEMENT

In most cases, patients may return to activities as symptoms resolve.

COMPLICATIONS

The most common complication after release of nerve entrapment is recurrence. Recurrence may be related to inadequate release in many cases. Failure to make the diagnosis also can lead to complications and inadequate pain relief. Infection, hematoma, wound dehiscence, and other problems also can occur.

RESULTS

With careful patient selection, approximately 80% of patients can expect to have a good result with release of nerve impingement.

REFERENCES

Beskin JL: Nerve entrapments of the foot and ankle. J Am Acad Orthop Surg 5:261–269, 1997.

Hunter RE (ed): Entrapment neuropathies and nerve lesions in athletes: Diagnosis and treatment. Op Tech Sports Med 4:1–60, 1994.

Mann RA: Entrapment neuropathies of the foot. In DeLee JC, Drez D Jr (eds): Orthopaedic Sports Medicine: Principles and Practice. Philadelphia, WB Saunders, 1994, pp 1831–1841.

Mann RA, Baxter DE: Diseases of the nerves. In Mann RA, Coughlin MJ (eds): Surgery of the Foot and Ankle. St. Louis, Mosby, 1993, pp 543–573.

Miller MD, Fu FH: Ankle and foot. In Johnson RJ, Lombardo J (eds): Current Review of Sports Medicine. Philadelphia, Current Medicine, 1994, pp 102–116.

CHAPTER 32

Foot and Ankle Arthrodesis

INTRODUCTION

Post-traumatic arthritis of several joints about the foot and ankle is probably relatively common in athletes, although its treatment is better managed by foot and ankle specialists.

HISTORY AND PHYSICAL EXAMINATION

Patients typically note progressive pain with activity. They may have noted a significant injury or injuries in the past. Loss of motion also is common. Swelling and deformity of the affected joint may be elicited. Examination with documentation of motion, crepitus, alignment, and other factors is crucial.

DIAGNOSTIC IMAGING

Similar to in the knee, standing radiographs are crucial in evaluating arthritis. Careful evaluation of alignment is essential. It also is necessary to critically evaluate adjacent joints before considering arthrodesis.

NONOPERATIVE MANAGEMENT

Activity modification, orthotic devices, nonsteroidal anti-inflammatory drugs (NSAIDs), and other measures are the mainstay of treatment.

RELEVANT ANATOMY

Relevant anatomy is related to the joint that is to be fused. Ankle fusions usually are approached from the lateral side because of the medial neurovascular structures. Tarsometatarsal fusions must take into account the location of the dorsalis pedis artery.

SURGICAL *TECHNIQUE*

Indications

Arthrosis with pain or deformity or both that is refractory to nonoperative measures and adversely affects the patient's lifestyle is an indication for arthrodesis. Patients must be informed about loss of motion inherent with these procedures. Ankle fusion typically results in approximately 50% reduction in dorsiflexion and 70% reduction in plantar flexion. Other fusions also significantly reduce motion.

Technique

Ankle Arthrodesis

Although many different methods have been proposed for this procedure, two methods are discussed.

Transfibular Approach

1. Positioning: The patient is placed supine with a bump under the ipsilateral hip. Attention is given to alignment during positioning.
2. Incision: A 15- to 20-cm curvilinear incision is made, centered on the distal fibula (Fig. 32–1). The sural nerve is lateral and the superficial peroneal nerve anterior to the incision. Thick flaps are created, and the bones are exposed.
3. Bony cuts: The fibula is osteotomized 2 cm proximal to the tibiotalar joint and beveled. The tibiotalar joint is exposed, and the distal tibia is cut perpendicular to the long axis of the tibia with a saw. The talar dome is cut parallel to the tibia, with as little bone as possible removed.
4. Arthrodesis: The foot is placed in 0° dorsiflexion and 5° valgus. Cuts are adjusted as necessary. If the medial malleolus is prominent, it is resected through a separate medial incision. Two 6.5-mm cancellous screws are placed obliquely from the sinus tarsi and lateral process into the tibia. Bone graft from the removed distal fibula can be placed if there is room.
5. Closure: The wounds are closed over a drain in standard fashion.

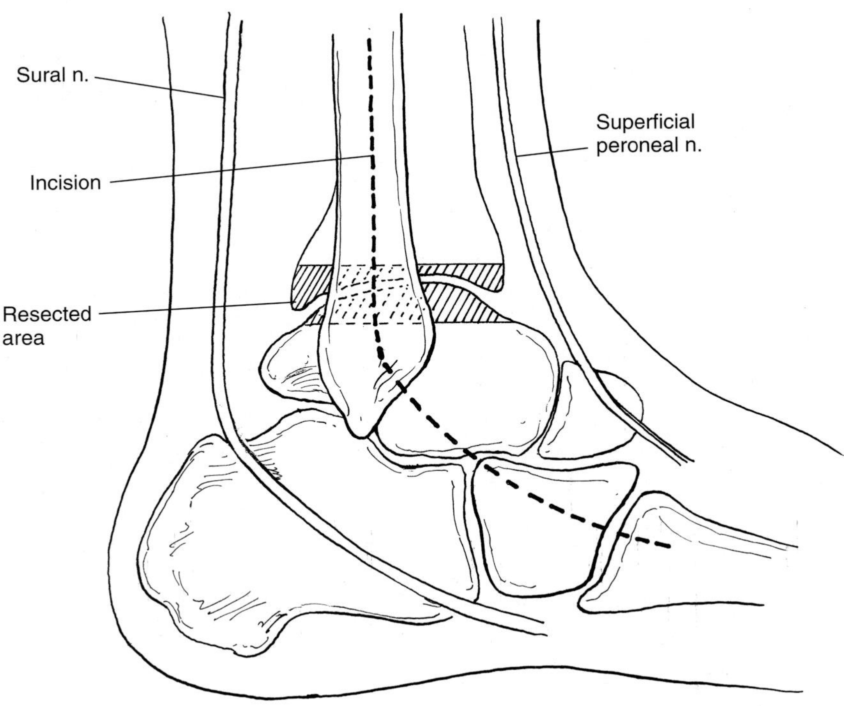

FIGURE 32–1. Surgical technique for transfibular ankle arthrodesis. *A*, Incision between the sural and superficial peroneal nerves.

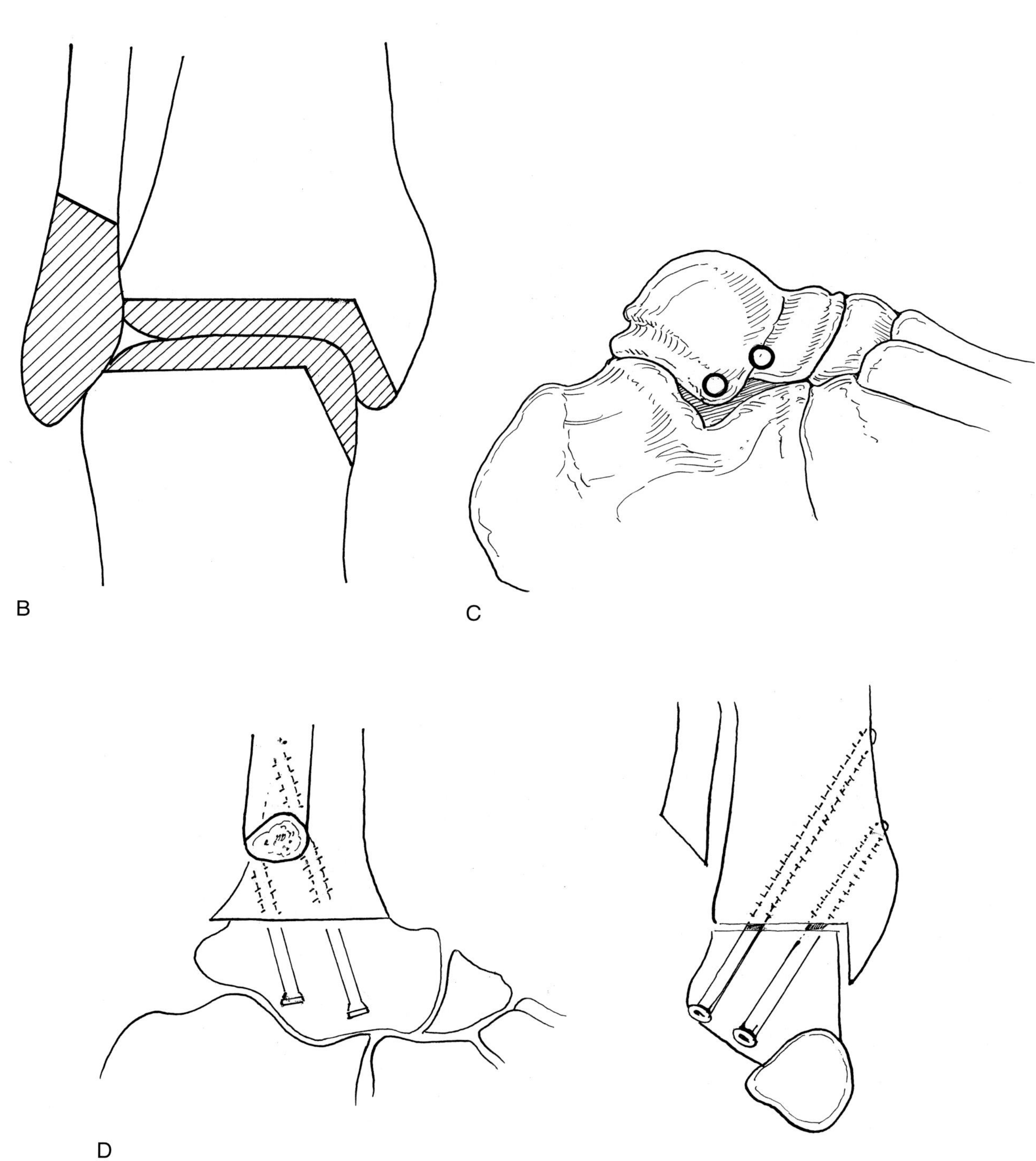

FIGURE 32–1 *Continued. B,* Oblique fibula cut and excision. *C,* Planned location of screws. *D,* Lateral and anteroposterior views of screw placement.

Arthroscopic Approach

1. Positioning: The patient is placed supine with a roll under the affected side. Distraction devices are optional.
2. The arthroscope is placed initially in the anterolateral portal, and a 4.5-mm shaver (followed by a 4-mm burr) is placed in the anteromedial portal. Remaining articular cartilage and dense subchondral bone are removed (Fig. 32–2).
3. A smaller (3-mm) burr is used to remove remaining cartilage in the medial gutter.
4. The scope is switched to the anteromedial portal, and a 4-mm burr is placed in the anterolateral portal and used to remove articular cartilage and subchondral bone from the lateral tibia and talar dome.
5. A smaller (3-mm) burr is used to remove remaining cartilage in the lateral gutter and syndesmosis.
6. The foot is positioned in neutral dorsiflexion with no varus or valgus angulation. Under fluoroscopic control, three 6.5-mm cancellous screws are placed. The first screw is placed from the tibia, just above the medial malleolus, to the talus, at a 45° angle. The second screw is placed from the fibula into the talus, also at a 45° angle. This second screw also is angled anteriorly approximately 15°. The third and final screw is placed from the anterior tibia (medial to the tibialis anterior tendon) into the talus at a 45° angle to the tibia in the sagittal plane. The threads of the screws are inspected carefully on radiographs to ensure that they are all within the talus and adjusted if necessary.
7. Wounds are closed with simple sutures, and the ankle is immobilized.

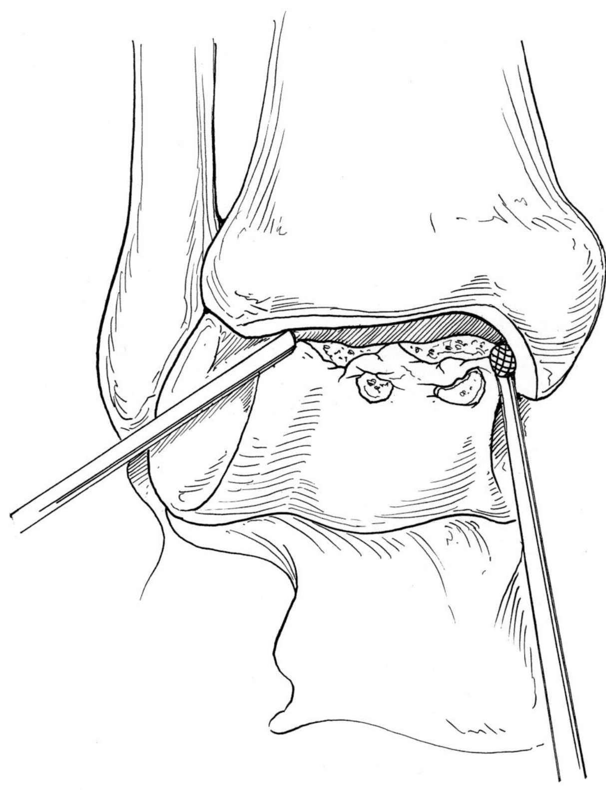

FIGURE 32–2. Arthroscopically assisted technique for tibiotalar fusion. *A*, With the arthroscope in the anterolateral portal and the burr in the anteromedial portal, any remaining articular cartilage is removed.

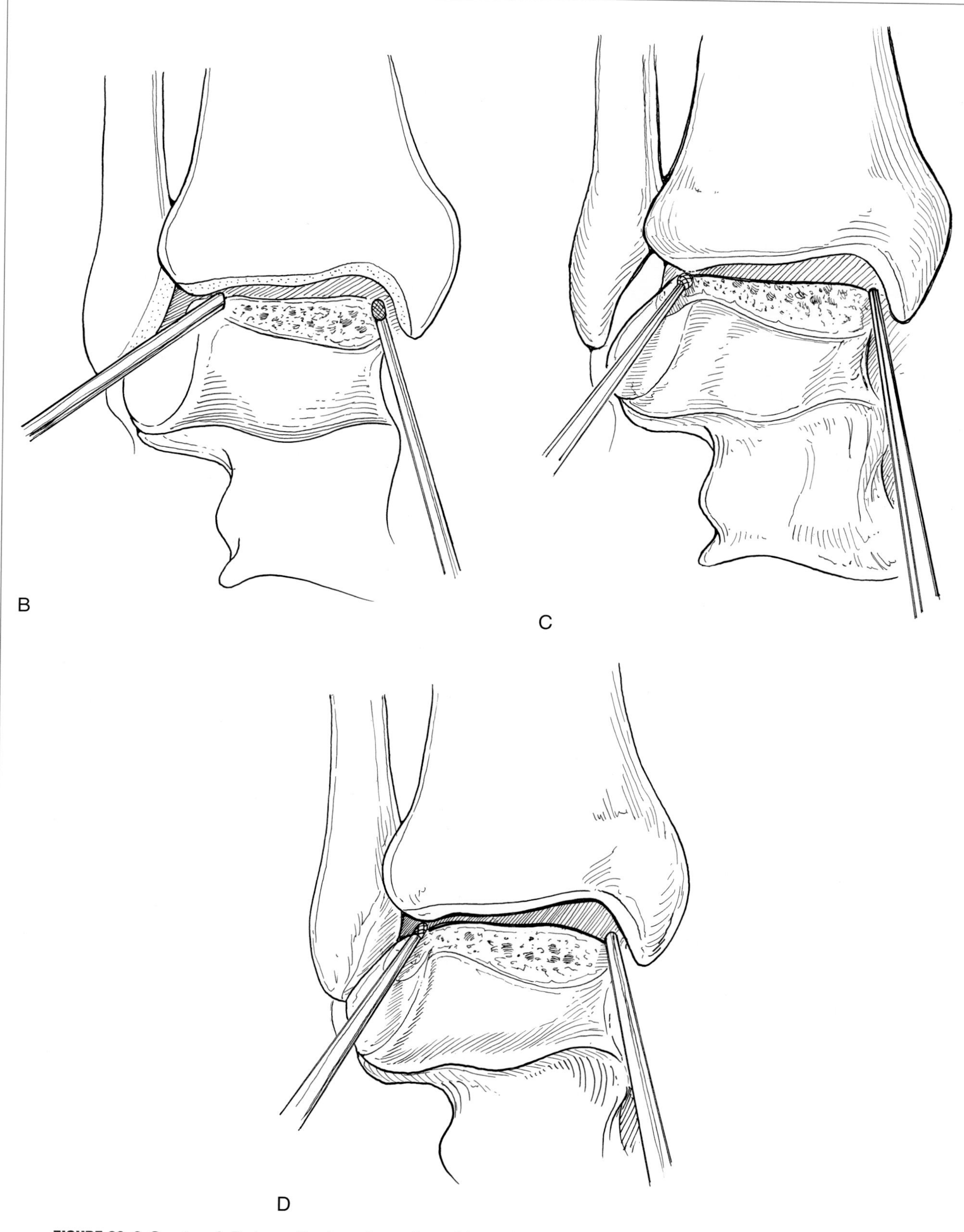

FIGURE 32–2 *Continued. B*, A smaller burr is used to address the medial gutter. *C* and *D*, The arthroscope and shaver/burr are switched into opposite portals, and the process is repeated.

Illustration continued on following page

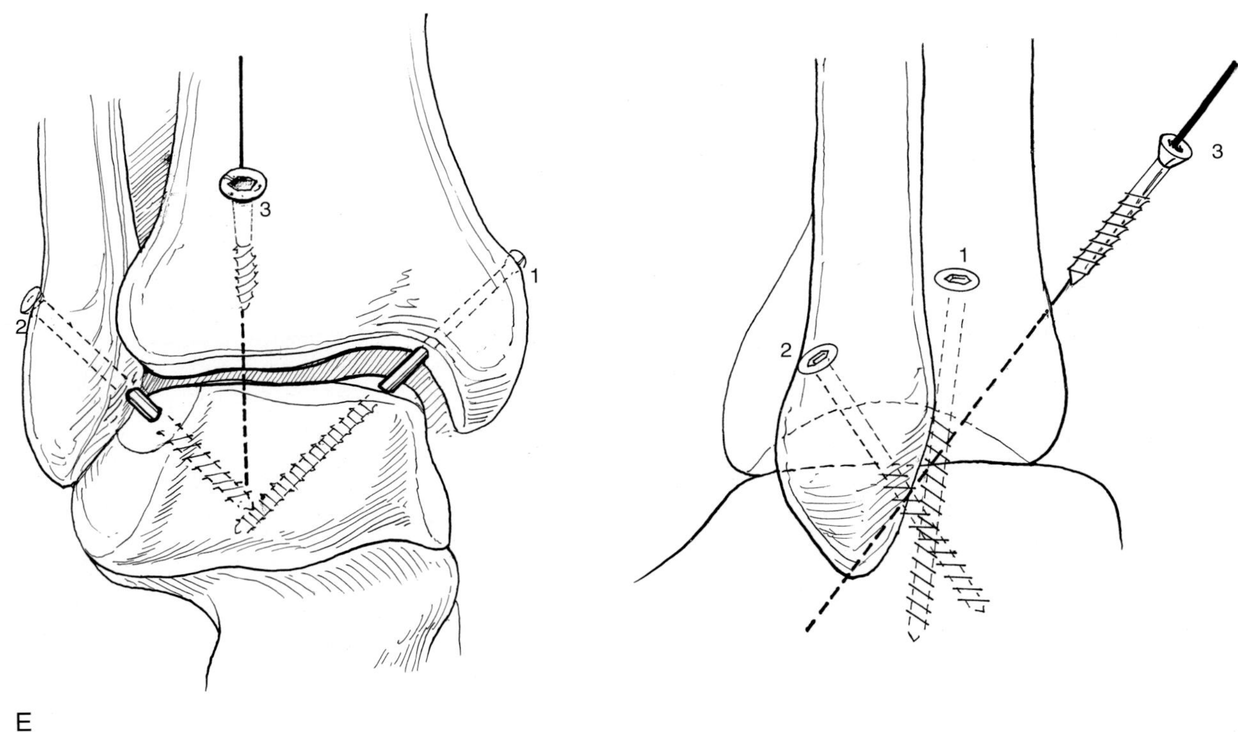

FIGURE 32–2 *Continued. E,* Anteroposterior and lateral views of cannulated screw placement.

Tarsometatarsal Arthrodesis

This condition typically involves the first metatarsocuneiform joint.

1. Incision: A 4- to 5-cm longitudinal dorsal incision is centered over the joint (Fig. 32–3).
2. Exposure: Care is taken to preserve cutaneous nerves. The interval between the extensor hallucis longus tendon and the tibialis anterior tendon (near its insertion) is approached, and the metatarsocuneiform joint is opened and exposed subperiosteally.
3. Preparation: Remaining articular cartilage, dense subchondral bone, and osteophytes are removed.
4. Fusion: A notch cut is made in the dorsal aspect of the proximal portion of the first metatarsal, and a compression screw is placed obliquely from the metatarsal into the cuneiform.

Metatarsophalangeal and Interphalangeal Arthrodesis

These procedures are similar to that described for tarsometatarsal arthrodesis and are approached through a dorsal incision. The procedures are illustrated in Figures 32–4 and 32–5.

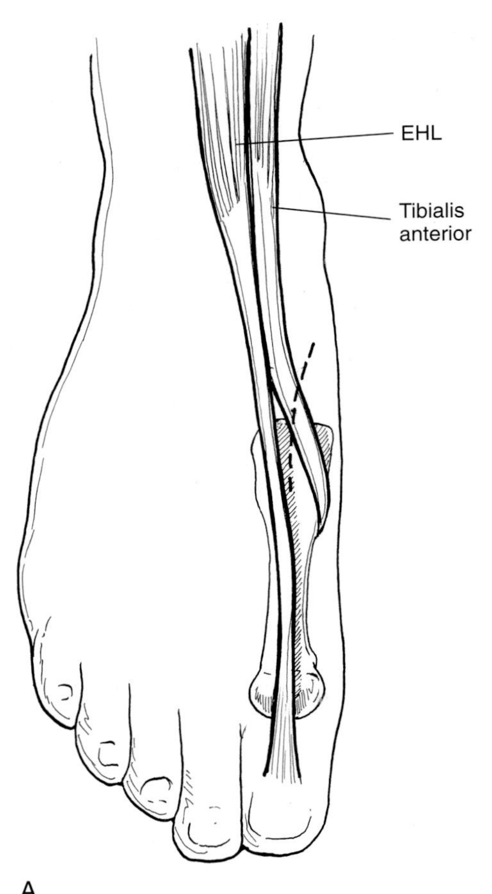

FIGURE 32–3. First metatarsocuneiform fusion. *A,* Incision and initial dissection between the extensor hallucis longus and tibialis anterior tendons. EHL, extensor hallucis longus tendon.

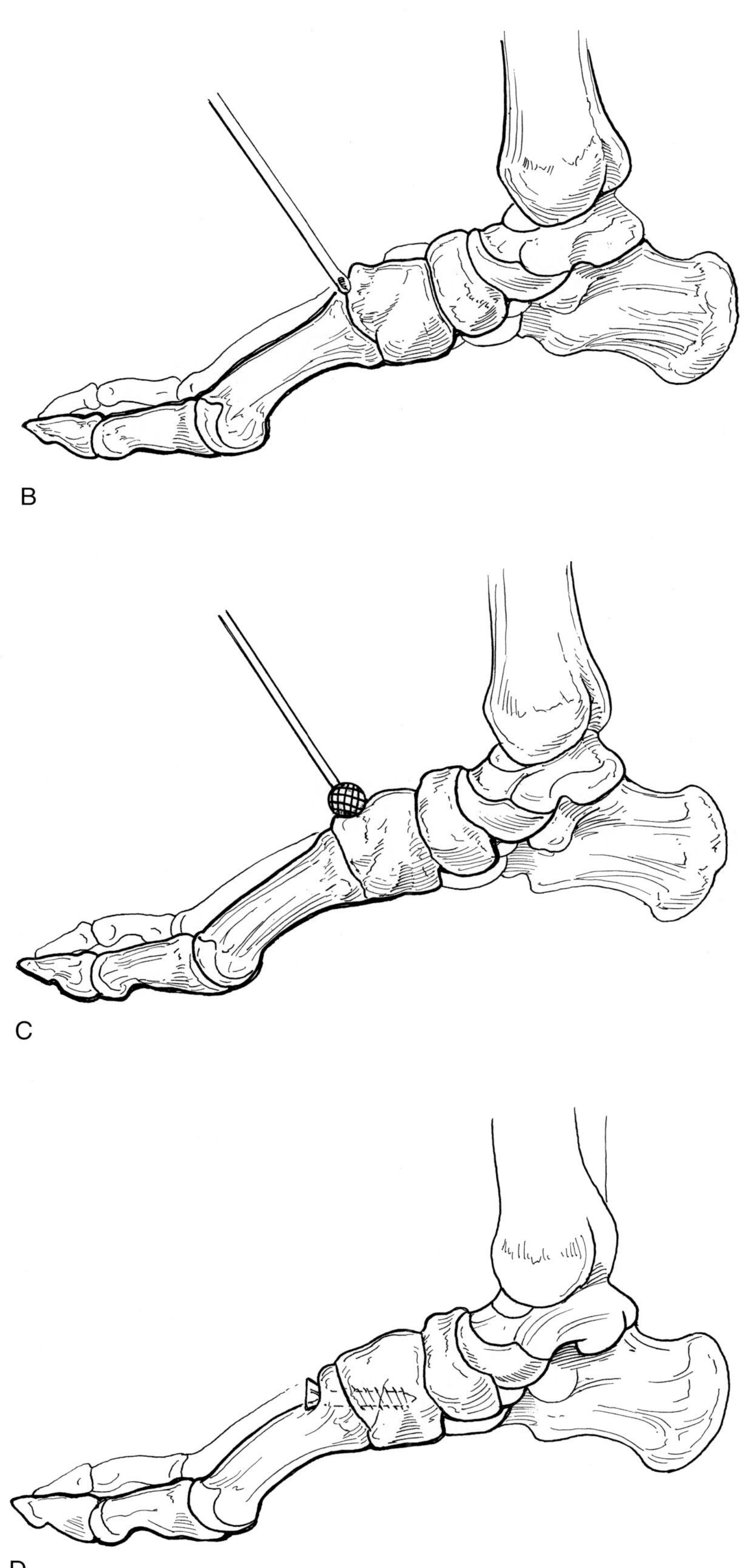

FIGURE 32–3 *Continued. B,* Curette used to remove remaining cartilage. *C,* Burr used to remove osteophytes and dense subchondral bone. *D,* Compression screw, placed through a notch in the dorsal cortex of the first metatarsal.

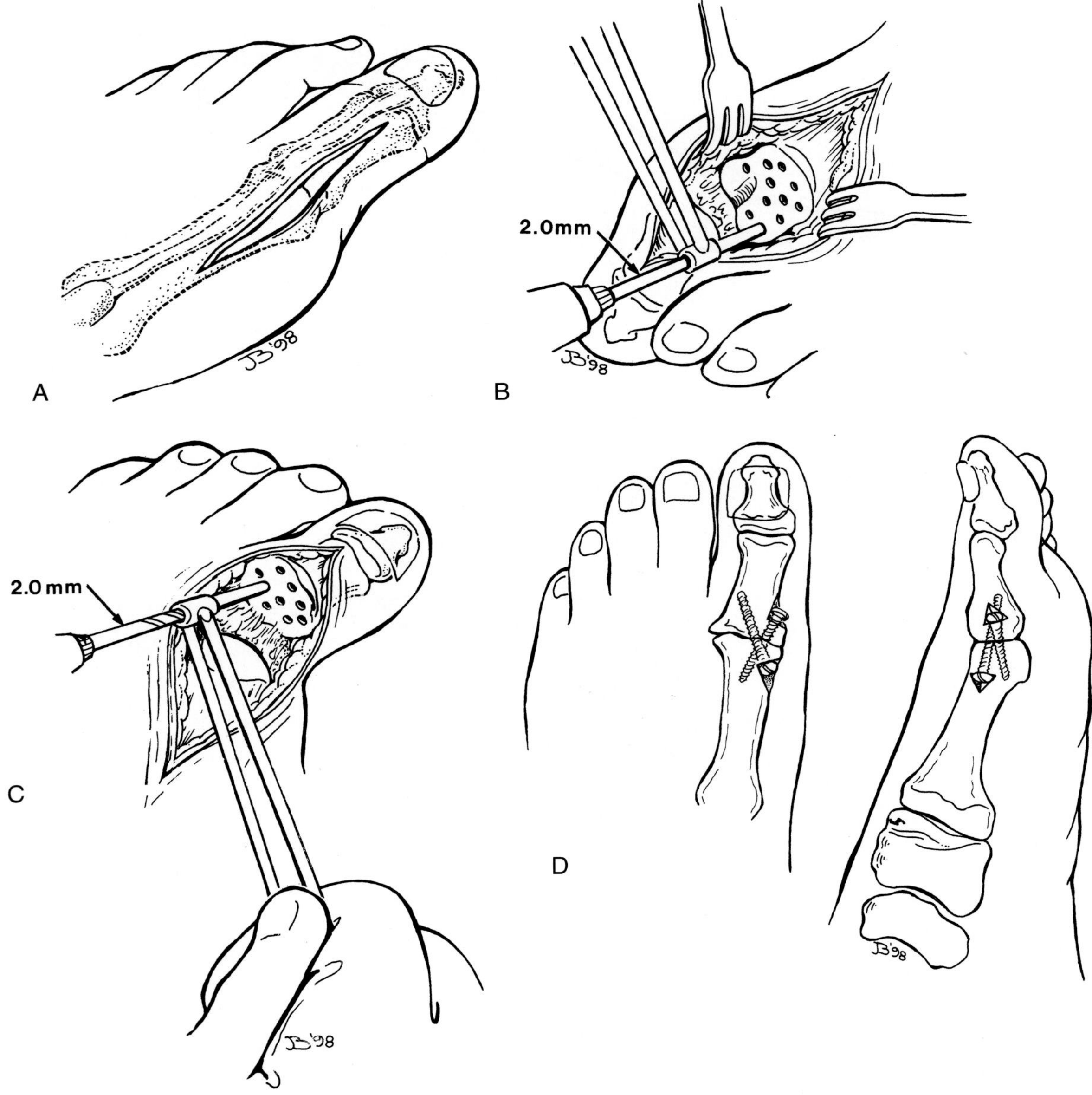

FIGURE 32–4. First metatarsophalangeal fusion. *A*, Skin incision 3 to 5 mm medial to the extensor hallucis longus tendon and centered over joint. *B* and *C*, Preparation with perforation of subchondral plates of both sides of the joint. *D*, Screw placement and final position of arthrodesis. (From Castro MD, Pomeroy GC: Arthrodesis for degenerative disease of the hallux metatarsophalangeal and interphalangeal joints. Op Tech Orthop 9:38–44, 1999.)

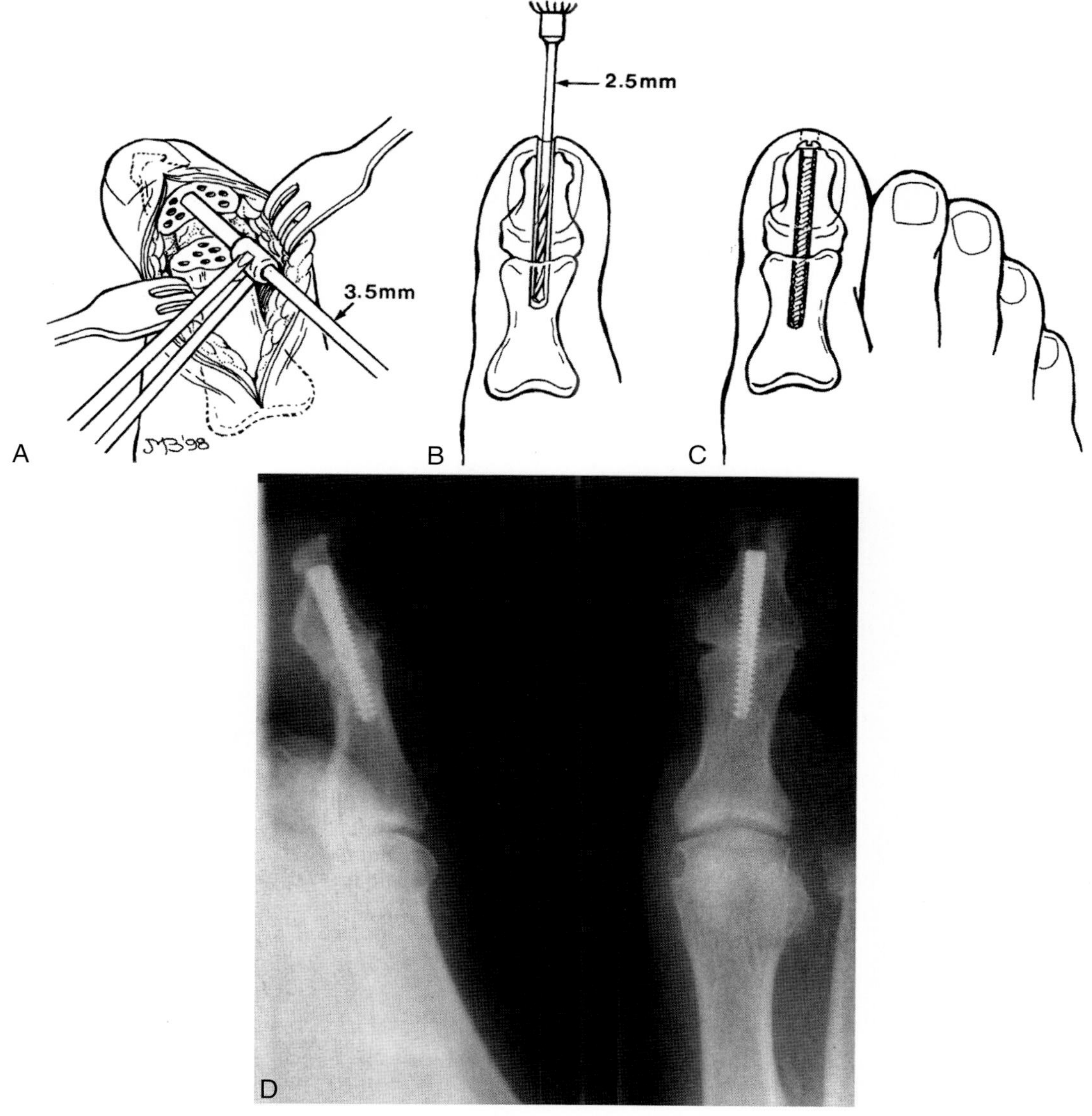

FIGURE 32–5. First interphalangeal joint fusion. *A*, After perforation of the subchondral plates of both sides of the joint, a 3.5-mm glide drill hole is placed proximal to distal through the distal phalanx. *B*, A 2.5-mm thread hole is drilled retrograde to the desired depth. *C*, A 3.5-mm cortical screw is used to fix the joint. *D*, Lateral and anteroposterior radiograph shows arthrodesis of first interphalangeal joint using a headless screw. (From Castro MD, Pomeroy GC: Arthrodesis for degenerative disease of the hallux metatarsophalangeal and interphalangeal joints. Op Tech Orthop 9:38–44, 1999.)

POSTOPERATIVE MANAGEMENT

Minimal weight bearing is allowed until signs of union are present radiographically (usually 2 to 3 months postoperatively). Progressive weight bearing is allowed at this point.

COMPLICATIONS

The most common complications after arthrodesis are nonunion and malunion. The risk of these complications can be reduced drastically with careful preoperative planning and surgical technique. Positioning the ankle and foot should be done carefully before fixation. Other complications, such as infection and wound problems, also can occur.

RESULTS

Mann reported 46 of 48 successful tibiotalar fusions with the transfibular technique. Ogilvie-Harris and associates reported successful arthrodesis in 17 of 19 patients with an arthroscopically assisted technique. Similar results have been reported with other arthrodesis procedures in the foot.

REFERENCES

Castro MD, Pomeroy GC: Arthrodesis for degenerative disease of the hallux metatarsophalangeal and interphalangeal joints. Op Tech Orthop 9:38–44, 1999.

Mann RA: Arthrodesis of the foot and ankle. In Mann RA, Coughlin MJ (eds): Surgery of the Foot and Ankle, 6th ed. St. Louis, Mosby, 1993, pp 673–713.

Ogilvie-Harris DJ, Lieberman L, Fitsialos D: Arthroscopically assisted arthrodesis for osteoarthritic ankles. J Bone Joint Surg [Am] 75:1167–1174, 1993.

CHAPTER 33

Treatment of Bunionette

INTRODUCTION

A bunionette, or *tailor's bunion*, is similar to hallux valgus but is on the lateral border of the foot. The prominent fifth metatarsal is painful with footwear.

HISTORY AND PHYSICAL EXAMINATION

Patients may complain of pain and irritation between the underlying bony abnormality and restricting footwear. Examination may show an inflamed bursa or keratosis.

DIAGNOSTIC IMAGING

Standing anteroposterior and lateral radiographs are obtained. The 4–5 intermetatarsal angle and metatarsophalangeal-5 angle are measured on the anteroposterior radiograph (Fig. 33–1).

NONOPERATIVE MANAGEMENT

Change in footwear is the first intervention that should be attempted. Padding of the prominent metatarsal head and shaving of the hypertrophic callus may give some relief. Orthotic devices sometimes can be helpful.

RELEVANT ANATOMY

Coughlin described three types of bunionette deformities (Fig. 33–2). Surgical treatment is based on this anatomy.

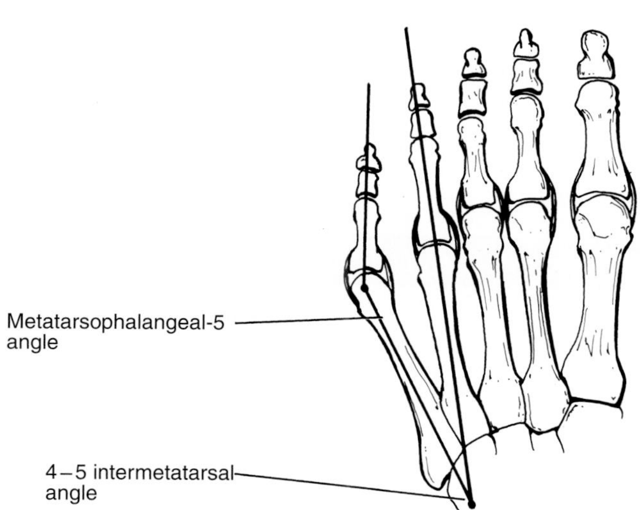

FIGURE 33–1. The 4–5 intermetatarsal angle and metatarsophalangeal-5 angle measurements. (From Coughlin MJ: Conditions of the forefoot. In DeLee JC, Drez D Jr [eds]: Orthopaedic Sports Medicine: Principles and Practice. Philadelphia, WB Saunders, 1994, pp 1842–1939.)

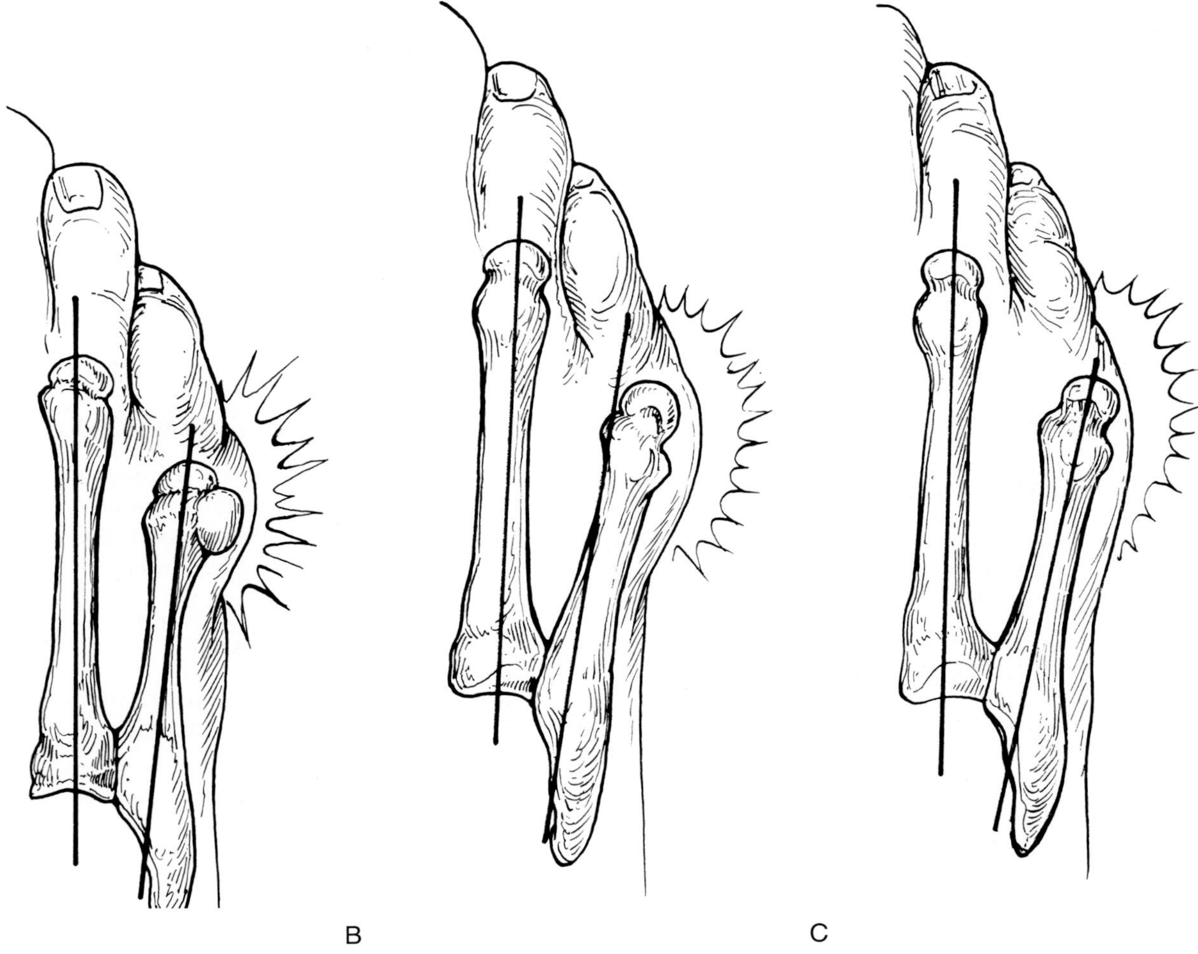

FIGURE 33–2. Three types of bunionettes. *A*, Type 1: Enlarged fifth metatarsal head/exostosis. *B*, Type 2: Lateral bow within fifth metatarsal. *C*, Type 3: Increased 4–5 intermetatarsal angle (>8° to 10°).

SURGICAL *TECHNIQUE*

Indications

Failure of the conservative measures outlined earlier is an indication for surgical treatment.

Technique

A variety of techniques have been described for the treatment of bunionette deformities, based on the pathoanatomy. Typically, type 1 bunionette deformities are correctable with a lateral condylectomy alone. Type 2 and mild type 3 (4–5 intermetatarsal angle <12°) bunionettes can be addressed with a distal chevron osteotomy. More severe type 3 bunionettes may require a midshaft osteotomy.

Lateral Condylectomy

1. Incision: A longitudinal incision is made laterally, centered on the metatarsophalangeal joint (Fig. 33–3). The dorsal lateral sensory nerve is identified and retracted. The capsule is exposed.
2. Capsulotomy: An inverted L capsular incision is made, and the capsule is sharply elevated from the lateral aspect of the metatarsal head.
3. Osteotomy: The lateral eminence is removed in line with the lateral border of the fifth metatarsal shaft using a microsagittal saw.
4. Balancing: If the fifth toe remains medially deviated, a medial capsular release is done.
5. Closure: The capsule and skin is closed, and a soft tissue dressing is applied.

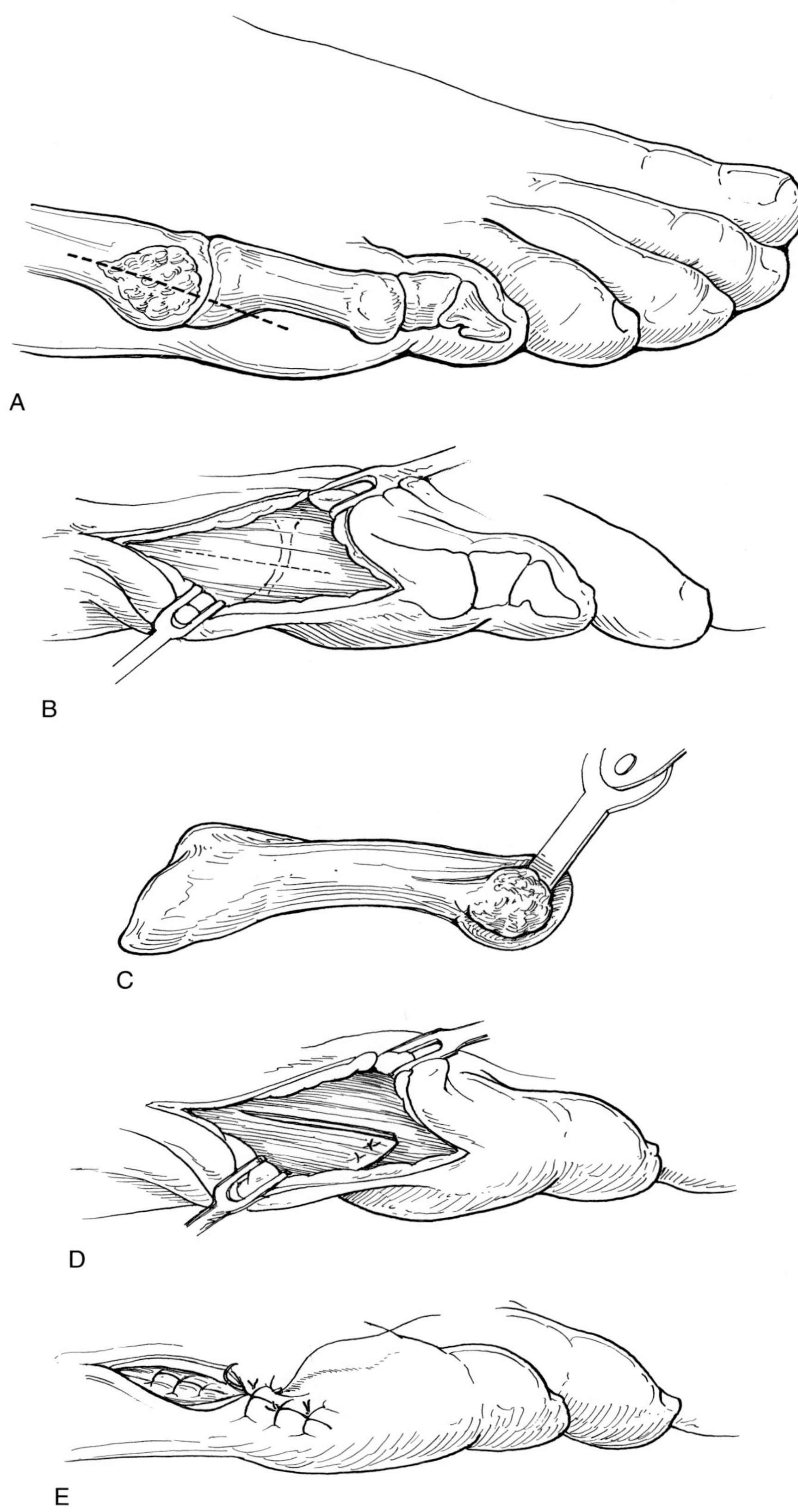

FIGURE 33–3. Lateral condylectomy. *A*, Lateral incision centered over the fifth metatarsophalangeal joint. *B*, L-shaped capsulotomy. *C*, Removal of lateral exostosis. *D*, Capsular imbrication. *E*, Wound closure.

Distal Chevron Osteotomy

1. Incision: A longitudinal incision is made as described for lateral condylectomy (Fig. 33–4).
2. Lateral condylectomy: This is done as described earlier.
3. Osteotomy: A chevron osteotomy is made with a sagittal saw at an angle of approximately 60°. The apex of the cut is the center of the metatarsal head. The distal fragment is displaced medially 3 to 4 mm. A K-wire is inserted from distal and medial to proximal and lateral to fix the osteotomy site.
4. Balancing: The overhanging lateral metatarsal neck is removed in line with the lateral border of the shaft with the microsagittal saw. Additional soft tissue balancing is done as necessary.
5. Closure: Closure is as described for lateral condylectomy.

Midshaft Osteotomy

1. Incision: A dorsal lateral longitudinal incision is made over the entire length of the fifth metatarsal (Fig. 33–5). The dorsolateral cutaneous nerve is isolated and

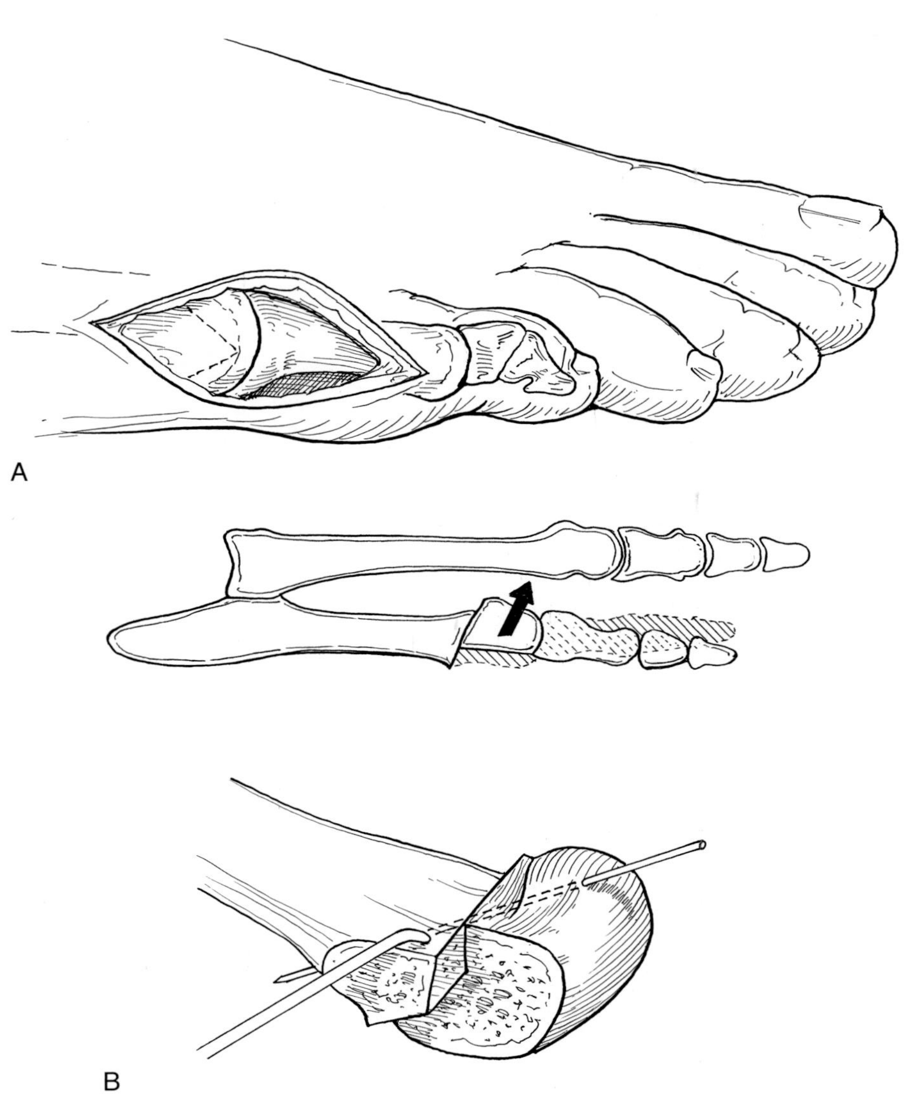

FIGURE 33–4. Distal chevron osteotomy. *A*, Osteotomy following lateral condylectomy. Note angle of approximately 60°. *B*, Neck/shaft is displaced laterally 3 to 4 mm.

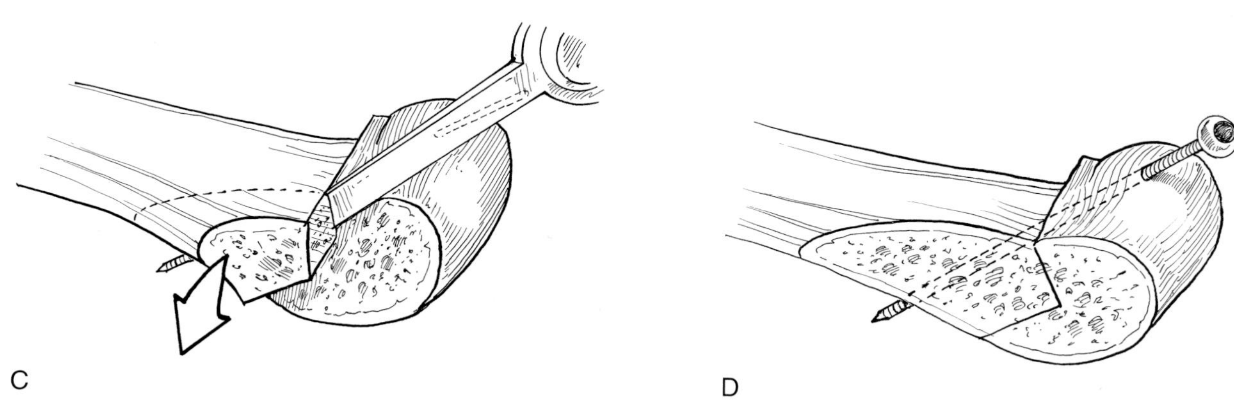

FIGURE 33–4 *Continued. C*, Removal of remaining overhang. *D*, Fixation with a K-wire.

protected. The abductor digiti quinti muscle is displaced plantarly, and the extensor tendon is displaced medially.

2. Lateral condylectomy: This is done as described earlier.
3. Osteotomy: After the shaft is exposed, a long oblique osteotomy is made with a sagittal saw from proximal dorsal to distal plantar at a 45° angle to the long axis. The distal fragment is rotated medially, and the osteotomy is fixed with an interfragmentary cortical screw from dorsal to plantar.
4. Balancing: Prominent bone over the lateral aspect of the osteotomy is removed, and soft tissue balancing is completed.
5. Closure: The periosteum is closed, and wounds are closed in standard fashion.

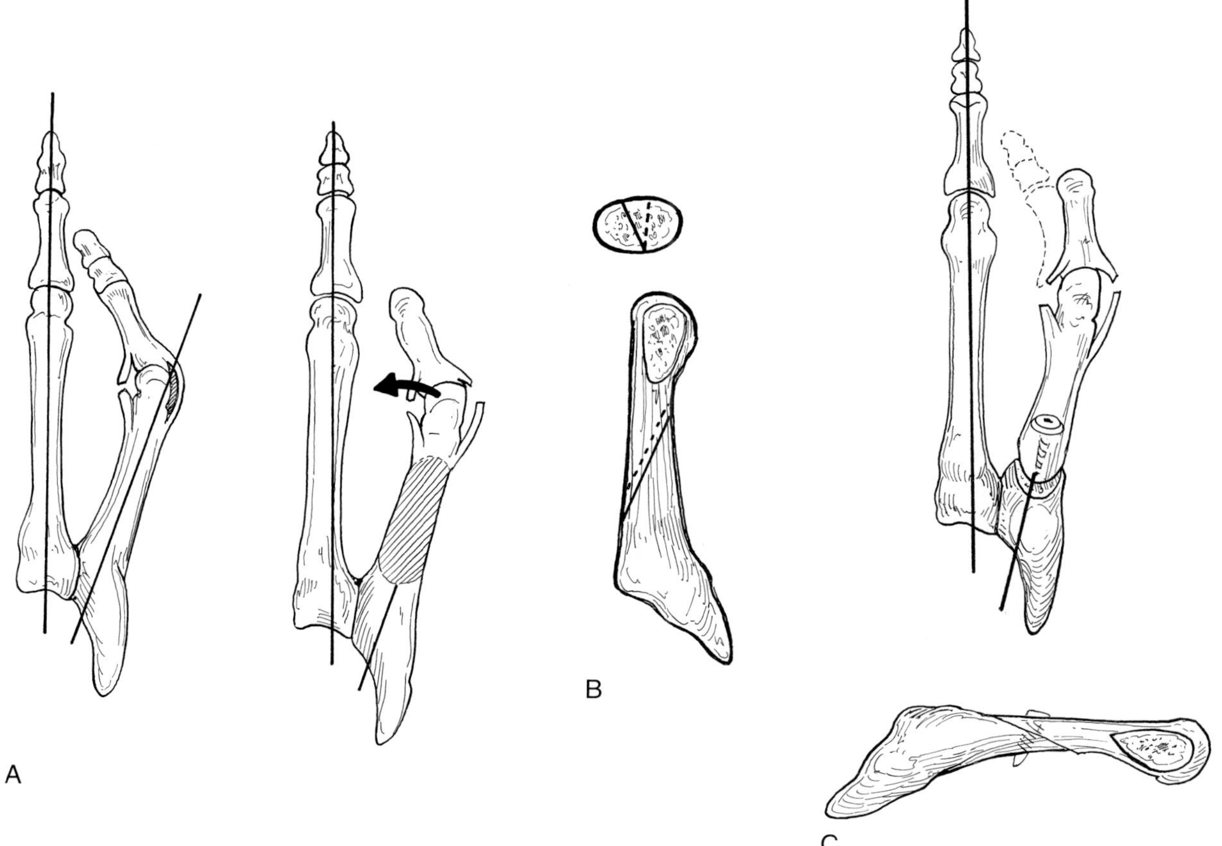

FIGURE 33–5. Midshaft osteotomy. *A*, Lateral condylectomy completed and osteotomy planned in patient with type 3 bunionette. *B*, Osteotomy completed at 45° angle. *C*, Rotation and fixation.

POSTOPERATIVE MANAGEMENT

Patients undergoing lateral condylectomy and distal chevron osteotomy can be managed in a wooden-soled postoperative shoe. A cast or fracture boot is used after midshaft osteotomies. Crutches are used for approximately 3 weeks. K-wires (if used) are removed at 4 to 5 weeks. Protective weight bearing is allowed after bony union.

COMPLICATIONS

Complications include delayed union, nonunion, malunion, metatarsophalangeal joint subluxation, metatarsalgia, and recurrence of the deformity.

RESULTS

Good results can be expected in about 85% of cases. Proper procedure selection is important.

REFERENCES

Coughlin MJ: Treatment of bunionette deformity with longitudinal diaphyseal osteotomy with soft tissue repair. Foot Ankle 11:195–203, 1991.

Coughlin MJ: Conditions of the forefoot. In DeLee JC, Drez D Jr (eds): Orthopaedic Sports Medicine: Principles and Practice. Philadelphia, WB Saunders, 1994, pp 1842–1939.

Sfera JJ, Shute GC: Treatment of the bunionette deformity. Op Tech Orthop 9:62–69, 1999.

CHAPTER 34

Treatment of Hallux Valgus and Rigidus

INTRODUCTION

Hallux valgus involves subluxation of the first metatarsophalangeal joint and is related to footwear. Hallux rigidus is a result of osteoarthritis of the first metatarsophalangeal joint. Neither hallux valgus nor hallux rigidus is peculiar to athletes, and these disorders are common.

HISTORY AND PHYSICAL EXAMINATION

Patients with hallux valgus typically present with a complaint of pain over the medial eminence, exacerbated by footwear. They present with a typical deformity (Fig. 34–1). Chronic hallux valgus can lead to lateral metatarsalgia with intractable plantar keratosis beneath the lesser metatarsal heads. Runners with hallux valgus can develop callosities on the medial border of the great toe or first metatarsal. Patients with hallux rigidus present with localized pain and loss of motion. The pain is worse with gait (especially during the toe-off phase). Hallux rigidus can follow chronic turf toe injuries.

Examination of hallux valgus and hallux rigidus includes observation of standing and walking. Other disorders about the foot are considered, and a complete neurovascular examination is completed. Range of motion is recorded (this may be markedly restricted, especially in dorsiflexion in patients with hallux rigidus). The axial grind test (similar to the test for evaluation of carpometacarpal arthritis of the base of the thumb) can elicit pain in patients with hallux rigidus (Fig. 34–2).

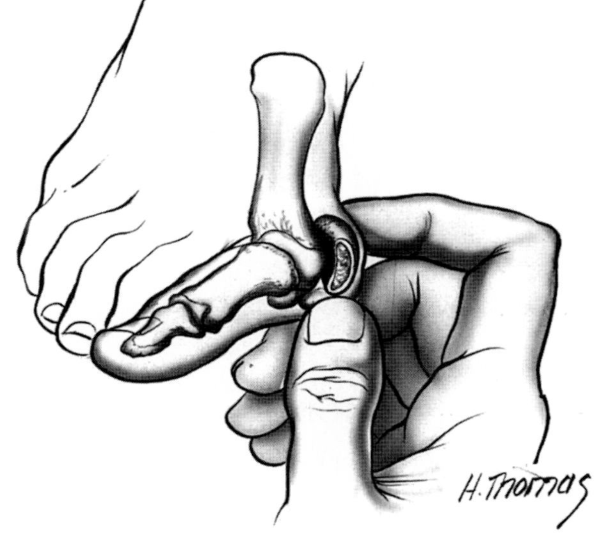

FIGURE 34–1. Typical medial prominence seen in patients with hallux valgus. (From Hoppenfeld S: Physical examination of the foot by complaint. In Jahss MH [ed]: Disorders of the Foot and Ankle, 2nd ed. Philadelphia, WB Saunders, 1991, pp 52–63.)

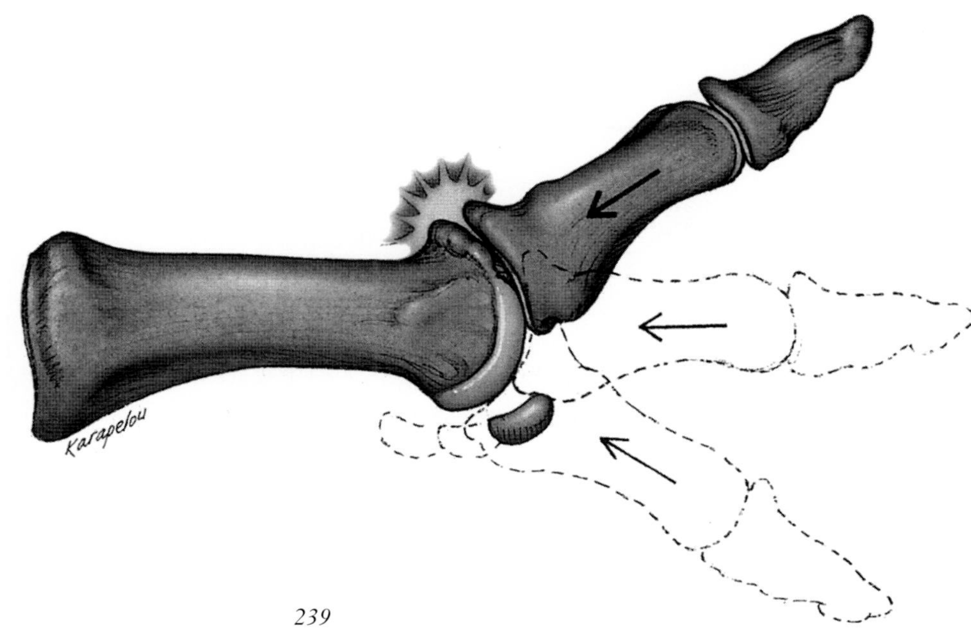

FIGURE 34–2. Axial grind test for hallux rigidus. The patient has pain with axial compression and dorsiflexion. (From Baumhauer JF: Dorsal cheilectomy of the first metatarsophalangeal joint in the treatment of hallux rigidus. Op Tech Orthop 9:26–32, 1999.)

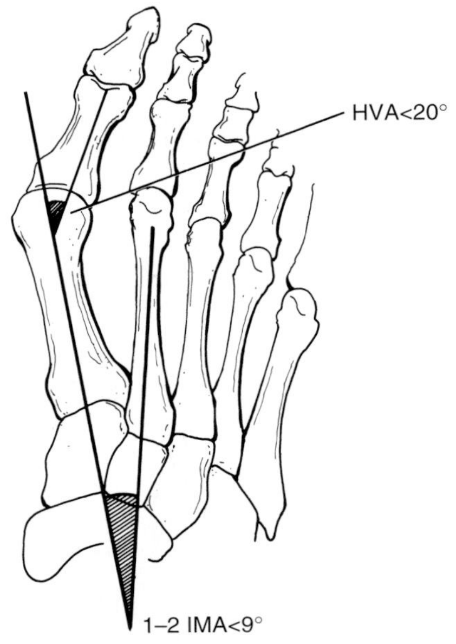

FIGURE 34–3. The hallux valgus angle (HVA) (normally <15° to 20°) is formed by lines bisecting the first metatarsal and proximal phalanx. The 1–2 intermetatarsal angle (1–2 IMA) (normally <9°) is formed by lines bisecting the first and second metatarsals. (From Coughlin MJ: Conditions of the forefoot. In DeLee JC, Drez D Jr [eds]: Orthopaedic Sports Medicine: Principles and Practice. Philadelphia, WB Saunders, 1994, pp 1842–1939.)

DIAGNOSTIC IMAGING

Weight-bearing radiographs are evaluated carefully. The hallux valgus angle and first and second intermetatarsal angles are measured (Fig. 34–3).

NONOPERATIVE MANAGEMENT

Footwear modification, orthotic devices, nonsteroidal anti-inflammatory drugs, and other measures are the mainstay of treatment. Athletes should consider surgery only as a last resort because of the likelihood of a reduced ability to run or dance. Hallux rigidus shoe modifications should include a rigid shank to decrease stress on the joint and limit motion.

RELEVANT ANATOMY

Variation in the head of the metatarsal can be related to development of hallux valgus (more rounded heads are susceptible). Structures that stabilize the first metatarsophalangeal joint include collateral ligaments and sesamoid ligaments (Fig. 34–4). Dynamic stabilizers include the flexor hallucis brevis tendons, which insert into the medial and lateral sesamoids, which in turn insert into the plantar plate; the abductor hallucis; the adductor hallucis; and the extensor hallucis longus. No tendons insert onto the metatarsal head, and the capsular ligaments stabilize the joint. With subluxation of the joint, the dorsal capsule and hood ligament become attenuated (Fig. 34–5).

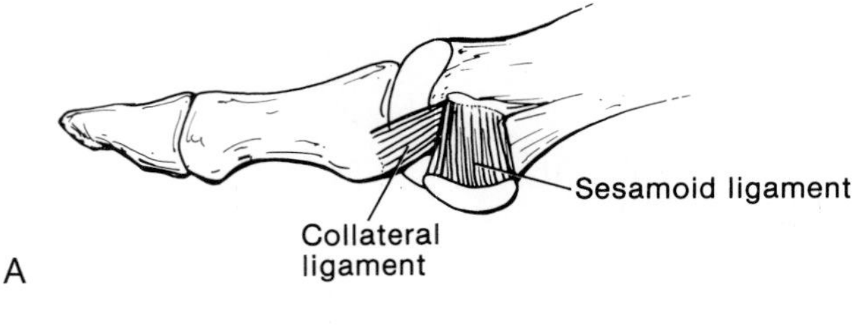

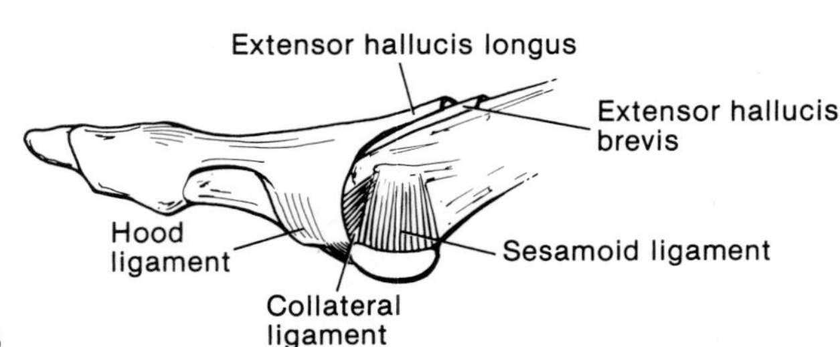

FIGURE 34–4. *A*, Collateral and sesamoid ligaments. *B*, The extensor hallucis longus inserts into the hood ligament. (From Coughlin MJ: Conditions of the forefoot. In DeLee JC, Drez D Jr [eds]: Orthopaedic Sports Medicine: Principles and Practice. Philadelphia, WB Saunders, 1994, pp 1842–1939.)

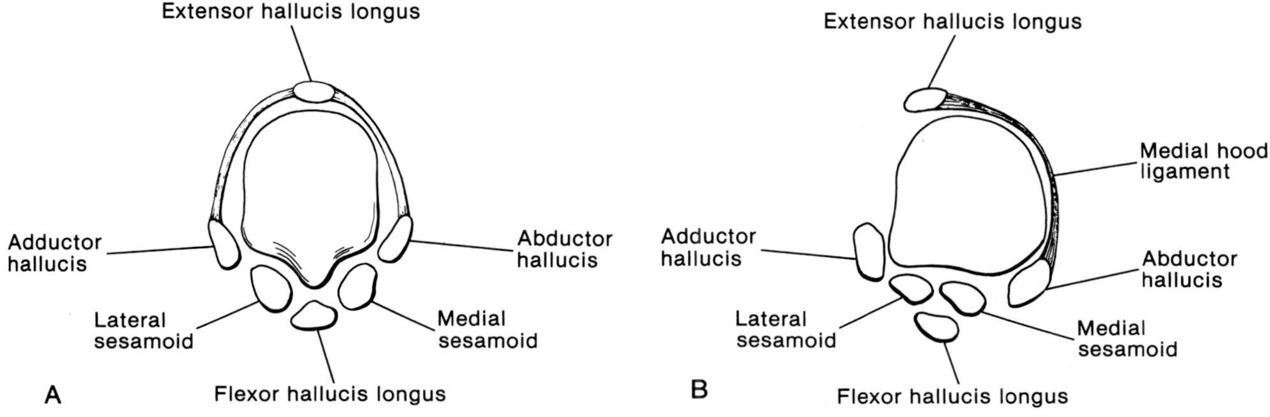

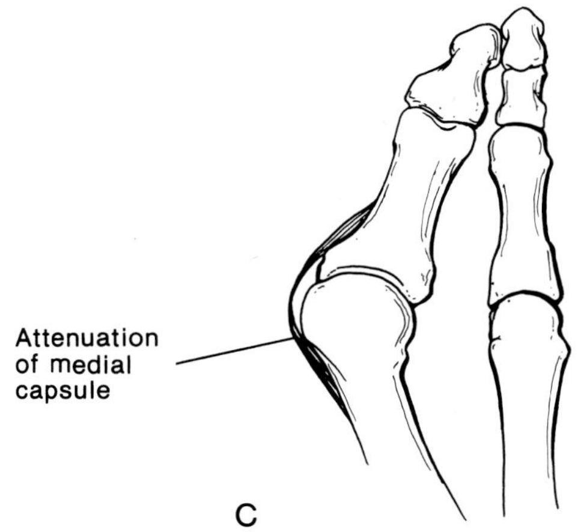

FIGURE 34–5. *A*, Cross-sectional view of normal tissues at the first tarsometatarsal joint. *B*, Subluxation of the joint causes disruption of these structures. *C*, Anteroposterior view of capsular attenuation. (From Coughlin MJ: Conditions of the forefoot. In DeLee JC, Drez D Jr [eds]: Orthopaedic Sports Medicine: Principles and Practice. Philadelphia, WB Saunders, 1994, pp 1842–1939.)

SURGICAL *TECHNIQUE*

Indications

Hallux valgus correction should be reserved for cases in which pain prohibits an athlete from performing. Dorsal cheilectomy is indicated in patients with isolated dorsal degenerative joint disease, limited toe motion, negative grind test in neutral or plantar flexion, and the absence of sesamoid disease.

Technique

A variety of techniques have been described for the treatment of hallux valgus, largely based on the degree of deformity (hallux valgus angle [HVA] and 1–2 intermetatarsal angles [IMA]) (Fig. 34–6). The following general guidelines usually are followed:

HVA	*IMA*	*Procedure*
<40°	<13° to 15°	Modified McBride or distal chevron osteotomy
<40°	>13° to 15°	Modified McBride and proximal osteotomy
>40°	>20°	Modified McBride and proximal osteotomy or arthrodesis

The modified McBride (distal soft tissue release and exostectomy), (distal) chevron osteotomy, and proximal metatarsal osteotomy are described. First metatarsophalangeal fusion is described in Chapter 32. Dorsal cheilectomy for hallux rigidus is described here.

Modified McBride Distal Soft Tissue Procedure

1. Incision: A 3-cm dorsal longitudinal incision is made in the first intermetatarsal web space (Fig. 34–7).
2. Adductor hallucis release: The adductor hallucis tendon is identified and incised approximately 1.5 cm proximal to its insertion. The stump of the insertion is tagged for later use, and the proximal tendon is allowed to retract.
3. Lateral capsule: The lateral sesamoid is freed, and the lateral capsule is perforated or torn. The lateral sesamoid is not excised as McBride originally described (making this the modified McBride procedure). The stump is used to reinforce the lateral capsule.
4. Medial eminence resection: A medial incision is made, capsular flap is created, and medial eminence is resected with an oscillating saw. The medial capsule is imbricated before closure.
5. Lateral capsule reinforcement: Absorbable sutures are used to approximate the first and second metatarsophalangeal capsules.
6. Wounds are closed, and a soft dressing is applied.

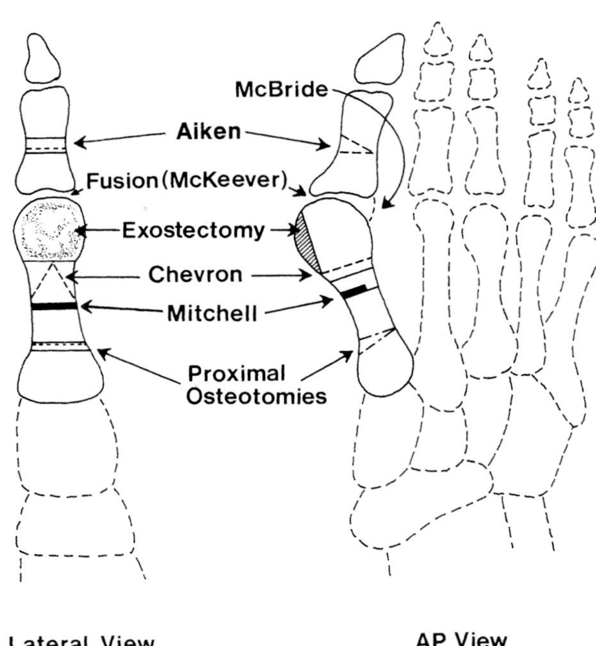

FIGURE 34–6. Common surgical procedures available for hallux valgus correction. (From Mizel MS, Sobel M, Ptaszek AJ: Disorders of the foot and ankle. In Miller MD [ed]: Review of Orthopaedics, 3rd ed. Philadelphia, WB Saunders, 2000, pp 279–303.)

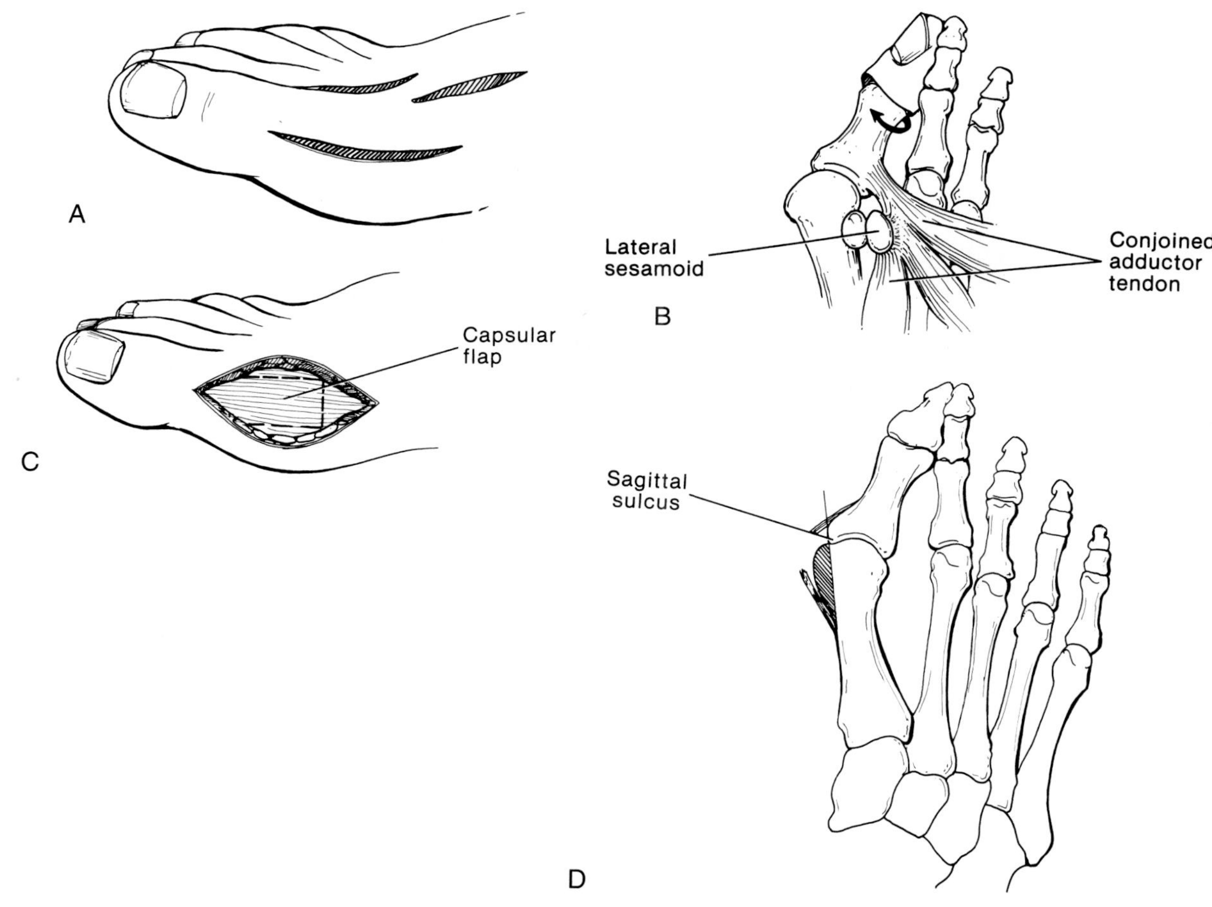

FIGURE 34–7. Modified McBride distal soft tissue release and medial exostosectomy. *A*, Two incisions are made, one in the first web space and one to expose the medial eminence. *B*, The conjoined adductor tendon is identified and incised, and the lateral sesamoid is freed. *C*, A U-shaped capsular flap is made to expose the medial eminence. *D*, The medial eminence is resected along a line parallel with the long axis of the medial cortex of the first metatarsal. (From Coughlin MJ: Conditions of the forefoot. In DeLee JC, Drez D Jr [eds]: Orthopaedic Sports Medicine: Principles and Practice. Philadelphia, WB Saunders, 1994, pp 1842–1939.)

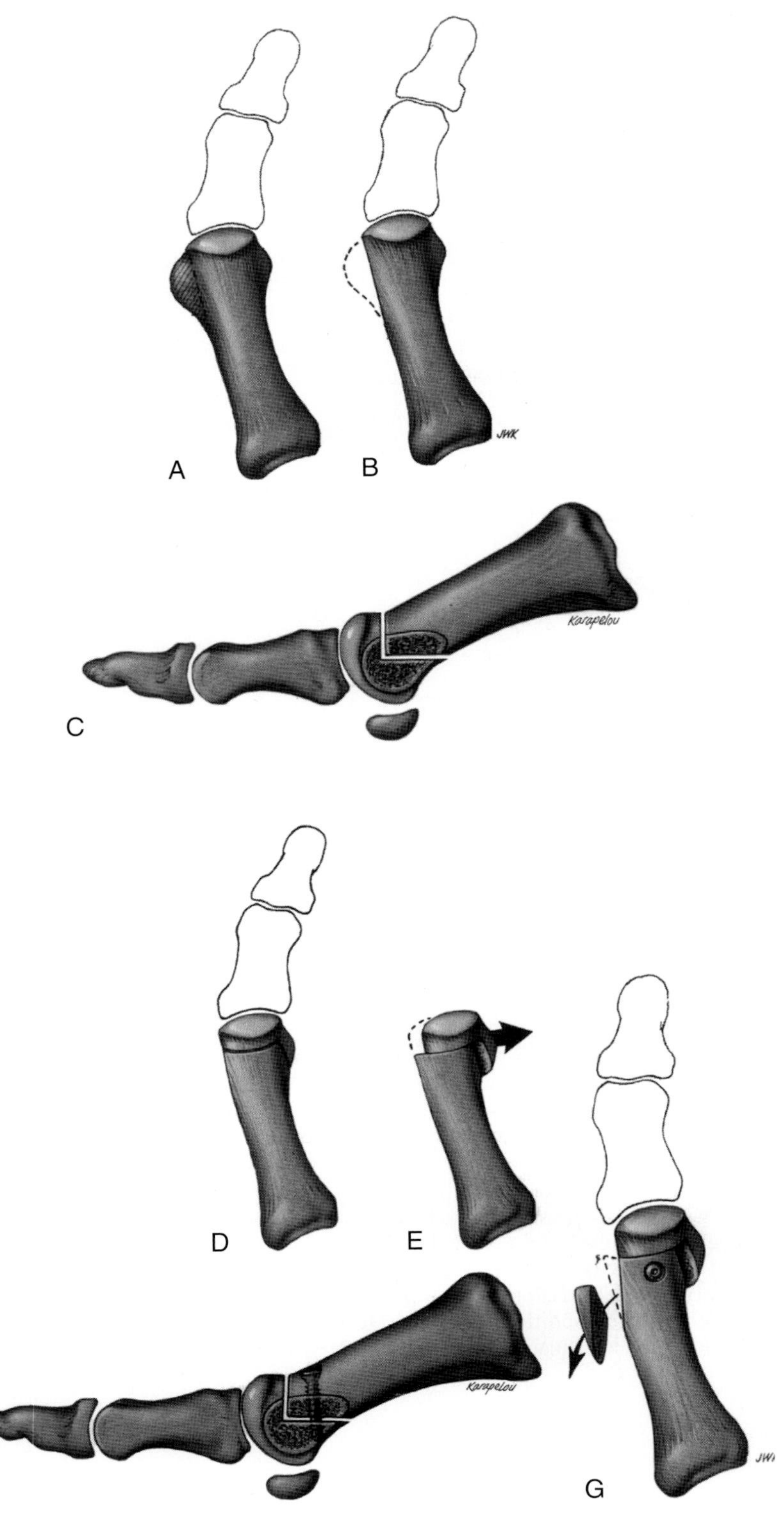

FIGURE 34–8. Distal chevron osteotomy. *A*, Planned exostosectomy. *B*, Completed exostosectomy. *C*, Lateral view of modified chevron osteotomy. The plantar portion of the osteotomy is longer and parallel with the plantar plane of the foot. *D*, Anteroposterior view of completed osteotomy. *E*, The capital fragment is shifted approximately 5 mm laterally. *F*, Interfragmentary compression screw placement. *G*, Completion of the procedure with removal of the medial overhang. (From Wright DG: Distal first metatarsal chevron osteotomy. Op Tech Orthop 9:15–18, 1999.)

Distal Chevron Osteotomy

1. Incision: A 5-cm medial midline incision is made over the distal aspect of the first metatarsal (Fig. 34–8). The dorsal sensory nerve is identified and protected.
2. Capsulotomy: An incision is made midline in the capsule. The sesamoids are mobilized.
3. Exostosectomy: A bunionectomy is done parallel to the medial border of the foot.
4. Chevron osteotomy: Using a microsagittal saw, a chevron cut is made in the metatarsal neck. The apex of the cut is in the center of the metatarsal head. The dorsal cut is short and oblique, and the plantar cut is long and parallel to the plane of correction.
5. Fixation: The dorsal surface of the metatarsal neck is exposed. The distal head fragment is shifted approximately 5 mm laterally, and a countersunk 3.5-mm cortical interfragmentary screw is placed from superior to inferior.
6. Balancing: Soft tissue releases are done as necessary to balance the sesamoids (as seen radiographically). The medial overhang is removed to create a smooth medial border.
7. Closure: The joint is irrigated and closed in layers, beginning with the capsule.

Proximal Metatarsal Osteotomy

There is more than one way to do a proximal metatarsal osteotomy. A chevron osteotomy, similar to the distal chevron osteotomy described earlier, can be done. Alternatively, lateral closing or medial opening wedge osteotomies are sometimes an option. A crescentic osteotomy sometimes is favored because it preserves first metatarsal length.

1. Incision: A 3-cm dorsal longitudinal incision is made over the dorsal aspect of the first metatarsal on the medial border of the extensor hallucis longus (Fig. 34–9).
2. Exposure: The metatarsal shaft is exposed, and the metatarsocuneiform joint is located. The osteotomy is planned approximately 1 cm distal to this joint.
3. Osteotomy: If a screw is planned for fixation, a 3.5-mm drill is used to predrill the pilot hole for the screw. This screw is inserted from distal to proximal, 1 cm distal to the osteotomy, and at an angle about 45° to the metatarsal shaft. A crescentic blade and saw is used to create the osteotomy with the apex proximally. It is checked with a freer to ensure that it is complete.
4. Alignment: The distal metatarsal is rotated into the proper alignment and held in place. A 2.5-mm drill is used to cross the osteotomy site, and the appropriately sized screw is placed from distal (dorsal) to proximal (plantar). Alternatively, the osteotomy site can be fixed with K-wires or a Steinmann pin.
5. Closure: Wounds are closed in standard fashion, and a bulky dressing is applied.

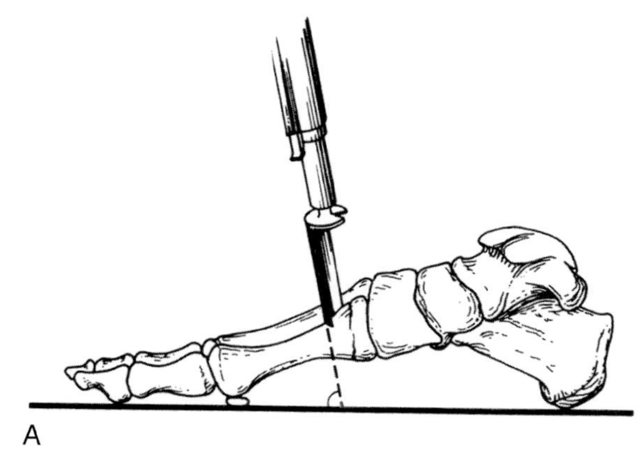

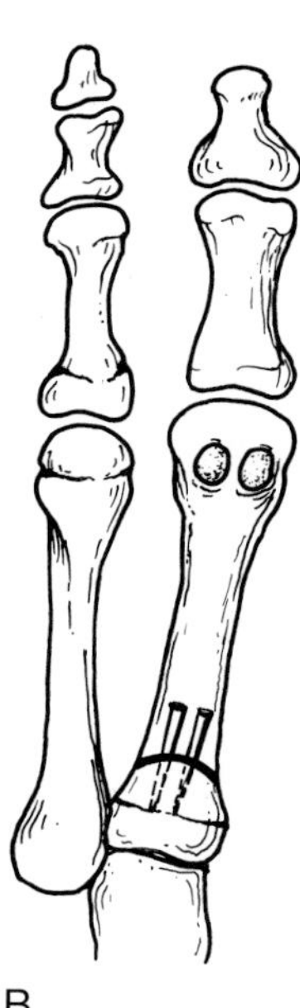

FIGURE 34–9. Proximal crescentic osteotomy. *A*, Osteotomy is made 1 cm distal to the metatarsocuneiform joint. *B*, The distal metatarsal is rotated laterally, and internal fixation is done with K-wires or a screw. (From Coughlin MJ: Juvenile bunions. In Mann RA, Coughlin MJ [eds]: Surgery of the Foot and Ankle, 6th ed. Mosby, St. Louis, 1993, pp 297–339.)

Dorsal Cheilectomy

1. Incision: A 3- to 5-cm dorsal medial incision is made, centered over the metatarsophalangeal joint (Fig. 34–10). The dorsal medial hallucis nerve is identified and protected.
2. Exposure: The extensor hallucis longus tendon is retracted laterally, and a capsulotomy is made. The distal metatarsal head and neck are exposed. The proximal phalanx is maximally flexed, and the dorsal osteophytes are seen.
3. Osteotomy: Beginning distally with a 0.5-inch sharp osteotome, an osteotomy of the dorsal third of the metatarsal head, including the cartilage-deficient area, is accomplished. The cut is angled so that the proximal extent ends at the junction of the shaft and metatarsal head. A rongeur or rasp is used to smooth the dorsal cortex. If necessary, an osteotome is used in a proximal-to-distal direction on the dorsal aspect of the base of the proximal phalanx if an osteophyte is present.
4. Closure: Wounds are irrigated and closed in normal fashion.

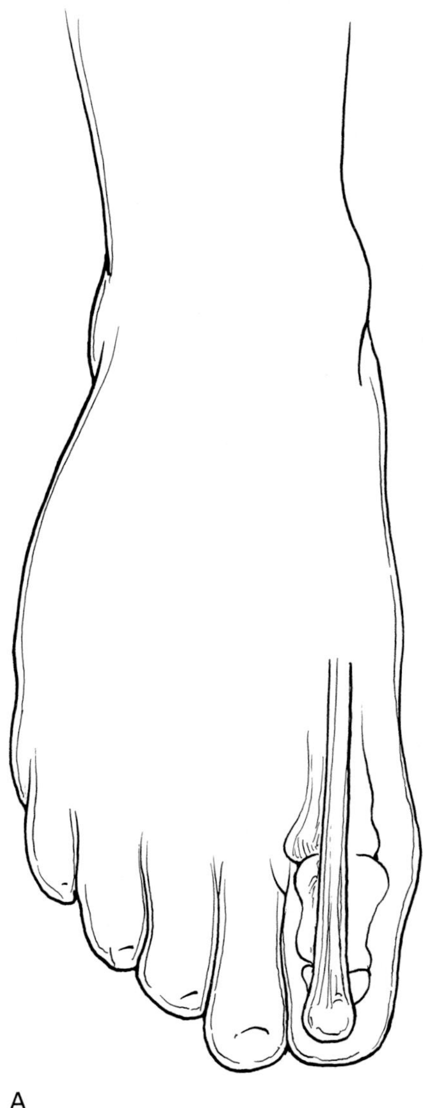

FIGURE 34–10. Dorsal cheilectomy. *A*, A 5-cm dorsomedial incision.

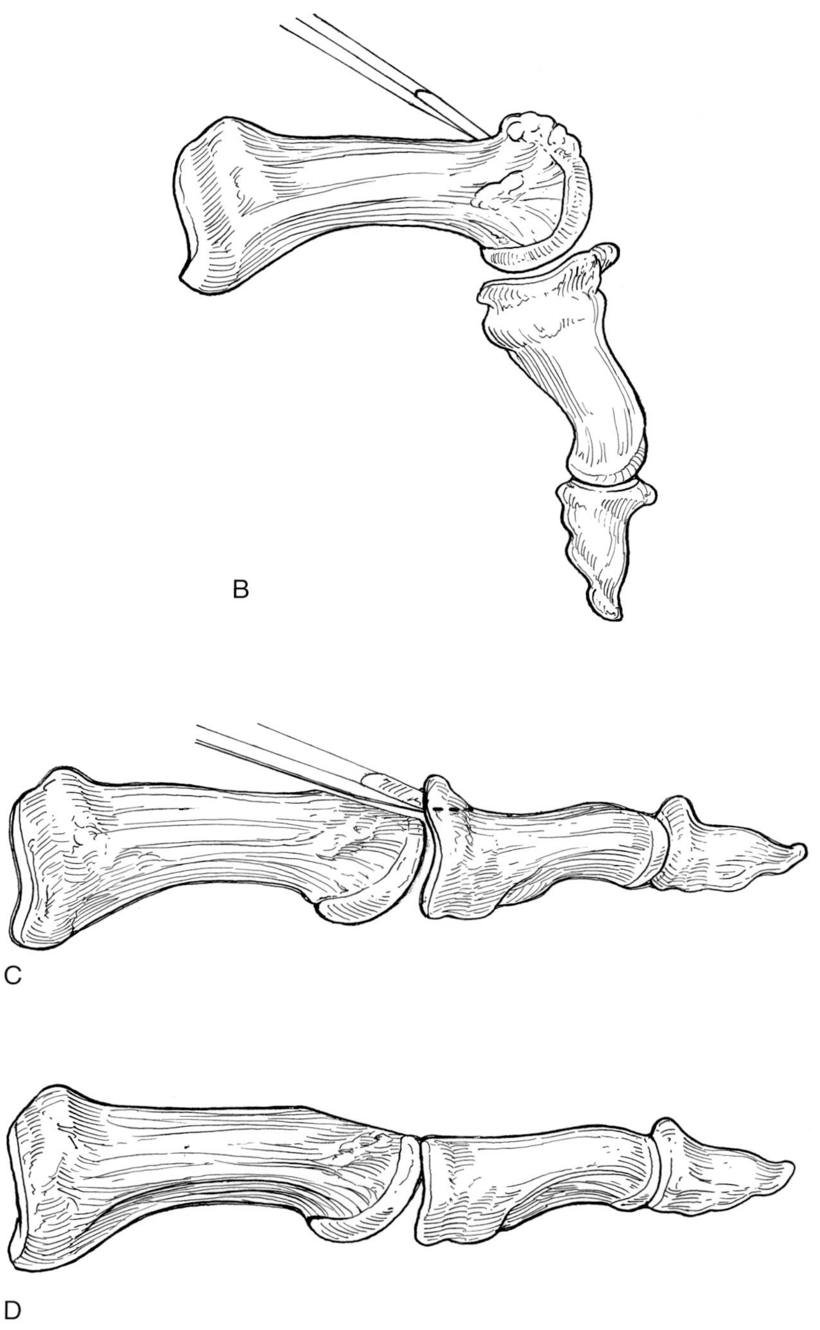

FIGURE 34–10 *Continued. B*, The dorsal third of the metatarsal head is removed with a 0.5-inch osteotome. *C*, If necessary, the dorsal osteophyte on the proximal metatarsal is removed from proximal to distal. *D*, Completed cheilectomy.

POSTOPERATIVE MANAGEMENT

In general, if any bony work is accomplished, most surgeons favor 4 to 6 weeks of minimal weight bearing.

COMPLICATIONS

Complications include nonunion, malunion, incomplete correction, and, for distal metatarsal procedures, avascular necrosis. Most authors do not recommend lateral soft tissue procedures at the same time as distal osteotomies. Hallux varus can be a complication after distal soft tissue repair, but the incidence is lower without sesamoid removal. Complications of dorsal cheilectomy involve inadequate or excessive resection.

RESULTS

Good results largely depend on proper patient and procedure selection. According to Mann and Coughlin, patient satisfaction is approximately 90% for distal soft tissue procedures and crescentic osteotomy and 80% for the distal chevron procedure. Good results have been reported in approximately 90% of patients undergoing dorsal cheilectomy.

REFERENCES

Abidi NA, Conti SF: Hallux valgus: Indications and technique of proximal chevron osteotomy combined with distal soft tissue release. Op Tech Orthop 9:8–14, 1999.

Baumhauer JF: Dorsal cheilectomy of the first metatarsophalangeal joint in the treatment of hallux rigidus. Op Tech Orthop 9:26–32, 1999.

Coughlin MJ: Conditions of the forefoot. In DeLee JC, Drez D Jr (eds): Orthopaedic Sports Medicine: Principles and Practice. Philadelphia, WB Saunders, 1994, pp 1842–1939.

Mann RA, Coughlin MJ: Adult hallux valgus. In Mann RA, Coughlin MJ (eds): Surgery of the Foot and Ankle, 6th ed. St. Louis, Mosby, 1993, pp 167–296.

Wright DG: Distal first metatarsal chevron osteotomy. Op Tech Orthop 9:15–18, 1999.

SECTION III

THIGH, HIP, AND PELVIS

CHAPTER 35

Hip Arthroscopy

INTRODUCTION

Hip arthroscopy is relatively new, and its indications are limited. Bony restraints make this procedure technically challenging, but as equipment and arthroscopic skills improve, there is a place for this procedure in the sports surgeon's armamentarium.

POSITIONING

There are two schools of thought regarding positioning: lateral decubitus, as popularized by Glick and colleagues, and supine, as recommended by Byrd (Fig. 35–1). In both positions, it is necessary to add traction to the affected leg (via a commercially available device or a simple footplate). Traction should be added until the proximal femur is distracted at least 1 cm as seen on fluoroscopy. The affected leg is abducted slightly for both positions.

PORTALS

Three portals are commonly used: anterior, anterolateral, and posterolateral. The two lateral portals are

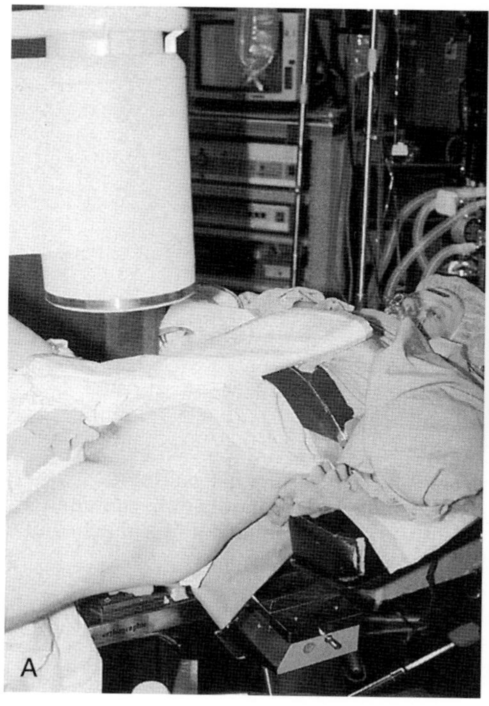

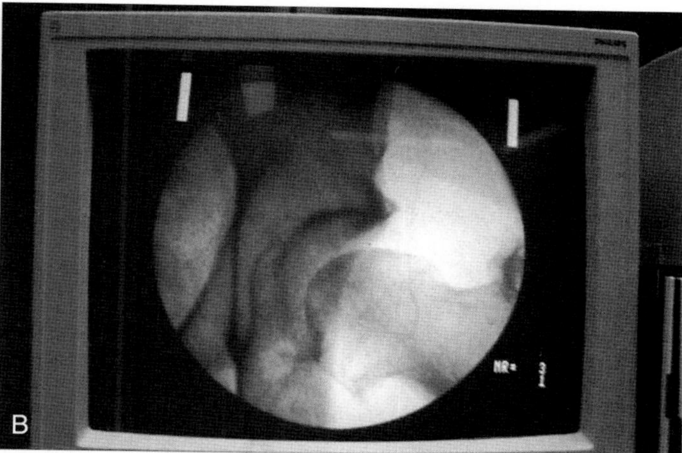

FIGURE 35–1. Supine position for hip arthroscopy. Note use of fluoroscopy. *A*, Setup. *B*, Fluoroscopic image with hip distracted. (From Miller MD, Osborne FR, Warner JJP, Fu FH: MRI-Arthroscopy Correlative Atlas. Philadelphia, WB Saunders, 1997, p 100.)

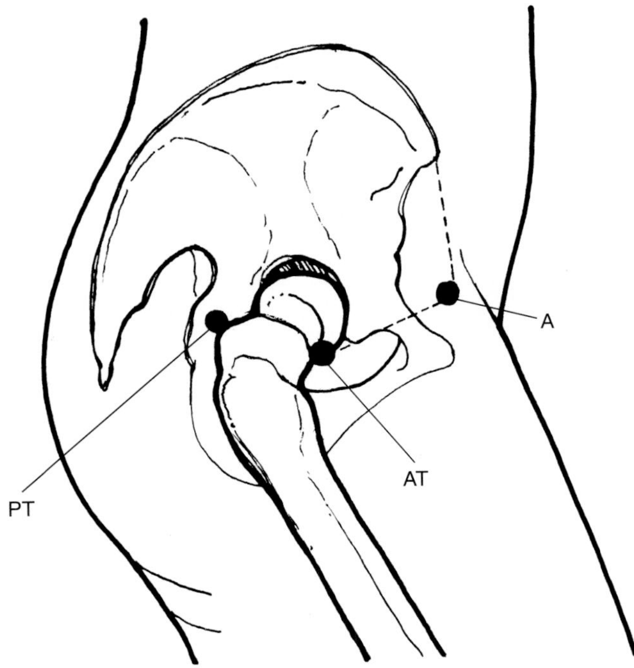

FIGURE 35–2. Portals for hip arthroscopy. A, anterior; AT, anterior trochanteric; PT, posterior trochanteric.

established anterior and posterior to the greater trochanter (Fig. 35–2). The anterior portal is located at the intersection of a sagittal line drawn distally from the anterior superior iliac spine and a transverse line across the superior margin of the greater trochanter. An arthroscopic cannula can be introduced in this portal in a direction 45° cephalad and 30° toward the midline. Branches of the lateral femoral cutaneous nerve are at risk with this portal, but a blunt dissection minimizes this risk.

Special extra-long cannulas and sheathes (5.25-inch) have been developed for hip arthroscopy (Fig. 35–3). Some of these instruments are cannulated and can be inserted with large-diameter spinal needles, which facilitates portal placement. Other instruments for use in hip arthroscopy are also available.

ARTHROSCOPIC ANATOMY

Most of the hip joint can be seen with the arthroscope (Fig. 35–4). Visualization can be improved with 70° scopes and use of various portals.

POSTOPERATIVE MANAGEMENT

Usually, patients are allowed to bear weight as tolerated and gradually return to activities as symptoms allow.

COMPLICATIONS

Perhaps the largest complication, which is underreported, is iatrogenic cartilage injury. Hip arthroscopy is challenging, and extreme care is necessary. Other risks include neurovascular injury (proper portal placement is essential) and traction palsies.

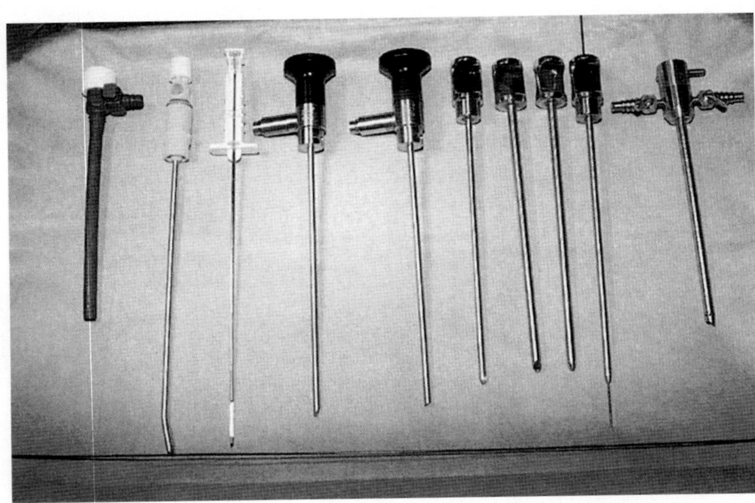

FIGURE 35–3. Instruments for hip arthroscopy. *Left to right,* Long disposable cannula, long curved shaver blade, 14-gauge spinal needle, 70° scope, 30° scope, cannulated cannulas with and without guide wires, arthroscopic sheath. (From Miller MD, Osborne FR, Warner JJP, Fu FH: MRI-Arthroscopy Correlative Atlas. Philadelphia, WB Saunders, 1997, p 101.)

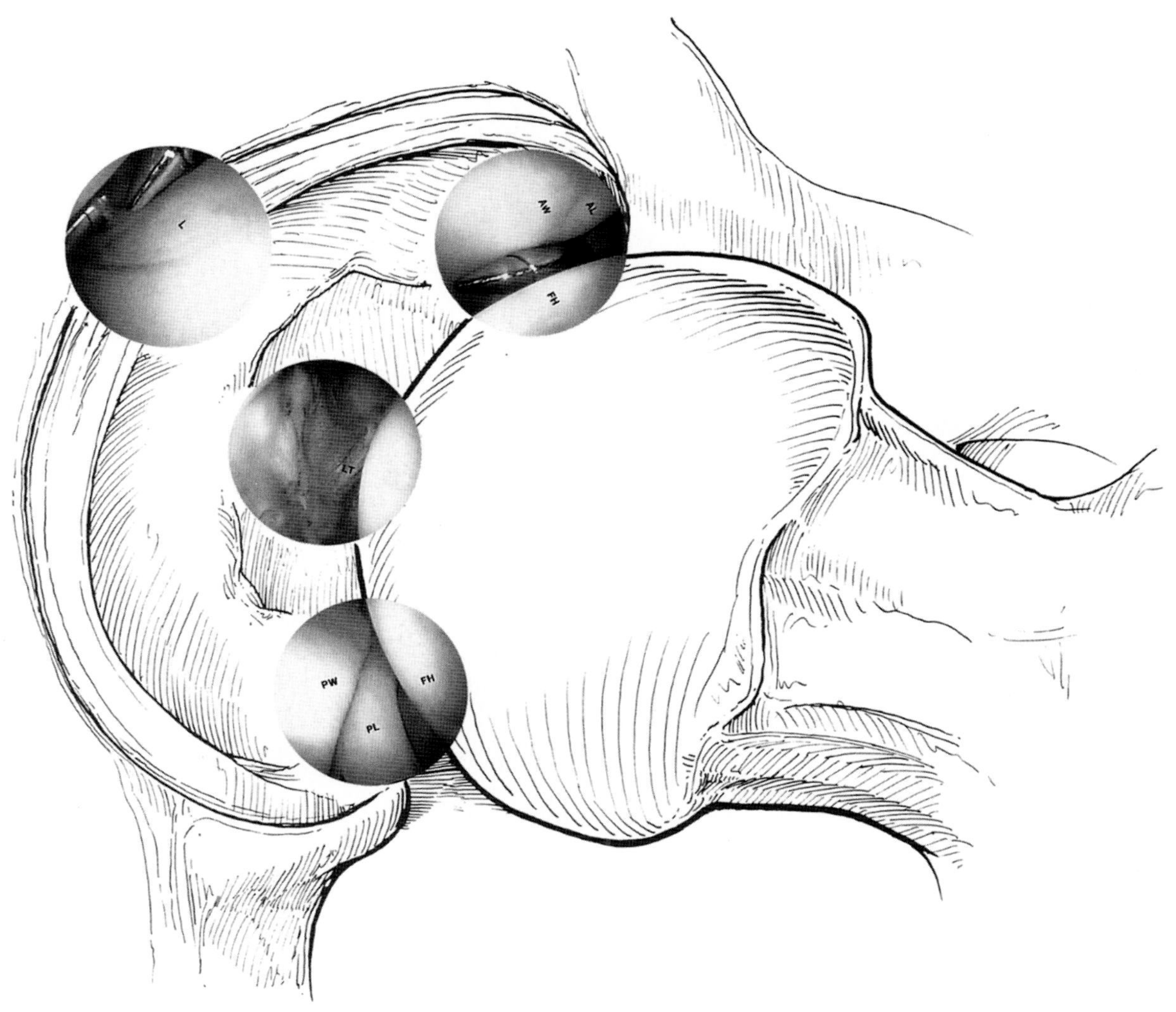

FIGURE 35–4. Arthroscopic anatomy of the hip. AL, anterior labrum; AW, acetabular wall; FH, femoral head; L, labrum; LT, ligamentum teres; PL, posterior labrum; PW, posterior wall. (From Miller MD, Osborne FR, Warner JJP, Fu FH: MRI-Arthroscopy Correlative Atlas. Philadelphia, WB Saunders, 1997, p 101.)

REFERENCES

Byrd JWT: Hip arthroscopy utilizing the supine position. Arthroscopy 10:275–280, 1994.

Glick J, Sampson T, Gordon R, et al: Hip arthroscopy by the lateral approach. Arthroscopy 37:223–231, 1987.

Keene GS, Villar RN: Arthroscopic anatomy of the hip: An in vivo study. Arthroscopy 10:392–399, 1994.

McCarthy JC, Day B, Busconi B: Hip arthroscopy: Applications and technique. J Am Acad Orthop Surg 3:115–122, 1995.

CHAPTER 36

Treatment of Snapping Hip

INTRODUCTION

Snapping hip, or *coxa saltans*, has several causes. Three categories usually are recognized: intra-articular (labral tears or loose bodies, discussed in Chapter 35), external, and internal. The external type is related to friction from the posterior aspect of the iliotibial band or the anterior edge of the gluteus maximus. Internal snapping is caused by the snapping of the iliopsoas over the femoral head and anterior capsule.

HISTORY AND PHYSICAL EXAMINATION

Patients complain of a painful snapping sensation either near the greater trochanter (external) or in the front of the hip (internal). They may be able to demonstrate this phenomenon. Examination should include range of motion and a complete neurovascular examination. Internal snapping may be elicited by flexing and extending (and sometimes simultaneously abducting and adducting) the hip while the patient lies supine. If pressure over the iliopsoas tendon at the level of the femoral head blocks the snapping, the diagnosis is confirmed. External snapping is elicited by having the patient lie on his or her side with the affected leg up and actively flex and extend the hip. Pressure over this area may block the snapping.

DIAGNOSTIC IMAGING

Plain radiographs should be reviewed to ensure that the patient does not have arthritis, hip dysplasia, and loose bodies. MRI may help rule out intra-articular lesions but generally is not helpful in the evaluation of external and internal snapping. Iliopsoas bursography can help make the diagnosis of internal snapping (Fig. 36–1).

NONOPERATIVE MANAGEMENT

Hip snapping may be a normal occurrence. Patients should be encouraged to modify their activities so that they do not produce snapping voluntarily. Therapy with an emphasis on stretching may be beneficial. Occasionally, injection of the affected area with steroids may be beneficial.

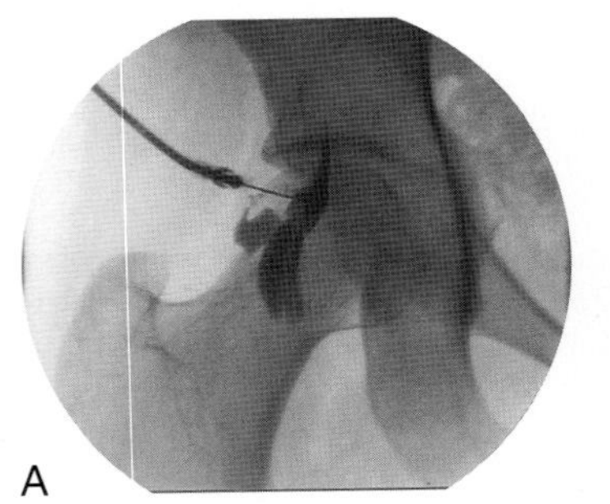

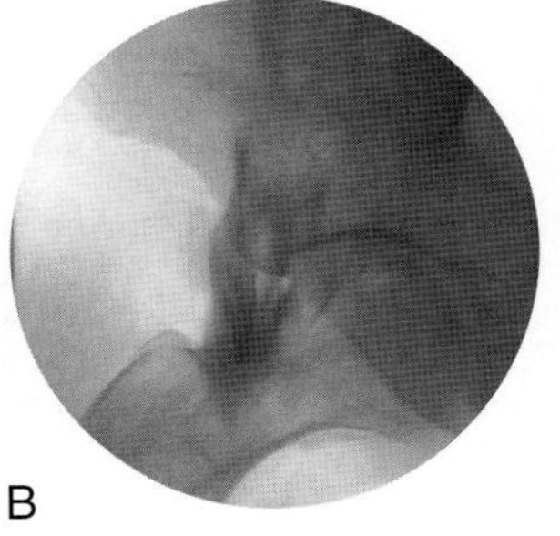

FIGURE 36–1. Iliopsoas bursogram shows snapping of the iliopsoas tendon (internal snapping). *A*, Normal location of the tendon in neutral position. *B*, The tendon snaps over the hip with external rotation. This phenomenon was even more remarkable when seen under fluoroscopy.

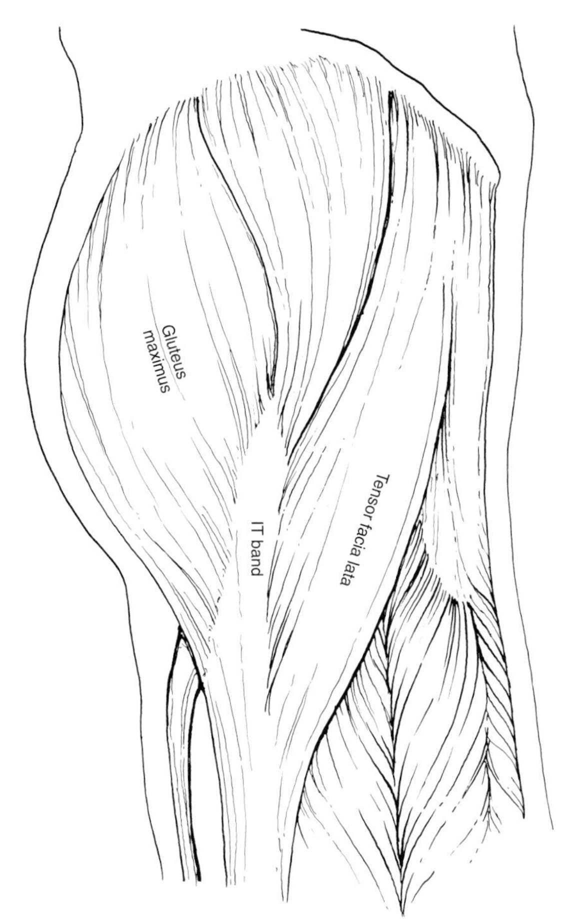

RELEVANT ANATOMY

External. The iliotibial tract has two musculotendinous attachments proximally: the tensor fascia lata anteriorly and the gluteus maximus posteriorly (Fig. 36–2). The iliotibial band remains taut throughout hip range of motion. Any disruption of either muscle or thickening of the band itself may lead to snapping.

Internal. The iliacus and psoas muscles converge after passing under the inguinal ligament. The musculotendinous junction occurs at the level of an osseous groove in the pelvis. The tendon remains in the groove with hip motion except that the hip moves from flexion to extension when the tendon shifts medially (Fig. 36–3).

FIGURE 36–2. Anatomic arrangement of iliotibial (IT) band, tensor fascia lata, and gluteus maximus.

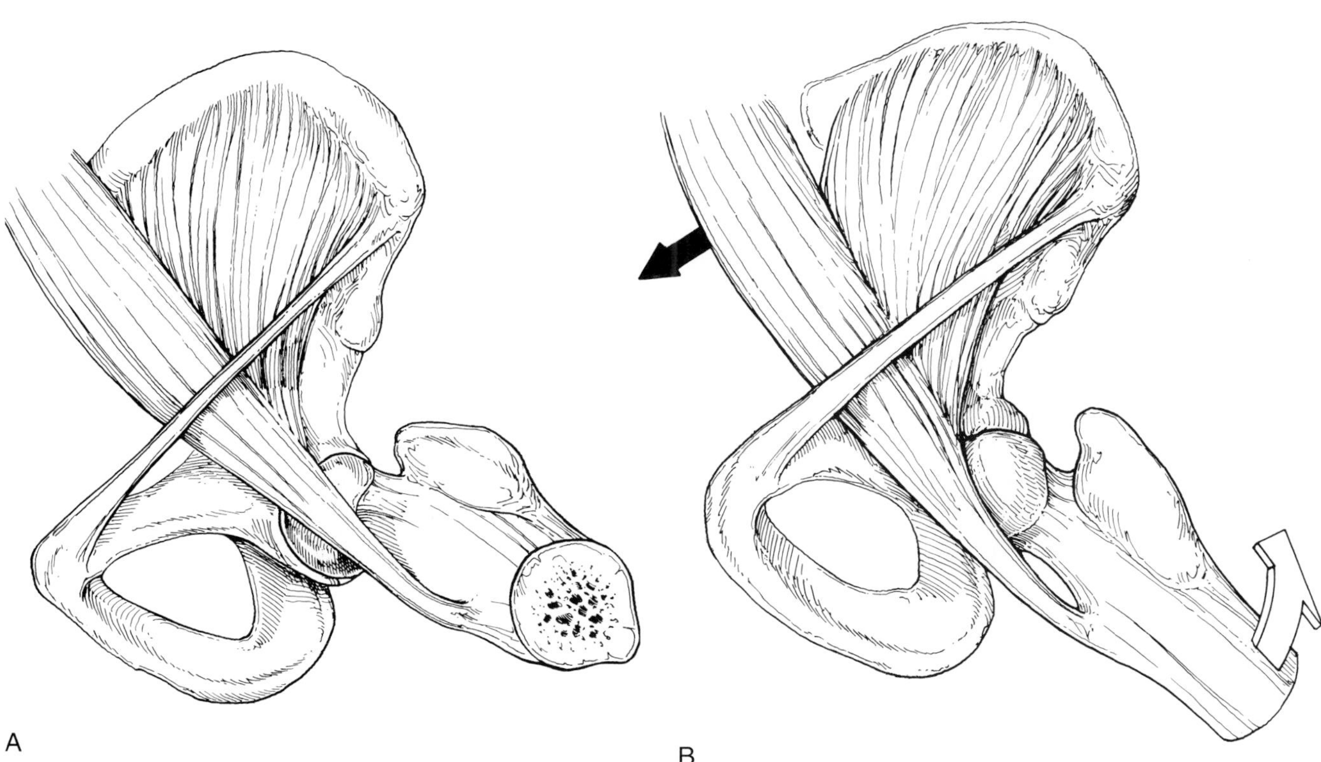

FIGURE 36–3. Iliopsoas tendon excursion. *A*, With flexion of the hip, the iliopsoas tendon is lateral, in its groove. *B*, With hip extension, the tendon shifts medially.

SURGICAL TECHNIQUE

Indications

Most patients with external or internal snapping get relief from nonoperative management or do not have enough symptoms to warrant surgical intervention. Occasionally, patients may present with refractory painful snapping that affects their lifestyle, and surgery is warranted.

Technique

External Snapping: Iliotibial Band Z-Plasty

1. Incision: A 10- to 15-cm straight lateral incision is made, centered on the greater trochanter (Fig. 36–4).
2. Dissection: The subcutaneous fat is incised, and the fascia lata and iliotibial band are exposed.
3. Z-Plasty: An 8-cm longitudinal incision is made in the fascia lata just anterior to the tight band that is palpated. A second incision is made at the proximal end of the first incision and directed anteriorly and distally. A third incision is made at the distal end of the first incision, cutting through the tight band posteriorly (and proximally). The flaps are dissected and transposed. The fascia lata is closed with absorbable suture. Alternatively, the iliotibial band simply can be released (Fig. 36–5).
4. Subcutaneous tissue and skin are closed in standard fashion.

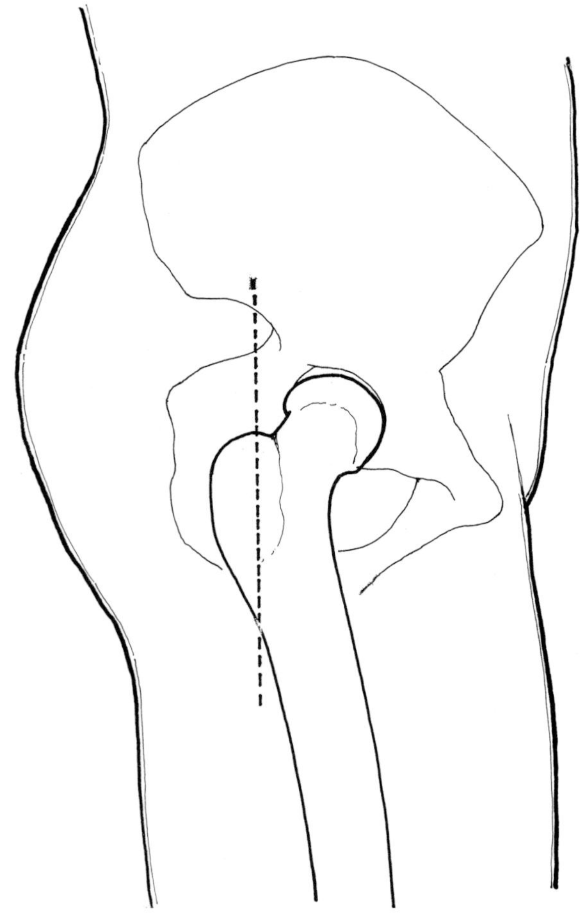

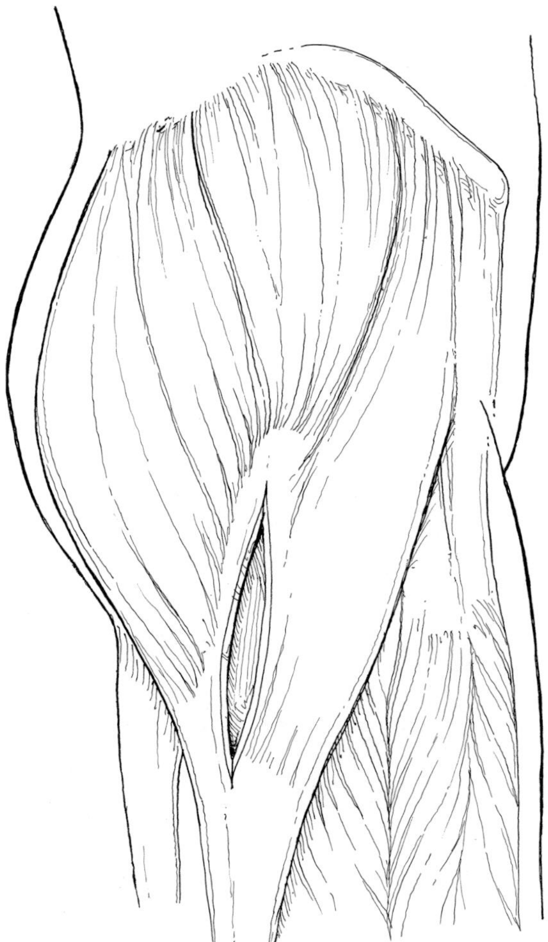

FIGURE 36–4. Z-Plasty of fascia lata and iliotibial band. *A*, Incision. *B*, Exposure of fascia lata and iliotibial band.

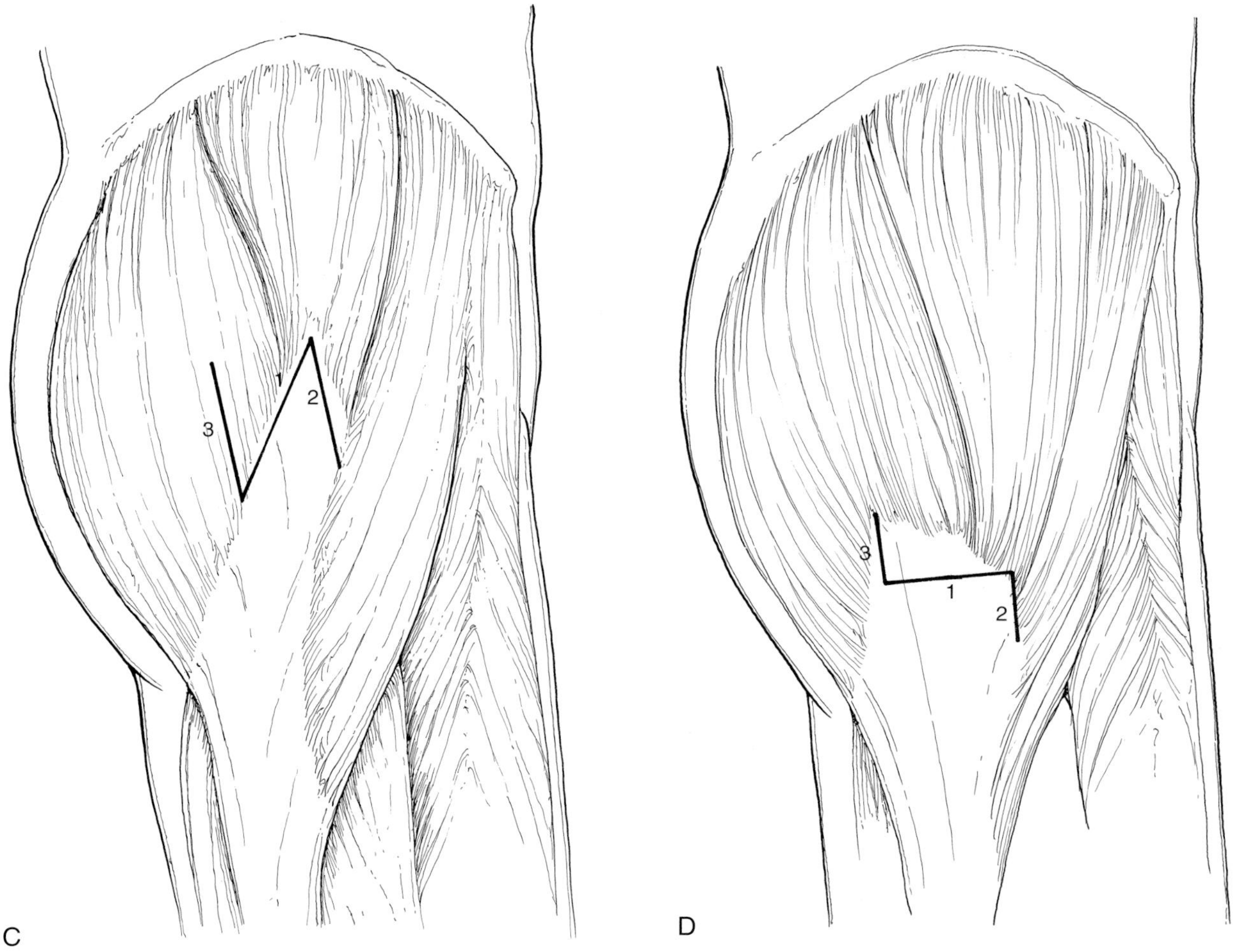

FIGURE 36–4 *Continued. C,* Z-Plasty before transposition. *D,* Z-Plasty after transposition.

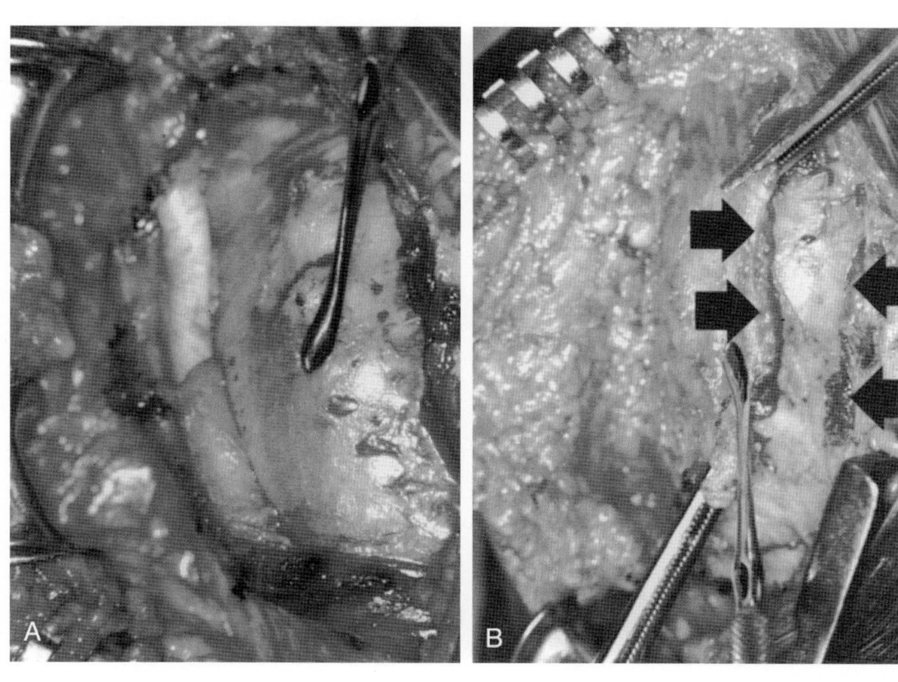

FIGURE 36–5. Proximal iliotibial band release. Before *(A)* and after *(B)* iliotibial release. *Arrows* show edge of the released band. (From Miller MD, Cooper DE, Warner JJP: Review of Sports Medicine and Arthroscopy. Philadelphia, WB Saunders, 1995, p 106.)

Internal Snapping: Iliopsoas Tendon Lengthening

1. Incision: An 8- to 10-cm incision is made in the ilioinguinal crease from 1 cm medial to the femoral artery (feel for pulse) to a point approximately 2 to 3 cm medial and distal to the anterior superior iliac spine (Fig. 36–6). The lateral femoral cutaneous nerve is identified and protected.
2. Dissection: Dissection is done along the medial border of the sartorius muscle. The femoral nerve is identified and protected. This approach exposes the iliopsoas from its lateral side. The entire iliopsoas is rotated so that its anterior border faces medially and its posterior border faces laterally. Then the posteromedial tendinous portion can be addressed.
3. Tenotomies: A series of step-cut tenotomies is made beginning distally. The initial tenotomy (depth 50% of tendon) is made approximately 2 cm proximal to the lesser tuberosity. Three or four additional tenotomies are made at 2-cm intervals until the musculotendinous junction is reached proximally. At this junction, the tendinous portion is released entirely, leaving only the muscle fibers and investing structures to preserve the continuity of the iliopsoas. The tendon is posterior (deep) to the muscle.
4. Closure: After hemostasis is ensured, the deep fascia is closed with interrupted sutures, and a subcuticular, cosmetic closure is completed.

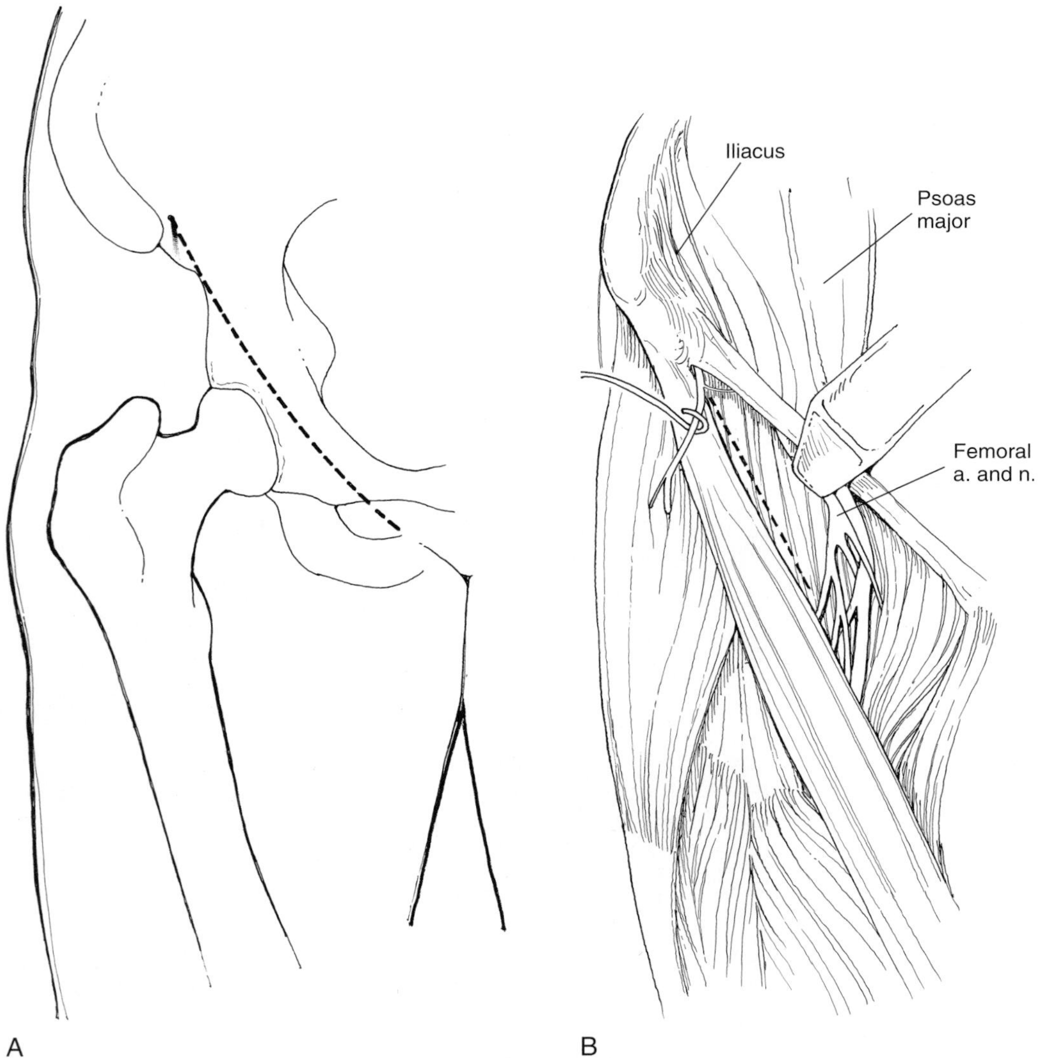

FIGURE 36–6. Iliopsoas tenotomy. *A*, Incision in inguinal crease. *B*, Dissection and exposure and protection of lateral femoral cutaneous nerve and femoral nerve. Dissection is carried out along the medial border of the sartorius.

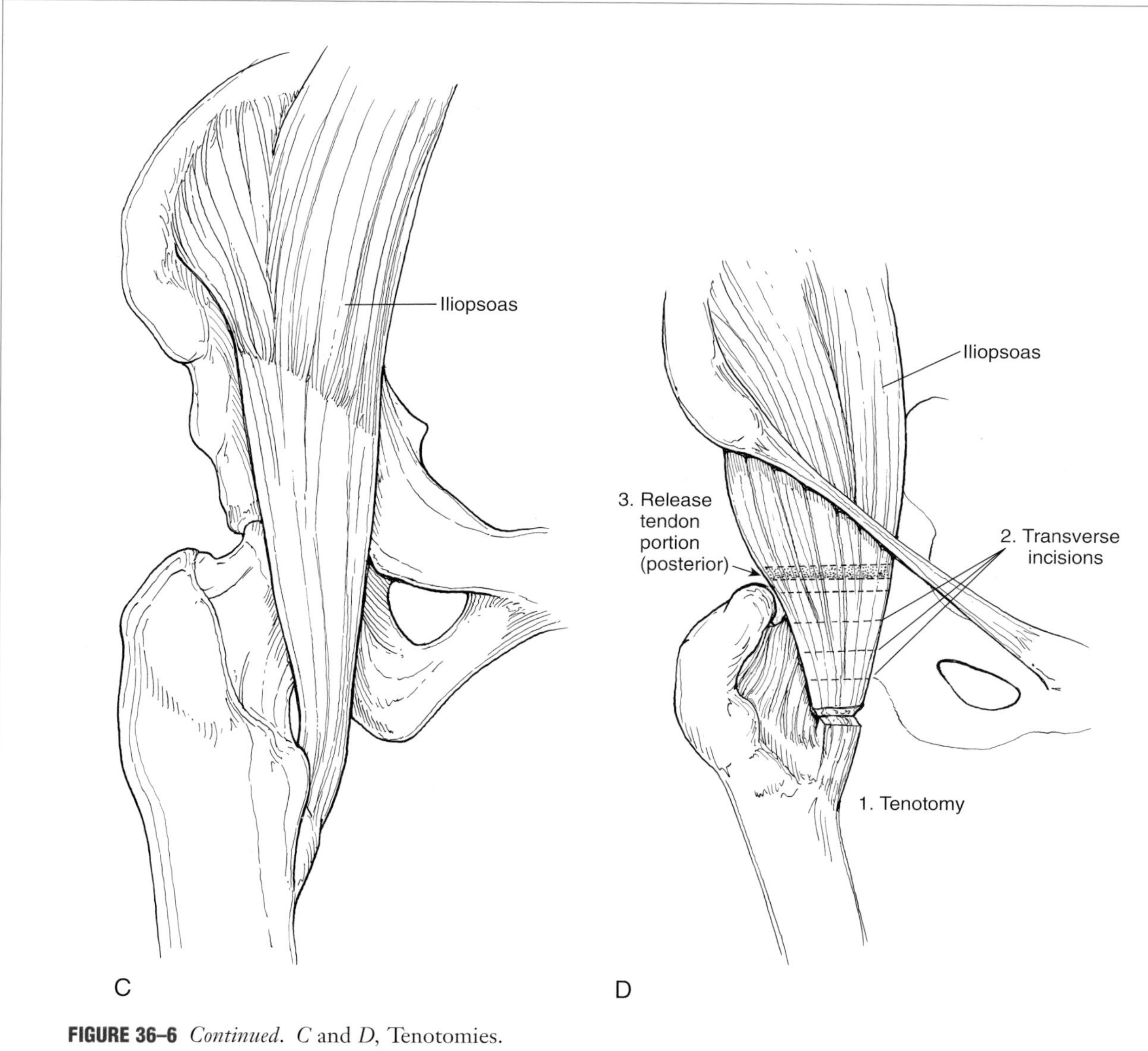

FIGURE 36–6 *Continued. C* and *D*, Tenotomies.

POSTOPERATIVE MANAGEMENT

A soft dressing is applied, and the patient is allowed to ambulate with crutches early. Early hip range of motion is encouraged. Progressive weight bearing is initiated at 2 weeks. Stretching and strengthening are begun approximately 6 weeks postoperatively.

COMPLICATIONS

Recurrence is perhaps the most common complication. Even if snapping returns, however, it is often less painful than the original symptoms. Neurovascular injury is possible without careful dissection during iliopsoas tenotomies.

RESULTS

In one study of external snapping, a Z-plasty relieved snapping in 8 of 8 hips. Occasional aching above the greater trochanter occurred with exercise in 3 of 8 hips. Internal snapping resolved in 14 of 20 hips, and marked reduction in snapping occurred in 5 of the remaining 6 hips in one study.

REFERENCES

Allen WC, Cope R: Coxa saltans: The snapping hip revisited. J Am Acad Orthop Surg 3:303–308, 1995.
Brignall CG, Stainsby GD: The snapping hip: Treatment by Z-plasty. J Bone Joint Surg [Br] 73:253–254, 1991.
Jacobson T, Allen WC: Surgical correction of the snapping iliopsoas tendon. Am J Sports Med 18:470–474, 1990.
Zoltan DJ, Clancy WG Jr, Keene JS: A new operative approach to snapping hip and refractory trochanteric bursitis in athletes. Am J Sports Med 14:201–204, 1986.

CHAPTER 37

Treatment of Hip Injuries

INTRODUCTION

Sports-related hip injuries have terminated several athletes' careers prematurely. Subluxation of the hip may disrupt the normal articulation temporarily but does not require reduction. Dislocation of the hip (usually posterior) may disrupt the ligaments, capsular structures, and blood supply and may be associated with fractures. Femoral neck stress fractures usually are related to overuse and must be followed closely.

HISTORY AND PHYSICAL EXAMINATION

An athlete who sustains a hip subluxation may note only groin pain and some difficulty walking. Hip dislocations are more dramatic. Posterior hip dislocations result in shortening, internal rotation, and adduction of the injured extremity. Femoral neck stress fractures are common among military recruits and in runners. They may present with activity-related groin pain that is relieved by rest. A recent increase in activity that is new, strenuous, and highly repetitious is a classic triad on presentation. Examination may show pain at extremes of motion and pain with active straight-leg raising and logrolling. Heel strike may cause pain.

DIAGNOSTIC IMAGING

Plain radiographs always should be obtained initially. With hip subluxation, these films often are normal. Later radiographs may show the sequelae of vascular compromise (head collapse and arthritis). Hip dislocations are obvious on plain radiographs; however, small osteochondral fragments may not be clear, especially after reduction. Plain radiographic findings in patients with stress fractures may be subtle or delayed. Bone scans, CT, and MRI may help to make the diagnosis (Fig. 37–1). MRI also can be helpful in the early diagnosis of avascular necrosis (Fig. 37–2).

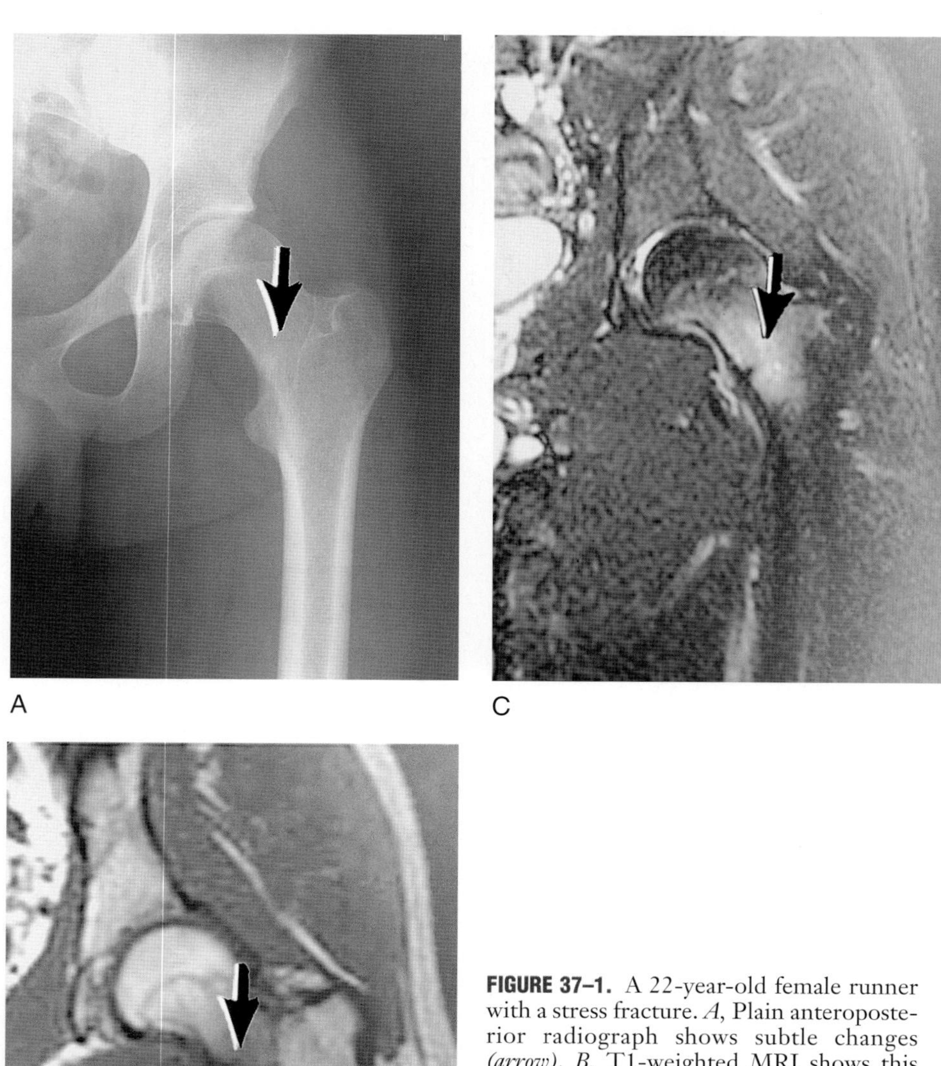

FIGURE 37–1. A 22-year-old female runner with a stress fracture. *A*, Plain anteroposterior radiograph shows subtle changes *(arrow)*. *B*, T1-weighted MRI shows this more clearly *(arrow)*. *C*, T2-weighted MRI shows a black line with surrounding edema *(arrow)*.

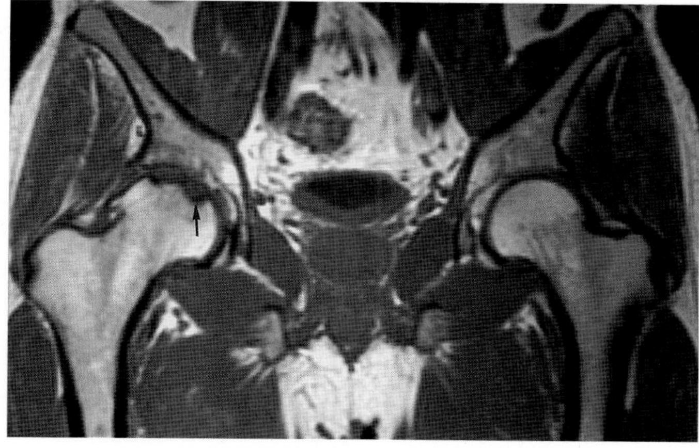

FIGURE 37–2. MRI shows avascular necrosis *(arrow)* in a patient with otherwise unsuspected injury.

NONOPERATIVE MANAGEMENT

Hip subluxations/dislocations with congruent reductions should be treated with an initial period of bed rest and skin traction followed by protected weight bearing for 2 months. Serial radiographs should be followed closely for signs of avascular necrosis, chondrolysis, and post-traumatic arthrosis. Stress fractures can be managed successfully nonoperatively if they are not complete and are nondisplaced. Prolonged protective weight bearing is necessary. Because displaced fractures have a poor prognosis, most authors advocate operative intervention for complete fractures.

RELEVANT ANATOMY

The tenuous blood supply to the femoral head arises primarily from branches of the medial femoral circumflex artery (Fig. 37–3). Injury to these branches may lead to avascular necrosis and collapse.

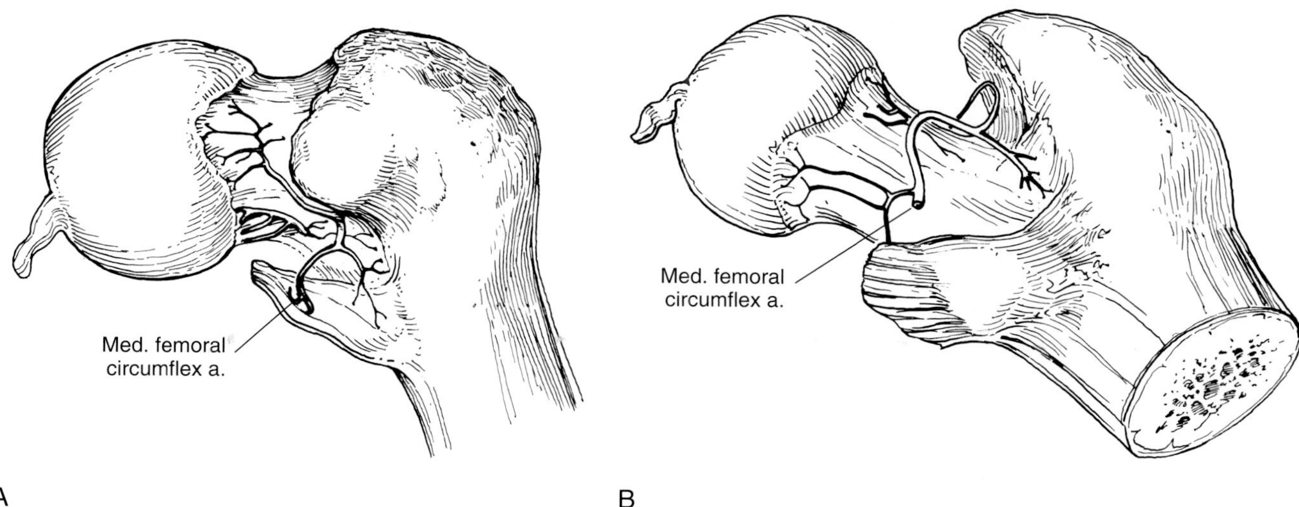

FIGURE 37–3. Anatomy of the blood supply to the femoral head. Anterior *(A)* and posterior *(B)* views.

SURGICAL *TECHNIQUE*

Indications

Hip dislocations must be reduced within 6 hours of injury—the earlier the better (to reduce incidence of avascular necrosis). Femoral neck stress fractures must be fixed if they are displaced or if they are at risk for displacement. Many authors recommend internal fixation for compression fractures (inferior neck) greater than 50% and most tension fractures (superior neck) because of the risk of completion and displacement.

Technique

Hip Dislocation

Prompt, gentle closed reduction should be accomplished as soon as practical. If closed reduction is not possible, open reduction should be accomplished. Interposed fragments should be removed, and significant fractures should be fixed.

Femoral Neck Stress Fractures

Several methods have been advocated for the treatment of femoral neck fractures. Percutaneous cannulated screws are usually adequate (Fig. 37–4).

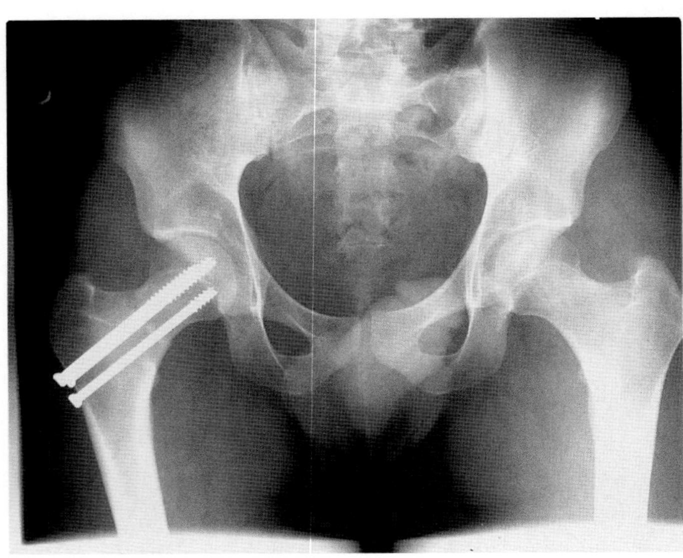

A

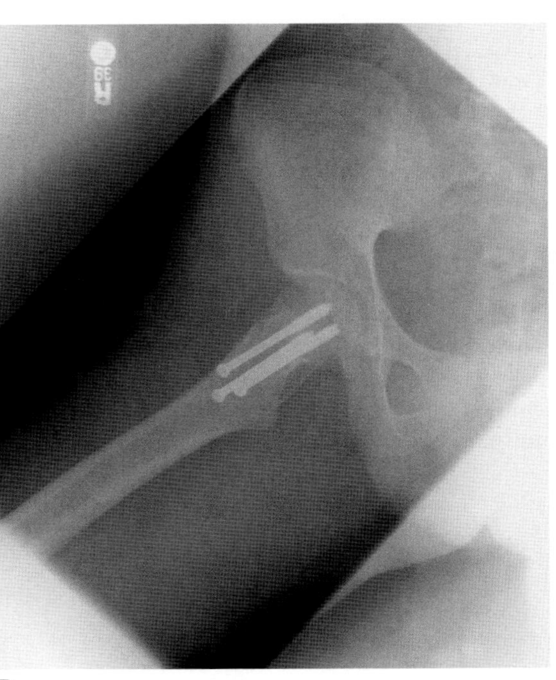

B

FIGURE 37–4. ORIF of femoral neck fracture as seen on plain radiographs. Anteroposterior *(A)* and lateral *(B)* radiographs.

POSTOPERATIVE MANAGEMENT

Prolonged protected weight bearing is required until signs of successful healing are present.

COMPLICATIONS

Hip subluxation/dislocation can lead to avascular necrosis of the femoral head, even if it is recognized and treated early. Post-traumatic arthrosis is also common. Completion and displacement of femoral neck fractures can be disastrous. Nonunion, varus malunion, avascular necrosis, and arthrosis are possible.

RESULTS

Early intervention is the key to obtaining successful results in the treatment of hip injuries.

REFERENCES

Burchfield DM, Finerman GAM: Hip and thigh injuries. In Johnson RJ, Lombardo J (eds): Current Review of Sports Medicine. Philadelphia, Current Medicine, 1994, pp 54–67.

Cooper DE, Warren RF, Barnes R: Traumatic subluxation of the hip resulting in aseptic necrosis and chondrolysis in a professional football player. Am J Sports Med 19:322–324, 1991.

Shin AY, Gillingham BL: Fatigue fractures of the femoral neck in athletes. J Am Acad Orthop Surg 5:293–302, 1997.

CHAPTER 38

Treatment of Muscle and Tendon Injuries

INTRODUCTION

Although most muscle and tendon injuries in the hip and thigh are treated nonoperatively, it is important to recognize and treat these injuries appropriately. Proximal hamstring injuries may require surgical intervention in select cases.

HISTORY AND PHYSICAL EXAMINATION

Quadriceps contusion can occur as a result of blunt trauma during participation in contact sports, and hamstring injury can be marked by acute pain in the posterior thigh in a middle-aged athlete during sprinting. Hamstring avulsion injuries can result from severe hip flexion with the knee in extension, classically during water-skiing (Fig. 38–1). Physical examination includes palpation of the hamstring origins with the patient in the prone position with the muscle bellies relaxed and tensed.

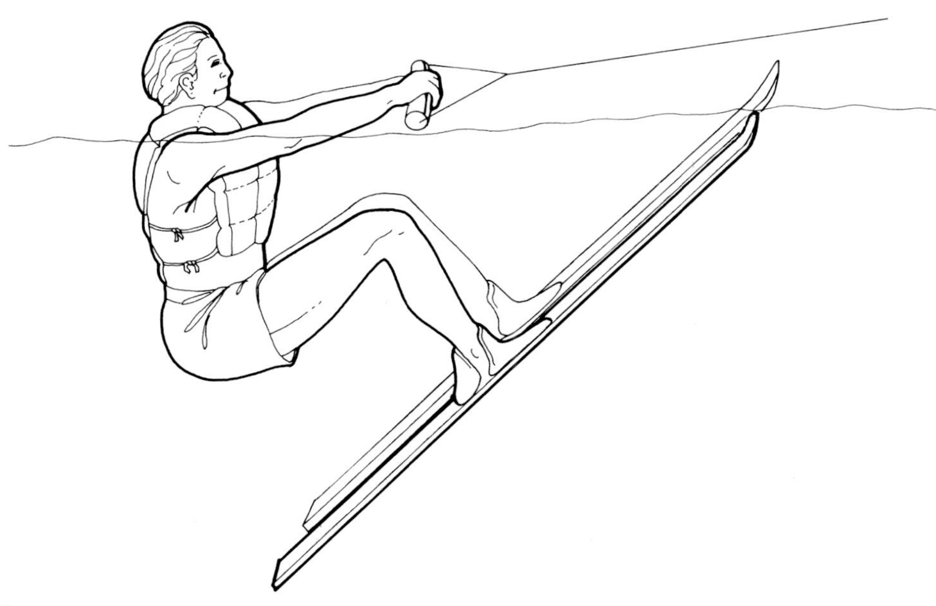

FIGURE 38–1. Mechanism of injury for proximal hamstring avulsion during water-skiing. The hip is hyperflexed, and the knee is extended with this injury. *A*, Starting position.

Illustration continued on following page

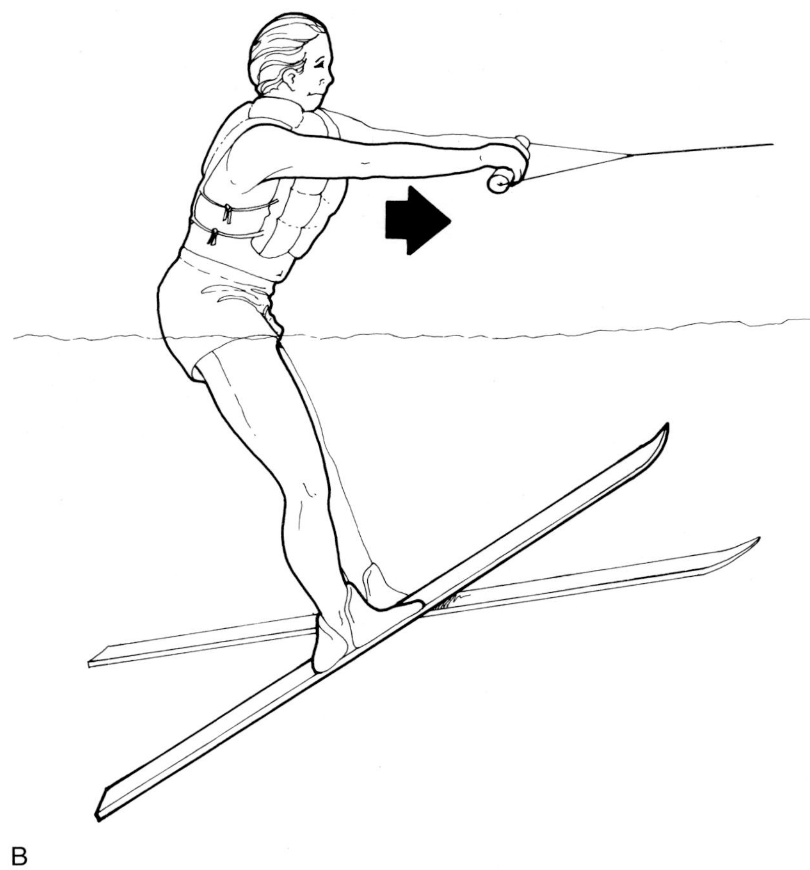

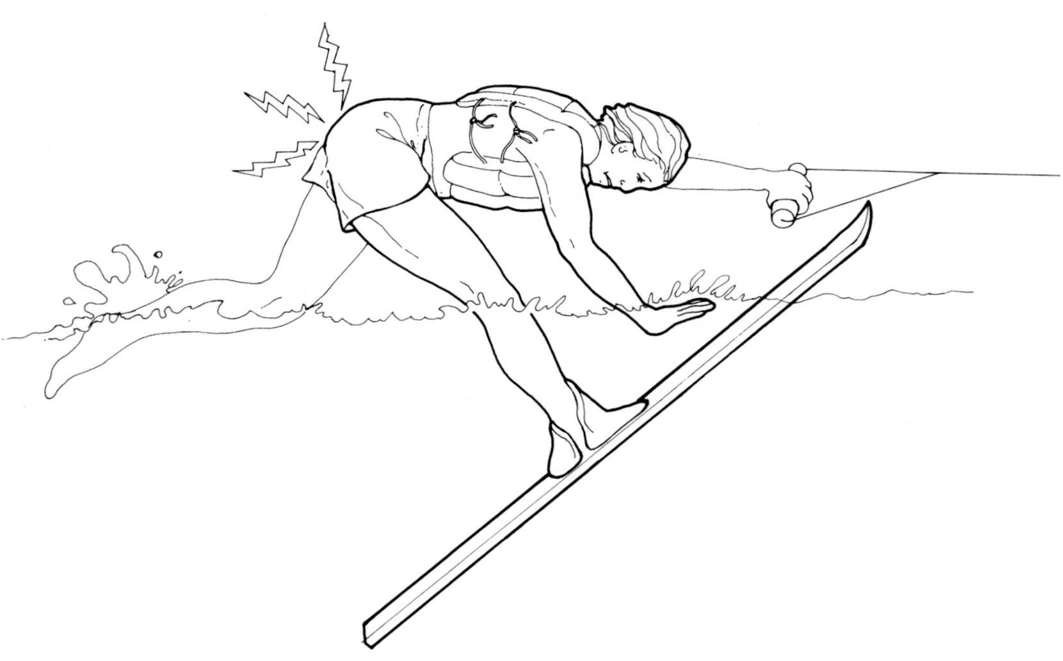

FIGURE 38–1 *Continued. B*, Skier loses control of left ski. *C*, Left ski catches and hyperextends hip, resulting in proximal hamstring avulsion injury.

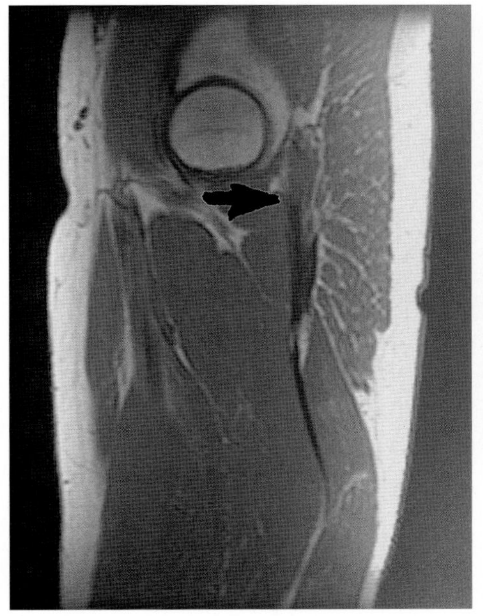

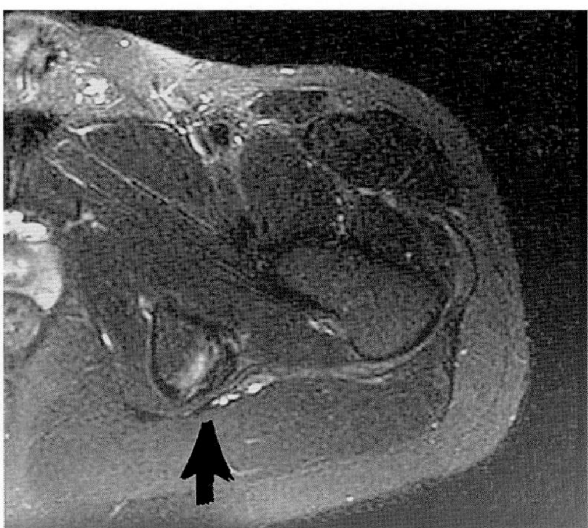

FIGURE 38–2. MRI of proximal hamstring avulsion. *A*, T1-weighted sagittal image shows edema and lack of definition of the proximal hamstring origin *(arrow)*. *B*, T2-weighted axial image shows tendinous injury in attrition in a patient with a chronic hamstring rupture *(arrow)*.

DIAGNOSTIC IMAGING

Unless there is a bony avulsion, plain radiographs are usually unremarkable. MRI often can be helpful in evaluating proximal injuries (Fig. 38–2).

Quadriceps contusions occasionally may result in myositis ossificans, which can be seen radiographically (Fig. 38–3). The important features that distinguish this from osteosarcoma are location, history of trauma, stabilization by 3 to 4 months, and mature bone occupying the periphery of the lesion.

NONOPERATIVE MANAGEMENT

Most hamstring injuries do well with nonoperative management. *R*est, *i*ce, *c*ompression, and *e*levation (RICE); nonsteroidal anti-inflammatory drugs; exercise; and stretching are the mainstays of treatment. Quadriceps contusions are treated best with early passive flexion and additional thigh padding after recovery.

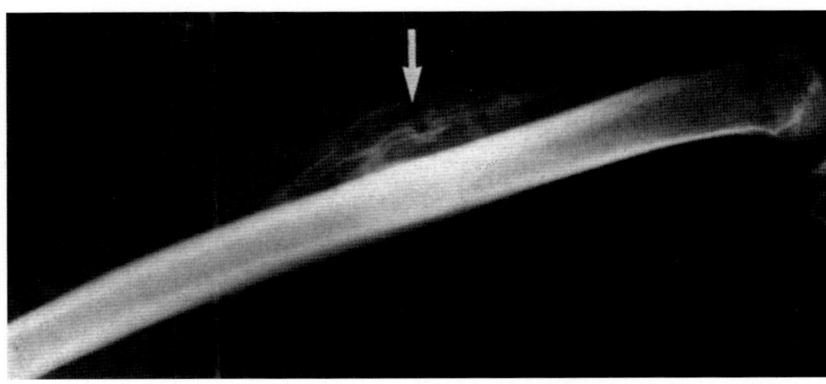

FIGURE 38–3. Lateral radiograph of a patient with myositis ossificans *(arrow)* 6 weeks after a quadriceps contusion. (From Brunet ME, Hontas RB: The thigh. In DeLee JC, Drez D Jr [eds]: Orthopaedic Sports Medicine, Principles and Practice. Philadelphia, WB Saunders, 1994, pp 1086–1112.)

RELEVANT ANATOMY

Because the hamstring tendons greatly overlap the muscle bellies (Fig. 38–4), the musculotendinous junction, where most hamstring injuries occur, can be almost anywhere in the posterior thigh. The hamstrings originate on the ischial tuberosity and insert on the proximal tibia and fibula. The anterior thigh is made up largely of the four quadriceps muscles, which do not become tendinous until their most distal extent (Fig. 38–5).

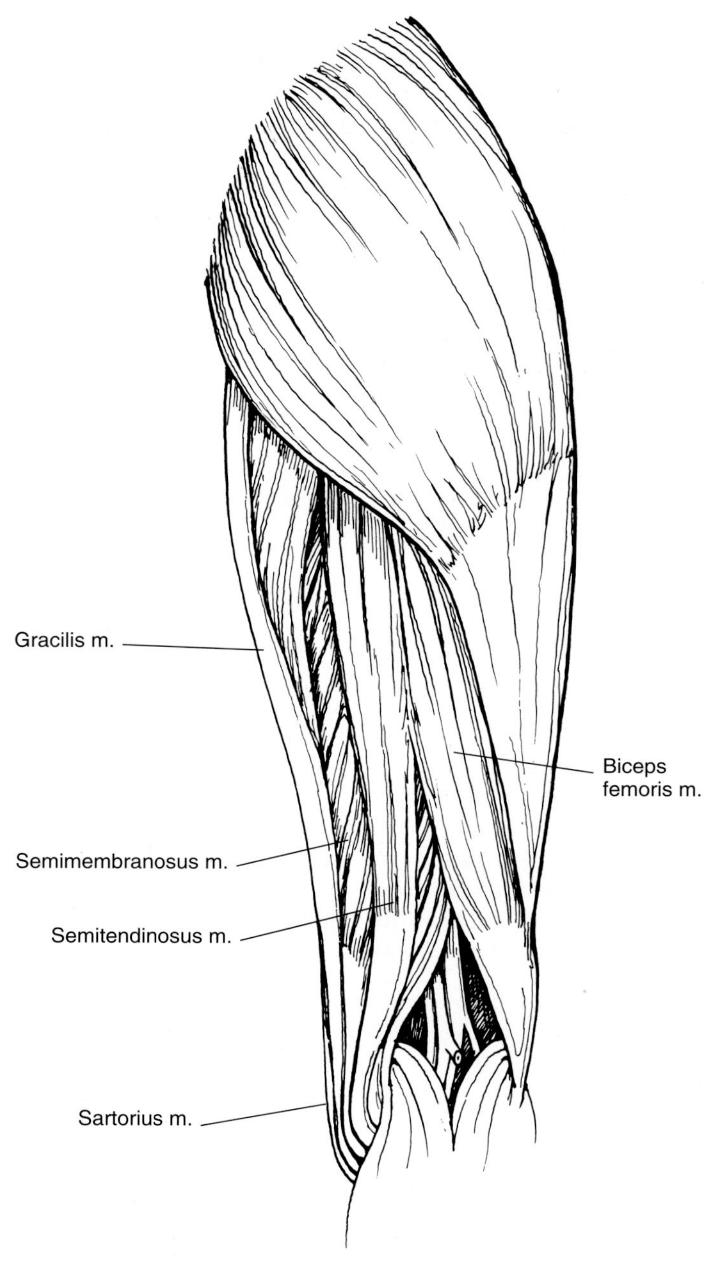

FIGURE 38–4. Superficial *(A)* and deep *(B)* muscles of the posterior thigh. The musculotendinous junctions are located throughout the thigh.

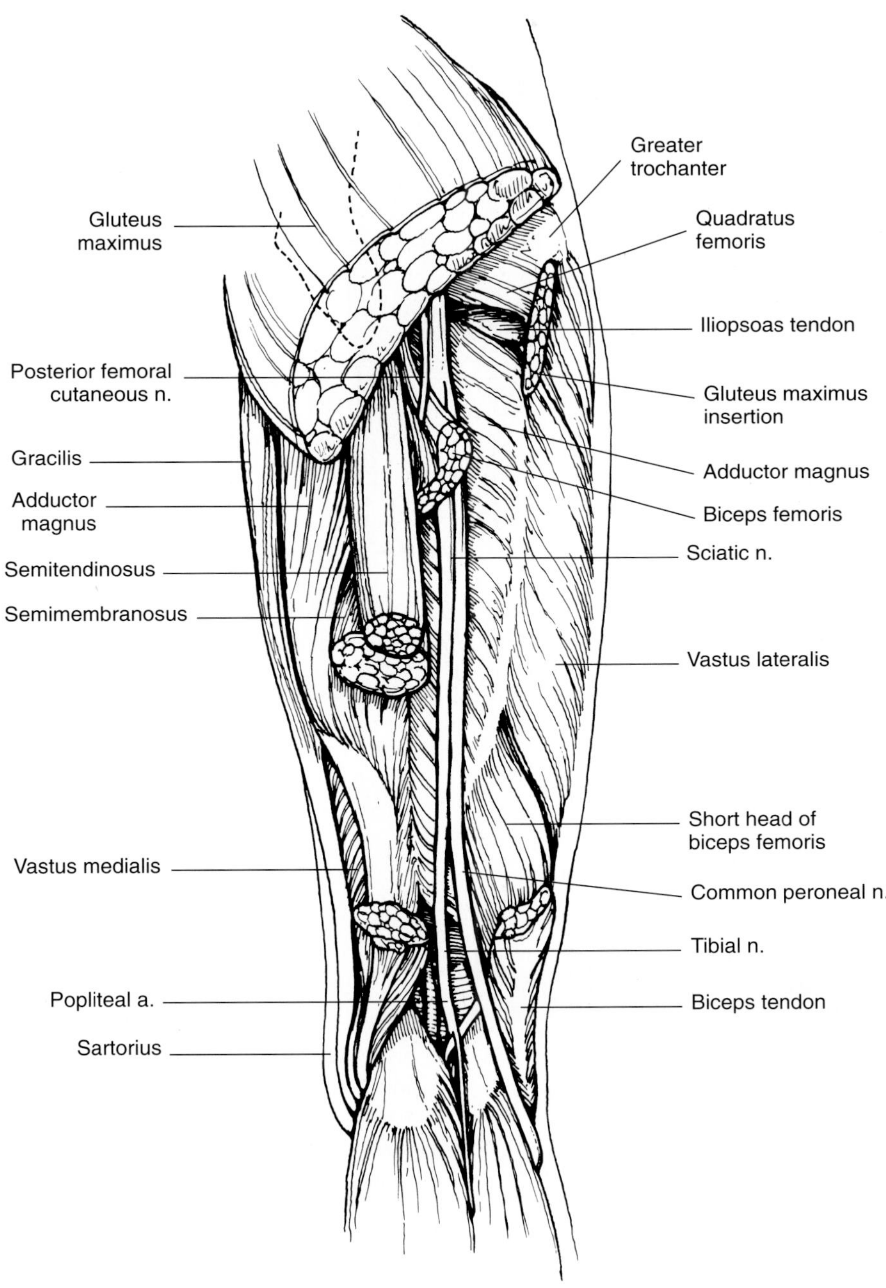

FIGURE 38–4 *Continued*

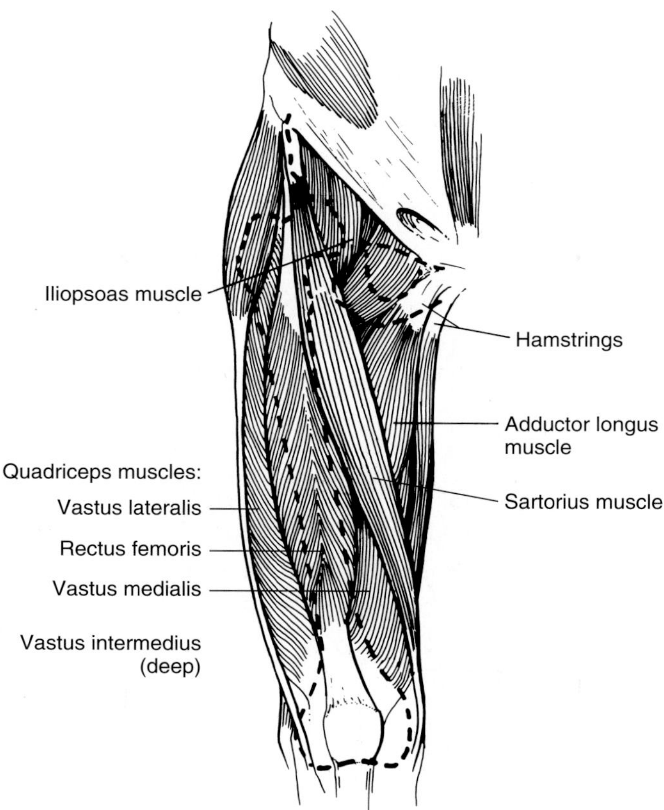

FIGURE 38–5. The four quadriceps muscles make up most of the anterior thigh. (From Brunet ME, Hontas RB: The thigh. In DeLee JC, Drez D Jr [eds]: Orthopaedic Sports Medicine, Principles and Practice. Philadelphia, WB Saunders, 1994, pp 1086–1112.)

SURGICAL TECHNIQUE

Indications

Most muscular injuries in the thigh are treated nonoperatively. The two exceptions are proximal hamstring avulsions and late quadriceps injuries with myositis ossificans. Most authors recommend a delay of at least 6 months between injury and excision of myositis ossificans, and then only if symptoms and disability persist.

Technique

Proximal Hamstring Avulsion

The patient is placed prone, and an extended longitudinal incision is made (Fig. 38–6). The sciatic nerve is identified and protected. The avulsed tendon is located, and traction sutures are placed in it. The ischial tuberosity is identified, and suture anchors are placed at the hamstring origin. The avulsed tendons are repaired using these suture anchors.

Myositis Ossificans Excision

Incisions and dissections must be carried out in a similar fashion as excisional biopsies for tumors. A longitudinal incision is made directly over the area of interest. Exposure and excision of the entire mass is accomplished. Meticulous hemostasis and atraumatic technique are necessary to prevent recurrence.

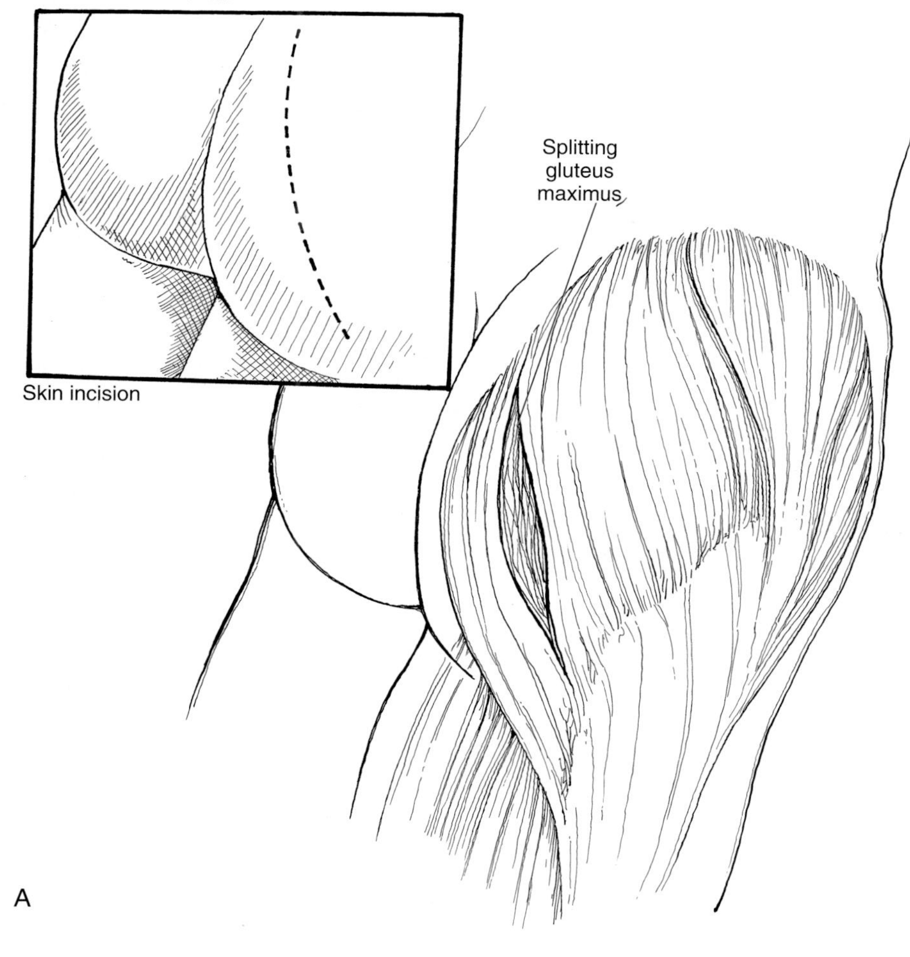

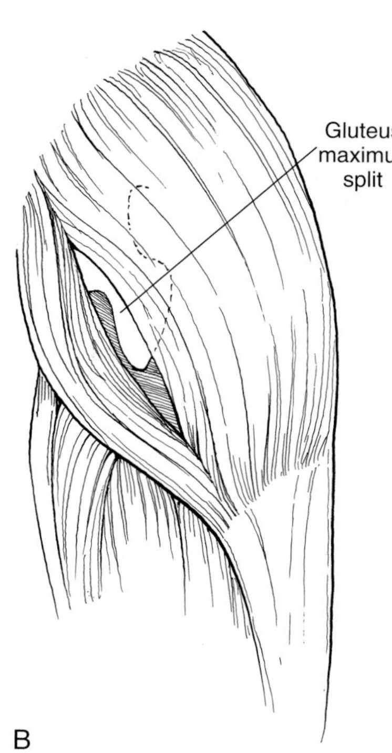

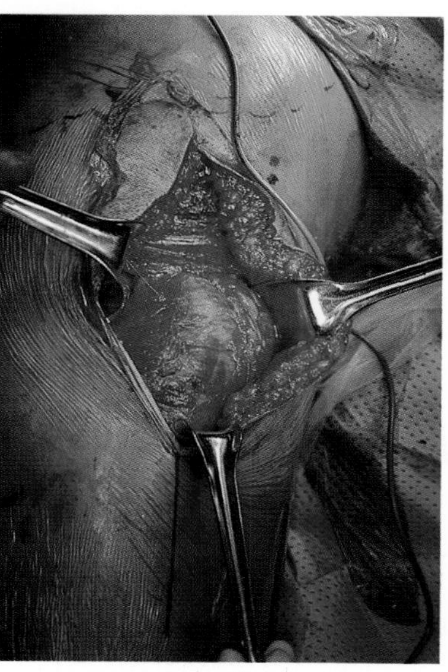

FIGURE 38–6. Proximal hamstring avulsion repair. *A*, Incision and initial dissection. *B*, The gluteus maximus is split, and the ischial tuberosity is exposed.

Illustration continued on following page

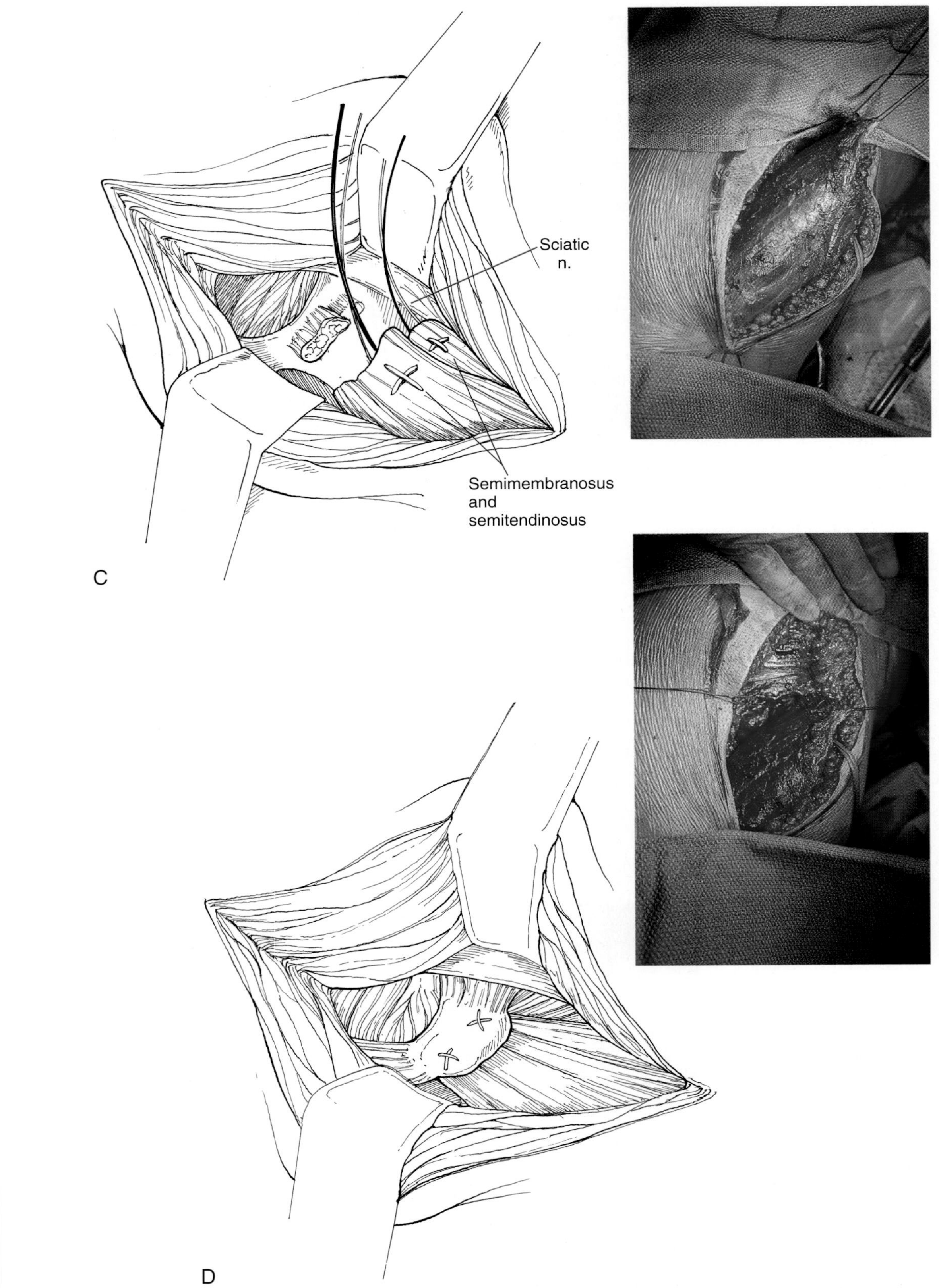

FIGURE 38–6 *Continued. C*, Sutures are placed in the proximal hamstring tendons, which are mobilized. *D*, Suture anchors are placed into the tuberosity, and the tendons are repaired to bone.

POSTOPERATIVE MANAGEMENT

The leg is immobilized in a hip-knee-foot orthosis with the hip in neutral and the knee in slight flexion for 6 weeks after proximal hamstring repair. A knee immobilizer and partial weight bearing for 3 weeks and treatment with indomethacin are recommended after myositis ossificans excision.

COMPLICATIONS

Recurrence is the biggest risk in the treatment of proximal hamstring repair. Myositis ossificans can also occur, requiring late excision. Sciatic nerve injury is an important concern with proximal hamstring repair.

RESULTS

Results with proximal hamstring repairs are satisfactory in only about two thirds of patients. Perhaps earlier recognition and treatment of these injuries would improve these results. Successful results can be expected with excision of myositis ossificans in most cases; however, early surgery for this condition can have disastrous results.

REFERENCES

Brunet ME, Hontas RB: The thigh. In DeLee JC, Drez D Jr (eds): Orthopaedic Sports Medicine, Principles and Practice. Philadelphia, WB Saunders, 1994, pp 1086–1112.

Clanton TO, Coupe KJ: Hamstring strains in athletes: Diagnosis and treatment. J Am Acad Orthop Surg 6:237–248, 1998.

Sallay PI, Friedman RL, Coogan PG, et al: Hamstring muscle injuries among water skiers: Functional outcome and prevention. Am J Sports Med 24:130–136, 1996.

CHAPTER 39

Treatment of Thigh Compartment Syndrome

INTRODUCTION

Acute compartment syndrome of the thigh is relatively rare but can be associated with femur fractures, blunt trauma, and other injuries.

HISTORY AND PHYSICAL EXAMINATION

Patients may present with an acute injury and pain. Findings of pain with passive motion of the knee and marked thigh tenderness and swelling necessitate compartment pressure measurement.

DIAGNOSTIC IMAGING

Plain radiographs and MRI are typically normal initially. Quadriceps injury with associated hematoma formation may be seen on MRI; however, compartment pressure measurement is the key to early management of this condition.

NONOPERATIVE MANAGEMENT

There is some controversy regarding nonoperative management of this condition. Initial treatment with ice, bed rest and lower extremity elevation, analgesics, and careful monitoring may be successful according to Robinson and associates; however, most authors recommend a more aggressive approach.

RELEVANT ANATOMY

There are three thigh compartments (anterior, posterior, and medial) divided by two thick intramuscular septa and a thinner posterior septum (Fig. 39–1). Similar to elsewhere in the body, excessive pressure in any confined compartment may lead to compartment syndrome.

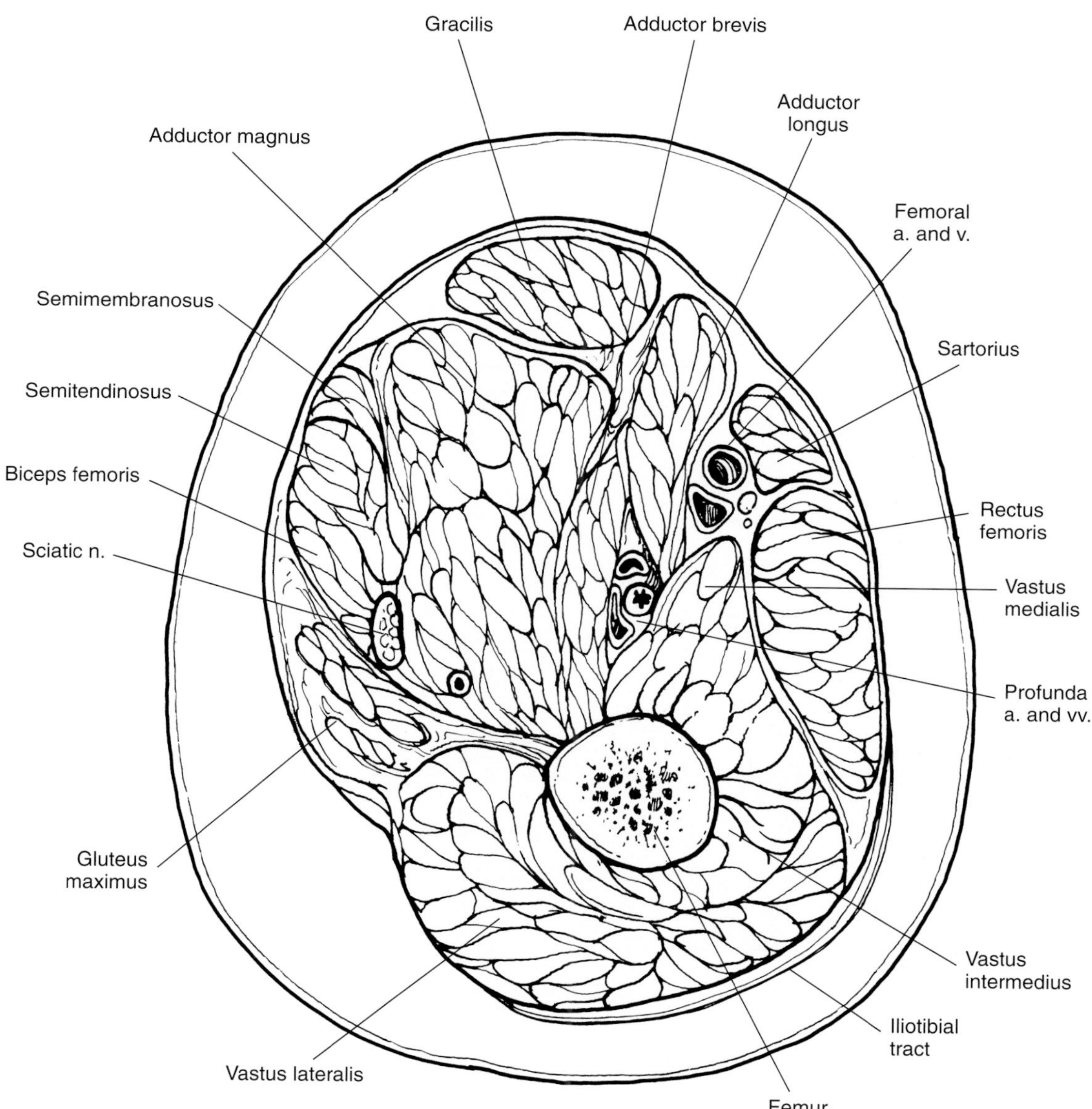

FIGURE 39–1. Cross-sectional anatomy of the thigh. Note thick lateral and medial intramuscular septa.

SURGICAL TECHNIQUE

Indications

Although there is some controversy, most authors recommend fasciotomy for acute thigh compartment syndrome. Typical compartment pressures associated with compartment syndrome of the thigh are within 30 to 50 mm Hg, or 10 to 30 mm of the patient's diastolic blood pressure. Compartment syndromes associated with fluid extravasation from arthroscopic pumps usually can be treated successfully without surgery.

Technique

A long lateral incision is made from the greater trochanter to the lateral epicondyle (Fig. 39–2). The anterior compartment is released by incision of the fascia lata. With retraction of the vastus lateralis medially, the intermuscular septum is exposed and incised, decompressing the posterior compartment. It is usually not necessary to release the medial compartment.

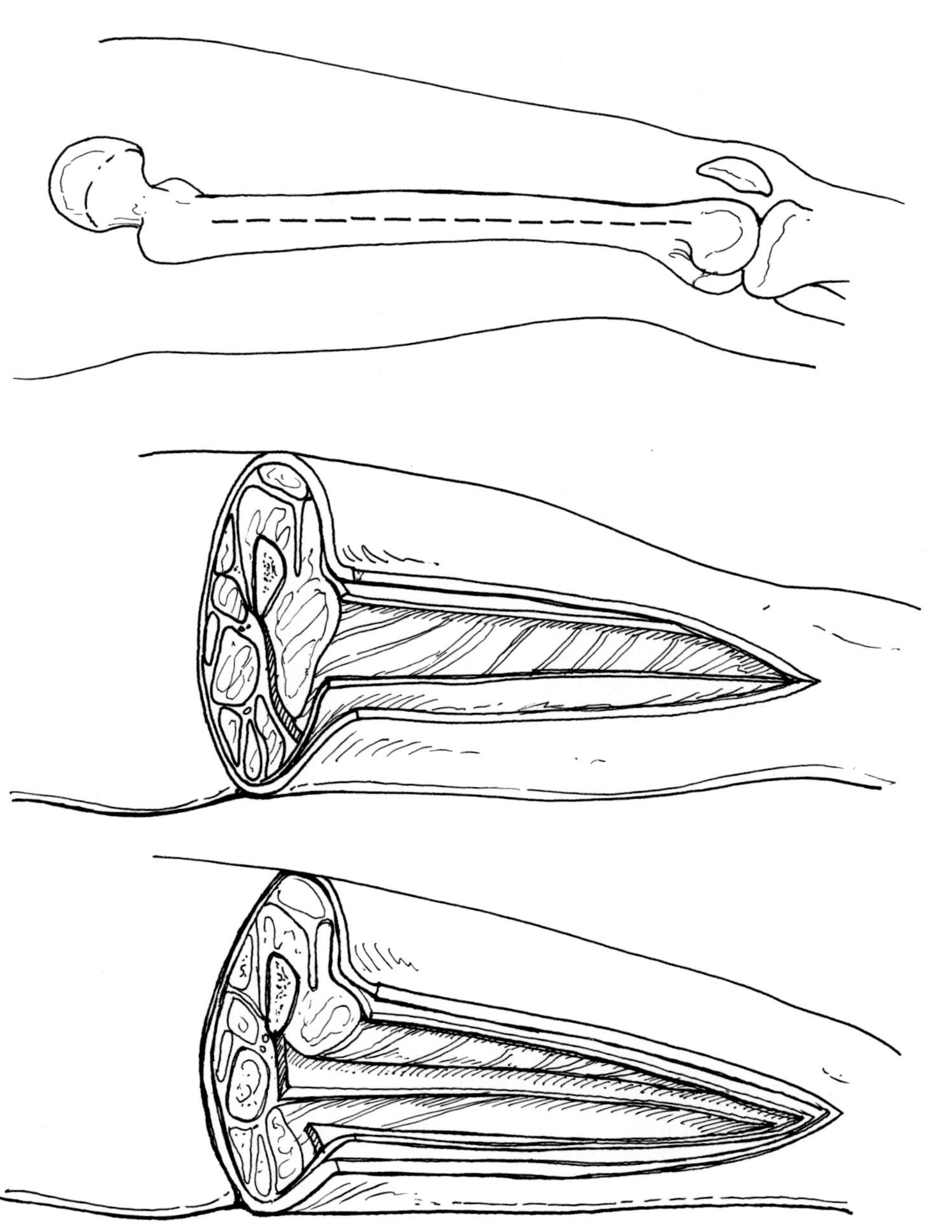

FIGURE 39–2. Compartment release.

POSTOPERATIVE MANAGEMENT

Sterile dressings are applied and changed on a regular basis. Delayed primary closure or split-thickness skin grafting can be accomplished after the fifth postoperative day.

COMPLICATIONS

Delay in recognition or treatment may result in muscle necrosis. Neurovascular injury must be avoided with proper incisions and releases.

RESULTS

In a report of athletic injury with acute thigh compartment syndrome by Rooser and associates, six of eight patients had a good or excellent result after fasciotomy. Nonoperative management also may yield good results according to Robinson and colleagues; however, some caution must be used with this approach.

REFERENCES

Robinson D, On E, Halperin N: Anterior compartment syndrome of the thigh in athletes: Indications for conservative treatment. J Trauma 32:183–186, 1992.

Rooser B, Bengtson S, Hagglund G: Acute compartment syndrome from anterior thigh contusion. J Orthop Trauma 5:57–59, 1991.

Schwartz JT, Brumback RJ, Lakatos R, et al: Acute compartment syndrome of the thigh: A spectrum of injury. J Bone Joint Surg [Am] 71:392–400, 1989.

Tarlow SD, Achterman CA, Hayhurst J, et al: Acute compartment syndrome of the thigh complicating fracture of the femur. J Bone Joint Surg [Am] 68:1439–1443, 1986.

CHAPTER 40

Treatment of Iliotibial Band Syndrome

INTRODUCTION

Iliotibial band syndrome is a painful condition involving the lateral aspect of the knee, particularly in endurance runners and cyclists.

HISTORY AND PHYSICAL EXAMINATION

Patients typically complain of gradual onset of pain in the lateral portion of their knee. Hill training and long distances are often factors. The pain occurs with active or passive motion of the knee between 20° and 80° of motion. Patients may have localized tenderness over the lateral epicondyle and not the joint line. The Renne test, in which the patient stands on the affected limb with the knee 30° to 40° flexed, may reproduce the pain. This test also may be done with the patient supine, with the knee flexed 90° and pressure applied directly to the iliotibial band over the lateral epicondyle. As the knee is extended, pain occurs at approximately 30° of knee flexion (Ober test).

DIAGNOSTIC IMAGING

Although radiographs should be obtained, they are rarely helpful.

NONOPERATIVE MANAGEMENT

Training modifications, cross-training, reduced activity, shoe modifications (for runners), and seat modifications (for cyclists) usually solve the problem. Nonsteroidal anti-inflammatory drugs, ice, and stretching also may be beneficial. Occasionally, injections may be beneficial.

RELEVANT ANATOMY

The iliotibial band is the thickened distal portion of the fascia lata. It inserts distally at Gerdy's tubercle on the proximal lateral tibia. The anterior two thirds typically is called the *iliotibial band* and the posterior one third the *iliotibial tract* in this region. The iliotibial tract lies anterior to the axis of knee flexion when the knee is in extension and posterior to the axis when the knee is in flexion. The lateral femoral epicondyle is posterior to the posterior edge of the iliotibial tract in extension and anterior to it in flexion. The irritation in this area is caused by friction between these structures with repetitive knee flexion and extension.

SURGICAL TECHNIQUE

Indications

Surgery is indicated for persistent pain refractory to nonoperative management as outlined earlier.

Technique

Two techniques have been described for this problem: release of the iliotibial tract and elliptical excision of the iliotibial band and tract. In both approaches, an 8- to 10-cm incision is made over the lateral epicondyle, the iliotibial band and tract are identified, and an elliptical excision of the affected area (Fig. 40–1) or release of the iliotibial tract (Fig. 40–2) is completed with the knee in 30° of flexion.

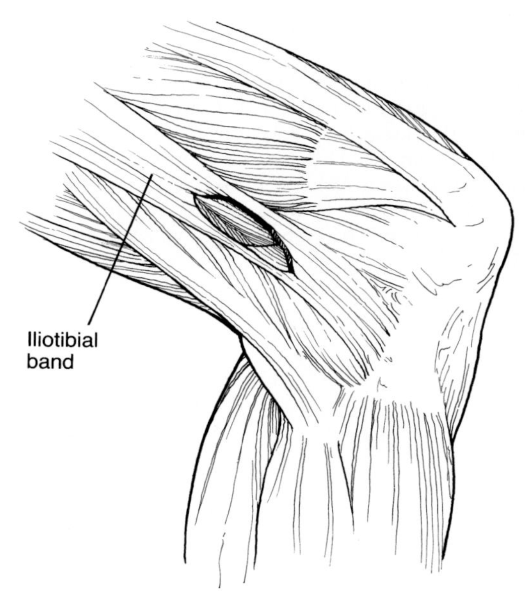

FIGURE 40–1. Elliptical excision of affected area of iliotibial band and tract. (From Miller MD, Cooper DE, Warner JJP: Review of Sports Medicine and Arthroscopy, 2nd ed. Philadelphia, WB Saunders, 2002, p 64.)

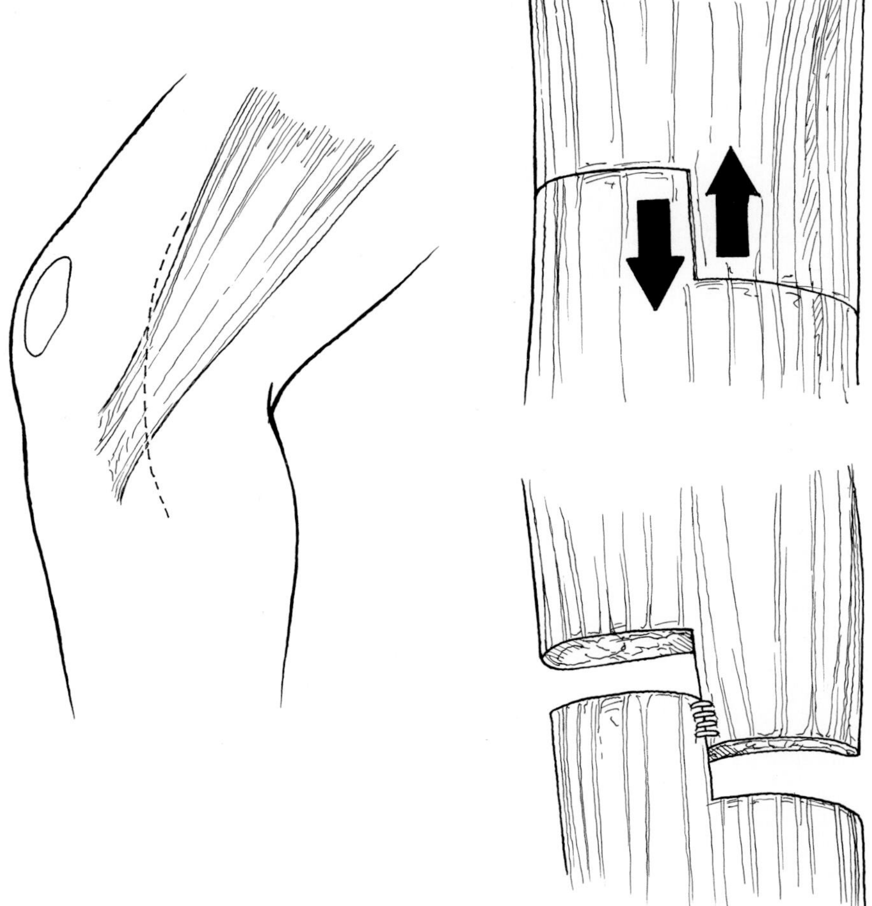

FIGURE 40–2. Release of distal extent of iliotibial tract.

POSTOPERATIVE MANAGEMENT

The leg is immobilized in extension for 1 week, and partial weight bearing is allowed immediately. Training is resumed gradually after 3 weeks. Isometric muscle strengthening is allowed in the early postoperative period.

COMPLICATIONS

Excessive steroid injections may weaken the tendon. Complications of operative intervention may include recurrence.

RESULTS

Martens and associates reported excellent surgical results in 19 of 19 cases. Other reports are equally successful.

REFERENCES

Burchfield DM, Finerman GAM: Hip and thigh injuries. In Johnson RJ, Lombardo J (eds): Current Review of Sports Medicine. Philadelphia, Current Medicine, 1994, pp 54–67.

Holmes JC, Pruitt AL, Whelan NJ: Iliotibial band syndrome in cyclists. Am J Sports Med 21:419–424, 1993.

Martens M, Libbrecht P, Burssens A: Surgical treatment of the iliotibial band friction syndrome. Am J Sports Med 17:651–654, 1989.

PART TWO

Upper Extremity

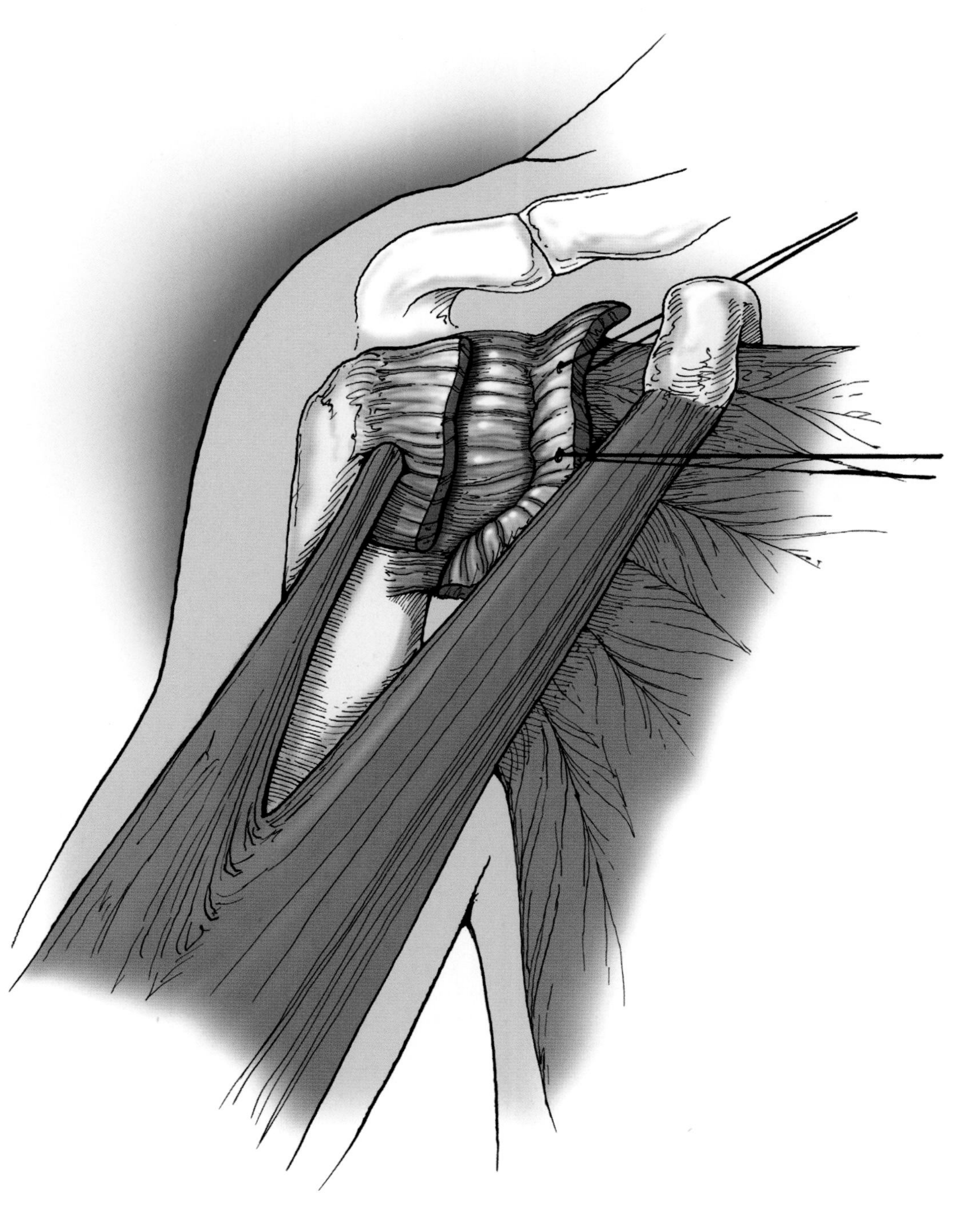

SECTION IV

SHOULDER

CHAPTER 41

Shoulder Arthroscopy

INTRODUCTION

Shoulder arthroscopy has changed over the past decade from a diagnostic tool to a therapeutic one. Indications vary, as do the procedures described in this chapter. Open procedures remain the "gold standard" against which arthroscopic procedures can be compared.

POSITIONING

Shoulder arthroscopy can be accomplished with the patient in either a lateral decubitus or a beach-chair position. There are strong advocates for both positions; however, we believe that the beach-chair position offers several advantages, including, among others, limited neurapraxia (from traction), better application of regional anesthesia, easier conversion to open procedures, and improved anatomic positioning. There are several commercially available beach-chair devices (Fig. 41–1).

PORTALS

The most commonly used portals are the posterior, anterosuperior, anteroinferior, and lateral portals. The superior, or Nevasier, portal and the posterolateral portal can be used for superior labral anterior to posterior (SLAP) repairs (Fig. 41–2).

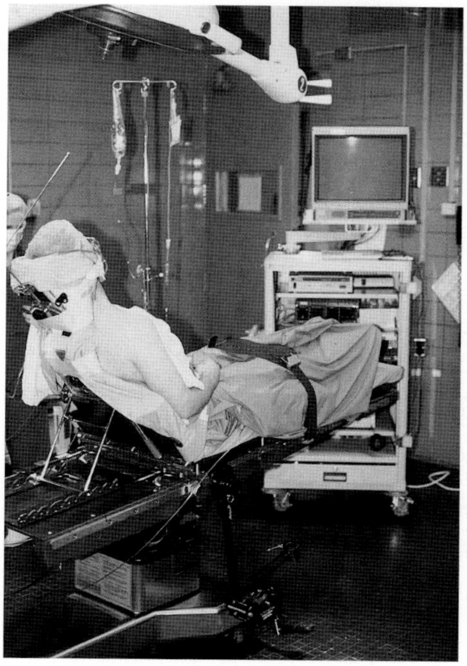

FIGURE 41–1. Positioning for shoulder arthroscopy in the beach-chair position.

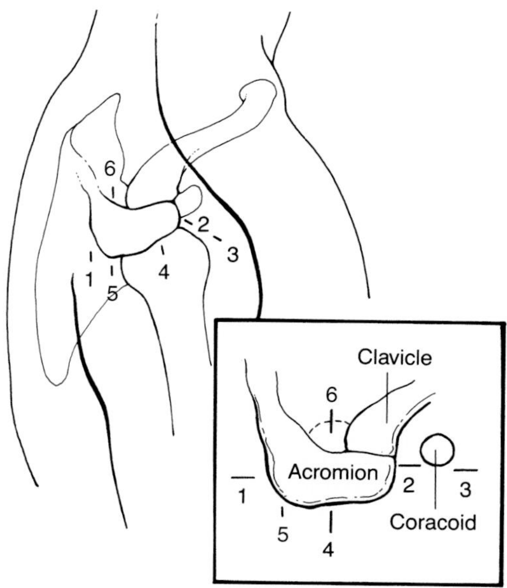

FIGURE 41–2. Portals for shoulder arthroscopy. 1, Posterior. 2, Anterosuperior. 3, Anteroinferior (placed just above the subscapularis tendon). 4, Lateral. 5, Port of Wilmington. 6, Supraspinatus (Nevasier). (Adapted from Miller MD, Cooper DE, Warner JJP: Review of Sports Medicine and Arthroscopy, 2nd ed. Philadelphia, WB Saunders, 2002, p 172.)

ARTHROSCOPIC ANATOMY

Following a specific sequence, the operator visualizes the biceps tendon, labrum, articular surfaces, glenohumeral ligaments, and rotator cuff. Subacromial bursoscopy should allow visualization of the superior surface of the rotator cuff, the inferior acromion, the coracoacromial ligament, and the distal clavicle/acromioclavicular joint (Figs. 41–3 and 41–4).

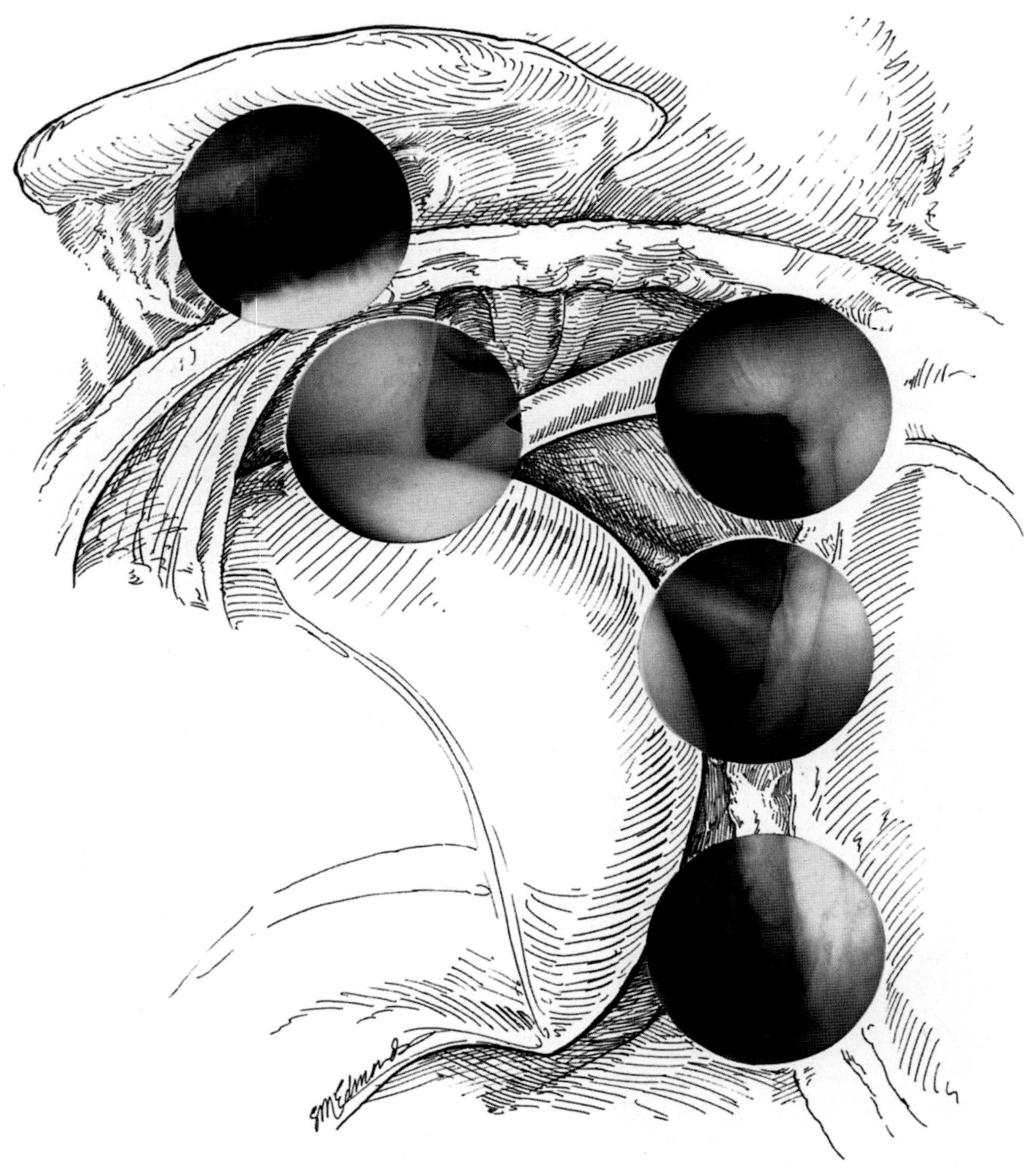

FIGURE 41–3. Arthroscopic anatomy of the shoulder. (From Miller MD, Osborne JR, Warner JJP, Fu FH: MRI-Arthroscopy Correlative Atlas. Philadelphia, WB Saunders, 1997, p 160.)

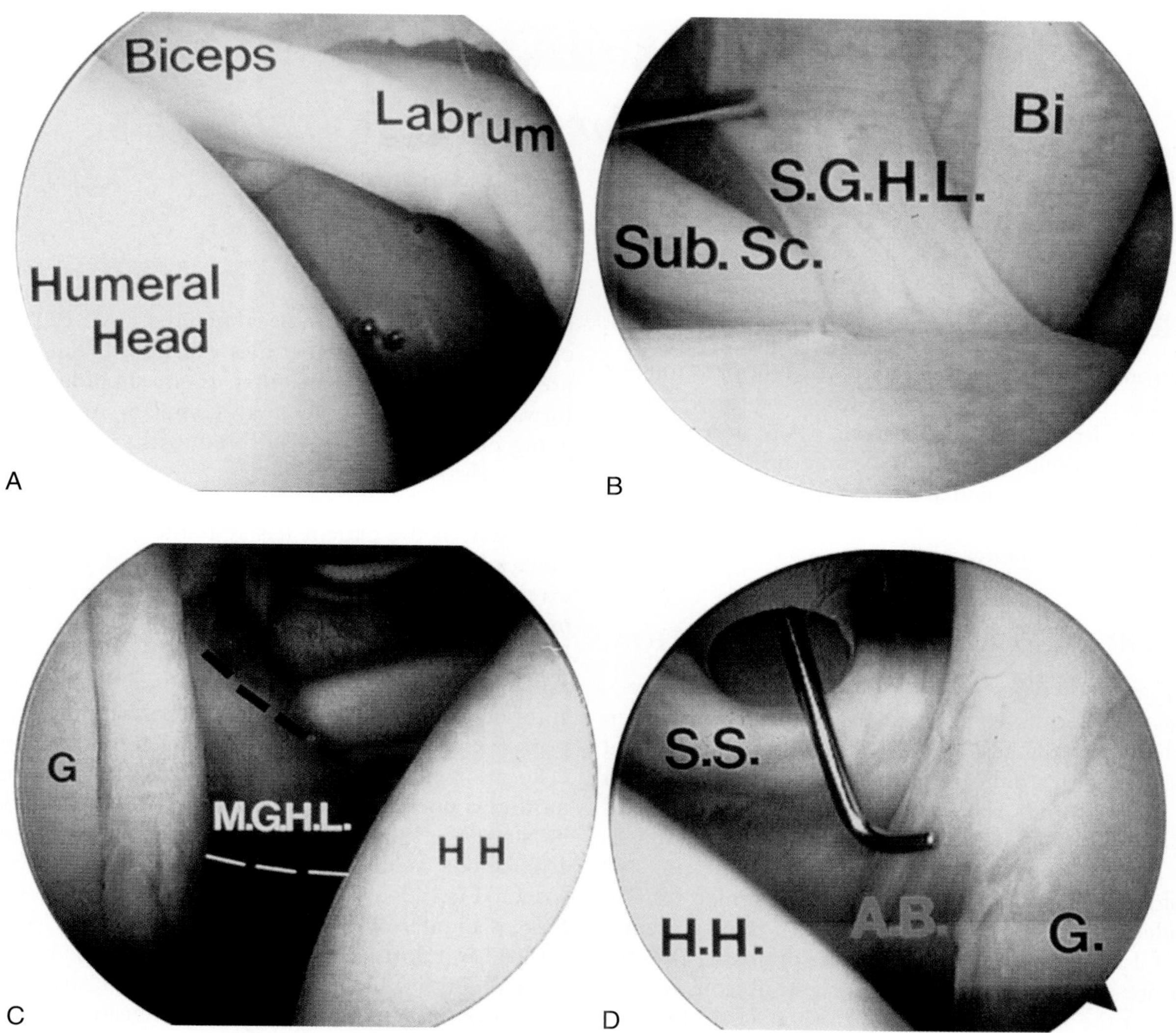

FIGURE 41–4. *A* and *B*, Arthroscopic view of the superior aspect of the glenohumeral joint. Note the normal relationship of the biceps tendon and labrum *(A)* and the position of the superior glenohumeral ligament (SGHL) between the biceps tendon (Bi) and the subscapularis tendon (Sub Sc) *(B)*. *C*, The middle glenohumeral ligament (MGHL) drapes over the subscapularis tendon between the glenoid (G) and the humeral head (HH). *D*, The anterior band (AB) of the inferior glenohumeral ligament complex attaches to the labrum and glenoid (G). SS, subscapularis. (From Miller MD, Cooper DE, Warner JJP: Review of Sports Medicine and Arthroscopy, 2nd ed. Philadelphia, WB Saunders, 2002.)

REFERENCES

Caborn DNM, Fu FH: Arthroscopic approach and anatomy of the shoulder. Op Tech Orthop 1:126–133, 1991.

Miller MD, Osborne JR, Warner JJP, Fu FH: MRI-Arthroscopy Correlative Atlas. Philadelphia, WB Saunders, 1997, p 160.

Warner JJP: Shoulder arthroscopy in the beach chair position: Basic setup. Op Tech Orthop 1:147–154, 1991.

CHAPTER 42

Treatment of Anterior Shoulder Instability

INTRODUCTION

Numerous procedures that address anterior shoulder instability have been described. Many of these procedures (e.g., Bristow, Magnusson-Stack) are nonanatomic and are not discussed here. Anatomic procedures (e.g., Bankart repair [open and arthroscopic] and inferior capsular shift) are very successful and well accepted; they are the focus of this chapter.

HISTORY AND PHYSICAL EXAMINATION

There are two types of anterior shoulder instability—traumatic dislocation and atraumatic subluxation. Matsen has characterized these as TUBS (*T*raumatic *U*nilateral dislocation with a *B*ankart lesion [anterior labral avulsion from the glenoid] that is amenable to *S*urgery) and AMBRI (*A*traumatic *M*ultidirectional instability that is often *B*ilateral and usually responds to *R*ehabilitation and occasionally requires surgery [*I*nferior capsular shift] if extended rehabilitation is unsuccessful). The presentation of TUBS patients is usually quite dramatic. Patients often present in significant pain with an obvious prominence (of the humeral head) anteriorly. Classically, they describe a history of an anterior force applied to their abducted, externally rotated arm, resulting in the arm's "popping out of its socket." After a preliminary examination, the shoulder is reduced; then a complete history and physical examination can be completed. AMBRI patients, on the other hand, sometimes can be difficult to diagnose. They may relate that their shoulder "slides" forward, or they simply may complain of their arm's going numb (dead arm syndrome) with certain activities such as throwing.

Before examining the shoulder, the clinician must determine if the patient has systemic laxity (e.g., finger metacarpophalangeal joint hyperextension, elbow hyperextension). Observation of the patient for prominences, muscle wasting, and use of the extremity is often helpful. Palpation, including checking for both sensation in the axillary nerve distribution (this nerve can be injured with anterior dislocations) and muscle weakness (rotator cuff tears are common in older patients following anterior dislocations), should also be accomplished. Range of motion is documented (external rotation can be affected by surgery). Inferior traction should be placed on the arm, and a sulcus sign (widening of the subacromial space) (Fig. 42–1*A*) should be elicited to determine if there is an inferior component to the instability. A drawer (or load and shift) test (Fig. 42–1*B*) can also be helpful for determining both anterior and posterior laxity. The key diagnostic examination is the apprehension and relocation test (Fig. 42–1 *C* and *D*). On abduction and external rotation, the patient becomes apprehensive that the shoulder is going to dislocate. Anterior pressure relocates the shoulder and gives the patient relief.

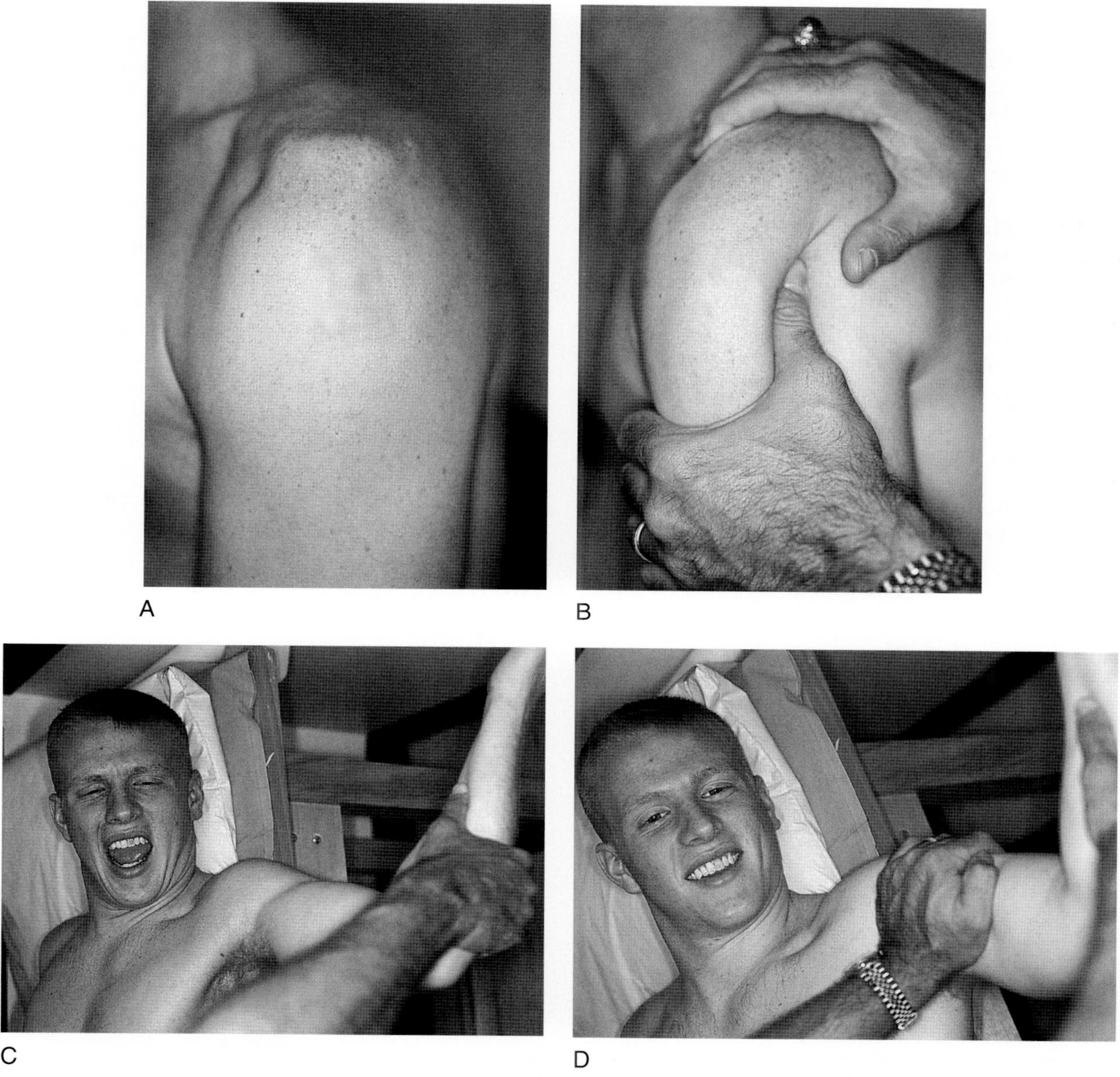

FIGURE 42–1. *A*, Sulcus sign. *B*, Drawer test. *C*, Apprehension test. *D*, Relocation test.

DIAGNOSTIC IMAGING

Standard anteroposterior (AP) and axillary lateral radiographs are usually adequate in the emergency room. A bony Bankart lesion (avulsion of the glenoid rim) can be visualized on a West Point view (prone axillary lateral with the beam angled 25° from midline and downward) or a Garth view (AP in the plane of the scapula with a 45° caudal tilt). A Hill-Sachs defect (an impression fracture of the humeral head) can best be visualized on a Stryker notch view (10° cephalic tilt with the arm held over the head), or an AP radiograph can be taken with the arm in internal rotation. MRI, especially with the addition of contrast material, can often be helpful in determining if there is a soft tissue Bankart lesion (Fig. 42–2).

NONOPERATIVE MANAGEMENT

A combination of reduction, immobilization, and rehabilitation has been the traditional method of treatment for anterior shoulder dislocation. This treatment is associated with an extremely high recurrence rate, however, especially in younger patients. Extended rehabilitation (rotator cuff strengthening program) is the mainstay of treatment for AMBRI patients.

RELEVANT ANATOMY

Bankart tears represent an avulsion of the anteroinferior labrum off the glenoid. The anterior band of the inferior glenohumeral ligament complex (IGHLC), an important constraint to anterior displacement, attaches to the labrum (and glenoid) at this location (Fig. 42–3).

The subscapularis muscle is intimately attached to the anterior shoulder capsule. An open approach to the capsule requires splitting or dissecting of this tendon off the capsule. The rotator interval, a variable opening in the anterosuperior capsule, is located deep to the upper border of the subscapularis.

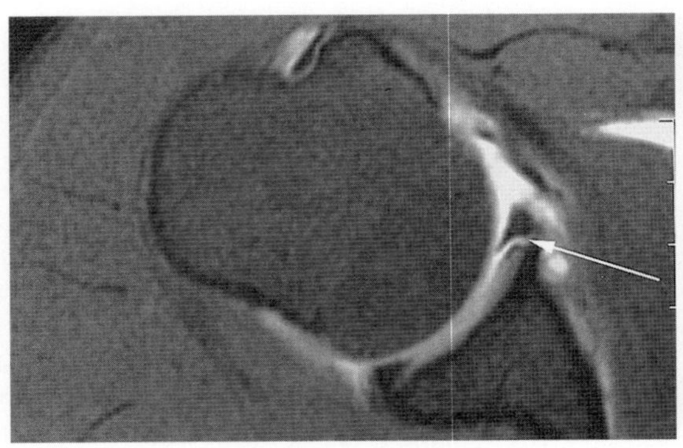

A

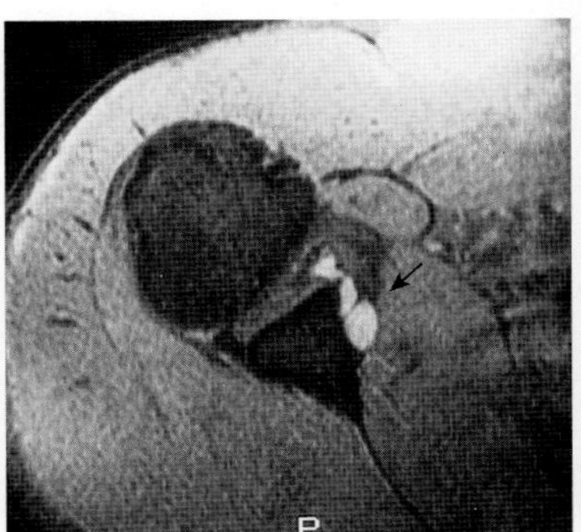

B

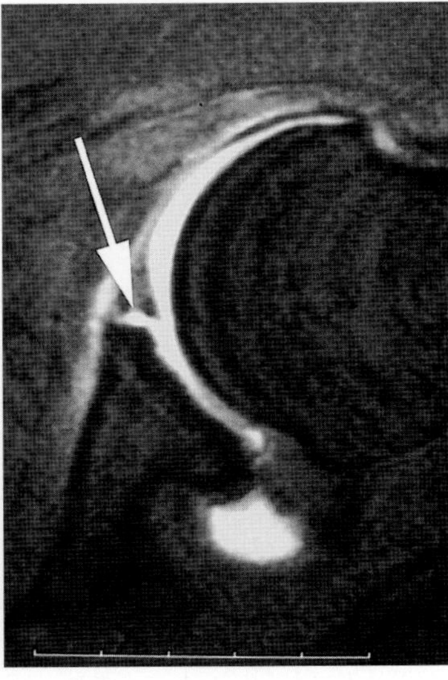

C

FIGURE 42–2. MRI-arthroscopy. *A*, Anterior labral tear (Bankart lesion) *(arrow)*. *B*, Capsular stripping *(arrow)*. *C*, Glenolabral articular disruption (GLAD) lesion *(arrow)*.

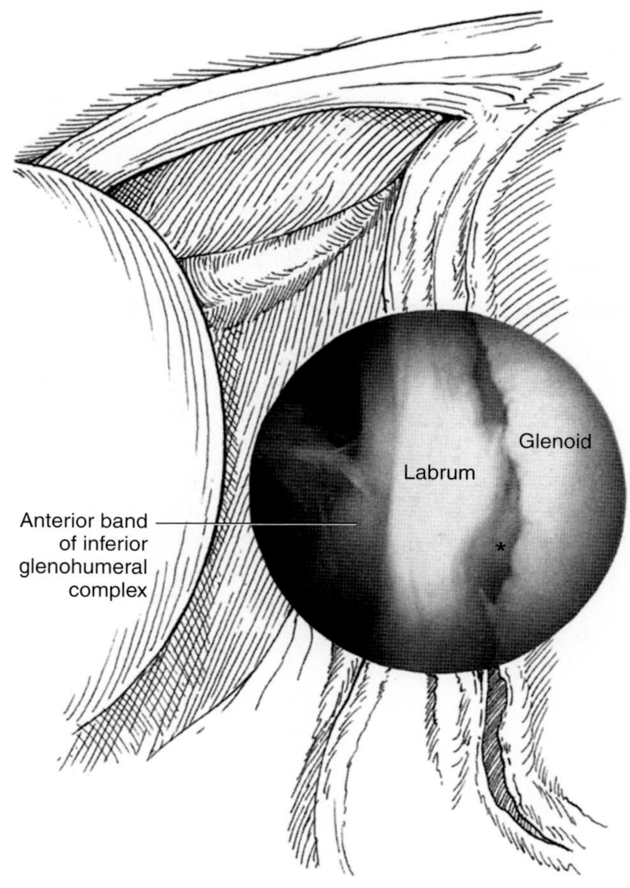

FIGURE 42–3. Expanded arthroscopic view of a Bankart tear. The labrum and anterior band of the glenohumeral ligament complex are torn (*) from the anterior glenoid. (From Miller MD, Osborne JR, Warner JJP, Fu FH: MRI-Arthroscopy Correlative Atlas. Philadelphia, WB Saunders, 1997, p 173.)

SURGICAL TECHNIQUE

Indications

Chronic: Defined as recurrent anterior instability that has failed nonoperative management and adversely affects the patient's lifestyle. For AMBRI patients, rehabilitation must be attempted for at least 3 to 6 months. Recurrent dislocations are often associated with both Bankart tears and capsular laxity; therefore, most surgeons perform a simultaneous Bankart repair and inferior capsular shift in this population.
Acute: Because of the high recurrence rate (up to 80% to 90% in younger patients) and improved arthroscopic procedures, many surgeons now consider performing an arthroscopic Bankart repair for patients with first-time traumatic dislocations.

Technique

Open Bankart Repair and Inferior Capsular Shift

1. Examination under anesthesia (EUA): After appropriate anesthesia is administered, the patient is examined. The degree of instability (Fig. 42–4) is quantified.
2. Positioning: The procedure is performed with the patient in a beach-chair position. Commercially available customized devices are available.
3. Diagnostic arthroscopy: A brief diagnostic arthroscopy can be helpful even when an open procedure is planned. The arthroscope is introduced into the posterior portal and a thorough evaluation of the joint is completed. Careful attention should be given to the anterior band of the IGHLC and labrum. A Hill-Sachs defect can also be visualized with external rotation of the arm.
4. Incision: A 5- to 7-cm incision is made inferior and lateral to the coracoid and is carried down to the axillary crease.
5. Approach: Flaps are made and subcutaneous fat is dissected to expose the underlying deltoid and pectoralis major muscles. The cephalic vein is identified (Fig. 42–5) and is usually retracted laterally with the deltoid. A deep self-retaining retractor is placed in the deltopectoral interval, and the underlying subscapularis is exposed (Fig. 42–6). Claviopectoral fascia is removed from this muscle; the subscapularis is carefully dissected off the underlying capsule by an incision that is made partway through the combined structures approximately 1 cm medial to the bicipital groove. Retention sutures are placed in the tendon; needle tip electrocautery and a small elevator are used to gently free the tendon from the underlying capsule (Fig. 42–7). A laterally based T incision is made in the capsule (Fig. 42–8), and the glenohumeral joint is exposed. A Fukuda (ring) retractor is helpful for exposing the glenoid. (*Note:* Alternative capsular incisions include horizontal and vertical incisions based on the planned capsular shift.)

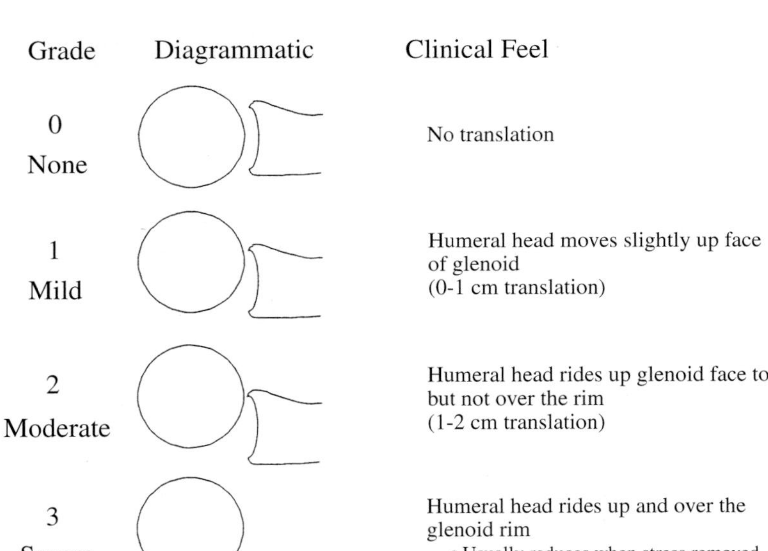

FIGURE 42–4. The grade of instability depends on the translation of the humeral head in relation to the glenoid rim. (From Hawkins RJ, Bokor DJ: Clinical evaluation of shoulder problems. In Rockwood CA Jr, Matsen FA III [eds]: The Shoulder, 2nd ed. Philadelphia, WB Saunders, 1998, p 185.)

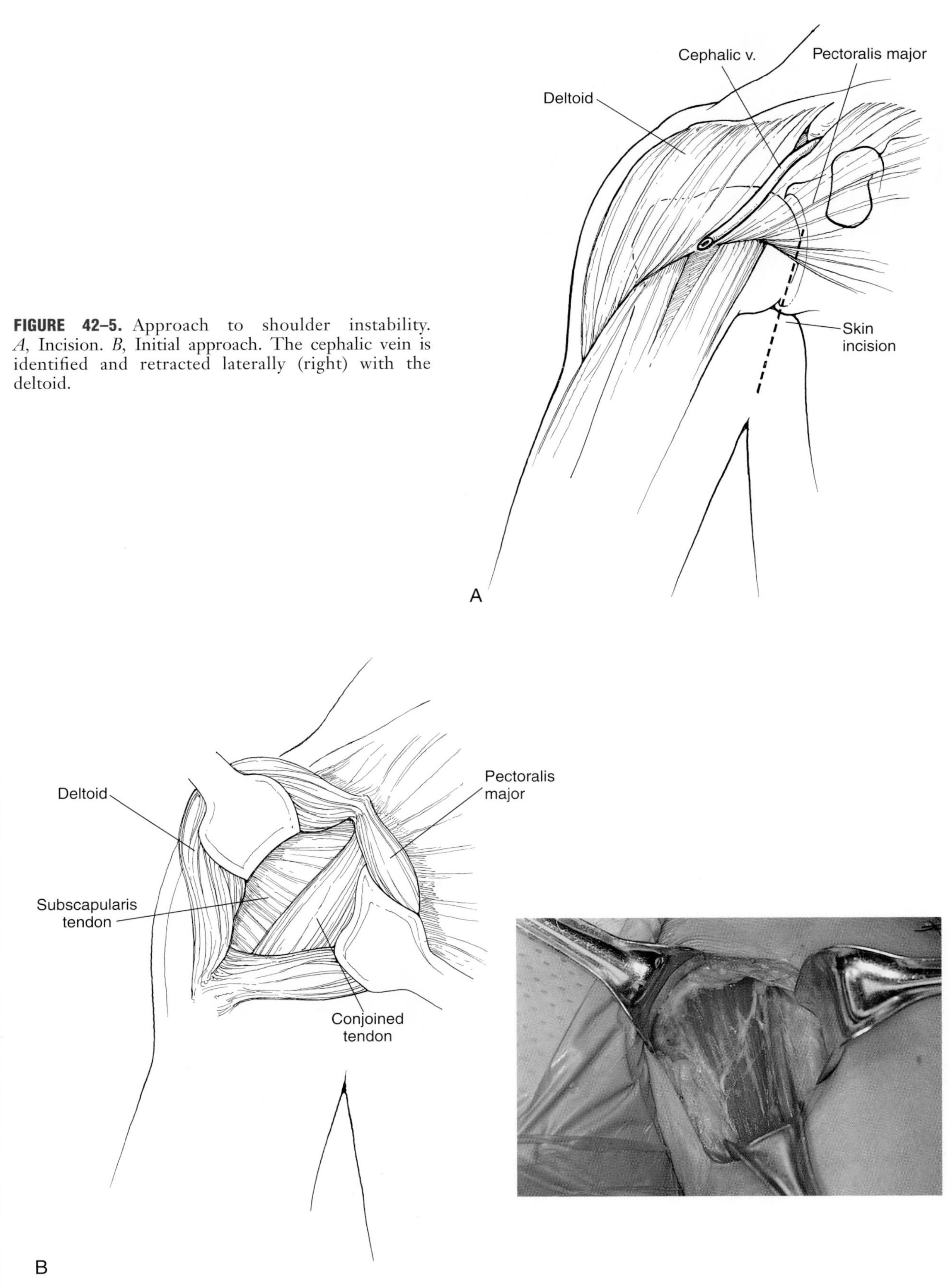

FIGURE 42–5. Approach to shoulder instability. *A*, Incision. *B*, Initial approach. The cephalic vein is identified and retracted laterally (right) with the deltoid.

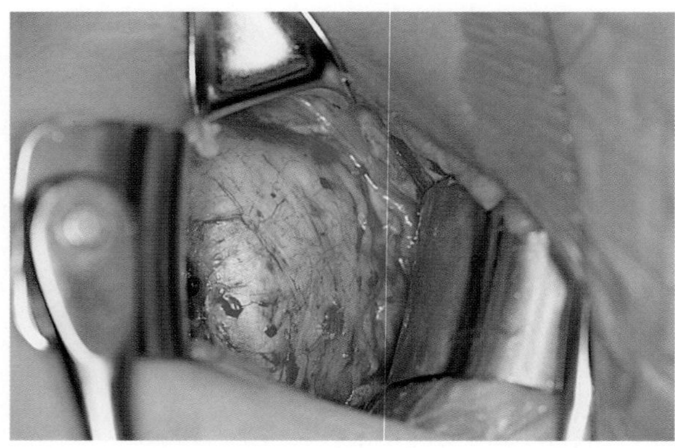

FIGURE 42–6. A self-retaining retractor is placed in the deltopectoral interval, and the clavipectoral fascia (superficial) and subscapularis tendon (deep) are exposed.

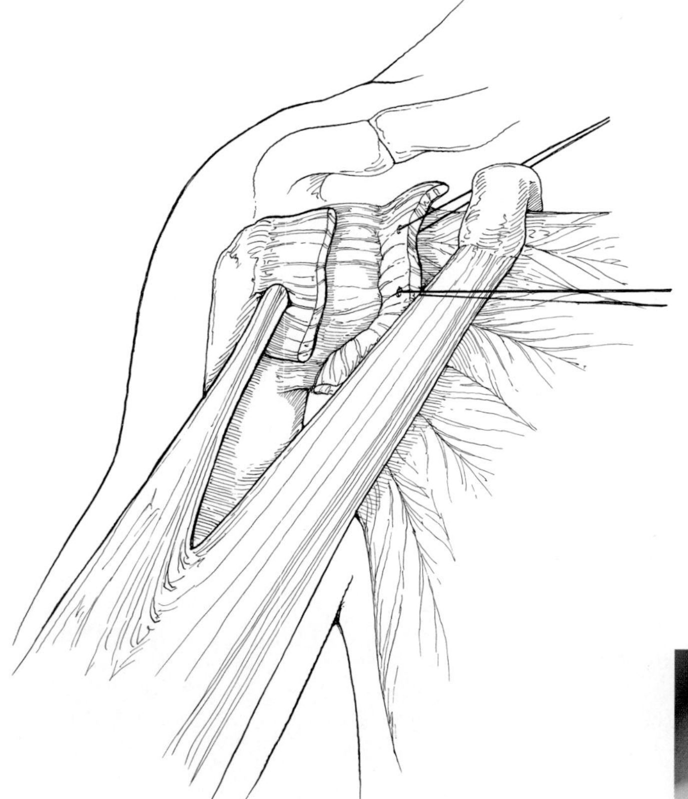

FIGURE 42–7. The subscapularis is carefully *teased* off the underlying capsule from lateral (left) to medial (right).

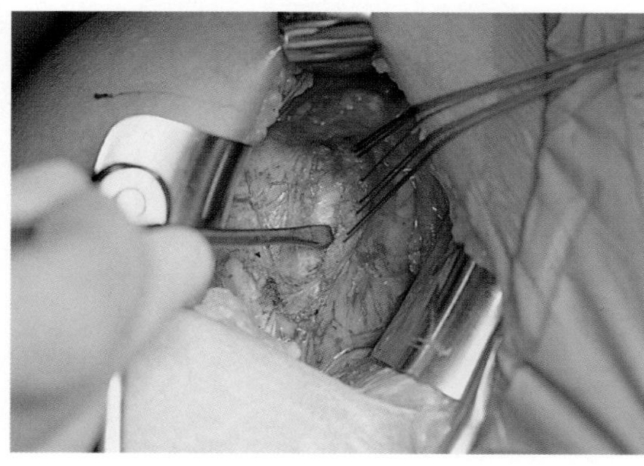

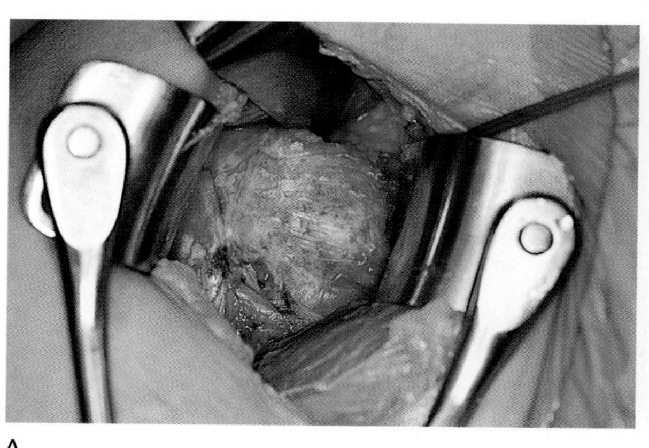
A

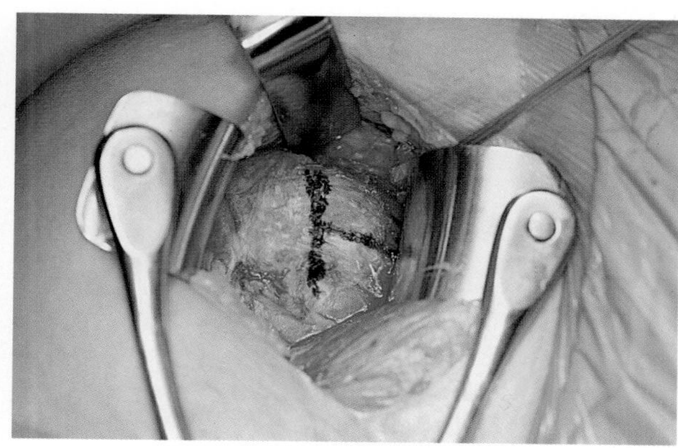
B

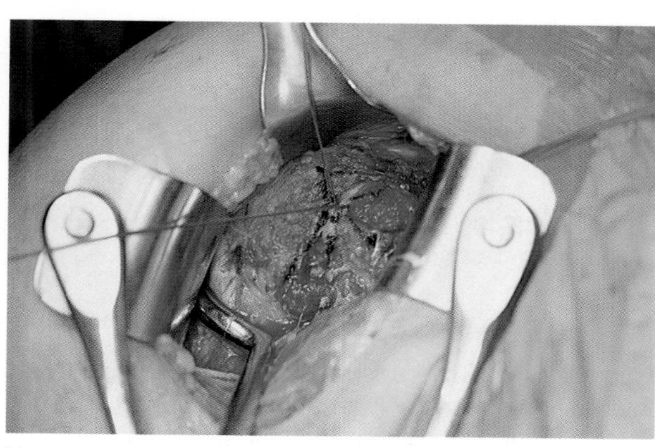
C

FIGURE 42–8. T-capsular incision. *A*, The subscapularis is retracted, and the capsule is exposed. *B*, A humeral-based T-capsular incision is planned. *C*, The incision is made, and shift is planned.

6. Bankart repair: If a Bankart lesion is identified, it is repaired back to the neck of the glenoid with sutures placed through drill holes or with suture anchors (Fig. 42–9).

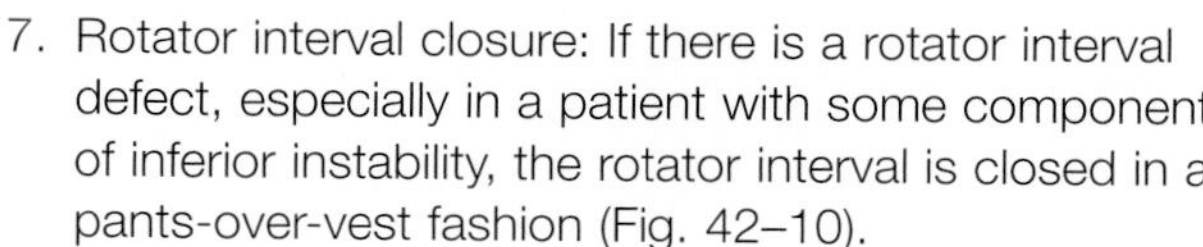

7. Rotator interval closure: If there is a rotator interval defect, especially in a patient with some component of inferior instability, the rotator interval is closed in a pants-over-vest fashion (Fig. 42–10).

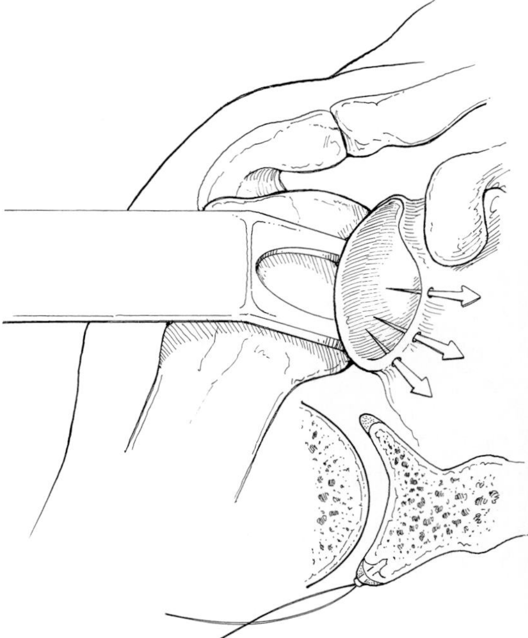

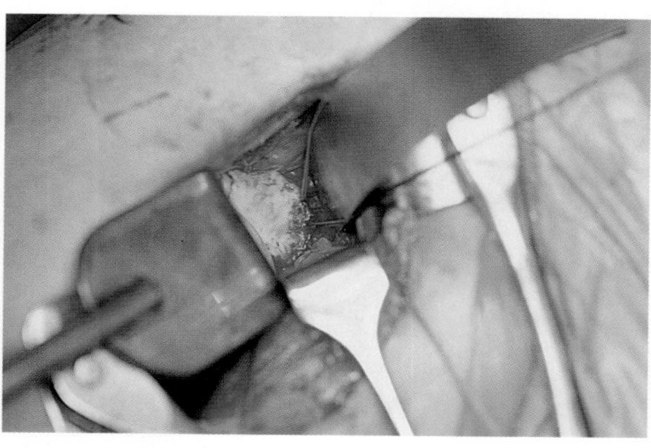

FIGURE 42–9. Bankart repair. A Fukuda retractor is placed into the glenohumeral joint, and the glenoid (and Bankart lesion) is inspected. Bankart repair is planned to restore the normal relationship of the labrum. The Bankart lesion can be repaired with sutures through drill holes *(top)* or with suture anchors *(bottom)*.

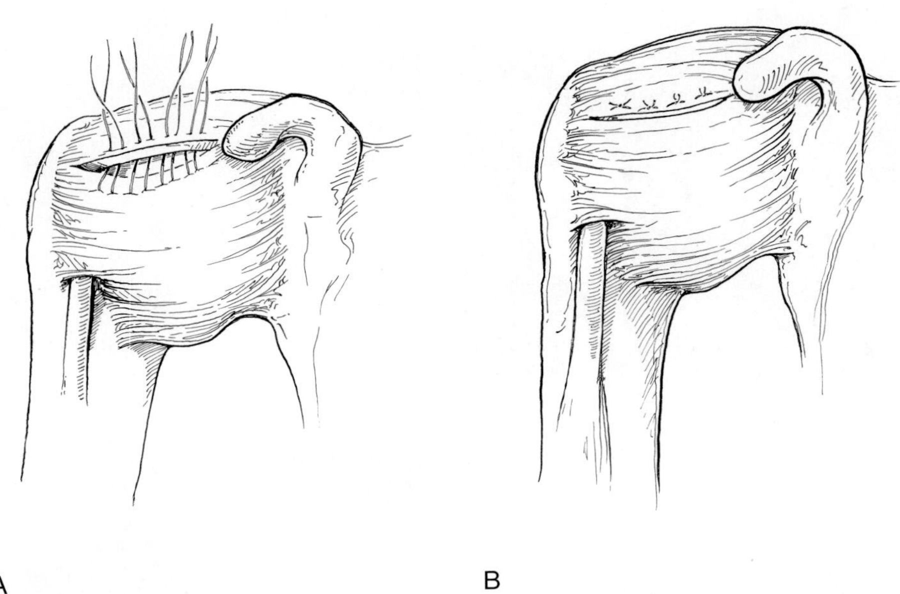

FIGURE 42–10. Rotator interval closure. *A*, Sutures are placed in a pants-over-vest fashion. *B*, Final repair eliminates inferior capsular laxity.

8. Capsular shift: The capsule is closed by shifting the inferior arm superiorly (with the arm in 30° to 45° of abduction and 30° to 45° of external rotation) and the superior arm inferiorly (with the arm in 0° of abduction and 30° to 45° of external rotation; Figs. 42–11 and 42–12).

9. Closure: The subscapularis is carefully reattached to its insertion (Fig. 42–13) with heavy nonabsorbable sutures. The deltopectoral interval is allowed to fall back into place (no sutures are necessary), and the subcutaneous tissues and skin are closed in the standard fashion.

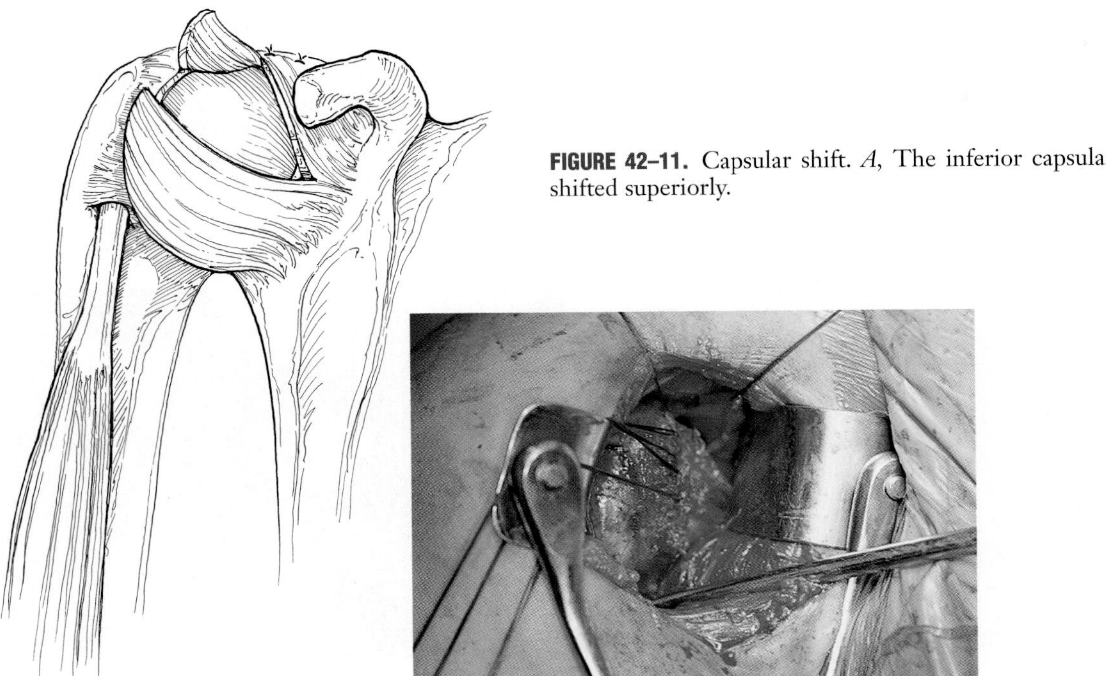

FIGURE 42–11. Capsular shift. *A*, The inferior capsular arm is shifted superiorly.

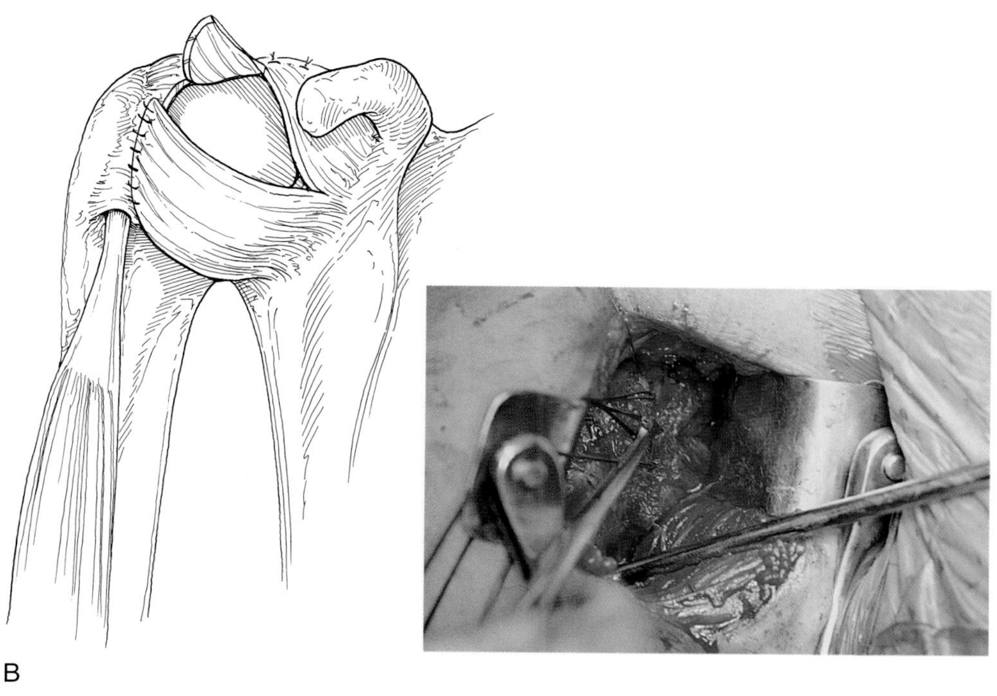

B

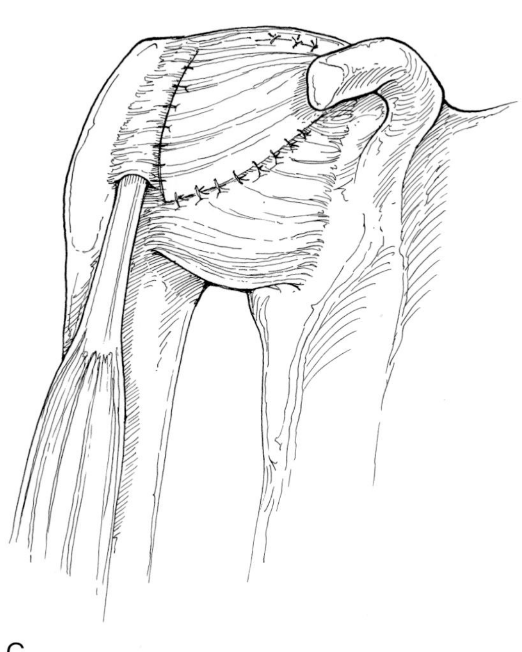

C

FIGURE 42–11 *Continued. B,* The superior capsular arm is shifted inferiorly. *C,* Final capsular shift markedly reduces capsular volume.

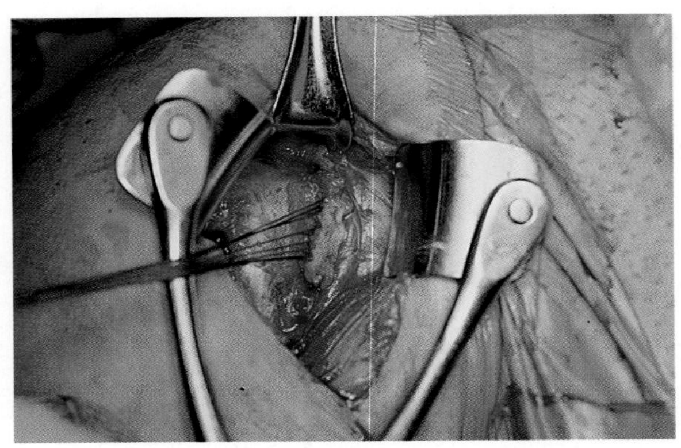

FIGURE 42–12. Subscapularis repair. The subscapularis is repaired with multiple strong nonabsorbable sutures back to its normal anatomic location.

Arthroscopic Bankart Repair (Suretac)

1. Positioning, EUA, and diagnostic arthroscopy are accomplished as discussed earlier.
2. Glenoid rim preparation: The glenoid rim is "freshened" with a sharp elevator and an arthroscopic shaver (Fig. 42–14).
3. The suture anchor or Suretac is placed with the use of an appropriate drill. The Suretac device uses a cannulated drill that captures the labrum (which can be pulled superiorly from the anterosuperior portal) and is drilled into the glenoid (Fig. 42–15).
4. The outer portion of the drill is removed and the Suretac device (Smith & Nephew Endoscopy, Andover, Mass) is placed over the guide wire (Fig. 42–16). (*Note:* For other anchors, the suture anchor is placed and the labrum is secured with arthroscopically placed knots.)
5. At least two, and sometimes three or more, devices are placed in similar fashion. After the repair is completed, it is inspected and probed (Fig. 42–17). The portals are closed with simple nylon or Prolene sutures, a dressing is applied, and the patient is placed in a shoulder immobilizer.

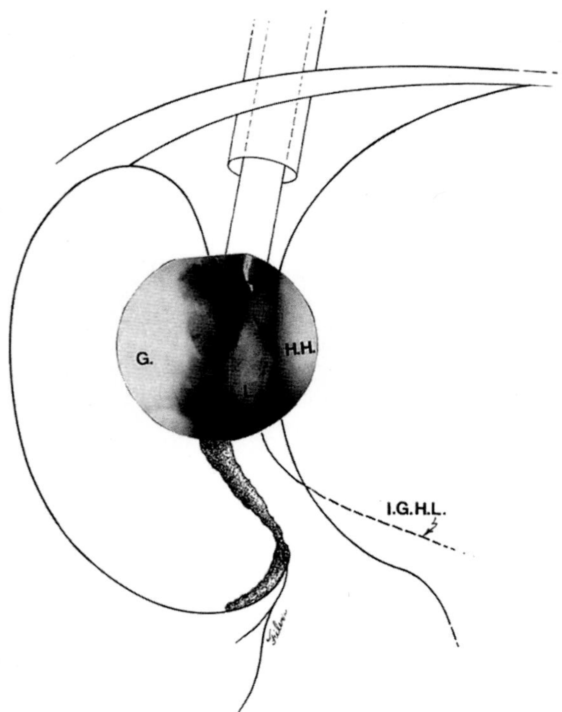

FIGURE 42–13. Artist's depiction of glenoid rim preparation. *Inset,* Arthroscopic view of glenoid rim preparation. G, glenoid; HH, humeral head; L, labrum; IGHL, inferior glenohumeral ligament. (From Warner JJP, Warren RF: Arthroscopic Bankart repair using cannulated, absorbable fixation device. Op Tech Orthop 1:192–198, 1991.)

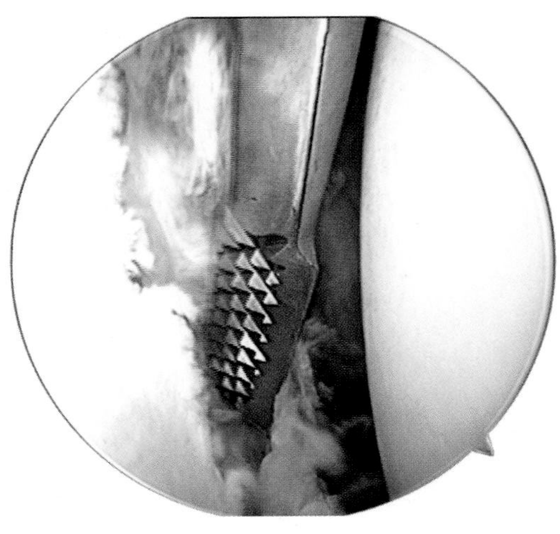

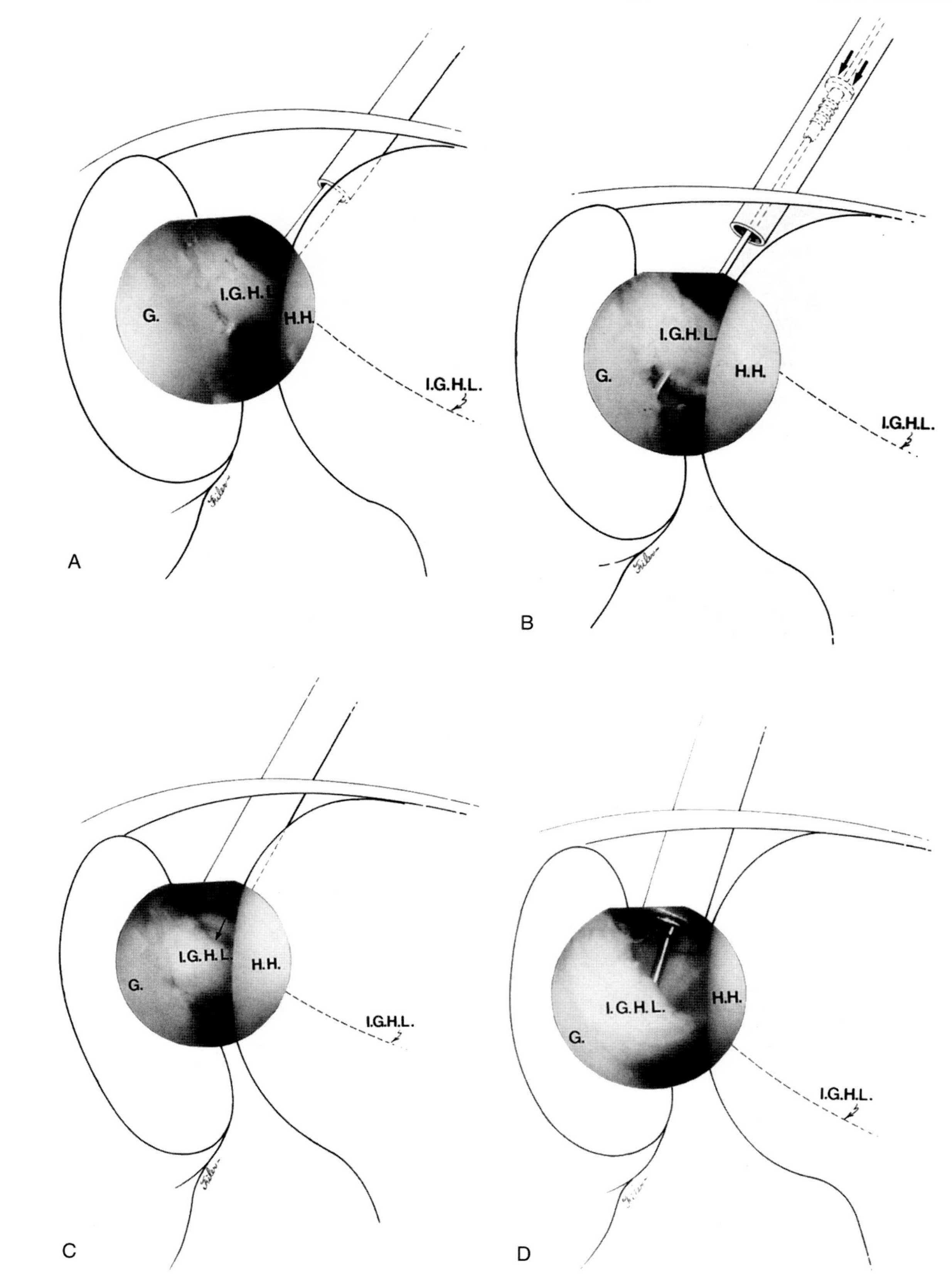

FIGURE 42–14. Drilling. G, glenoid; HH, humeral head; IGHL, inferior glenohumeral ligament. (From Warner JJP, Warren RF: Arthroscopic Bankart repair using cannulated, absorbable fixation device. Op Tech Orthop 1:192–198, 1991.)

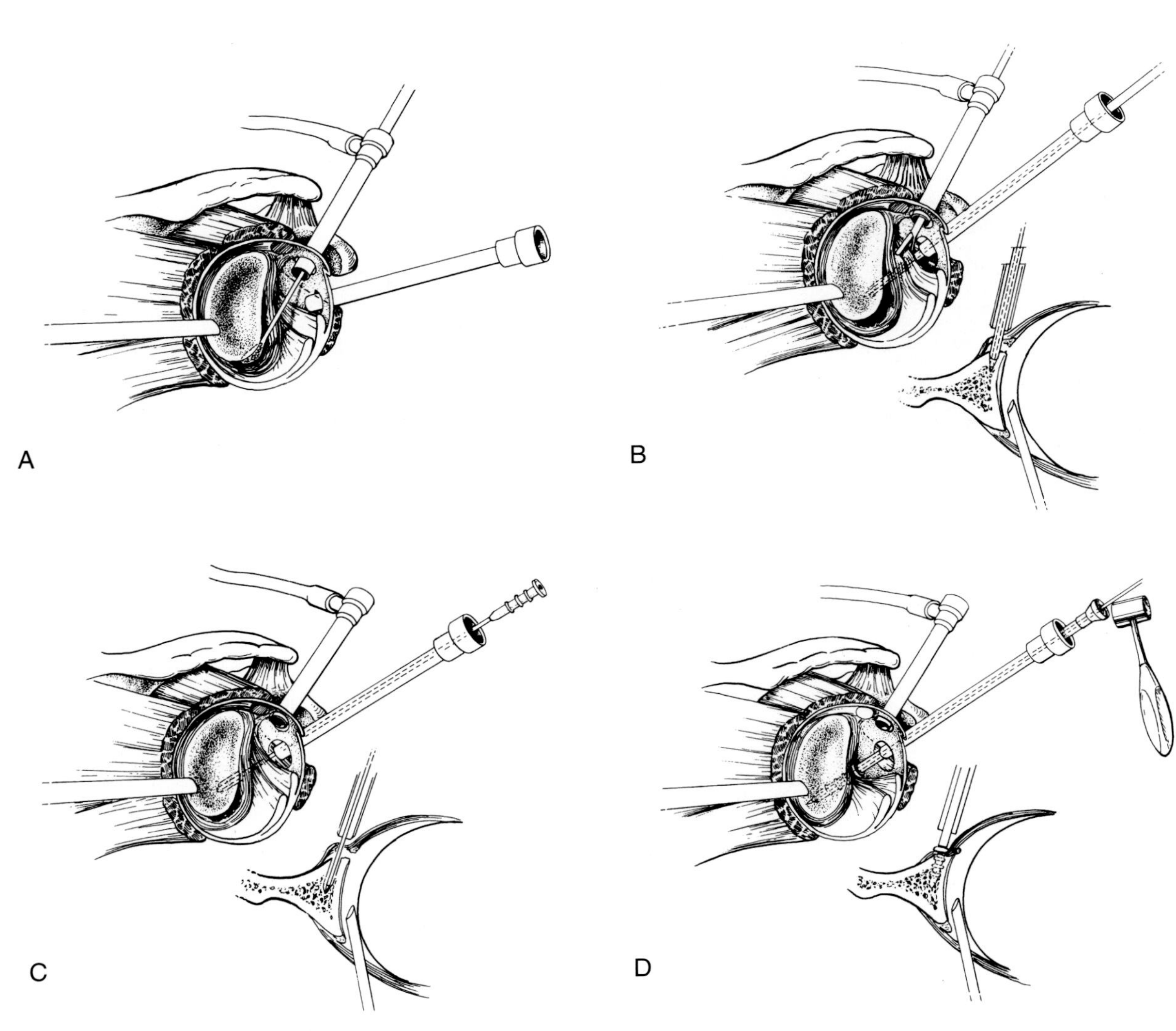

FIGURE 42–15. Tack placement. *A*, Rasping of the glenoid neck. *B*, Drilling. *C*, Tack is placed over guide wire. *D*, Tack is tapped into place. (From Warner JJP, Warren RF: Arthroscopic Bankart repair using cannulated, absorbable fixation device. Op Tech Orthop 1:192–198, 1991.)

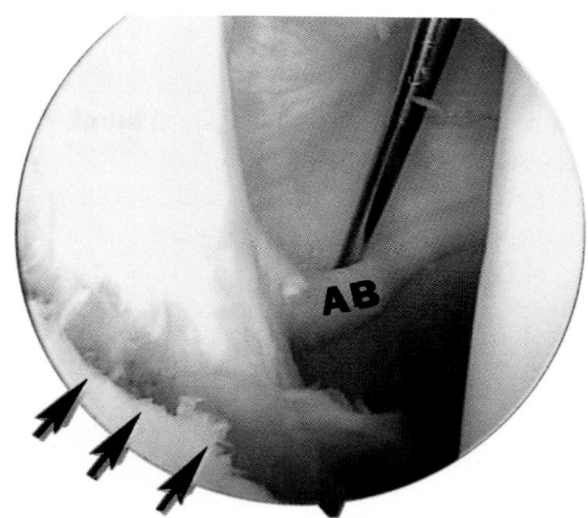

A

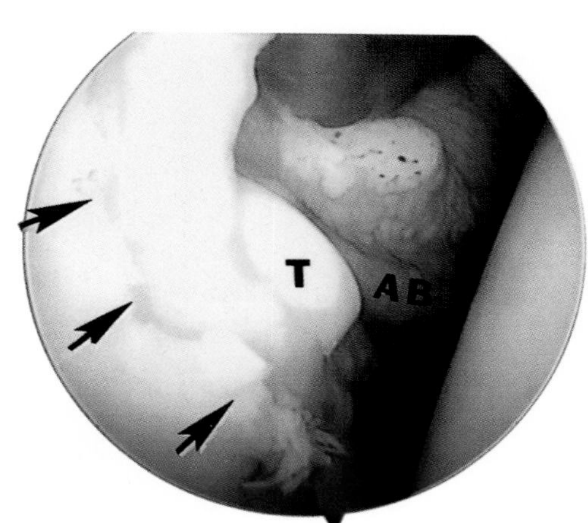

B

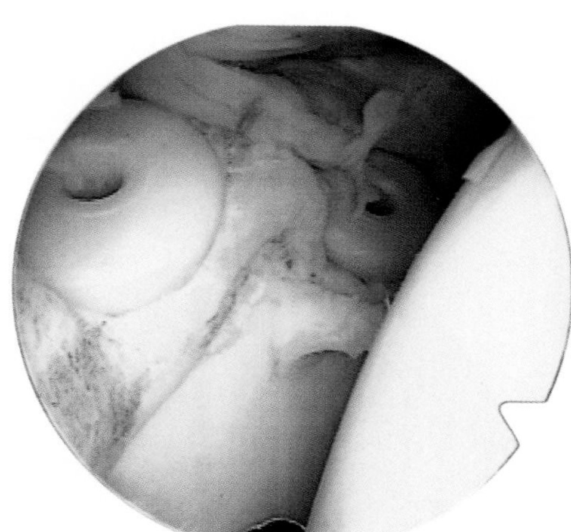

C

FIGURE 42–16. *A*, Bankart lesion. *Arrows* show location of the Bankart lesion. *B*, After tack (T) placement. *Arrows* show restored labrum adjacent to the glenoid. Note re-creation of the normal lip of labrum after Suretac placement. *C*, Final tack placement as viewed from the anterior-superior portal. AB, anterior band of the inferior glenohumeral ligament complex.

Suture Anchors

Positioning and glenoid rim preparation are similar to those described earlier. Occasionally, a burr is helpful for this step. A suture anchor is placed at the edge of the glenoid, and sutures and arthroscopic knots are used to reapproximate the labrum using a variety of techniques (see Fig. 42–17).

Knotless Anchors

This technique (Fig. 42–18) uses a unique device that does not require arthroscopic knot tying. Tension is applied to the labral repair based on the depth of the anchor. The attached loop is captured by the anchor, which is placed into a drill hole.

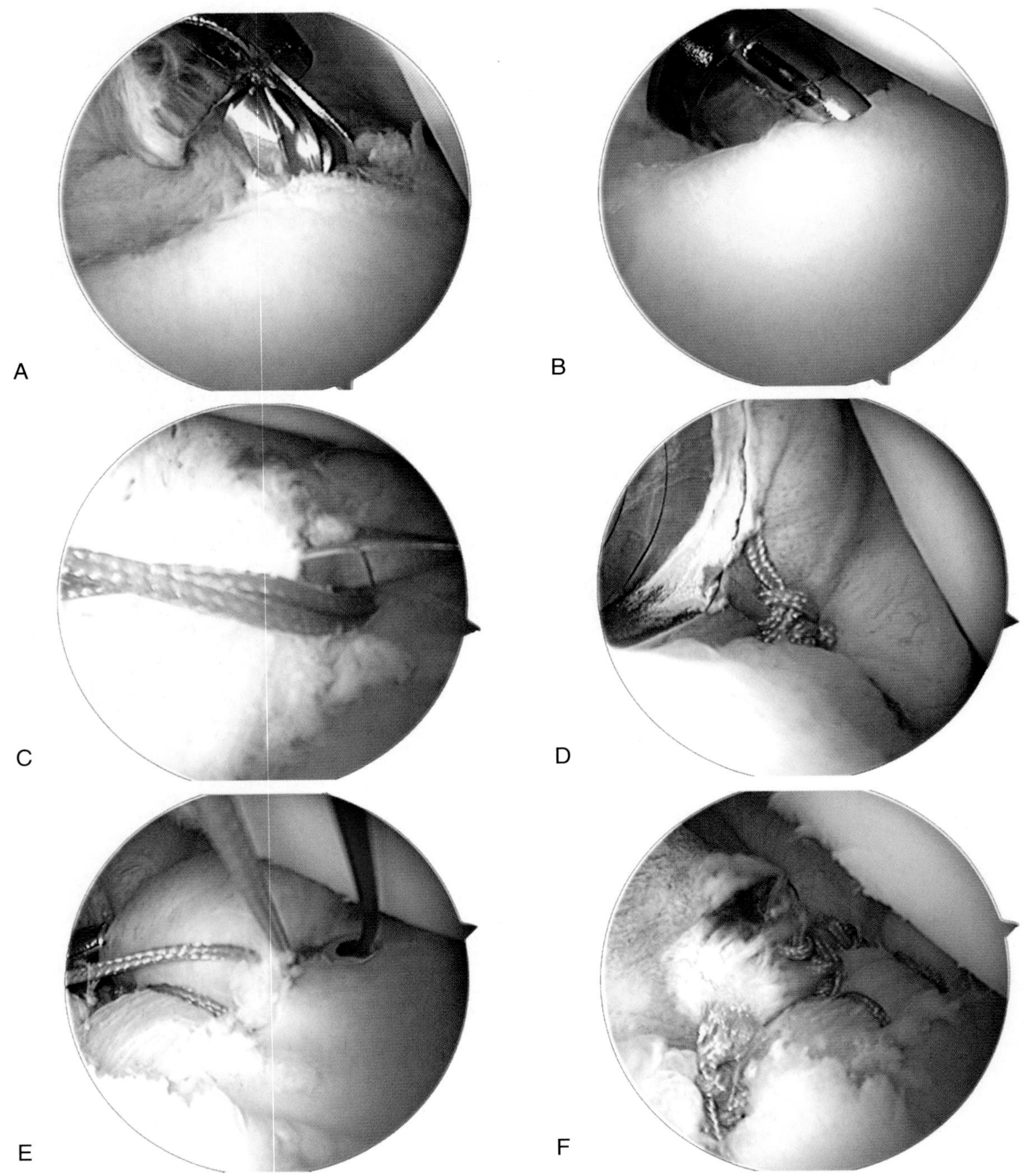

FIGURE 42–17. Arthroscopic Bankart lesion repair with conventional suture anchors. *A*, Glenoid rim preparation. *B*, Anchor placement as viewed from the anterosuperior portal. *C*, Suture retriever pierces the capsule and labrum and is used to retrieve one arm of the suture. *D*, Knot is tied arthroscopically. *E*, A retriever is used to shuttle another suture arm. *F*, Final repair. (From Cole BJ, Katolik LI: Shoulder. In Miller MD, Cooper DE, Warner JJP [eds]: Review of Sports Medicine and Arthroscopy, 2nd ed. Philadelphia, WB Saunders, 2002.)

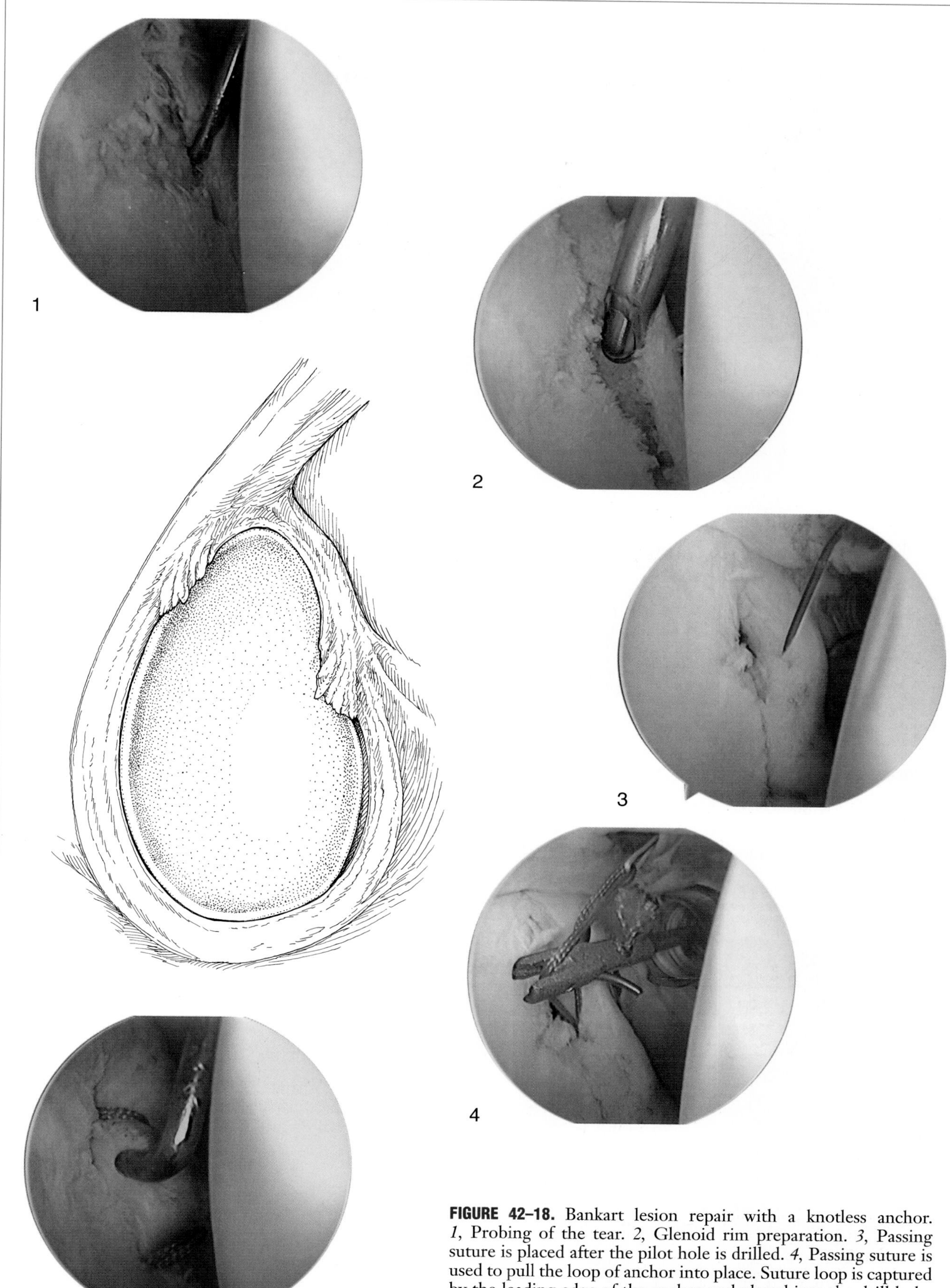

FIGURE 42–18. Bankart lesion repair with a knotless anchor. *1*, Probing of the tear. *2*, Glenoid rim preparation. *3*, Passing suture is placed after the pilot hole is drilled. *4*, Passing suture is used to pull the loop of anchor into place. Suture loop is captured by the leading edge of the anchor and placed into the drill hole. *5*, Final repair. (Courtesy of David R. Diduch, MD.)

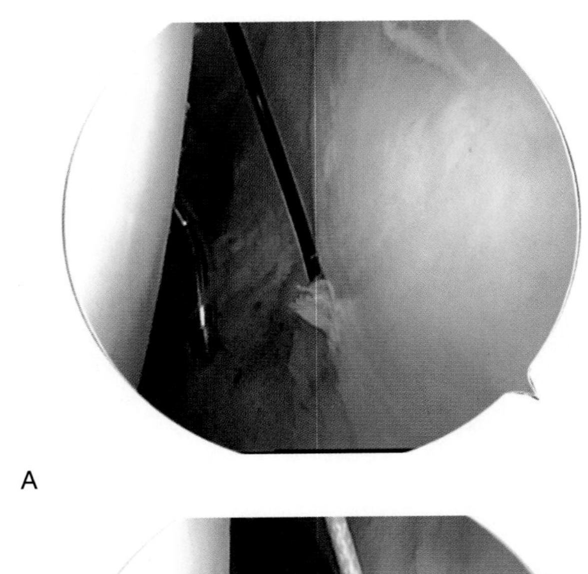

A

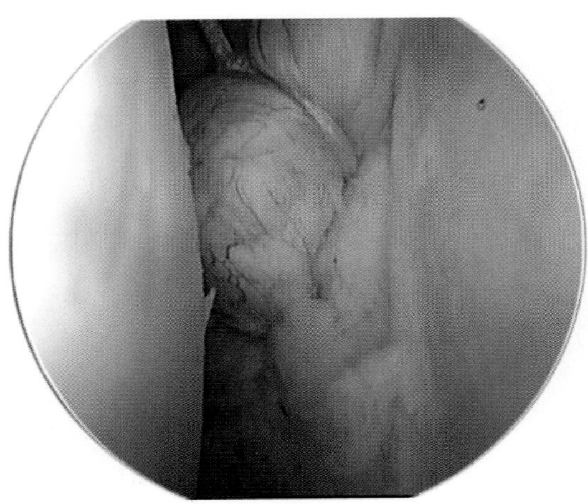

B

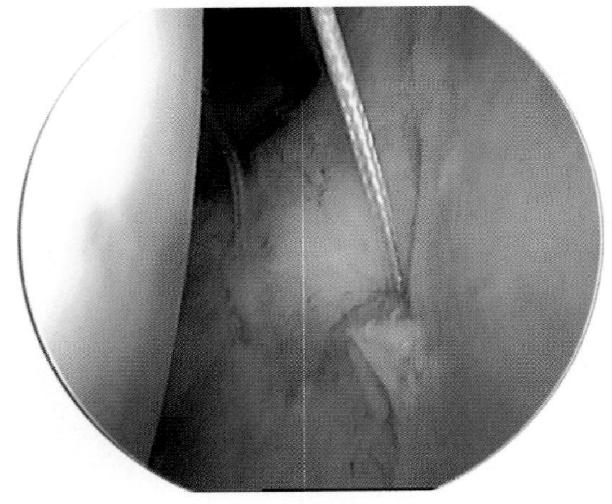

C

FIGURE 42–19. Arthroscopic capsular imbrication. *A*, Shuttle is used to capture redundant tissue. *B*, Suture is passed. *C*, Suture is tied with arthroscopic knots. (Courtesy of Brian J. Cole, MD.)

Arthroscopic Capsular Imbrication

Capsular volume can be reduced in small amounts with the use of arthroscopically imbricated capsules (Fig. 42–19). This technique can be applied for patients with small amounts of capsular redundancy.

Thermal Capsulorrhaphy

Although the indications are still being refined, a special heat probe with radiofrequency heat energy can be used to reduce capsular laxity (Fig. 42–20). Unfortunately, high failure rates and tissue necrosis have been reported with this device.

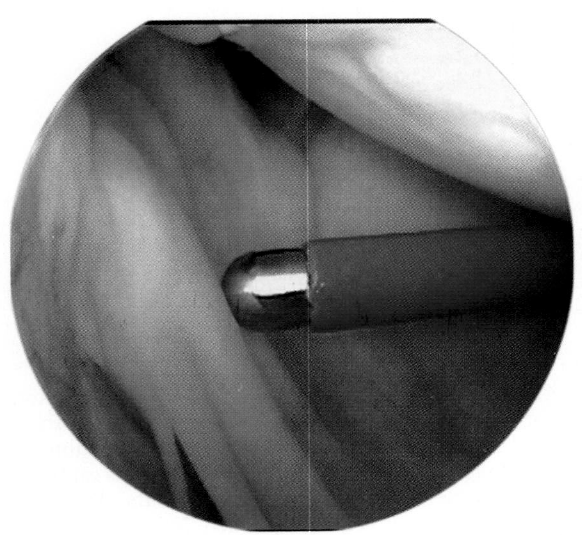

FIGURE 42–20. Thermal probe used for radiofrequency heat shrinkage. (Courtesy of Brian J. Cole, MD.)

POSTOPERATIVE MANAGEMENT

Open Capsular Shift

Patients are managed with a sling for comfort and early passive motion. Elbow range-of-motion and pendulum exercises are instituted immediately postoperatively. Gentle passive range of motion is begun at approximately 2 weeks postoperatively. More aggressive motion (active-assisted and active) is added 6 weeks postoperatively. Rotator cuff strengthening is begun after full motion is achieved. Return to sports is delayed until 6 months postoperatively.

Arthroscopic Bankart Repair (Suretac)

Postoperative management is dictated by the fixation device that is used. The Suretac device is not very strong biomechanically, and because it is bioabsorbable it gets weaker with time. Therefore, *patients in whom this device is used must be absolutely immobilized for a period of 4 weeks.* They must be instructed not to move the arm at all, including for personal hygiene. After this 4-week period, first passive and then active range of motion are initiated (patients may be quite stiff, but they will quickly regain motion with supervised therapy). Rotator cuff rehabilitation is begun after motion is achieved. Return to sports is allowed 4 to 6 months postoperatively. Arthroscopic Bankart repair (suture anchors) is similar to that for open capsular shift.

COMPLICATIONS

Complications include infection and recurrent instability (both less than 5% in most reports). Loss of motion can also occur (especially of external rotation). Significant external rotation loss may require Z-lengthening of the subscapularis tendon. Another complication is neurovascular injury (e.g., to the musculocutaneous nerve from vigorous retraction of the conjoined tendon, to the axillary nerve from inferior retraction or direct injury). Complications resulting from migration of hardware are also well known.

RESULTS

In most series, the results of open Bankart repair and capsular shift are excellent. Recurrence rates of less than 5% can be expected. Initial results with arthroscopic repairs are also encouraging; although they are less successful than open methods, recurrence rates of 10% or less can be anticipated in properly selected individuals.

REFERENCES

Litner SA, Speer KP: Traumatic anterior glenohumeral instability: The role of arthroscopy. J Am Acad Orthop Surg 5:233–239, 1997.

Lusardi DA, Wirth MA, Wurtz D, et al: Loss of external rotation following anterior capsulorrhaphy of the shoulder. J Bone Joint Surg [Am] 75:1185–1192, 1993.

Neer CS II, Foster CR: Inferior capsular shift for involuntary inferior and multidirectional instability of the shoulder. A preliminary report. J Bone Joint Surg [Am] 62:897–908, 1980.

Warner JJP, Johnson DL, Miller MD, et al: Techniques for selecting capsular tightness in repair of anterior inferior shoulder instability. J Shoulder Elbow Surg 4:352–364, 1995.

Warner JJP, Miller MD, Marks P, Fu FH: Arthroscopic Bankart repair with Suretac device. Part I: Clinical observations. Arthroscopy 11:2–13, 1995.

Warner JJP, Miller MD, Marks P: Arthroscopic Bankart repair with Suretac device. Part II: Experimental observations. Arthroscopy 11:14–20, 1995.

CHAPTER 43

Treatment of Posterior Shoulder Instability

INTRODUCTION

Posterior shoulder instability is much less common than anterior instability, accounting for only about 3% of all shoulder dislocations. Because of its rarity and its less than obvious clinical presentation and findings on anteroposterior (AP) radiographs, the diagnosis is missed initially on a regular basis. Similar to anterior shoulder instability, posterior instability can be classified according to degree (dislocation or subluxation), direction (subacromial is the most common), and cause (traumatic or atraumatic).

HISTORY AND PHYSICAL EXAMINATION

Frank dislocation can be caused by a direct blow to the shoulder from the front or, more commonly, as a result of indirect injury. The most widely recognized indirect injury follows seizures and shock; the internal rotators of the shoulder girdle overpower the external rotators, resulting in a posterior dislocation. Repetitive forces to the extended upper extremity (e.g., interior linemen in football) result in posterior instability; this occurs more commonly among athletes.

The patient with an acute posterior shoulder dislocation presents with an internal rotation deformity and limited external rotation of the arm. Abduction is usually limited to less than 90°. Posterior prominence, or loss of anterior contour and prominence of the coracoid, may be seen in thinner individuals (Fig. 43–1). Additionally, the patient is unable to supinate the forearm fully with the arm forward flexed.

In patients with posterior subluxation, the posterior drawer (or push-pull) test (Fig. 43–2) may demonstrate significant posterior displacement of the humerus in relation to the glenoid. Additionally, the jerk test (Fig. 43–3) may demonstrate a jerk when the shoulder displaces posteriorly near midline or, more commonly, a jerk as it reduces anteriorly while it is passively returned to the starting position.

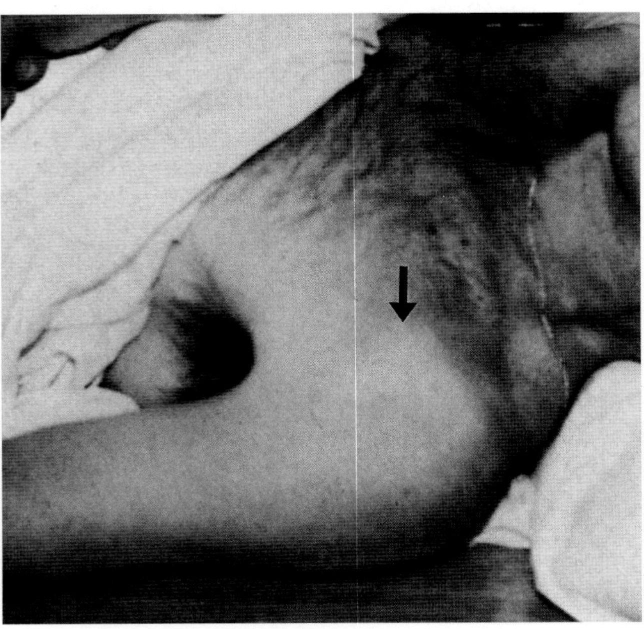

FIGURE 43–1. Prominence of the coracoid *(arrow)* is noted in this patient with a posterior shoulder dislocation. (From Pagnani MJ, Galinat BJ, Warren RF: Glenohumeral instability. In DeLee JC, Drez D Jr [eds]: Orthopaedic Sports Medicine: Principles and Practice. Philadelphia, WB Saunders, 1994, pp 580–622.)

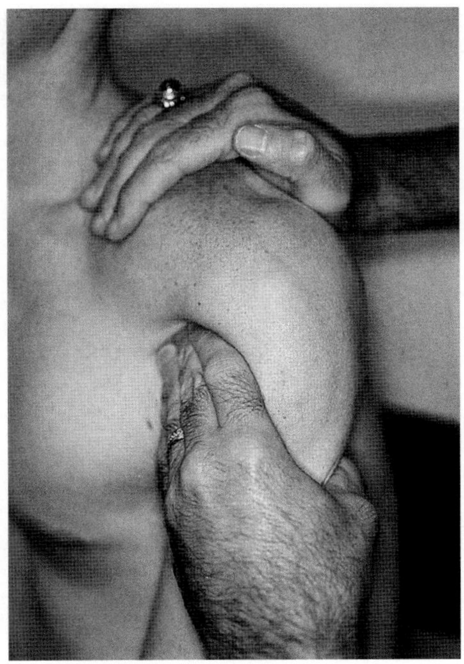

FIGURE 43–2. Posterior drawer test. One hand stabilizes the scapula, and the shoulder is passively displaced posteriorly.

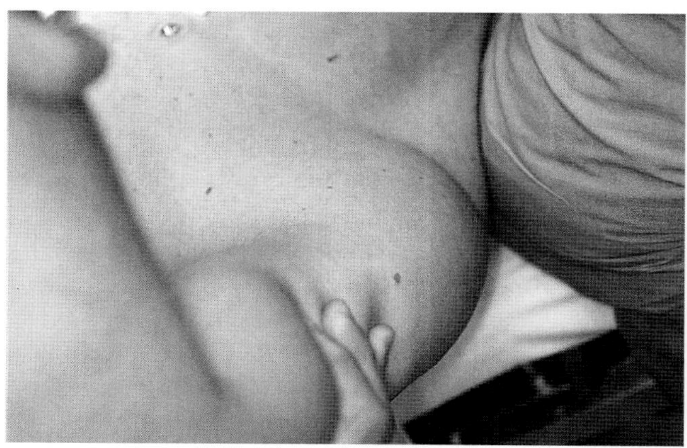
A

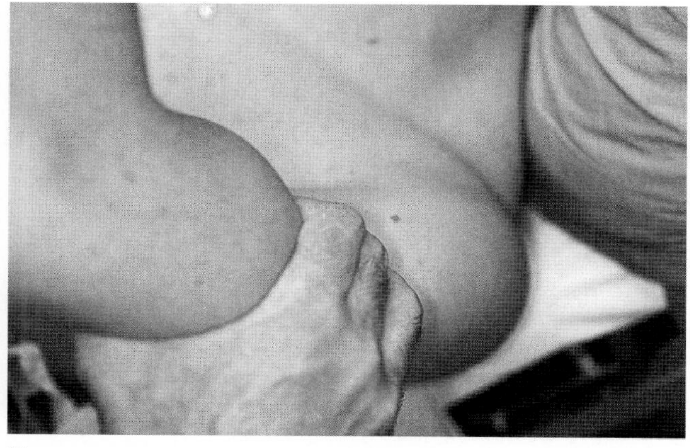
B

FIGURE 43–3. Jerk test for posterior instability. The patient is evaluated in the supine position with the arm internally rotated and forward flexed 90°. *A*, The examiner grasps the arm and axially loads the humerus. *B*, With axial load maintained, the arm is passively moved horizontally across the body, producing a jerk as it approaches midline.

DIAGNOSTIC IMAGING

As was indicated earlier, one of the main reasons for missing the diagnosis of posterior shoulder dislocation acutely is the failure to obtain adequate radiographs. Anteroposterior radiographs alone are not adequate! Several subtle signs may be seen on these views, including the so-called vacant glenoid sign and the light bulb sign; however, an axillary lateral view makes the diagnosis obvious (Fig. 43–4). It is important to also look carefully for the presence of a reverse Hill-Sachs deformity on the axillary lateral view. Large reverse Hill-Sachs impression fractures must be treated with subscapularis transfer procedures or a hemiarthroplasty. MRI may be beneficial in patients with established posterior instability (Fig. 43–5).

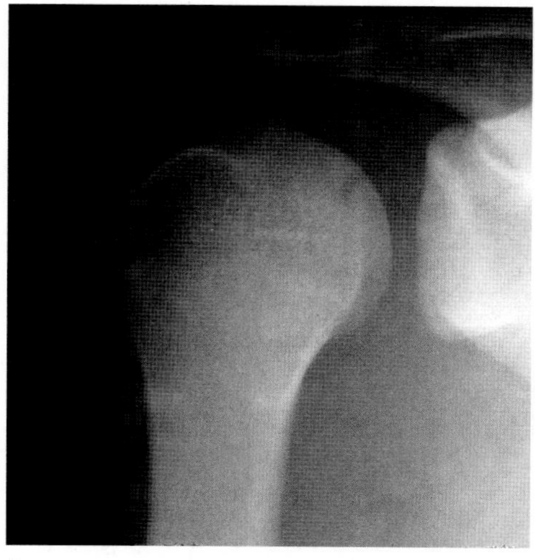
A

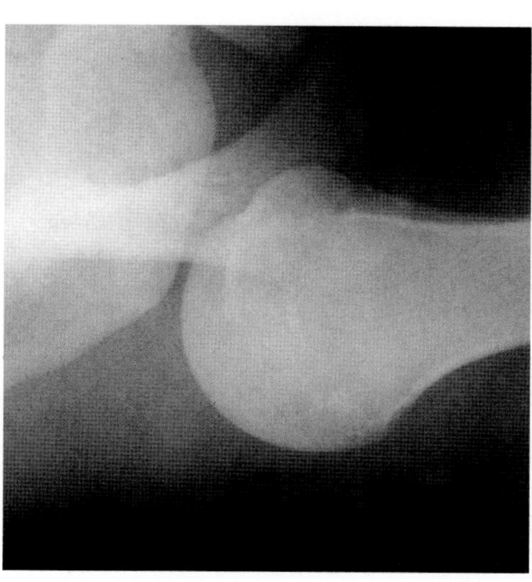
B

FIGURE 43–4. Posterior shoulder instability. *A*, Anteroposterior view. *B*, Lateral view.

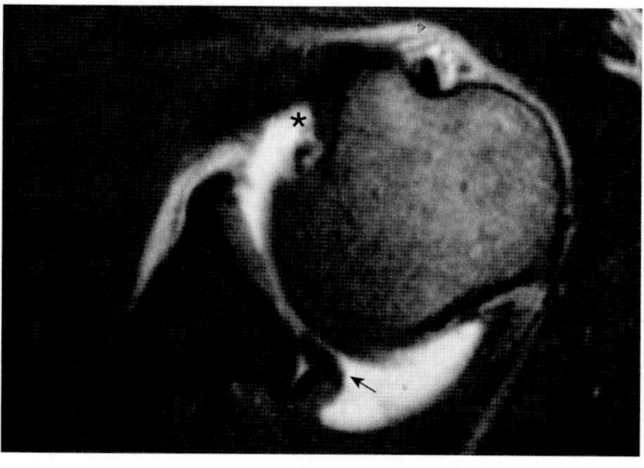

FIGURE 43–5. MRI view of a posterior Bankart lesion *(arrow)* and a reverse Hill-Sachs deformity (*).

NONOPERATIVE MANAGEMENT

If an acute posterior shoulder dislocation is recognized and is reduced immediately, recurrent posterior instability is unusual unless there is a large reverse Hill-Sachs lesion. Following reduction (lateral traction and gentle internal rotation followed by posterior pressure and external rotation), most authors recommend immobilization in a "gunslinger"-type brace (0° to 20° of external rotation, 0° of abduction, and slight extension) for 4 to 6 weeks, followed by aggressive physical therapy that emphasizes strengthening of external rotators. Most patients with recurrent posterior subluxation also benefit from strengthening of external rotators.

RELEVANT ANATOMY

The posterior deltoid overlies the infraspinatus muscle, which usually has a prominent fat stripe that divides this muscle in two. Below the infraspinatus muscle is the teres minor. It is critical to dissect above this muscle during treatment because distal to it is the quadrangular space, which contains the axillary nerve. Excessive medial retraction may jeopardize the suprascapular nerve.

SURGICAL TECHNIQUE

Indications

Failure to achieve a stable reduction, recurrent posterior dislocation following rehabilitation, and recurrent posterior subluxation with pain or unintentional instability following extended rehabilitation are all indications for surgery. Additionally, patients with pain during activities of daily living and competitive athletes with symptoms during strenuous activity may be surgical candidates.

Technique

1. Positioning: Following examination under anesthesia, the patient is placed in a lateral decubitus position, or in a beach-chair position with a bump under the affected shoulder.
2. Incision: A 6-cm vertical incision is made midway between the posterolateral corner of the acromion and the posterior axillary crease. The deltoid muscle is split to expose the underlying rotator cuff muscles (Fig. 43–6).

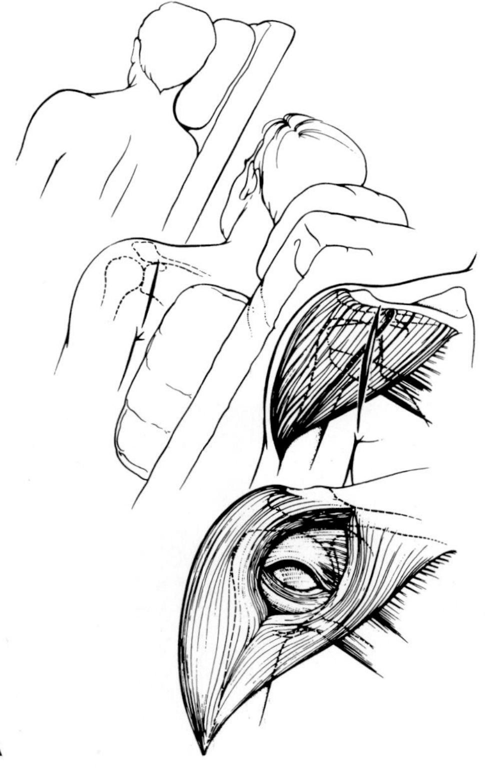

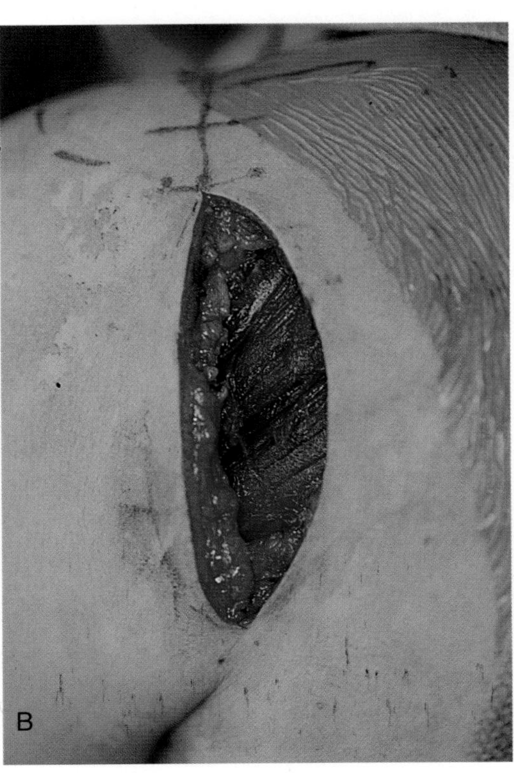

FIGURE 43–6. *A*, Positioning and initial approach for posterior capsular shift. *B*, Incision and initial deltoid exposure. Note orientation of posterior deltoid fibers, which can be split easily. (*A* from Pagnani MJ, Galinat BJ, Warren RF: Glenohumeral instability. In DeLee JC, Drez D Jr [eds]: Orthopaedic Sports Medicine: Principles and Practice. Philadelphia, WB Saunders, 1994, pp 580–622.)

3. Approach: The capsule may be approached by three different methods: (1) The infraspinatus can be dissected off the capsule, much as the subscapularis is approached during anterior procedures (Fig. 43–7); (2) the infraspinatus can be split, using the fat stripe as a landmark (Fig. 43–8); or (3) the interval between the infraspinatus and the teres minor can be developed (Fig. 43–9).

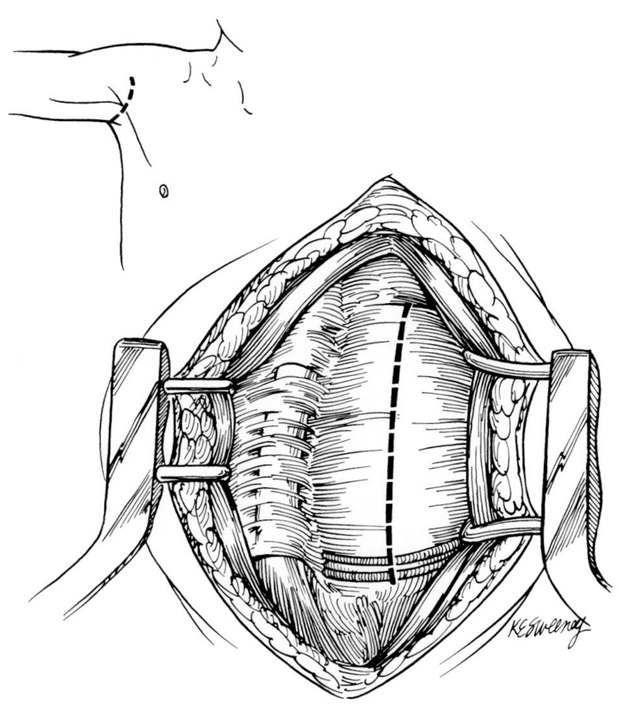

FIGURE 43–7. A posterior approach for treatment of posterior glenohumeral instability. An incision is centered over the posterior glenoid rim *(inset)*. Note the deltoid-splitting approach to minimize the amount of deltoid origin that must be released. Also note the incision in the infraspinatus and teres minor tendons. (From Matsen FA, Thomas SC: Glenohumeral instability. In Evarts CM [ed]: Surgery of the Musculoskeletal System, 2nd ed. New York, Churhill Livingstone, 1989.)

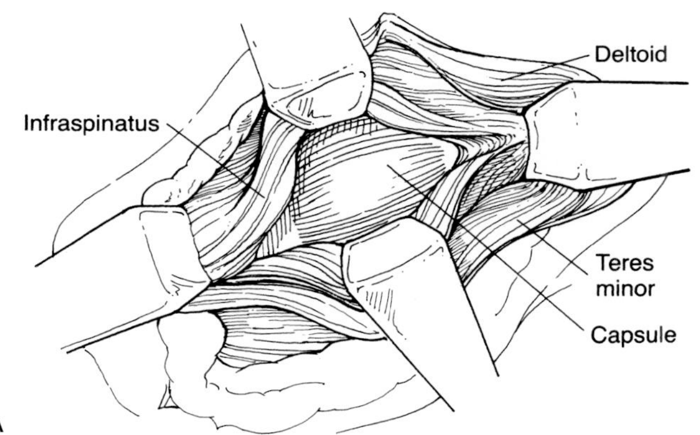

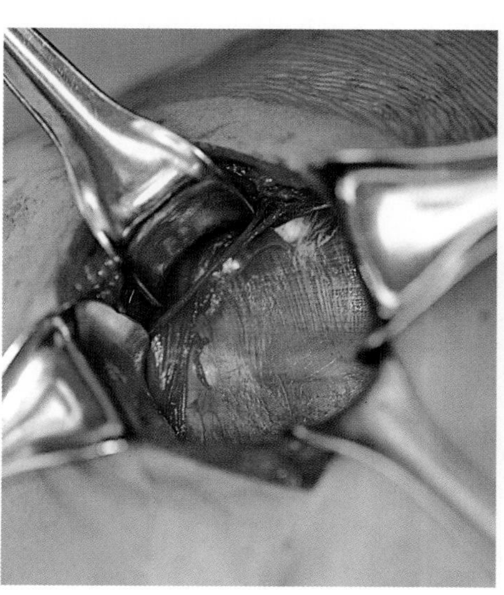

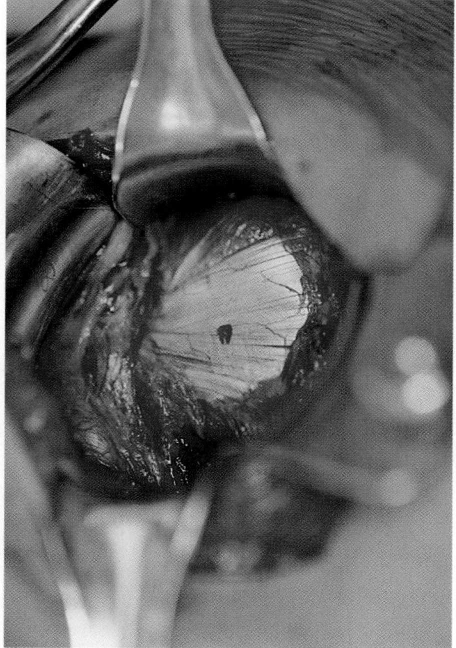

FIGURE 43–8. Infraspinatus splitting approach. *A*, Illustration showing approach. *B*, Interval is identified by fat stripe. *C*, The capsule is exposed. (*A* from Miller MD, Cooper DE, Warner JJP: Review of Sports Medicine and Arthroscopy. Philadelphia, WB Saunders, 1995, p 144.)

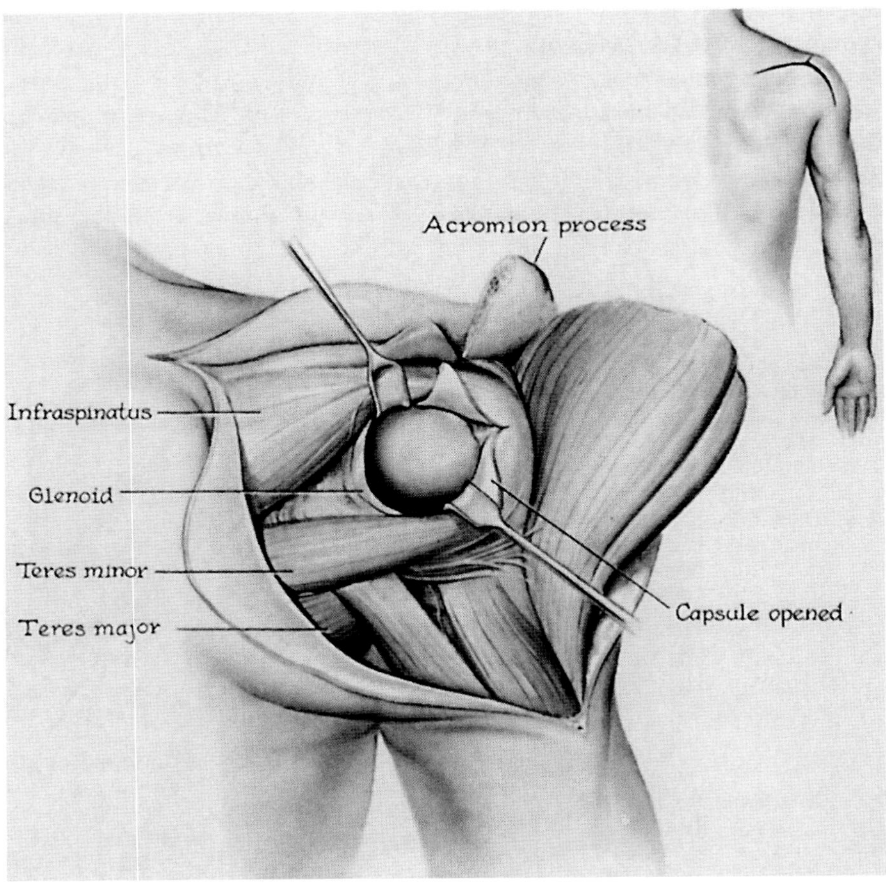

FIGURE 43–9. Posterior approach through the infraspinatus teres minor interval. (From Kaplan EB: Surgical Approaches to the Neck, Cervical Spine, and Upper Extremity. Philadelphia, WB Saunders, 1966, p 61.)

4. Capsular shift: Likewise, the shift can be accomplished with several different techniques: (1) A T-capsular shift can be based on the glenoid (Fig. 43–10); (2) a T-capsular shift can be based on the humerus (Fig. 43–11); (3) an H-capsular shift can be made (Fig. 43–12); or (4) a vertical capsular shift can be accomplished midway between the humeral and glenoid attachments of the capsule (Fig. 43–13).

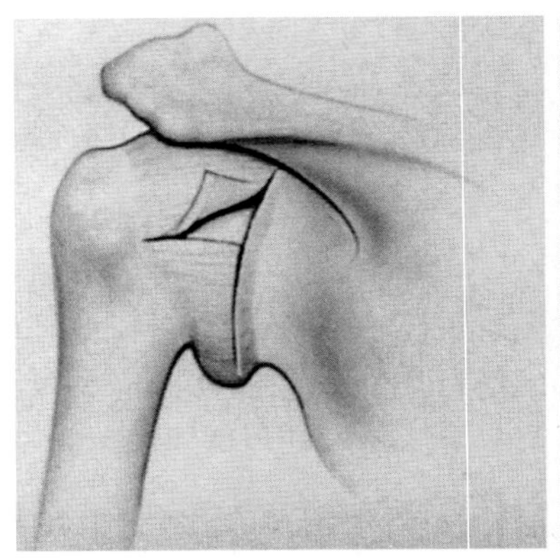

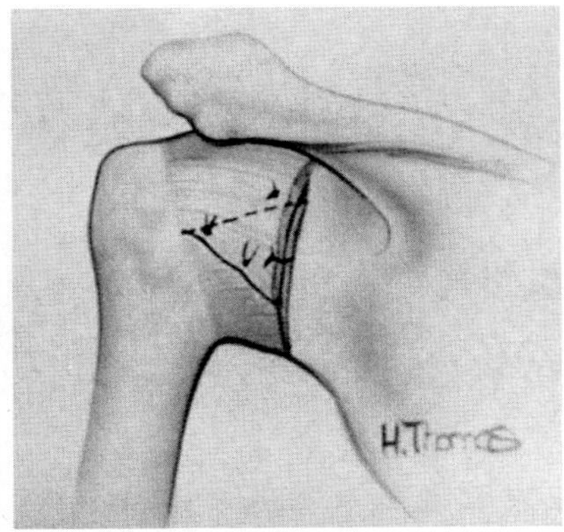

FIGURE 43–10. Glenoid-based T-capsular shift. *A*, Capsular incision. *B*, Capsular shift. (From Schwartz E, Warren RF, O'Brien SJ, et al: Posterior shoulder instability. Orthop Clin North Am 18:409–419, 1987.)

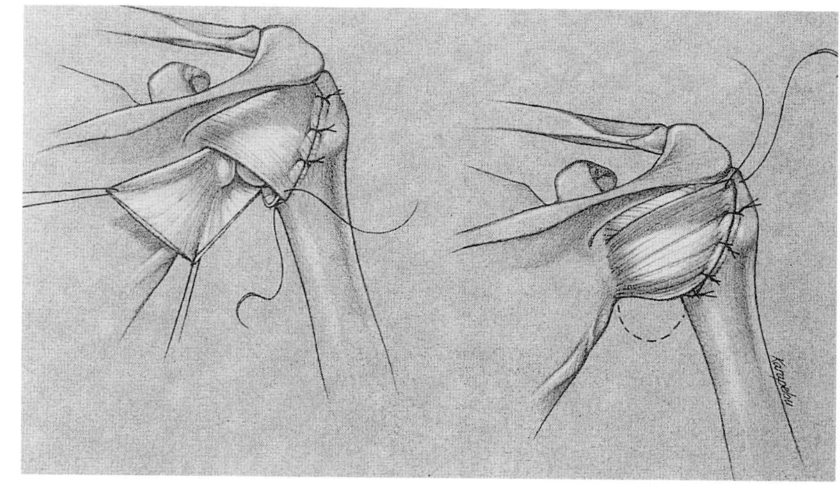

FIGURE 43–11. Humeral-based T-capsular shift. *A*, Capsular incision. *B*, Capsular shift.

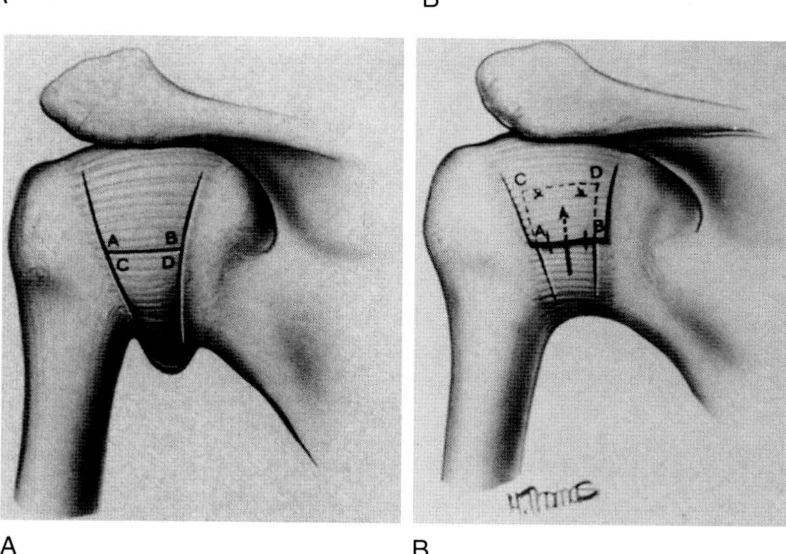

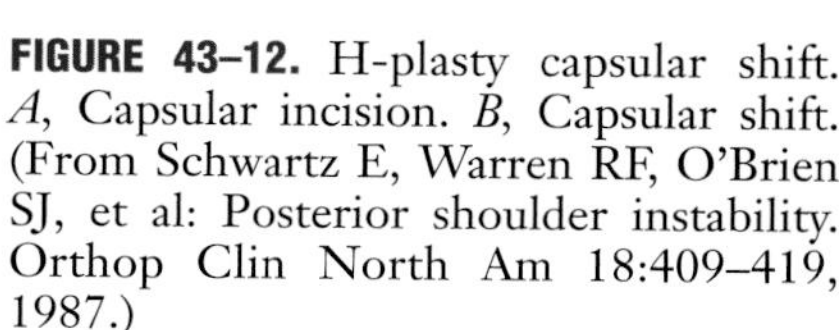

FIGURE 43–12. H-plasty capsular shift. *A*, Capsular incision. *B*, Capsular shift. (From Schwartz E, Warren RF, O'Brien SJ, et al: Posterior shoulder instability. Orthop Clin North Am 18:409–419, 1987.)

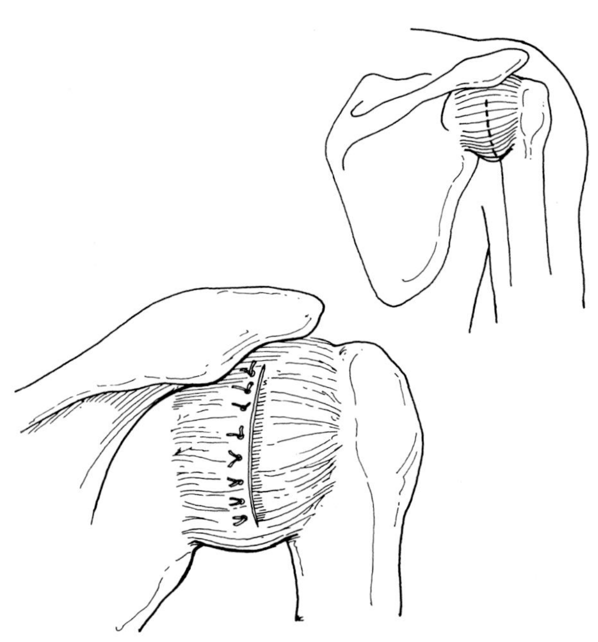

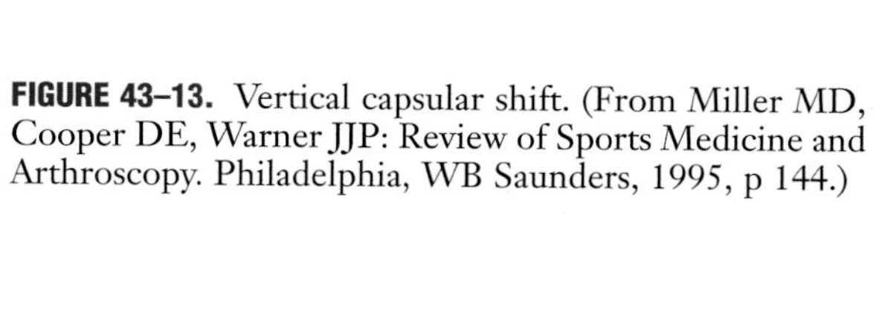

FIGURE 43–13. Vertical capsular shift. (From Miller MD, Cooper DE, Warner JJP: Review of Sports Medicine and Arthroscopy. Philadelphia, WB Saunders, 1995, p 144.)

5. Posterior bone block: Rarely, a posterior bone block can be used to supplement the repair or to address posterior glenoid deficiency. A tri-cortical bone block is obtained from the scapular spine or the iliac crest and is placed so that it is contiguous with the curvature of the glenoid (Fig. 43–14). It is important to ensure that the humeral head does not impinge on the bone block. The bone block is placed at the posteroinferior aspect of the glenoid and secured with a cancellous screw.
6. Closure: Depending on the approach taken, all layers are closed. It is not necessary to close the deltoid split. Skin closure is done in routine fashion, and the patient is placed in a gunslinger brace following dressing of the wound.

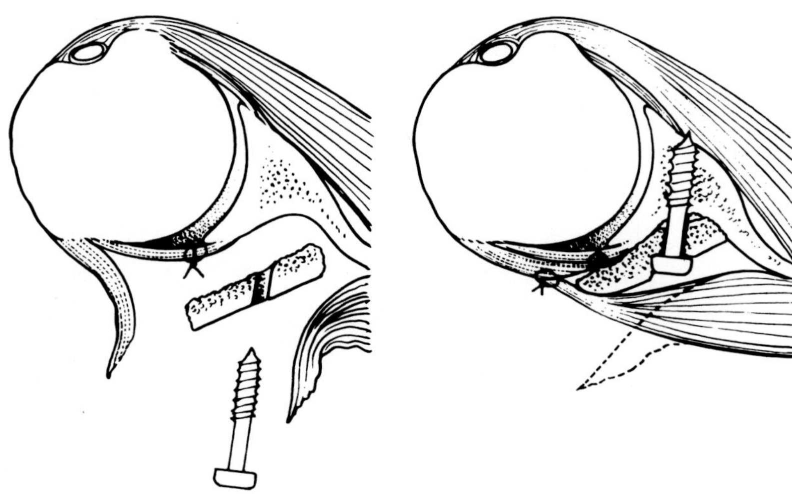

FIGURE 43–14. Posterior bone block. (From Pagnani MJ, Galinat BJ, Warren RF: Glenohumeral instability. In DeLee JC, Drez D Jr [eds]: Orthopaedic Sports Medicine: Principles and Practice. Philadelphia, WB Saunders, 1994, pp 580–622.)

POSTOPERATIVE MANAGEMENT

The patient is kept in a gunslinger brace for a period of 6 weeks. After this, passive range of motion followed by active range of motion and strengthening is allowed. Contact sports should be avoided for 6 months.

COMPLICATIONS

By far the biggest complication following posterior capsular shift is recurrence, which happens at a rate of up to 50% in some series. However, with proper patient selection and the use of appropriate techniques, this rate can be reduced to approximately 10%. Other problems such as neurovascular injury can be avoided by the use of proper technique.

RESULTS

As was indicated earlier, results are mixed. Successful results have been reported in several recent series.

REFERENCES

Fuchs B, Jost B, Gerber C: Posterior-inferior capsular shift for the treatment of recurrent, voluntary posterior subluxation of the shoulder. J Bone Joint Surg [Am] 82:16–25, 2000.

Pagnani MJ, Galinat BJ, Warren RF: Glenohumeral instability. In DeLee JC, Drez D Jr (eds): Orthopaedic Sports Medicine: Principles and Practice. Philadelphia, WB Saunders, 1994, pp 580–622.

Schwartz E, Warren RF, O'Brien SJ, et al: Posterior shoulder instability. Orthop Clin North Am 18:409–419, 1987.

CHAPTER 44

Superior Labral Anterior to Posterior (SLAP) Repair

INTRODUCTION

Superior labral anterior to posterior (SLAP) lesions, which were first described in 1990, can be difficult to diagnose, identify, and treat. These lesions, originally classified by Snyder and associates and whose classification was later modified by Maffett and colleagues, are divided into eight (or more) types (Fig. 44–1).

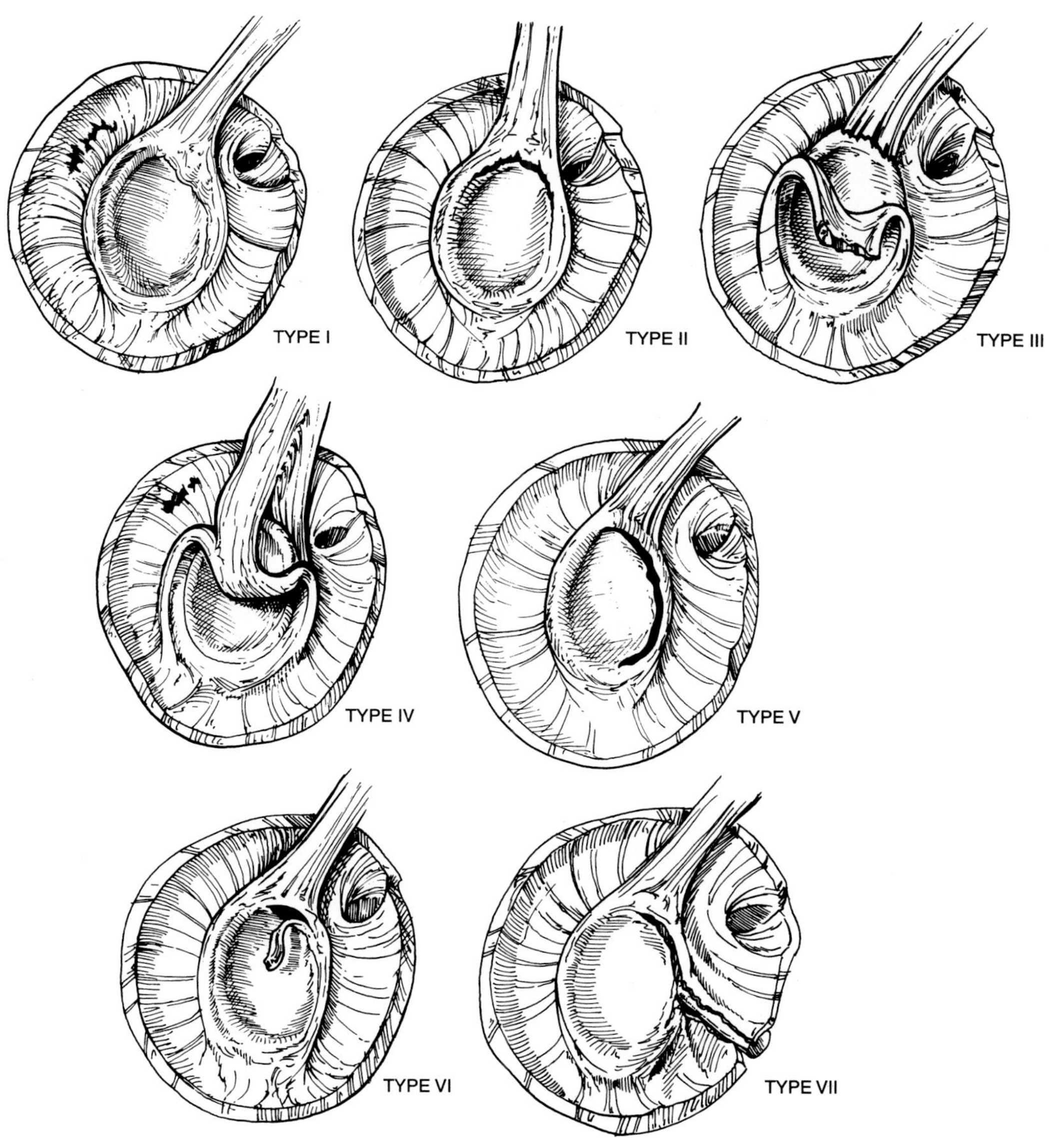

FIGURE 44–1. Maffett and colleagues' modification of Snyder and colleagues' classification of SLAP tears. (From Miller MD, Osborne JR, Warner JJP, Fu FH [eds]: MRI-Arthroscopy Correlative Atlas. Philadelphia, WB Saunders, 1997.)

HISTORY AND PHYSICAL EXAMINATION

Although the patient may relate a history of a fall or sudden traction to the affected arm, more commonly a mechanism of injury is difficult to elucidate. SLAP tears are common among baseball pitchers, perhaps because of repetitive microtrauma. Patients complain of pain; sometimes they may relate a history of catching or clicking of the affected shoulder.

A complete physical examination should include observation, palpation, and range-of-motion measurements, which are commonly normal in this population. Affected individuals may have bicipital groove tenderness, which is usually exacerbated by Speed's test (resisted forward flexion of a supinated arm) or Yergason's test (resisted supination with the elbow flexed 90°). Compression and rotation (the so-called crank or clunk test) may also elicit pain and/or popping. Finally, O'Brien has recently described a test in which the arm is flexed 90° and internally rotated; when this maneuver is performed, patients develop pain that is relieved with external rotation (Fig. 44–2).

DIAGNOSTIC IMAGING

Plain films are usually normal. SLAP tears may be associated with impingement or instability; therefore, appropriate films should be reviewed for subacromial spurs, acromioclavicular arthrosis, bony Bankart lesions, and Hill-Sachs deformities. MRI, especially with the addition of gadolinium contrast, is often helpful in identification of these injuries (Fig. 44–3).

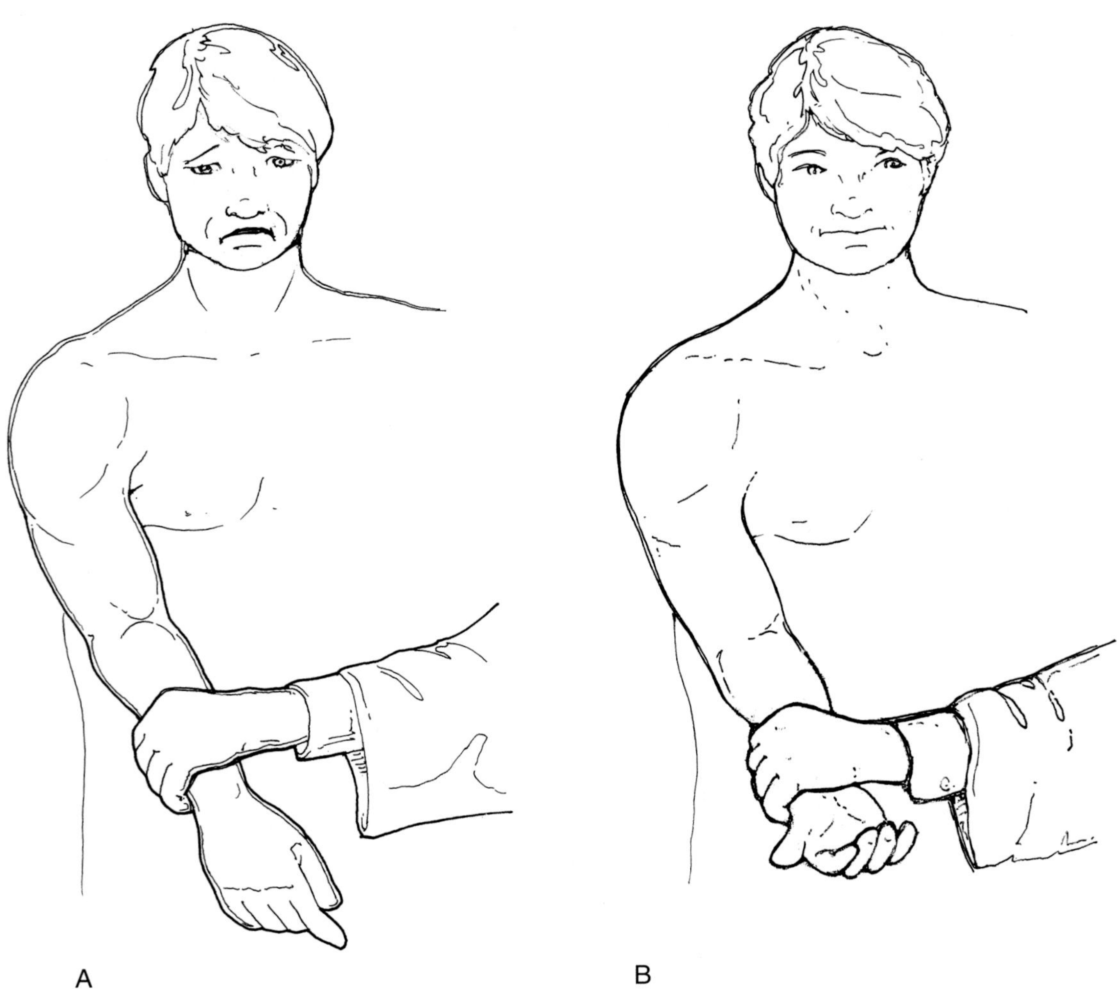

FIGURE 44–2. Active compression test for diagnosing SLAP tears as described by O'Brien. *A*, The patient experiences pain with resisted elevation with the forearm fully pronated. *B*, With the forearm supinated, the patient is asymptomatic.

NONOPERATIVE MANAGEMENT

Activity modification and rest may be helpful, although diagnosis is often delayed. Physical therapy may be beneficial.

RELEVANT ANATOMY

There is significant variability in the placement of the superior labrum. It may attach directly to the glenoid, or it may be attached more peripherally (Fig. 44–4). Additionally, it is common to have an anterosuperior foramen that may separate the anterosuperior labrum from the rim. This normal variant normally does not involve the biceps anchor.

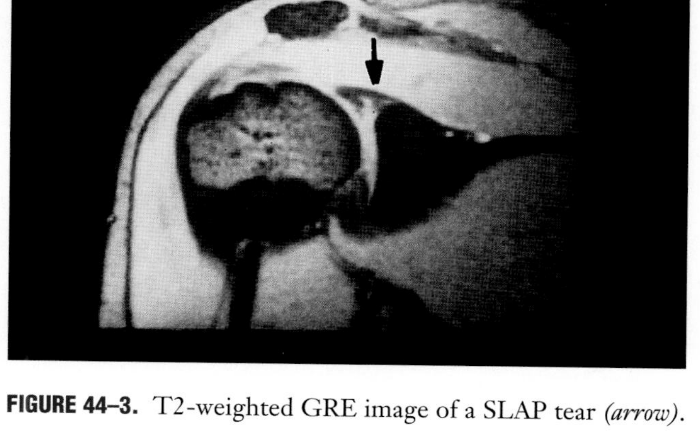

FIGURE 44–3. T2-weighted GRE image of a SLAP tear *(arrow)*.

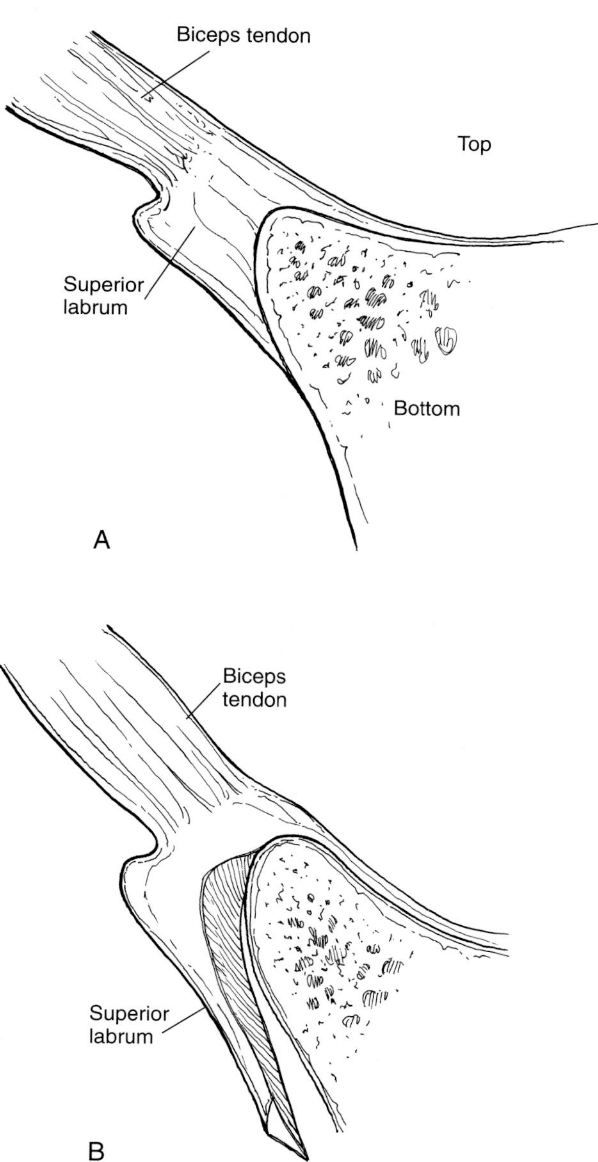

FIGURE 44–4. There is significant variability of the superior labrum. *A*, Most often, the superior labrum is attached to the margin of the glenoid. *B*, Occasionally, the superior labrum has a leaflike free edge that overhangs the articular surface similar to a knee meniscus. This must be probed carefully to ensure that it is a normal variant and not a SLAP tear.

SURGICAL TECHNIQUE

Indications

Surgery is indicated for the symptomatic patients with a suspected SLAP tear. Occasionally, the diagnosis is not suspected preoperatively; treatment must be individualized.

Technique

1. Examination under anesthesia (EUA), positioning, and diagnostic arthroscopy are carried out as described in Chapter 41.
2. The superior labrum is carefully probed, and the integrity of the biceps anchor is assessed. If the biceps is still intact, simple débridement is all that is required. If the anchor is detached from the superior labrum, repair is indicated.
3. The sublabral bone is decorticated with a rasp, shaver, or burr (Fig. 44–5).
4. An additional portal is established. Usually, the so-called port of Wilmington (1 cm anterior to the posterolateral corner of the acromion) is used. Before this portal is created a spinal needle is introduced to confirm that access to the posterosuperior labrum can be obtained (Fig. 44–6).
5. A suture anchor is placed into the sublabral bone, and the surgeon secures the labrum by passing sutures into the superior labrum and securing them with arthroscopically placed knots. Alternatively, an absorbable tack can be used by skewering the superior labrum immediately adjacent to the biceps tendon with a cannulated drill bit and placing a tack over the guide wire (Figs. 44–7 and 44–8).
6. The process is repeated on the anterosuperior aspect of the biceps anchor using the anterior superior portal.
7. Arthroscopic portals are closed with simple sutures.

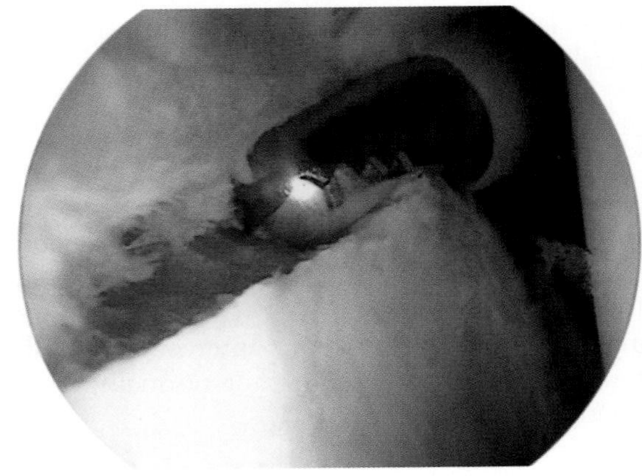

FIGURE 44–5. Preparation of the superior glenoid bed.

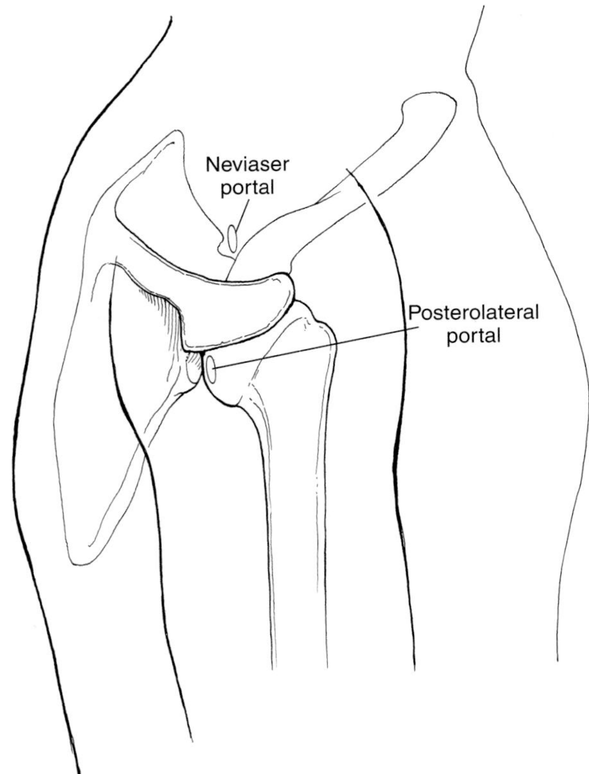

FIGURE 44–6. Accessory portals for SLAP repair include the port of Wilmington and the Nevasier portal.

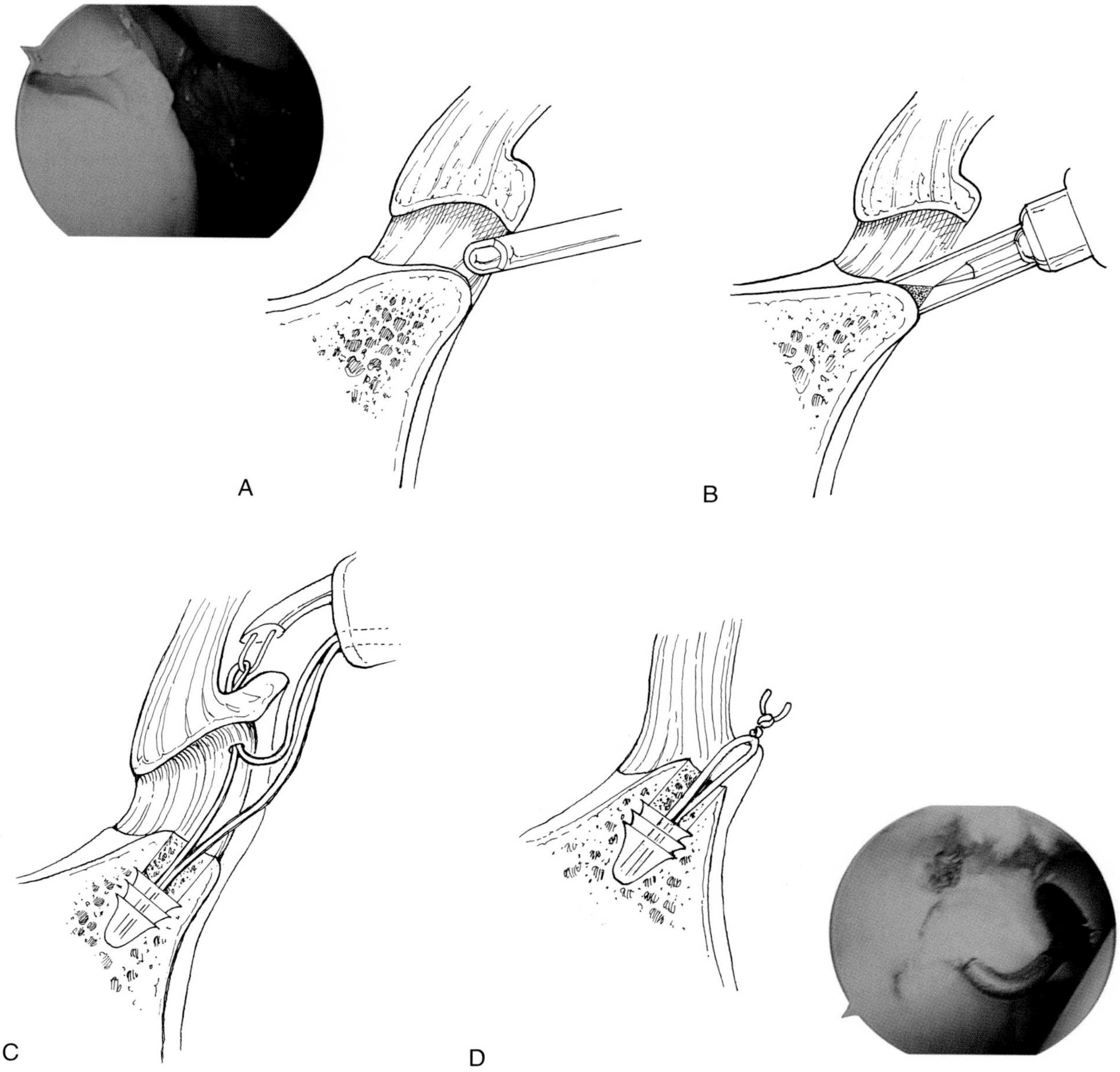

FIGURE 44–7. Suture anchor repair of SLAP tear. *A*, Glenoid rim preparation and passage of shuttle *(inset)*. *B*, Suture anchor placement. *C*, Passage of suture through labrum. *D*, Final repair.

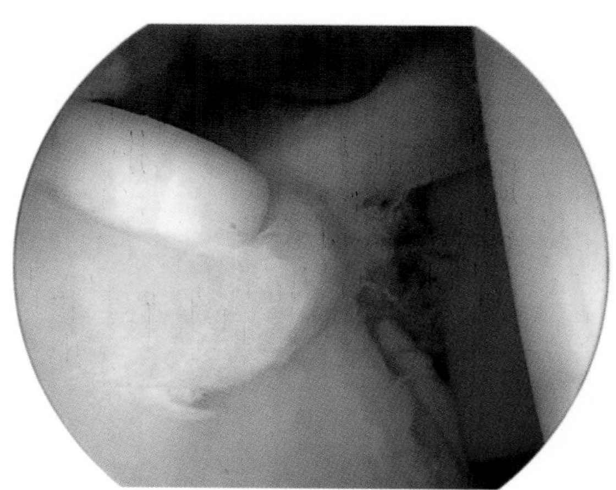

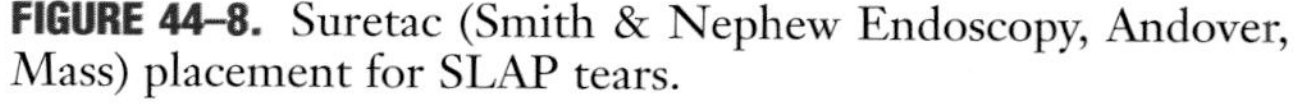

FIGURE 44–8. Suretac (Smith & Nephew Endoscopy, Andover, Mass) placement for SLAP tears.

POSTOPERATIVE MANAGEMENT

Postoperative management depends on the fixation device used. If an absorbable tack is used, strict immobilization for 4 weeks is recommended. Early motion may be possible with other devices.

COMPLICATIONS

Complications can include recurrence, articular damage, biceps tendon laceration, and other technical pitfalls. Postoperative problems can include stiffness and pain.

RESULTS

Initial results with simple débridement of SLAP lesions were encouraging; however, these results deteriorated with time. Better preliminary results have been reported with SLAP repairs.

REFERENCES

Cooper DE, Arnoczky SP, O'Brien SJ, et al: Anatomy, histology, and vascularity of the glenoid labrum. J Bone Joint Surg [Am] 74:46–52, 1992.

Maffett MW, Gartsman GM, Moseley B: Superior labrum-biceps tendon complex lesions of the shoulder. Am J Sports Med 23:93–98, 1995.

Mileski RA, Snyder SJ: Superior labral lesions in the shoulder: Pathoanatomy and surgical management. J Am Acad Orthop Surg 6:121–131, 1998.

O'Brien SJ, Pagnani MJ, Fealy S, et al: The active compression test: A new and effective test for diagnosing labral tears and acromioclavicular joint abnormality. Am J Sports Med 26:610–613, 1998.

Snyder SJ, Karzel RP, Del Pizzo W, et al: SLAP lesions of the shoulder. Arthroscopy 6:274–279, 1990.

Urban WP Jr, Caborn DNM: Management of superior labral anterior to posterior lesions. Op Tech Orthop 5:223–232, 1995.

CHAPTER 45

Biceps Tenodesis

INTRODUCTION

Isolated disorders of the biceps tendon are uncommon. More often, lesions of the biceps tendon are secondary to rotator cuff disease. Lesions of the biceps tendon have been classified by Slatis and Aalto into three types: type A, impingement tendonitis; type B, subluxation of the biceps tendon; and type C, attritional tendonitis. Biceps tenodesis may be used in the management of any of these etiologies. A careful history and physical examination of patients with biceps tendonitis most often reveal coexistent disease of the rotator cuff. The technique of biceps tenodesis is reviewed in this section without discussion of management of rotator cuff disease. See Chapter 46 for discussion of this topic.

HISTORY AND PHYSICAL EXAMINATION

The history and physical findings of biceps tendonitis vary with the underlying disease process. The majority of patients develop biceps tendonitis secondary to impingement syndrome. Patients complain of anterior shoulder pain that is aggravated with overhead use of the hand. The pain is localized to the anterior shoulder in the subdeltoid region. Often, the pain radiates to the arm in the region of the biceps muscle belly. Those with biceps subluxation complain of a similar pain pattern, although, in addition to the pain, they may have painful popping in the anterior shoulder associated with abduction and rotation of the joint. Patients with proximal biceps tendon rupture complain of an acute painful deformity of the arm with associated weakness of elbow flexion.

Physical examination of the biceps tendon reveals tenderness over the bicipital groove. The groove is located by internally rotating the arm 10° to 15° and palpating directly anterior and 2 to 3 inches inferior to the anterior acromion. Speed's test often reproduces the pain of biceps tendonitis. The test is performed by flexing the shoulder against resistance; forward flexion of the shoulder is at 90°, with the elbow extended and the forearm supinated. Yergason's test may also be positive. This test is performed with the elbow flexed to 90° and the arm at the side in neutral rotation; the forearm is fully pronated. A positive test occurs when pain is produced at the bicipital groove by resisted supination. The biceps instability test is used to reproduce biceps subluxation. This test is performed by positioning the arm in 90° of abduction and at full external rotation. The shoulder is internally rotated from this position while the region of the bicipital groove is palpated. A positive test results when a palpable or audible click occurs as the biceps tendon is forced over the lesser tuberosity. Finally, Ludington's test is useful when the deformity of biceps rupture is not readily apparent. With this test, the patient places the hands behind the head and flexes the biceps muscle. Differences in the contour of the muscles are best appreciated with the patient in this position.

DIAGNOSTIC IMAGING

Routine plain films of the shoulder are usually normal. The Fisk view may be used to visualize the bicipital groove. In addition, the 30° caudal tilt anteroposterior and scapular outlet views of the shoulder assist in the visualization of subacromial spurring. Shoulder arthrography may be useful for demonstrating irregularity in the tendon or tendon subluxation, but it does not provide the quality and quantity of information that can be obtained from MRI. Ultrasonography is useful in assessing tendon irregularity and subluxation, but it is extremely operator dependent, and sonographers experienced in shoulder assessment are not available in most centers.

MRI is useful for assessing the biceps tendon along its entire course. In addition, associated cuff disease and labral lesions can be assessed. Biceps tendon subluxation and dislocation are readily apparent on axial MRI views of the bicipital groove (Fig. 45–1).

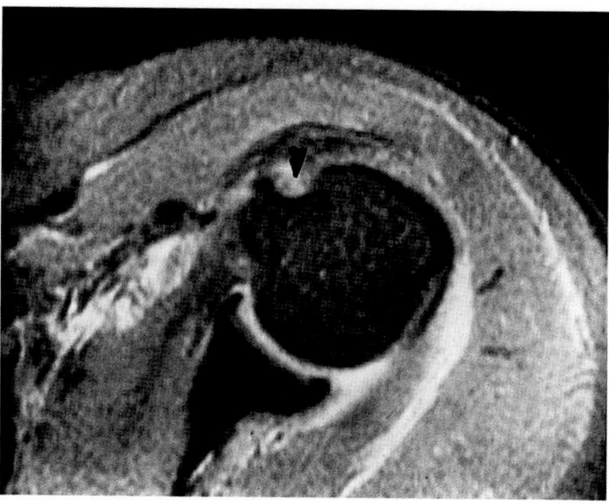

FIGURE 45–1. MRI shows displacement of the biceps tendon out of the groove *(arrowhead)*.

NONOPERATIVE MANAGEMENT

The selection of management options depends on the underlying cause. Biceps subluxation is unlikely to improve with conservative measures, and operative treatment is most often indicated. However, for lesions secondary to impingement or intrinsic tendonitis, nonoperative management is usually successful. Surgical management is recommended only after at least 6 months of nonoperative treatment. In cases of biceps rupture, the functional deficit may be slight. A majority of patients have minimal loss of elbow flexion strength and supination strength. Cybex testing of patients with chronic biceps rupture has failed to demonstrate any statistically significant loss of strength and only a 10% loss of supination power. Thus, patients who do not object to the cosmetic appearance and muscle weakness of the proximal rupture biceps tendon should be managed conservatively.

The program that we recommend is identical to that used in the management of impingement. The initial emphasis is on regaining full range of motion. Once motion is restored, a progressive rotator cuff–strengthening program is initiated. In addition, scapular stabilizer muscles are exercised.

RELEVANT ANATOMY

The long head of the biceps tendon originates at the supraglenoid tubercle of the glenoid, where it blends with the glenoid labrum. The anatomy of the insertion may vary in biceps contribution to the anterior or posterior glenoid labrum. The tendon travels intra-articularly toward the biceps groove 45° to the coronal plane of the humeral head. The tendon enters the groove formed by the lesser tuberosity anteriorly and the greater tuberosity posteriorly. The depth of the groove may vary. Shallow grooves have been associated with biceps subluxation. The transverse humeral ligament spans the tuberosities to form the roof of the groove. Some authors have suggested that the role of the ligament is to stabilize the tendon in the groove. However, others have shown that the biceps tendon will not sublux if the ligament is transected and the rotator cuff is intact. Thus, the main restraint to biceps subluxation is the sheath around the tendon formed by the rotator cuff in the proximal bicipital groove. The biceps tendon is enveloped by the cuff tendons near their insertion to the tuberosity. The supraspinatus tendon fibers blend with fibers of the subscapularis tendon to form the deep surface of the biceps groove. The roof of the groove is formed by the supraspinatus tendon. The supraspinatus tendon blends with the superior glenohumeral ligament insertion to the lesser tuberosity and the coracohumeral ligament insertion to the greater tuberosity (Fig. 45–2). Once the tendon is within the groove, the primary structure stabilizing it is the falciform ligament, which is an extension from the sternocostal portion of the pectoralis major insertion.

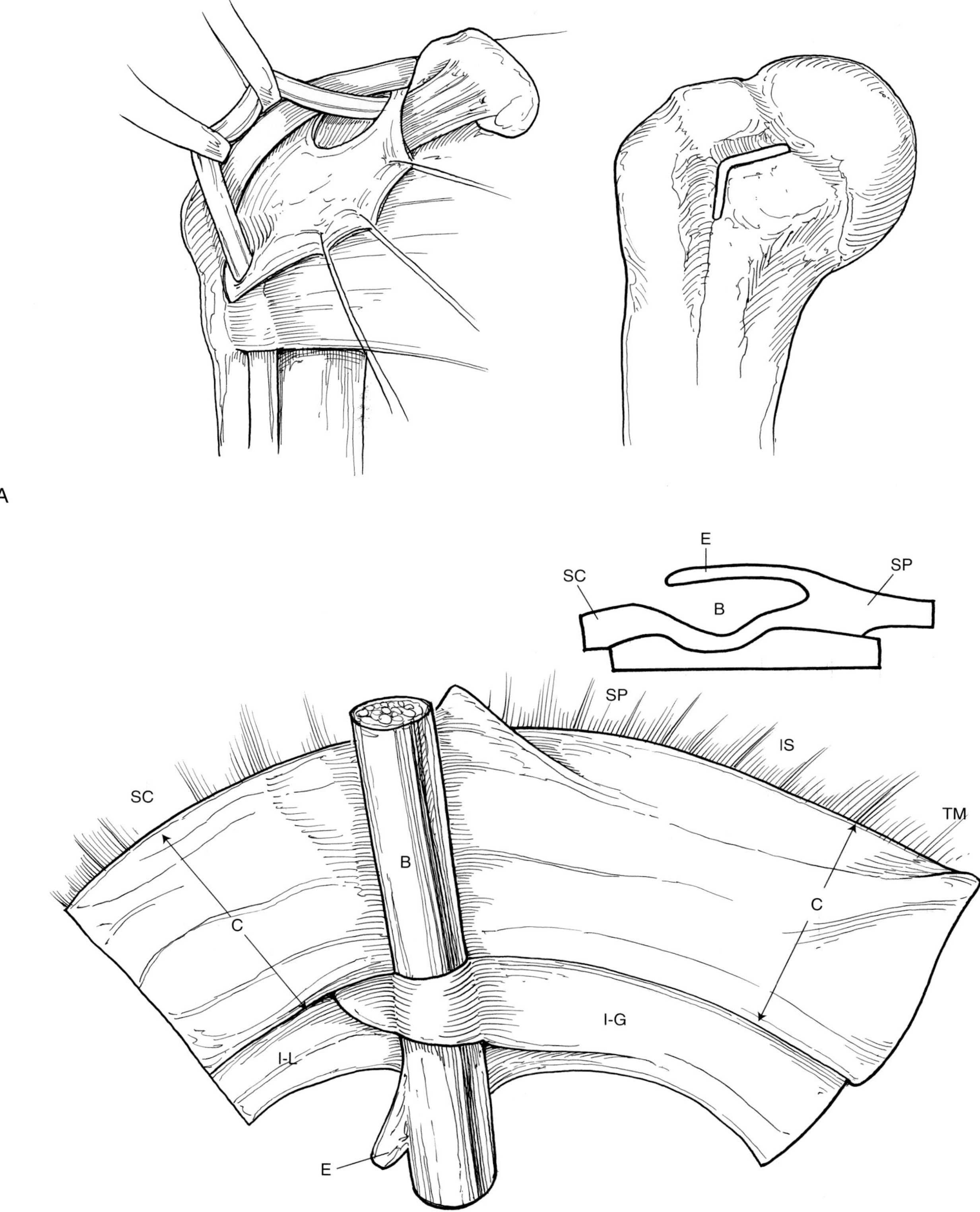

FIGURE 45–2. *A*, The rotator interval is opened to show the soft tissues stabilizing the tendon in the proximal biceps groove. *B*, This intra-articular view of the rotator cuff at the biceps groove illustrates the layering of the soft tissues restraining the tendon in the groove. Note the relationship of the capsule (C), insertion to the lesser tuberosity (I-L), insertion to the greater tuberosity (I-G), subscapularis (SC), supraspinatus (SP), slip from the supraspinatus (E), infraspinatus (IS), teres minor (TM), and biceps (B).

SURGICAL TECHNIQUE

Indications

Biceps tenodesis is indicated for proximal biceps rupture in active patients younger than 50 years of age who require full elbow flexion power and supination power. It is also indicated for biceps subluxation when the soft tissue restraints of the proximal biceps groove cannot be reconstructed. In addition, attrition of the tendon in stage II and stage III impingement should be managed with biceps tenodesis.

Technique

Arthroscopy

Diagnostic arthroscopy may confirm the diagnosis of biceps tendon pathology (Fig. 45–3). Although arthroscopic techniques for biceps tenodesis have been described, they have not gained wide acceptance.

FIGURE 45–3. Arthroscopic view from the posterior portal shows a complete avulsion and fraying of the biceps tendon *(arrow)*.

Keyhole

1. Position: The beach-chair position is used in this procedure.
2. Incision: For tenodesis of the intact biceps tendon, the incision is placed in Langer's lines and extends from the anterolateral acromion distally for a distance

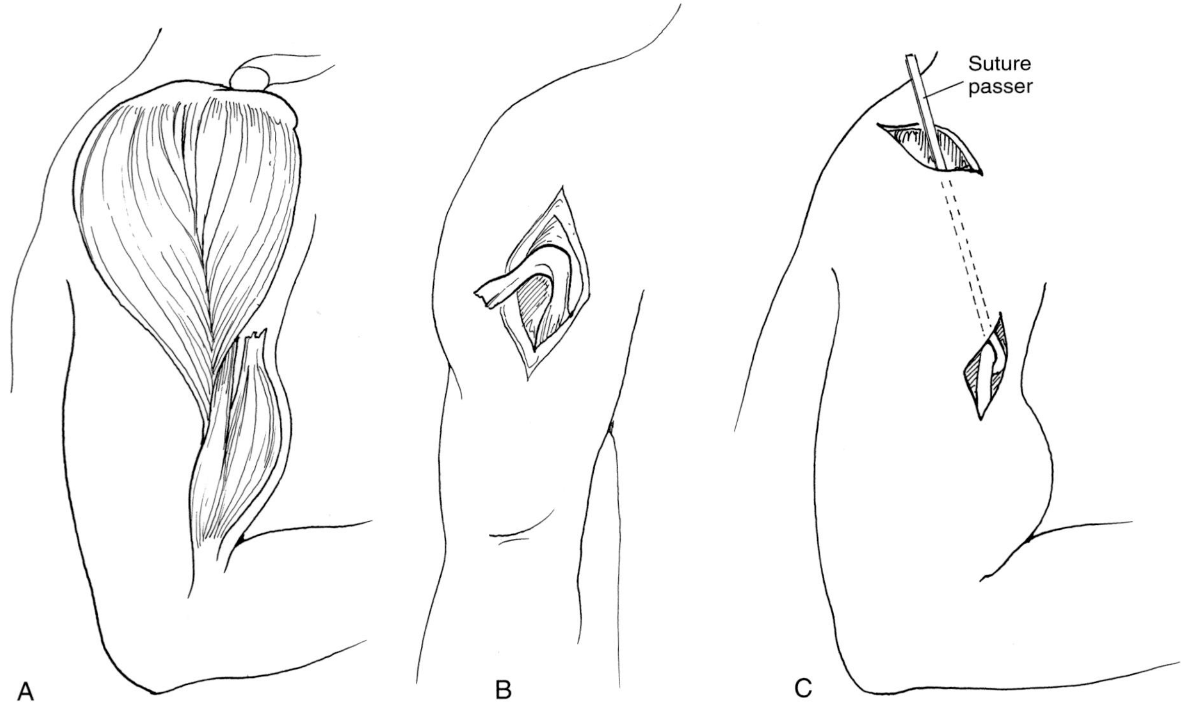

FIGURE 45–4. A second incision is required if the biceps ruptures. The incision is placed over the proximal biceps muscle belly. Several centimeters are all that is required to expose the retracted tendon stump. The tendon is passed from inferior to the superior incision using a suture passer. *A*, Distal retraction of torn biceps. *B*, Appropriate tension must be restored. *C*, Sometimes two separate incisions may be made, and the tendon can be passed proximally with a suture passer.

of 5 cm. If the tendon is ruptured, a second incision is created over the palpable proximal end of the biceps muscle (Fig. 45–4). The deltoid is split longitudinally in line with its fibers on a line over the anterolateral corner of the acromion. The deltoid split should not extend beyond 5 cm from the acromion. Subperiosteal dissection is used to reflect the deltoid anteriorly if acromioplasty or cuff repair is planned. (See Chapter 46.) A self-retaining retractor is placed in the deltoid split. The shoulder is flexed and rotated to deliver the bicipital groove into the exposure. The bicipital groove is opened longitudinally, preserving the soft tissue flaps for later closure.

3. Tendon release: In cases of biceps rupture, this step is eliminated. The tendon is marked in the groove with a suture. This suture marker serves as a reference point when the biceps is tenodesed with the appropriate tension on the tendon. In addition, the suture prevents retraction of the tendon into the arm after proximal release. The biceps tendon is released intra-articularly with the arthroscope or under direct vision through the rotator interval.
4. Keyhole: A 6-mm burr is used to trephine the cortex of the humerus in the bicipital groove inferior to the superior aspect of the lesser tuberosity. The keyhole is positioned in such a way that the tendon can be knotted and placed inside the keyhole with the marking suture lying at the inferior aspect of the keyhole. A 1-cm slot is cut with the burr to create the keyhole (Fig. 45–5). A generous bone defect is required for the tendon to be accepted.
5. Tenodesis: The tendon is knotted and sutured to itself with No. 2 braided, nonabsorbable suture. The end of the knot lies at the previously placed marking suture. The knotted tendon is placed into the keyhole, and the tendon is firmly wedged into the slot. The soft tissue flaps are sutured over and to the tendon with No. 2 braided sutures.

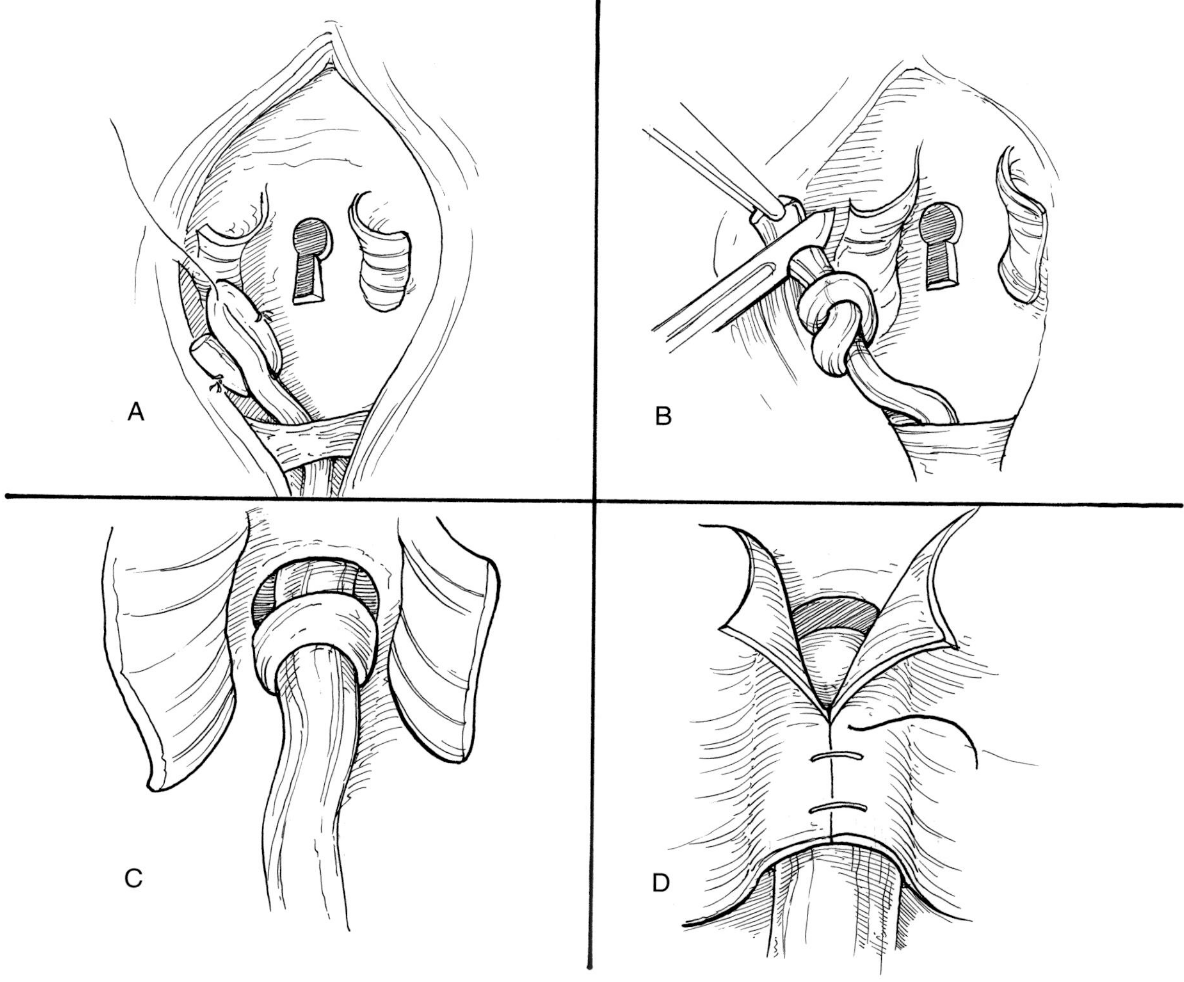

FIGURE 45–5. The keyhole technique of biceps tenodesis. The deltoid muscle should not be split more than 5 cm from the acromion. *A*, Keyhole. *B*, Proximal biceps tendon is knotted. *C*, Tendon insertion into the keyhole. *D*, Closure of the ligament.

POSTOPERATIVE MANAGEMENT

Appropriate postoperative management is dictated by the associated disease treated at the time of tenodesis. For biceps tenodesis without other procedures, the tenodesis is protected by having the patient avoid lifting more than 5 pounds at a time for 1 month. Then, a graduated increase in activity is allowed over the next 6 weeks. After 6 weeks, a progressive strengthening program is initiated. Return to full activity is permitted at 3 months.

COMPLICATIONS

The most common complication is failure to treat the associated disease. Careful preoperative and intraoperative assessments help to prevent this problem. We have not seen failure of a tenodesis, but this could occur with poor surgical technique or an overly aggressive postoperative rehabilitation program. The axillary nerve is at risk of injury because there is a tendency for the surgeon to split the deltoid beyond the recommended 5 cm when working in the biceps groove. The shoulder should be flexed to deliver the groove into the operative field, thereby avoiding this tendency. In addition, a suture can be placed at the apex of the deltoid split to avoid inadvertent extension of the split.

RESULTS

The results of biceps tenodesis depend on the coexistent disease. The results parallel those described in Chapter 46. Generally, 90% of patients are satisfied and would choose to have the procedure again in the same circumstances. Persistent problems after tenodesis most often result from unresolved rotator cuff disease.

REFERENCES

Berlemann U, Bayley I: Tenodesis of the long head of biceps brachii in the painful shoulder: Improving results in the long term. J Shoulder Elbow Surg 4:429–435, 1995.

Burkhart SS, Fox DL: SLAP lesions in association with complete tears of the long head of the biceps tendon: A report of two cases. Arthroscopy 8:31–35, 1992.

Curtis AS, Snyder SJ: Evaluation and treatment of biceps tendon pathology [review]. Orthop Clin North Am 24:33–43, 1993.

Dines D, Warren RF, Inglis AE: Surgical treatment of lesions of the long head of the biceps. Clin Orthop (164):165–171, 1982.

Grauer JD, Paulos LE, Smutz WP: Biceps tendon and superior labral injuries. Arthroscopy 8:488–497, 1992.

Warren RF: Lesions of the long head of the biceps tendon. Instr Course Lect 34:204–209, 1985.

CHAPTER 46

Impingement and Rotator Cuff Repair

INTRODUCTION

Impingement syndrome is a continuum with mild tendonitis on one end and massive rotator cuff tears on the other. Symptoms result from encroachment of the acromion, coracoacromial ligament, coracoid process, and/or acromioclavicular joint on the underlying rotator cuff. These problems commonly require surgery, and both arthroscopic and open techniques are well defined, especially for impingement syndrome. It is important that the sports medicine/shoulder surgeon be familiar with both arthroscopic and open techniques.

HISTORY AND PHYSICAL EXAMINATION

Except in a throwing athlete, impingement syndrome is a disease of middle age. Most often, patients do not relate a history of a specific injury, but instead complain of an insidious onset of pain with overhead activities. Stiffness and catching are also common complaints. Local or referred pain, usually to the deltoid insertion, is common. Night pain is common among patients with rotator cuff tears but is less frequent with impingement alone. Patients with complete rotator cuff tears may complain of weakness as well as pain.

The physical examination, including inspection for atrophy, palpation, and assessment of range of motion, is accomplished. Internal rotation may be limited in patients with impingement syndrome. Classic diagnostic tests include the impingement sign/test (Neer) and the impingement reinforcement test (usually credited to Hawkins or Fowler). The impingement sign is pain that is elicited by forcible elevation of the arm when the critical area of the supraspinatus tendon impinges against the anterior inferior acromion. This pain is typically relieved following administration of 10 mL of lidocaine (Xylocaine) into the subacromial space. Impingement reinforcement (Hawkins' test) consists of flexing the humerus 90° and forcibly internally rotating the shoulder, which also causes pain when the cuff is impinged (Fig. 46–1). It is critical to check for weakness in the supraspinatus (weakness with abduction), subscapularis (weakness with internal rotation), and infraspinatus (weakness with external rotation).

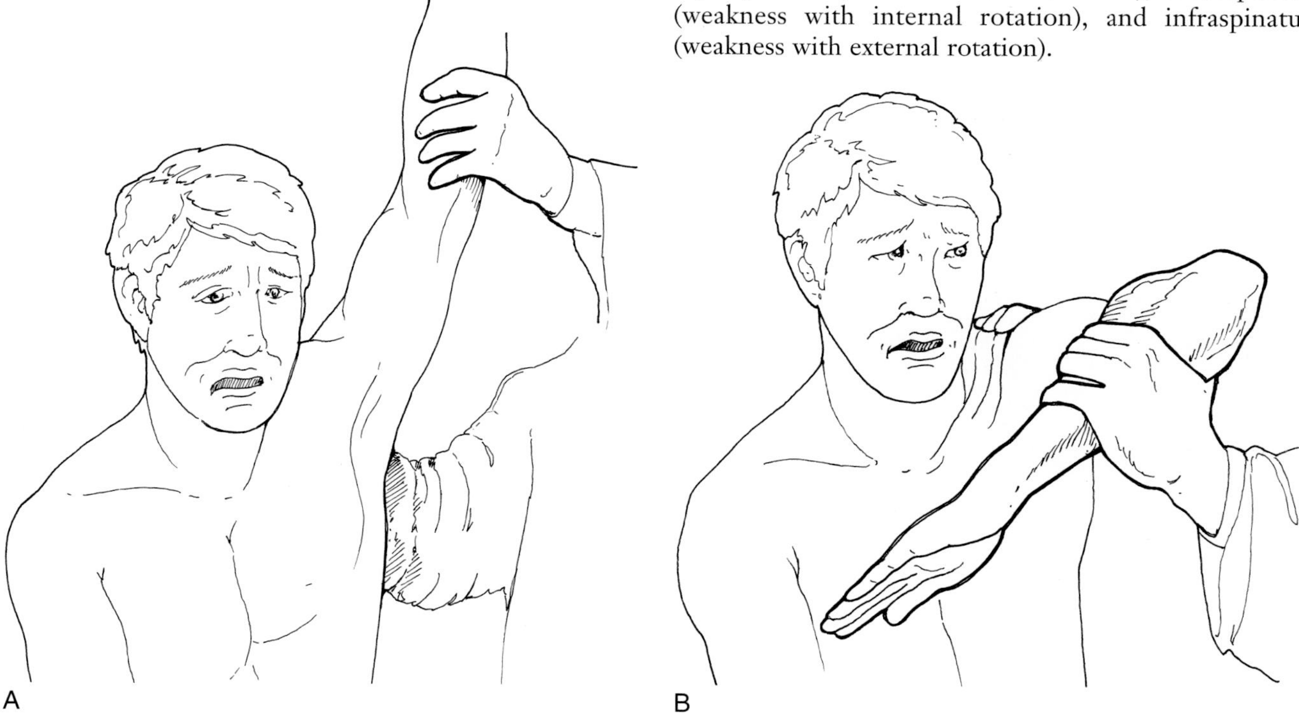

FIGURE 46–1. *A*, Impingement sign. *B*, Impingement reinforcement sign. Both tests become less painful after subacromial injection of lidocaine (impingement test).

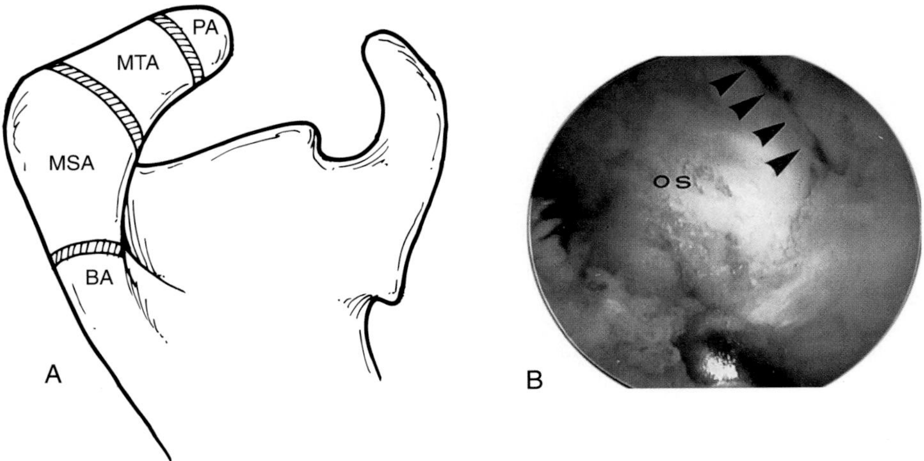

FIGURE 46–2. *A*, Os acromiale represents failure of ossification, typically between the mesoacromion (MSA) and meta-acromion (MTA) (most common) or the preacromion (PA) and meta-acromion. BA, Basiacromion. *B*, Arthroscopic image shows os acromiale *(arrowheads)* (*A* redrawn from Butters KP: The scapula. In Rockwood CA Jr, Matsen FA III [eds]: The Shoulder. Philadelphia, WB Saunders, 1990, p 343.)

DIAGNOSTIC IMAGING

Plain films can often be helpful. On the standard anteroposterior (AP) radiograph, the position of the humeral head should be evaluated (long-standing cuff tears can be associated with proximal migration of the head). Subacromial sclerosis (sourcil or eyebrow sign) may also be seen on these films. An axillary lateral view should also be obtained to reveal if an os acromiale is present (Fig. 46–2). A supraspinatus (scapular) outlet view (Bigliani; scapulolateral Y with caudal tilt) and a 30° caudal tilt view (Rockwood) can be helpful in characterizing the shape of the acromion (Fig. 46–3). Ultrasonography and arthrography can be helpful in the visualization of cuff tears; however, these techniques have largely been replaced by MRI in most centers. It must be emphasized, however, that MRI is not necessary in most cases because the diagnosis is often clear before additional diagnostic studies are considered.

NONOPERATIVE MANAGEMENT

Nonoperative management is the mainstay of treatment for this disorder. Patients are typically given nonsteroidal anti-inflammatory medications, rotator cuff–strengthening exercises (to help depress the humeral head away from the impinging area), and suggested means of activity modification. A limited number of subacromial injections of corticosteroids can also sometimes be helpful, although some studies have shown these not to be efficacious.

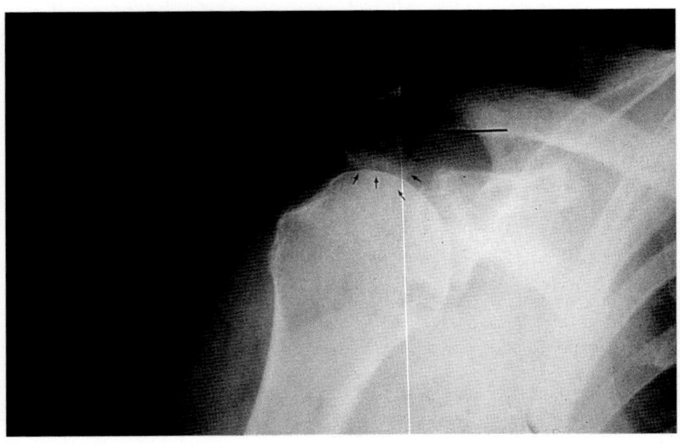

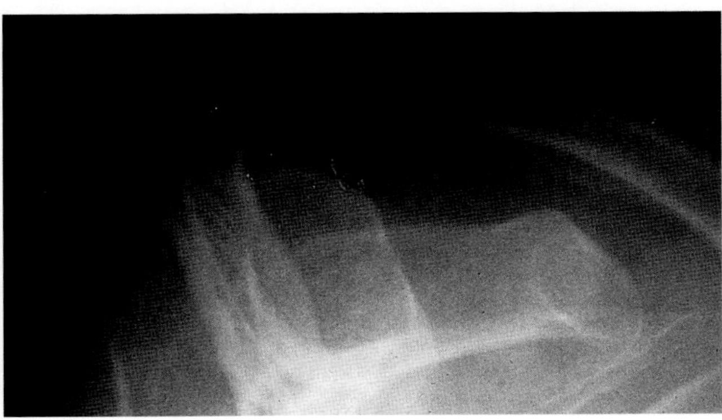

FIGURE 46–3. *A*, 30° caudal tilt and *B*, supraspinatus outlet views show large subacromial view (*arrows* demonstrate os acromiale spur.)

RELEVANT ANATOMY

The coracoacromial arch, made up of the coracoid, the coracoacromial ligament, and the anterior inferior acromion (Fig. 46–4), can impinge the subacromial bursa, the long head of the biceps, the rotator cuff (especially the supraspinatus), and the proximal humerus. Large inferior spurs off the acromion or the acromioclavicular joint and distal clavicle can also result in impingement. The rotator cuff muscles consist of the supraspinatus, infraspinatus, teres minor, and subscapularis (SITS). The supraspinatus and the upper portion of the infraspinatus are most often involved in impingement-related rotator cuff tears. The deltoid attaches to the acromion along the anterior surface and top of the acromion. Appropriate preservation or repair of this muscle is important during the performance of surgical procedures in this area.

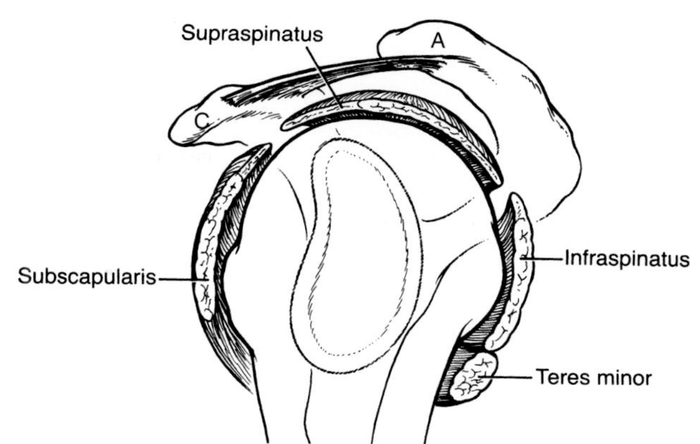

FIGURE 46–4. Sagittal cross section shows the rotator cuff tendons and coracoacromial arch. A, acromion; C, coracoid. (Modified from Matsen FA III, Arntz CT: Subacromial impingement. In Rockwood CA Jr, Matsen FA III [eds]: The Shoulder. Philadelphia, WB Saunders, 1990, p 625.)

SURGICAL *TECHNIQUE*

Indications

Surgical decompression or rotator cuff repair is considered in patients who have failed extended nonoperative management (usually 6 months). If an acute rotator cuff tear is suspected, some surgeons consider early surgery, especially in younger patients. Although distal clavicle resection (Mumford) is not discussed in this section, this procedure is often accomplished, in addition to addressing the acromion, in patients with acromioclavicular (AC) arthrosis and AC/distal clavicle impingement. This can also be accomplished with open or arthroscopic techniques. Treatment of patients with an associated os acromiale is controversial. Acromioplasty may not provide complete relief for these patients because the acromion is still "hinged" at the os. For a discussion of techniques that address this problem, see an article by Warner and associates (see References); this procedure is outside the scope of this text.

Technique

Open Acromioplasty

1. Positioning: The patient is placed in a beach-chair position.
2. Incision: A 5-cm incision is made in Langer's lines centered over the acromion and extending anteriorly.
3. The deltoid is subperiostally dissected off the acromion. Care is taken to create flaps that can be repaired to bone at the completion of the case (Fig. 46–5).

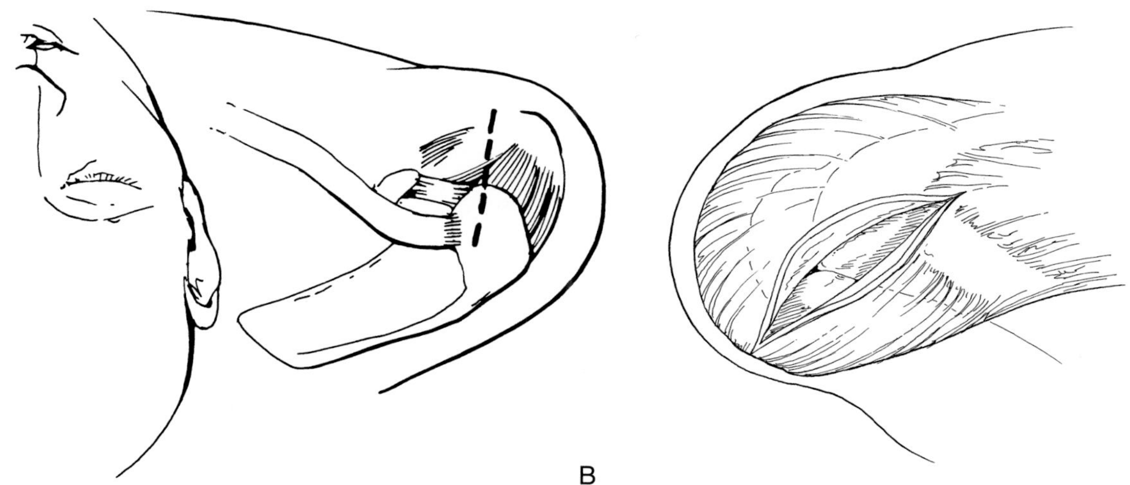

FIGURE 46–5. Incision *(A)* and subperiosteal dissection *(B)* of the deltoid off the acromion. (*A* from DeLee JC, Drez D Jr [eds]: Orthopaedic Sports Medicine: Principles and Practice. Philadelphia, WB Saunders, 1994.)

4. The coracoacromial ligament is identified and removed using electrocautery. Specific attention must be directed to maintaining homeostasis because the acromial branch of the thoracoacromial artery can cause bleeding during this step (Fig. 46–6).
5. An anterior and inferior acromioplasty is accomplished with the use of a saw or an osteotome (Fig. 46–7). A burr or rasp is used to smooth the undersurface of the acromion following this step.
6. The rotator cuff is carefully inspected and palpated by changing the position of the arm to inspect different parts of the cuff (Fig. 46–8).
7. The deltoid is carefully reapproximated; sutures are placed through the acromion to secure the cuff back to its original anatomic position.
8. The subcutaneous tissue and skin are closed in standard fashion, and a soft dressing is applied.

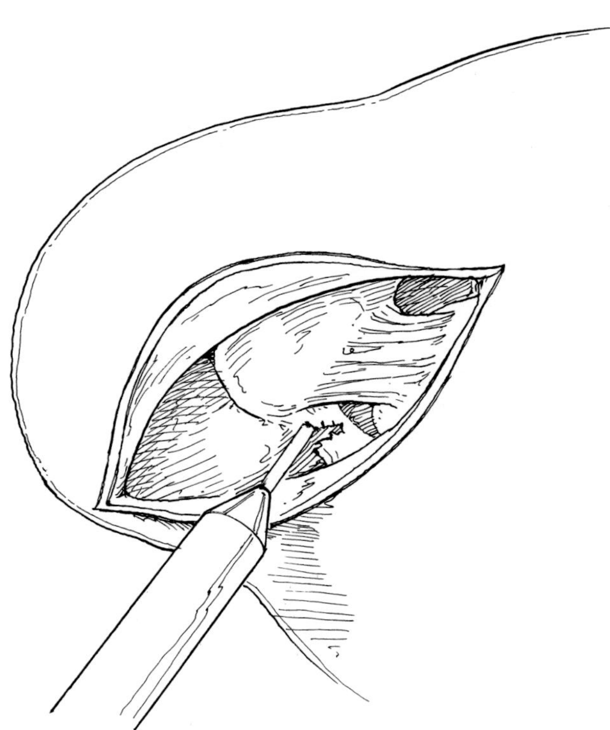

FIGURE 46–6. Division of the coracoacromial ligament with electrocautery.

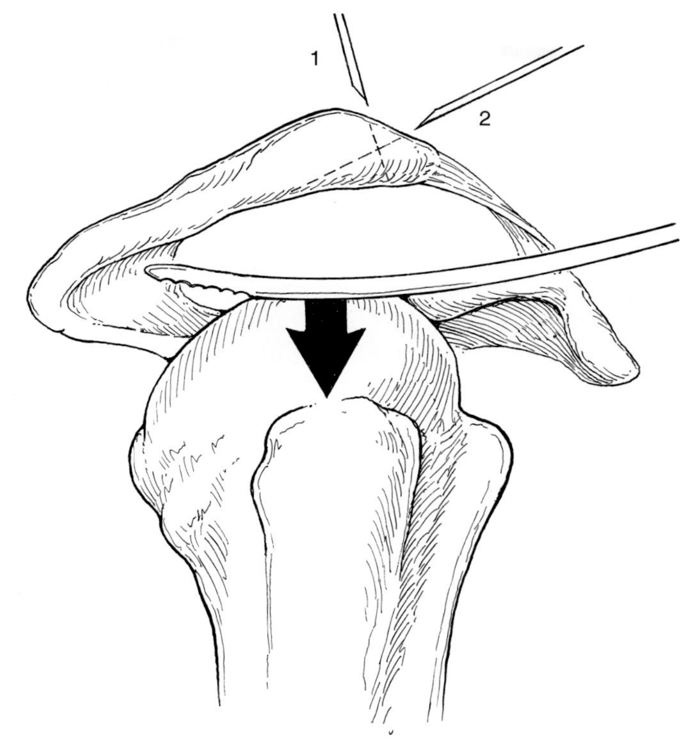

FIGURE 46–7. A broad flat retractor is used to protect and depress *(arrow)* the humeral head and rotator cuff. An anterior (1) and inferior (2) acromioplasty is then accomplished with a saw or osteotome.

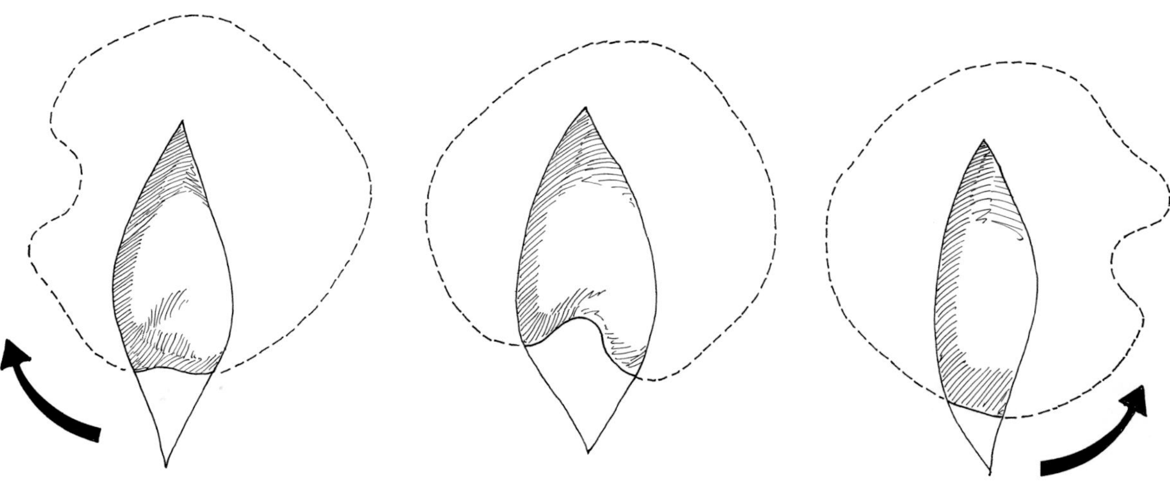

FIGURE 46–8. Inspection of the rotator cuff is possible by internally and externally rotating the arm in various positions of abduction.

Arthroscopic Acromioplasty

1. Positioning: The patient is placed in beach-chair position, and diagnostic arthroscopy is completed.
2. Bursoscopy: The arthroscope is removed from the glenohumeral joint and is reinserted into the subacromial space. The same posterior portal is used, and the blunt introducer is inserted into the scope cannula and aimed superiorly. The undersurface of the acromion is contacted and the cannula is advanced anteriorly out through the anterior portal (Fig. 46–9). It is often necessary to stretch the skin to allow the scope to exit anteriorly. A commercially available disposable plastic cannula can then be placed over the end of the scope cannula and introduced into the subacromial space. The arthroscope is attached and is carefully backed out of the cannula and into the subacromial space. A shaver, electrocautery, or other ablative devices can be introduced through the disposable cannula or through a lateral portal.
3. Lateral portal placement: This portal is typically located about midway between the anterior and posterior borders of the acromion. A spinal needle is placed into the bursa and is visualized arthroscopically so that the ideal location for this portal can be assessed. Once this has been established, the majority of the actual acromioplasty is accomplished through this portal.

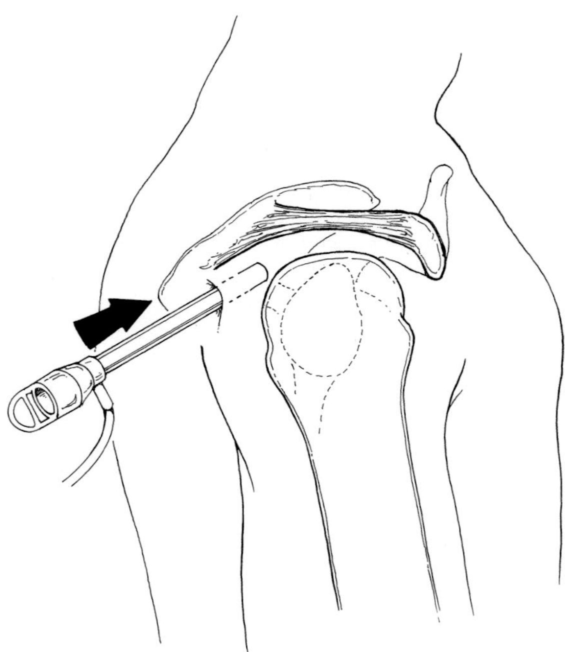

A

FIGURE 46–9. Arthroscopic subacromial decompression. *A*, After glenohumeral arthroscopy, the arthroscope is extracted and repositioned more superiorly, above the supraspinatus and under the acromion.

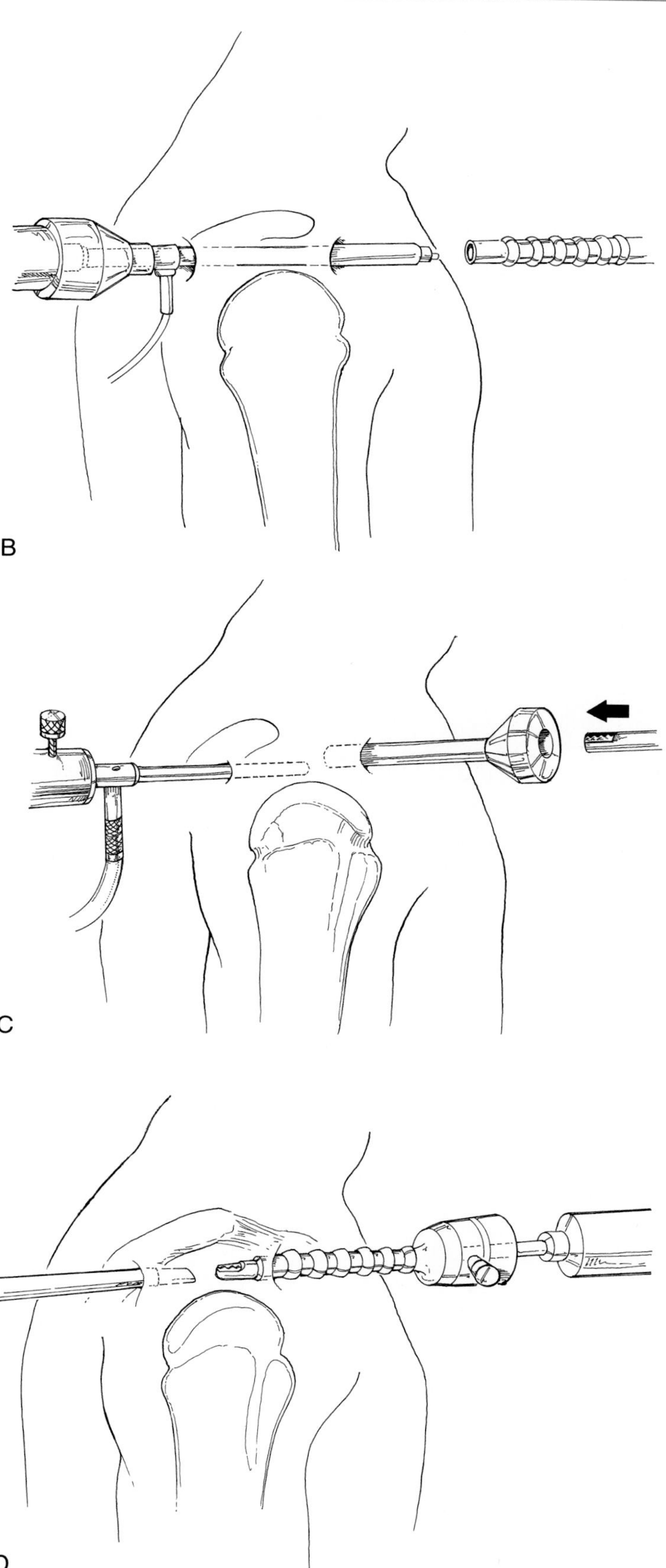

FIGURE 46–9 *Continued. B,* The scope is placed out the anterior portal, and a disposable cannula is placed over the tip of it. *C,* The scope is retracted, and the end of the cannula is visualized. *D,* A shaver and cautery device is introduced initially through the anterior portal, then through a lateral portal, and the acromioplasty is initiated.

4. Acromioplasty: The surgeon proceeds to remove the tissue that covers the undersurface of the acromion and the coracoacromial ligament with electrocautery (or a similar device) and a shaver. Liberal coagulation ("blitzkrieg") is recommended before shaving, especially near the coracoacromial ligament and the distal clavicle (Fig. 46–10). Various sequences have been recommended; however, it is important to remove the impinging area.
5. Distal clavicle resection: The undersurface of the distal clavicle, or the distal centimeter of the entire clavicle, can also be resected arthroscopically. See Chapter 50.
6. Assessment: The arthroscope is placed through the lateral portal and an impingement test is done arthroscopically, as described by Warner and colleagues. Alternatively, a portal can be extended and a finger used to palpate the end of the acromion. A rasp or burr can often be inserted blindly to remove any remaining impingement areas.

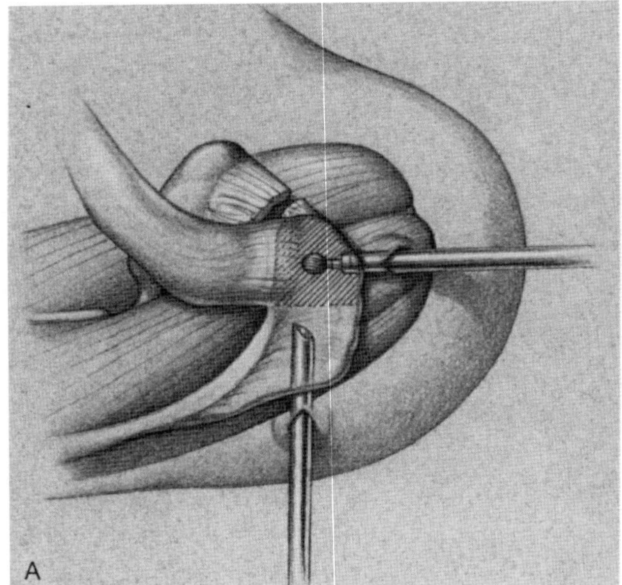

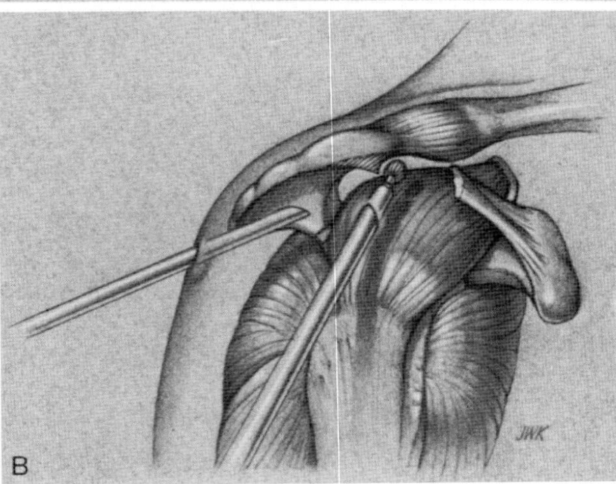

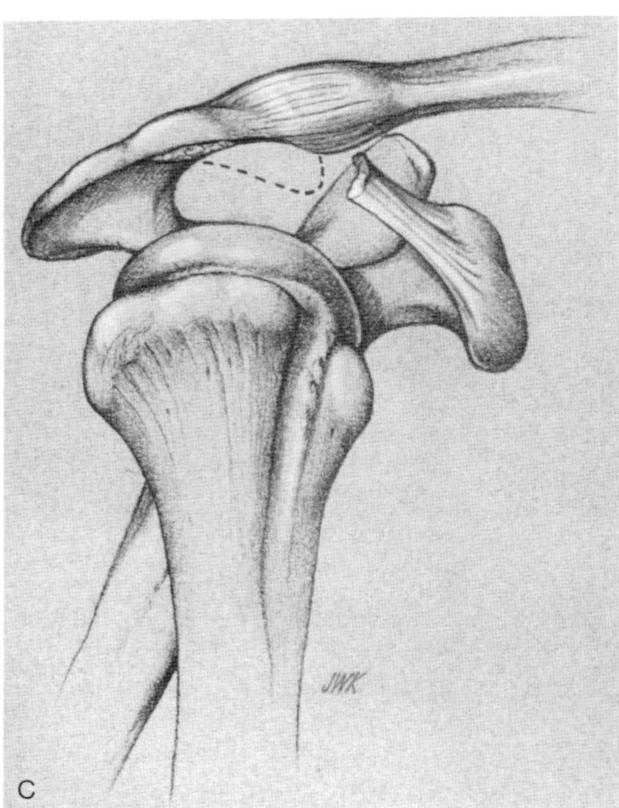

FIGURE 46–10. Technique for arthroscopic acromioplasty. *A*, Superior view. Shaded area represents extent of resection. *B*, Lateral view shows decompression. *C*, Completion results in conversion to a type I (flat) acromion. (From Harner CD: Arthroscopic subacromial decompression. Op Tech Orthop 1:220–234, 1991.)

Open Rotator Cuff Repair

1. Incision: The incision used for open acromioplasty can be used for cuff repair. Alternatively, a lateral incision, or an extension of the lateral portal used for arthroscopic acromioplasty, can be used. It is important not to extend any incision more than 5 cm lateral to the acromion because of risk to the axillary nerve.
2. Cuff exposure: Subperiosteal dissection of the deltoid off the acromion allows adequate visualization of the cuff. Resection of the distal clavicle often improves visualization. The lateral incision uses a deltoid-splitting approach; although it is sometimes difficult to visualize the cuff through this incision, this incision provides excellent exposure of the proximal humerus, thereby assisting the physician in securing sutures in the cuff (Fig. 46–11).
3. Mobilization: The edge of the cuff tear is visualized, explored, and freshened. Traction sutures are placed in the cuff, and the cuff itself is mobilized. Blunt dissection is helpful. The coracohumeral ligament sometimes must be released. Occasionally, it is necessary to free the cuff from the glenoid labrum.
4. Cuff sutures: A strong repair stitch, using heavy nonabsorbable suture (at least No. 2), is planned (Fig. 46–12). Usually, four to six sutures are placed in this fashion.

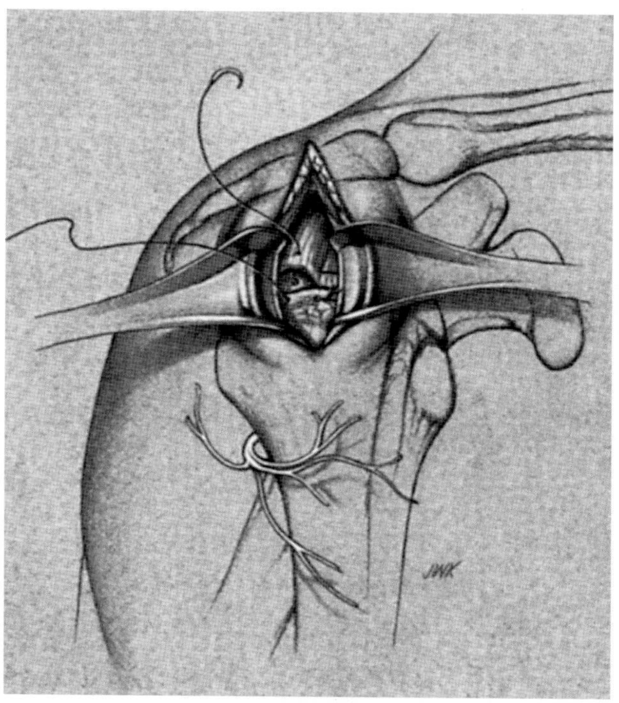

FIGURE 46–11. Lateral incision for rotator cuff repair. The incision cannot be extended beyond 5 cm because of the risk of injury to the axillary nerve. (From Harner CD: Arthroscopic subacromial decompression. Op Tech Orthop 1:220–234, 1991.)

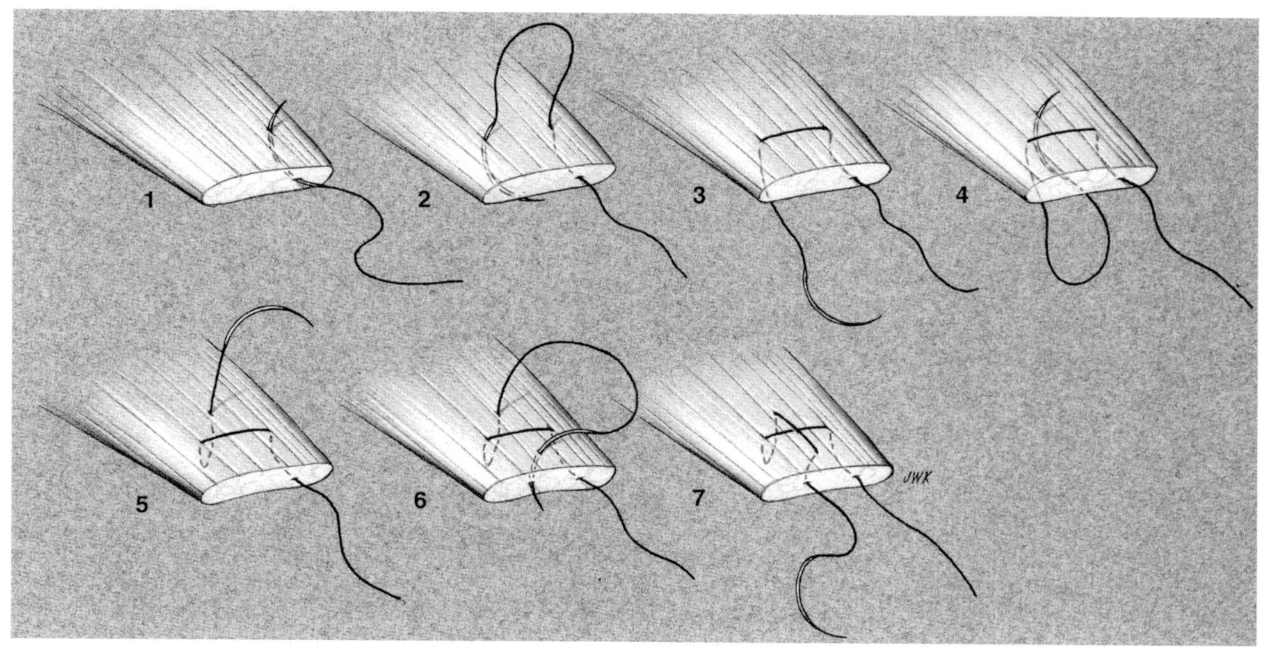

FIGURE 46–12. Modified Mason-Allen suture for rotator cuff repair. (From Griggs S, Williams GR, Ianotti JP: Surgical management of full-thickness rotator cuff tears. Op Tech Orthop 8:205–217, 1998.)

5. Repair: With the use of an osteotome or a burr, a trough is made in the proximal humerus just medial to the greater tuberosity. Sutures are passed into the trough with the use of a variety of commercially available devices (Fig. 46–13). These sutures are secured to each other on the lateral surface of the humerus. It is important that these sutures be placed distally or augmented with patches, buttons, or other devices in osteopenic bone.
6. Closure: Again, care is taken to repair the deltoid anatomically through drill holes into the bone. Subcutaneous tissues and skin are closed in standard fashion.

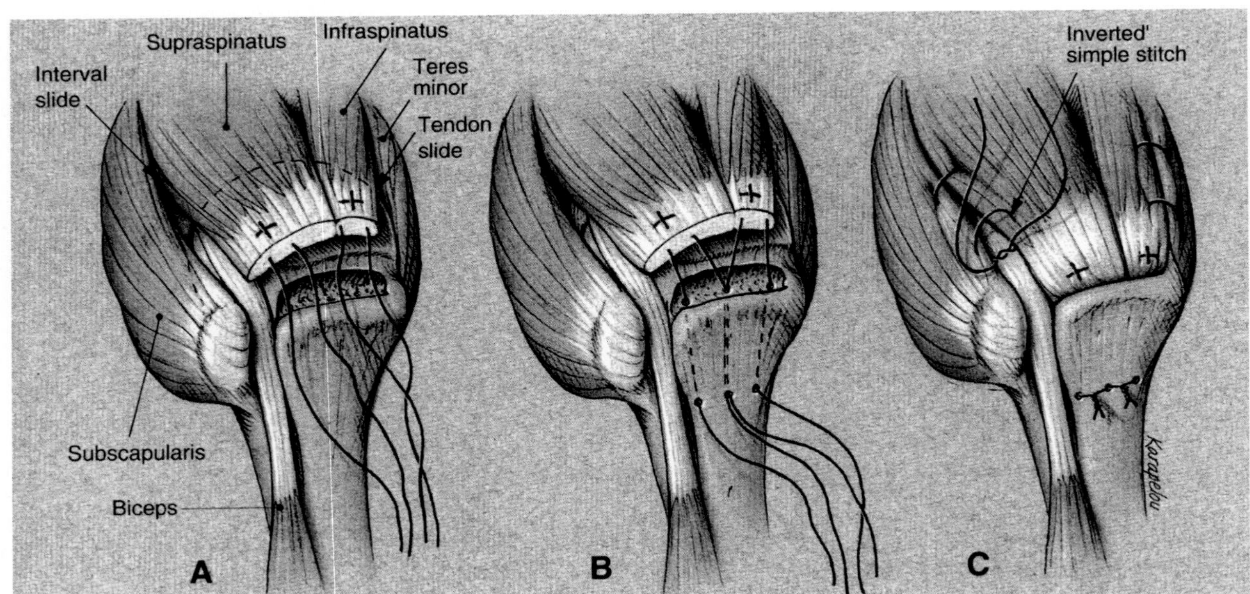

FIGURE 46–13. Mini-open rotator cuff repair. *A*, Modified Mason-Allen sutures are placed in the edge of the torn cuff. *B*, These sutures are pulled into a bony trough. *C*, Sutures are tied over the lateral cortex of the humerus. The rotator interval is closed after cuff repair. (From Griggs S, Williams GR, Ianotti JP: Surgical management of full-thickness rotator cuff tears. Op Tech Orthop 8:205–217, 1998.)

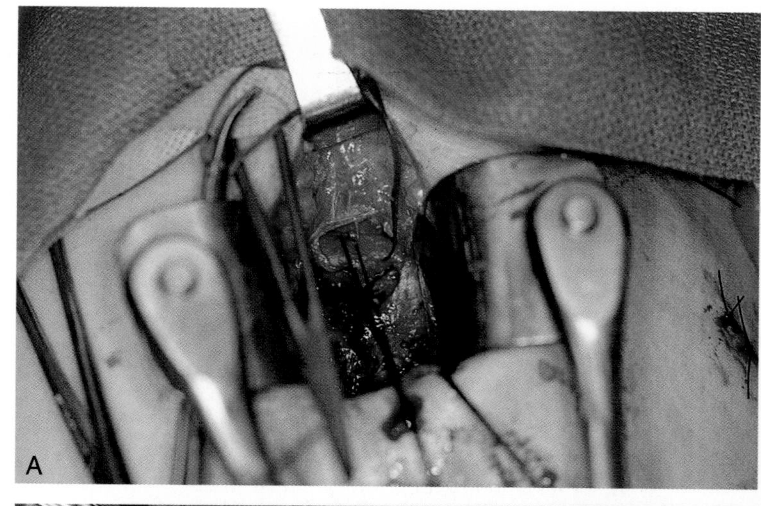

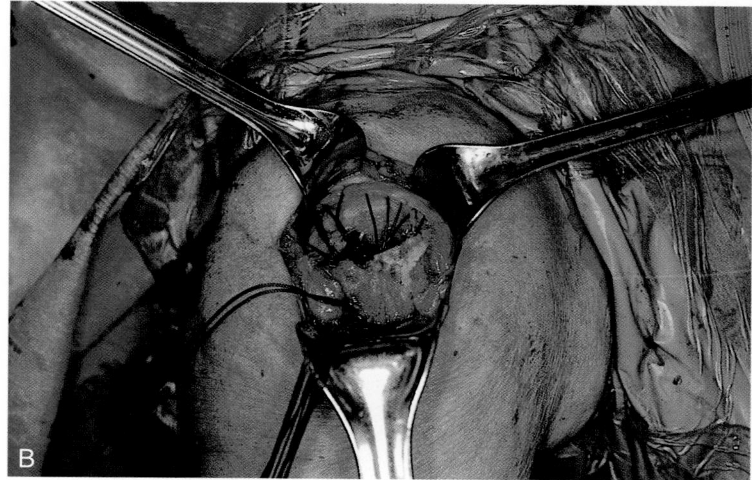

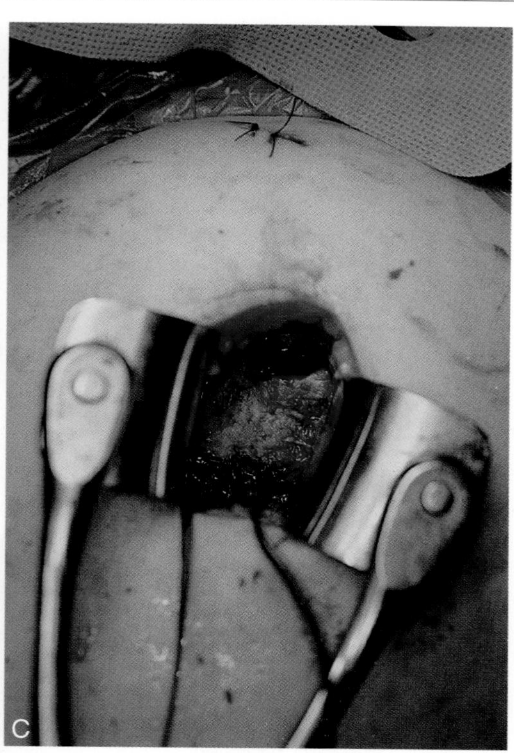

FIGURE 46–13 *Continued*

Arthroscopic Rotator Cuff Repair

Following identification of the tear and arthroscopic acromioplasty (Fig. 46–14), suture anchors are placed medial to the greater tuberosity. With the use of a variety of commercially available suture punches, hooks, and "relay" systems, sutures are placed into the edge of the cuff, and knots are tied on the superior surface of the cuff (Figs. 46–15 and 46–16).

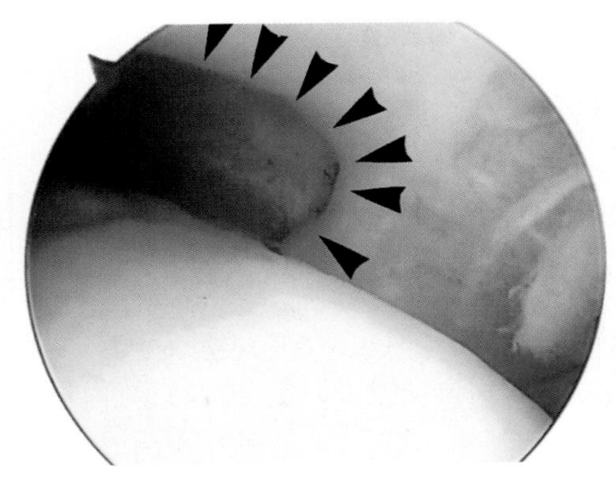

FIGURE 46–14. Arthroscopic view of rotator cuff tear *(arrowheads)*.

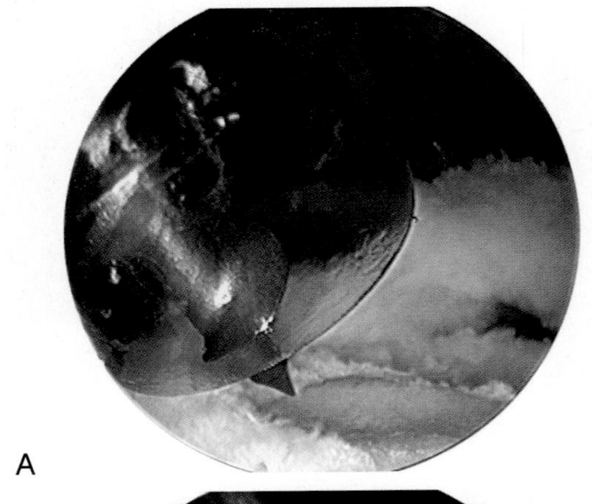

A

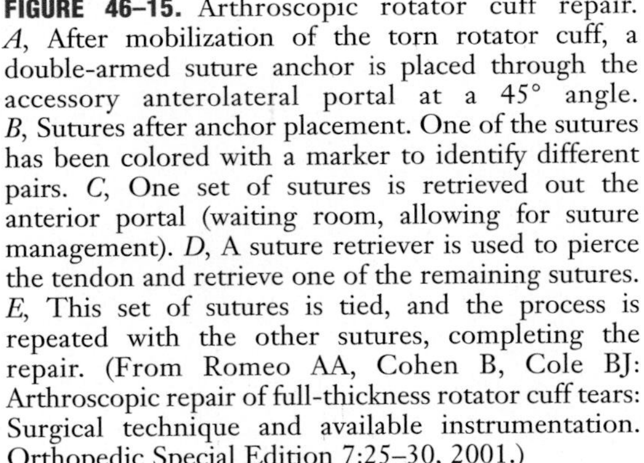

C

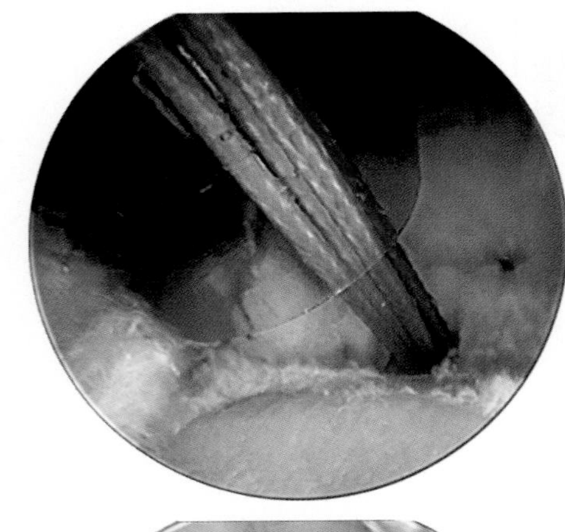

B

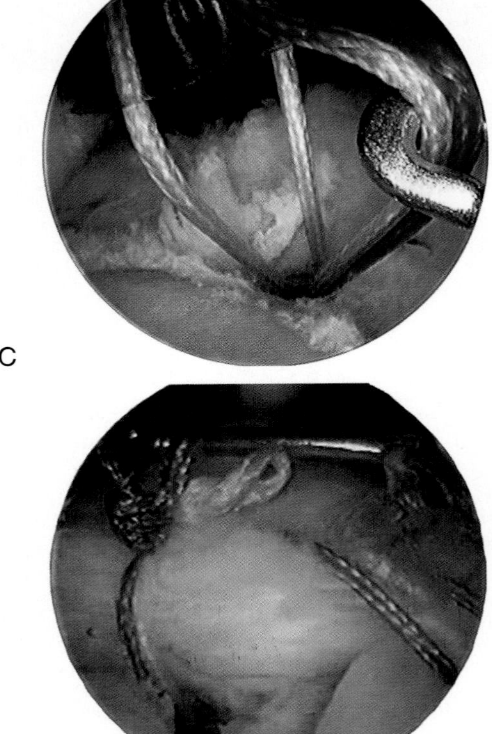

E

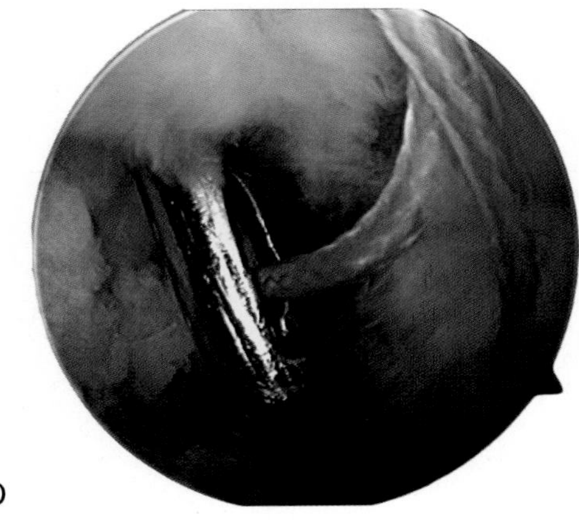

D

FIGURE 46–15. Arthroscopic rotator cuff repair. *A*, After mobilization of the torn rotator cuff, a double-armed suture anchor is placed through the accessory anterolateral portal at a 45° angle. *B*, Sutures after anchor placement. One of the sutures has been colored with a marker to identify different pairs. *C*, One set of sutures is retrieved out the anterior portal (waiting room, allowing for suture management). *D*, A suture retriever is used to pierce the tendon and retrieve one of the remaining sutures. *E*, This set of sutures is tied, and the process is repeated with the other sutures, completing the repair. (From Romeo AA, Cohen B, Cole BJ: Arthroscopic repair of full-thickness rotator cuff tears: Surgical technique and available instrumentation. Orthopedic Special Edition 7:25–30, 2001.)

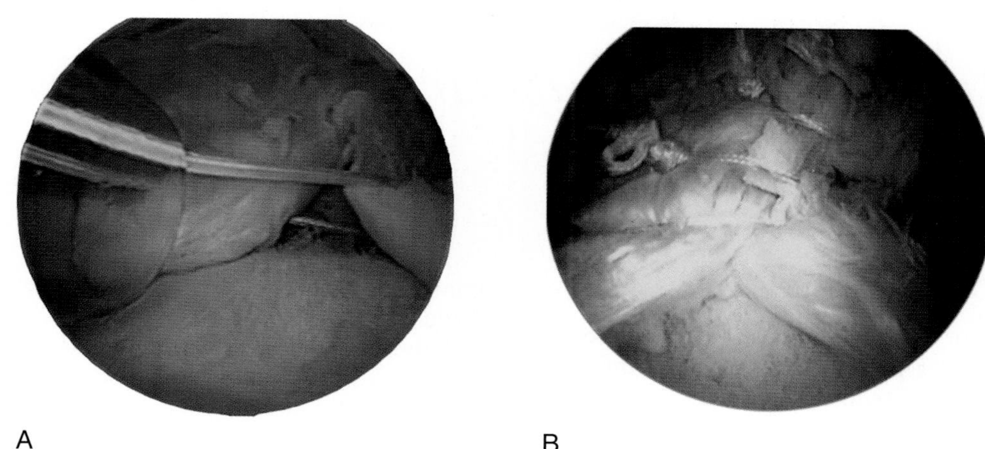

FIGURE 46–16. For larger tears, the edges of the tear are reapproximated before repairing the edge. Sutures are placed *(A)* and tied *(B)*, allowing convergence of the tear margins. (From Romeo AA, Cohen B, Cole BJ: Arthroscopic repair of full-thickness rotator cuff tears: Surgical technique and available instrumentation. Orthopedic Special Edition 7:25–30, 2001.)

POSTOPERATIVE MANAGEMENT

Early mobilization is ideal but dependent on the strength of the deltoid or rotator cuff repair. Arthroscopic acromioplasty spares the majority of the deltoid insertion, and free range of motion is allowed very early. Some caution is necessary following arthroscopic rotator cuff repair because the suture in the tendon is the "weak link" of the repair. Like other shoulder procedures, the rehabilitation sequence consists of passive motion followed by active motion, then strengthening.

COMPLICATIONS

1. Arthroscopic acromioplasty: fluid extravasation, excessive bleeding that obscures visualization, incomplete or inadequate acromioplasty, and loss of motion/scarring.
2. Open acromioplasty: fracture, deltoid injury or late avulsion, rotator cuff injury, and loss of motion/scarring.
3. Open rotator cuff repair: recurrence, loss of motion, deltoid detachment, denervation of deltoid or cuff, and failure to adequately secure the cuff (e.g., poor technique, mistaking the bursa for the cuff tendon, osteopenic bone).
4. Arthroscopic cuff repair: technical difficulty, anchor migration or pullout, recurrence, and loss of motion.

RESULTS

Long-term results of open acromioplasty are excellent. Early reports of arthroscopic acromioplasty are also encouraging. Open rotator cuff repairs are successful in approximately 80% of supraspinatus repairs. Long-term results of arthroscopic rotator cuff repair are unknown at present.

REFERENCES

Altchek DW, Carson EW: Arthroscopic acromioplasty: Indications and technique. Instr Course Lect 47:21–28, 1998.

Bell RH: Arthroscopic distal clavicle resection. Instr Course Lect 47:35–41, 1998.

Bigliani LU, Levine WN: Subacromial impingement syndrome—Current concepts. J Bone Joint Surg [Am] 79: 1854–1868, 1997.

Caldwell GL, Warner JJP, Miller MD, et al: Strength of fixation with transosseous sutures in rotator cuff repair. J Bone Joint Surg [Am] 79:1064–1067, 1997.

Gartsman GM: Arthroscopic management of rotator cuff disease. J Am Acad Orthop Surg 6:258–266, 1998.

Neer CS II: Anterior acromioplasty for the chronic impingement syndrome in the shoulder. A preliminary report. J Bone Joint Surg [Am] 54:41–50, 1972.

Rockwood CA, Lyons FA: Shoulder impingement syndrome: Diagnosis, radiographic evaluation, and treatment with a modified Neer acromioplasty. J Bone Joint Surg [Am] 75:1593–1605, 1993.

Warner JJ, Beim GM, Higgins L: The treatment of symptomatic os acromiale. J Bone Joint Surg [Am] 80:1320–1326, 1998.

CHAPTER 47

Treatment of Subscapularis Tendon Avulsion

INTRODUCTION

Isolated rupture of the subscapularis tendon was first recognized in 1835 in a postmortem specimen. Infrequent clinical cases were subsequently reported in the literature. In the recent literature, three large studies on isolated rupture of the subscapularis tendon have been published. Subsequently, this injury has been recognized with increased frequency as awareness of the diagnosis has improved. In addition, the advent of high-resolution MRI of the shoulder has improved diagnostic accuracy. This injury is probably more common than has been reported in the literature, and it continues to be underrecognized.

HISTORY AND PHYSICAL EXAMINATION

Avulsion of the subscapularis can occur as an isolated injury when the shoulder is violently externally rotated or hyperextended. In addition, anterior dislocation of the shoulder in patients over the age of 30 years is associated with a significant incidence of subscapularis avulsion. Patients typically complain of anterior shoulder pain and pain with forward flexion and external rotation of the shoulder, as well as shoulder weakness. In addition, painful popping may be present secondary to biceps tendon subluxation, which often coexists with this diagnosis.

Physical examination in the acute setting may reveal a hematoma of the anterior inferior axilla. The most consistent physical finding is increased passive external rotation of the shoulder on the affected side. In addition, the lift-off test may be positive. The lift-off test is performed by having the patient place the back of his or her hand against the lumbar spine and push away from the spine against the resistant force of the examiner's hand. A positive test is indicated by the patient's inability to hold the hand away from the lumbar spine (Fig. 47–1). Pain may inhibit some patients' ability to place the hand over the lumbar spine. In this situation, the abdominal compression test may be helpful. The patient is asked to compress the palm of the affected hand against the abdomen, while maintaining the arm at the side. In the absence of the subscapularis tendon, the shoulder must be extended to compensate for the inability to internally rotate the shoulder. Thus, in a negative test, the patient is able to maintain the humerus parallel to the trunk line. In a positive test, the humerus extends as the hand is pushed into the abdomen. Careful assessment of the anterior stability of the shoulder should be performed because anterior instability of the shoulder may coexist with subscapularis rupture.

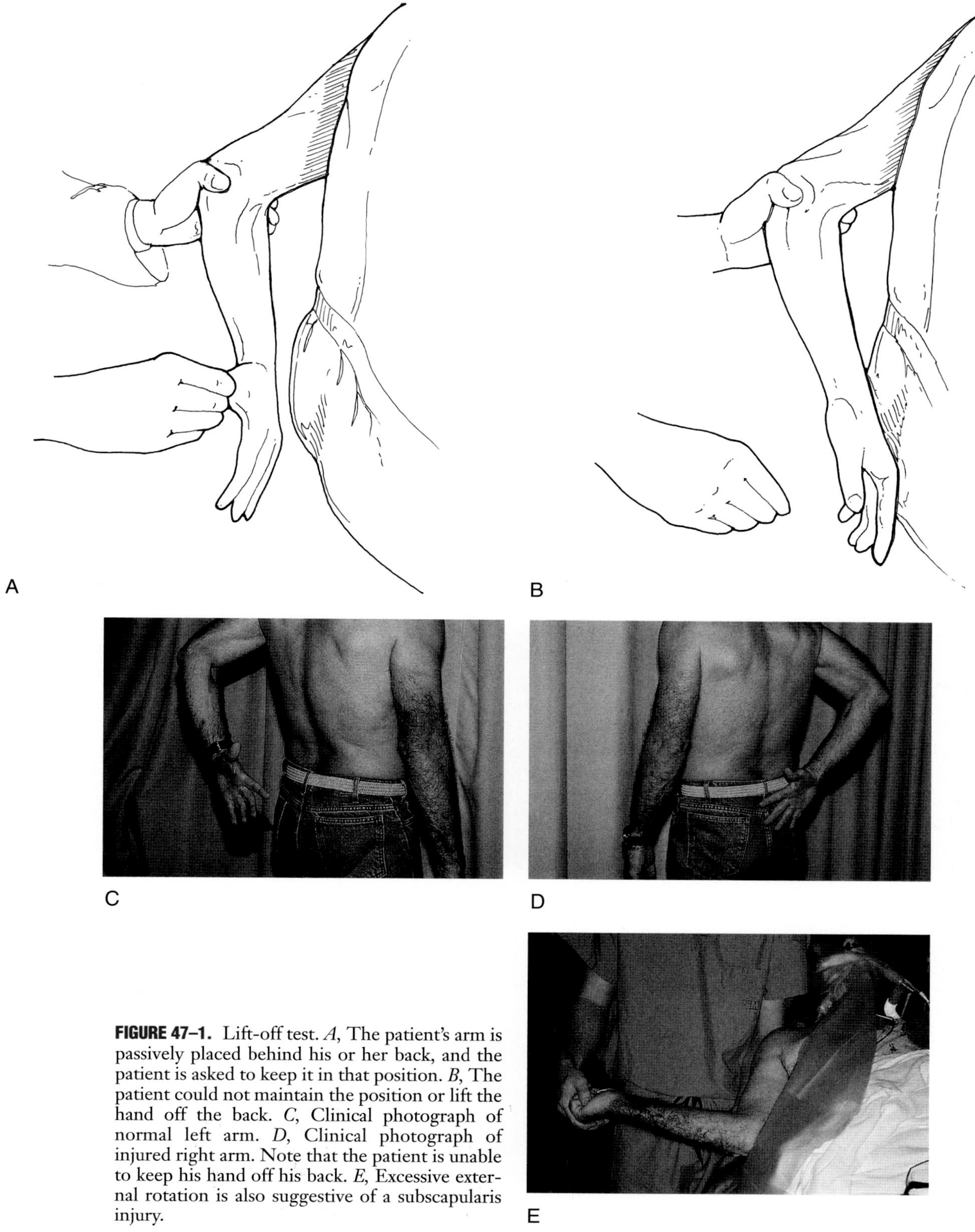

FIGURE 47–1. Lift-off test. *A*, The patient's arm is passively placed behind his or her back, and the patient is asked to keep it in that position. *B*, The patient could not maintain the position or lift the hand off the back. *C*, Clinical photograph of normal left arm. *D*, Clinical photograph of injured right arm. Note that the patient is unable to keep his hand off his back. *E*, Excessive external rotation is also suggestive of a subscapularis injury.

DIAGNOSTIC IMAGING

Anteroposterior (AP) and axillary radiographs of the shoulder are obtained routinely. X-rays are usually not helpful in establishing the diagnosis, although occasionally axillary review reveals an avulsed fragment of bone from the lesser tuberosity, thus confirming the diagnosis. In patients in whom the diagnosis remains unclear, MRI is very helpful. In addition, MRI assists in identification of incomplete ruptures of the subscapularis tendon, which can be managed nonoperatively (Fig. 47–2).

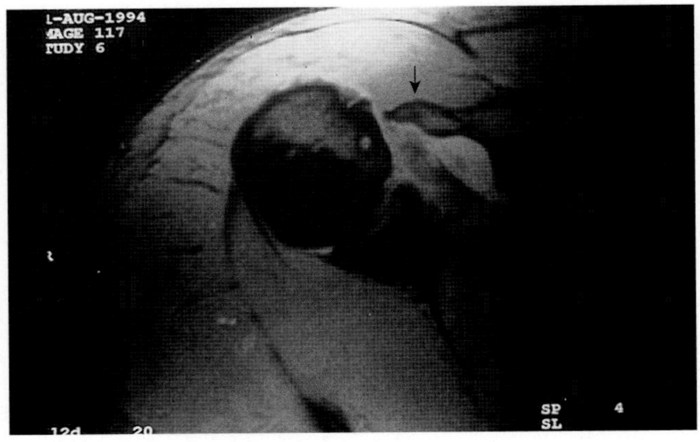

FIGURE 47–2. MRI shows ruptured subscapularis tendon *(arrow)*.

NONOPERATIVE MANAGEMENT

In the low-demand patient with minimal symptoms and no evidence of anterior instability of the shoulder, a nonoperative approach to management is reasonable. In addition, patients who may incur significant morbidity from surgical procedures owing to multiple medical problems should be considered for nonoperative care. Nonoperative management consists of a standard rotator cuff rehabilitation program that emphasizes early stretching and range-of-motion exercises followed by progressive resistive exercises after full mobility is restored. The patient should be monitored closely for development of symptoms of biceps tendon subluxation or anterior instability.

RELEVANT ANATOMY

The subscapularis muscle is the anterior rotator cuff. The muscle originates from the entire anterior surface of the scapula and inserts onto the lesser tuberosity of the humerus. The lower third of the subscapularis insertion on the humerus is primarily muscular with minimum intervening tendinous tissue. The muscle is multipennate and is dually innervated by the upper and lower subscapular nerves. This dual innervation allows the muscle to be split in line with its fibers from the lateral insertion with minimal risk of denervation. The axillary nerve and artery are intimately associated with the anterior inferior surface of the muscle as they pass around the inferior border of the subscapularis to enter the quadrilateral space (Fig. 47–3). The anterior humeral circumflex artery passes along the anterior inferior surface of the subscapularis and arborizes on the humerus near the subscapularis tendon insertion. Near the tendon's insertion on the lesser tuberosity, the anterior capsule of the glenohumeral joint is intimately attached to the subscapularis tendon. Blood supply to the muscle is provided from branches that extend from the axillary and subscapular arteries.

It is most critical for the surgeon to understand the relationship between the axillary nerve and the subscapularis tendon. The nerve is especially at risk in operative repair of subscapularis tendon avulsions because the tendon retracts in a way that involves the axillary nerve and may be obscured by hematoma secondary to the avulsion. When chronic ruptures are repaired subsequently, the nerve may be found incarcerated in scar with the tendon stump. It is critical that the nerve be directly identified in all cases of subscapularis rupture repair.

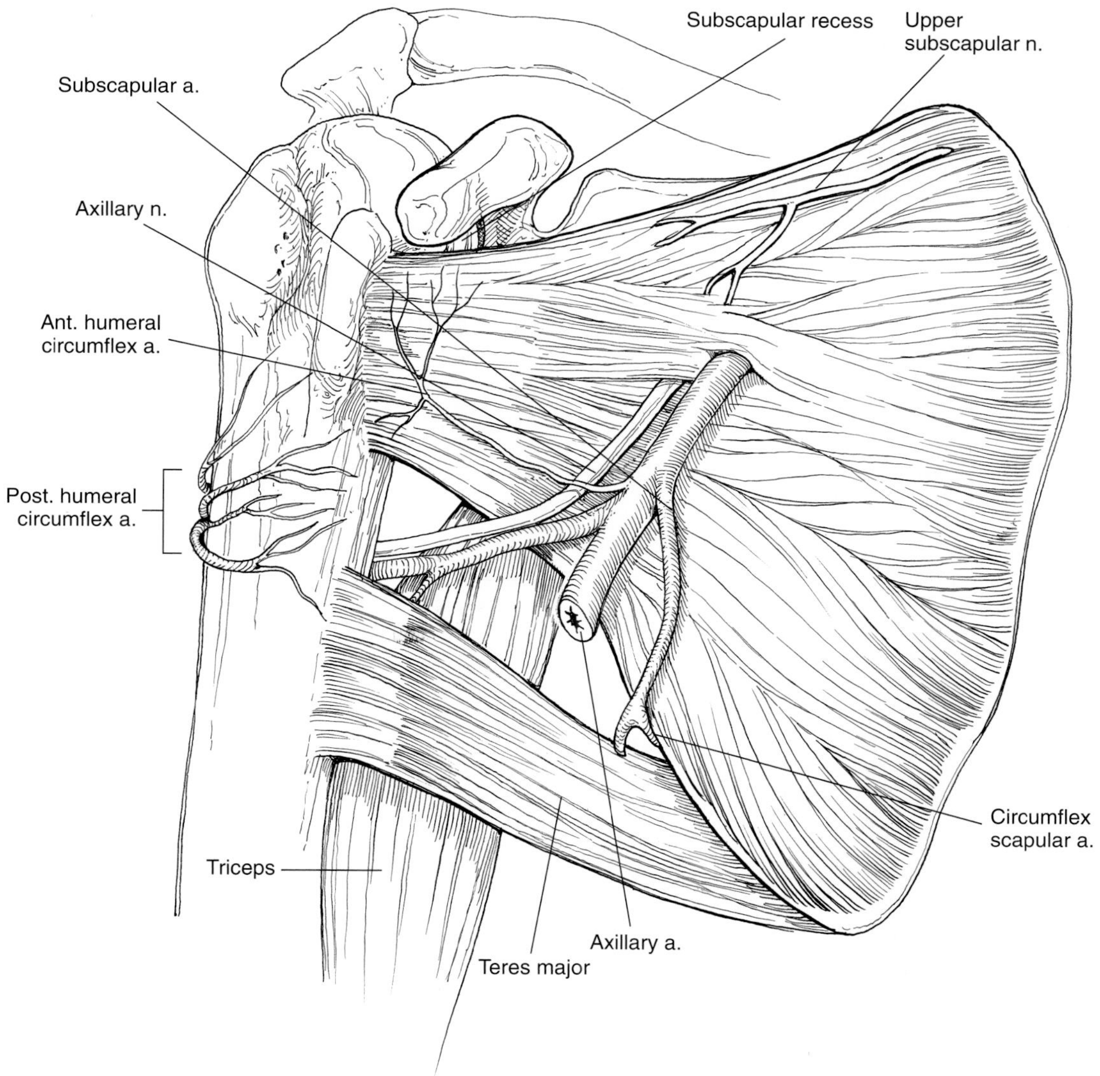

FIGURE 47–3. The axillary nerve and artery lie directly on the anterior surface of the subscapularis muscle. The nerve and artery may become incarcerated in the scar formed by the retracted tendon in a chronic rupture.

SURGICAL *TECHNIQUE*

Indications

Repair of the acutely ruptured subscapularis tendon should be considered in all physically active patients for whom no contraindication to repair exists. Late repair is problematic owing to scarring of the tendon stump and potential involvement of the axillary nerve. Therefore, we favor immediate repair in the absence of contraindications. In addition, repair of a symptomatic partial rupture that fails to improve with conservative care should be considered. Similar to the experience with chronic pectoralis major ruptures, we have noted significant symptom improvement with repair of late ruptures (existing longer than 3 months) of the subscapularis.

Technique

1. Positioning: A standard beach-chair position is used. The entire shoulder girdle and arm are sterilely prepped, and the arm is draped.
2. Incision: A deltopectoral incision is used. The cephalic vein is identified in the deltopectoral interval. The vein is mobilized and retracted either medially or laterally based on ease of dissection. As a deep plane is developed, self-retaining retractors are placed between the pectoralis major and the deltoid.
3. Tendon repair: As the deep plane of the dissection is developed, the glenohumeral joint is frequently visible when the subscapularis is completely avulsed. If difficulty is encountered in identifying the stump of the tendon, it most frequently retracts to a point immediately inferior to the coracoid process. Dissection of this region frequently reveals the tendon stump. Release of the conjoined tendon insertion to the coracoid process may sometimes be needed for additional exposure. The axillary nerve and artery are identified and protected. The tendon stump is grasped with a Kocher or Allis forceps, and blunt dissection is used to mobilize the tendon stump. The tendon stump is then repaired with multiple No. 2 braided, nonabsorbable sutures using a Mason-Allen stitch (Fig. 47–4).

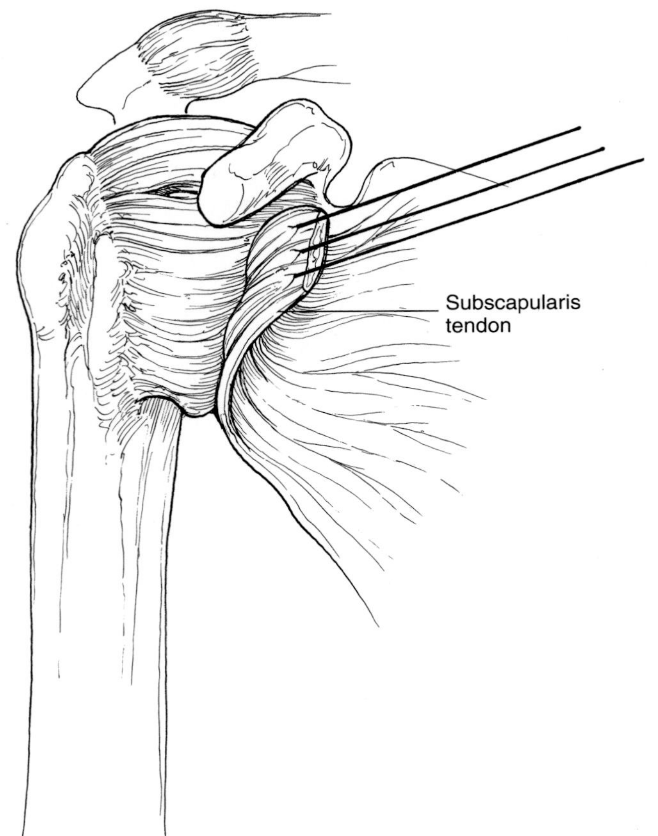

FIGURE 47–4. The subscapularis tendon is mobilized until adequate excursion of the tendon is observed when traction is applied to the tendon stump.

Tension is then held on the sutures to allow the contracted muscle to relax and pull out to full length. The tendon is adequately mobilized when it demonstrates a normal bounce test. The bounce test is performed by tugging on the previously placed sutures and demonstrating adequate musculotendinous excursion for external rotation of the shoulder. The lesser tuberosity is now exposed and prepared for tendon fixation. If a large fragment of the lesser tuberosity is avulsed, fixation can be obtained with multiple cancellous screws. It has been our experience that the thin cortical bone of the lesser tuberosity frequently provides insufficient purchase for the screws in the lesser tuberosity fragment; therefore, we routinely favor suture repair of the tendon. The tendon can then be reattached through drill holes, as was described in Chapter 46, or multiple suture anchors can be placed into the proximal humerus in the region of the lesser tuberosity. The arm is held in extreme internal rotation as the sutures are tied, advancing the tendon stump to the bone (Fig. 47–5).

If the tendon rupture appears to be chronic and adequate immobilization of the subscapularis tendon is not possible, the pectoralis major insertion may be mobilized and inserted onto the lesser tuberosity, as has been described by Wirth and Rockwood.

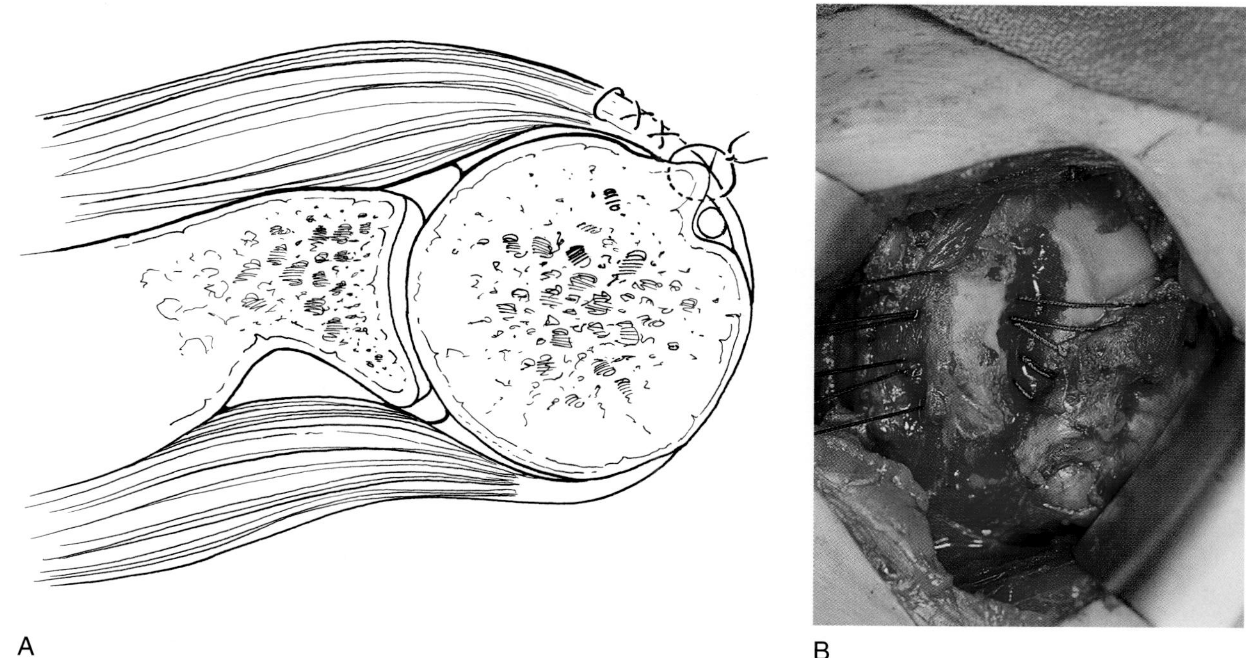

FIGURE 47–5. *A*, The subscapularis is sutured back to bone through drill holes. *B*, The subscapularis can be repaired into a trough, as shown here, or repaired with suture anchors.

POSTOPERATIVE MANAGEMENT

Patients are placed in a sling and swathe during the immediate postsurgical period. After 5 to 7 days, the dressing is changed to a light dressing and Codman exercises are initiated. Patients are cautioned to avoid external rotation beyond 30°. After 4 weeks, patients are instructed to discontinue the sling, and gentle active range of motion is initiated. At 6 weeks, a progressive active and passive motion program is begun. Once full motion is restored, a gentle resistive exercise program is initiated. Patients are maintained on light activities until 3 months postoperatively. From 3 months to 6 months postoperatively, progressive strengthening and increased resistance are allowed, with return to full activity after 6 months.

COMPLICATIONS

Complications of subscapularis repair include rupture of the repair, axillary nerve palsy, anterior shoulder capsular contracture, and frozen shoulder. Axillary nerve palsy is the most significant risk, and meticulous attention to detail is required during the surgical dissection. Anterior capsular contracture is best avoided by careful soft tissue balancing at the time of repair. During the repair of chronic ruptures, Z-lengthening of the subscapularis tendon stump may be required to restore adequate external rotation. In cases in which repair results in excessive anterior capsular tightening, consideration should be given to lengthening the subscapularis; if this is not possible, a pectoralis major transfer should be considered. Arthrofibrosis is best avoided by careful attention to detail during the postoperative physical therapy program.

RESULTS

In general, the results of repair of subscapularis tendon avulsion are rewarding. A majority of patients are returned to normal function and motion when repair is performed in the acute setting. Chronic ruptures often are associated with residual loss of internal rotation; however, they consistently result in marked improvement in function. Gerber and associates reported 13 of 16 patients with good to excellent results at an average follow-up of 43 months. The capacity of these patients to do their occupations improved from an average 59% preoperatively to 95% postoperatively.

REFERENCES

Deutsch A, Altchek DW, Veltri DM, et al: Traumatic tears of the subscapularis tendon. Clinical diagnosis, magnetic resonance imaging findings, and operative treatment [see comments]. Am J Sports Med 25:13–22, 1997.

Gerber C, Hersche O, Farron A: Isolated rupture of the subscapularis tendon. J Bone Joint Surg [Am] 78:1015–1023, 1996.

Ticker JB, Warner JJ: Single-tendon tears of the rotator cuff. Evaluation and treatment of subscapularis tears and principles of treatment for supraspinatus tears. Orthop Clin North Am 28:99–116, 1997.

Warren RF: Lesions of the long head of the biceps tendon. Instr Course Lect 34:204–209, 1985.

Wirth MA, Rockwood CA Jr: Operative treatment of irreparable rupture of the subscapularis. J Bone Joint Surg [Am] 79:722–731, 1997.

CHAPTER 48

Treatment of Pectoralis Major Rupture

INTRODUCTION

Rupture of the pectoralis major tendon is an uncommon injury. Patissier first described this relatively rare injury in 1822. Fewer than 150 cases have been reported in the world literature, and half of these cases have been reported over the past 10 years. This injury is probably underrecognized. A vast majority of these injuries occur in weight lifters; however, numerous other traumatic mechanisms have been described. Surgical repair remains the mainstay of treatment.

HISTORY AND PHYSICAL EXAMINATION

In cases of acute rupture of the pectoralis major, patients complain of severe onset of sharp pain in the anterior chest wall. Rupture of the pectoralis major happens most frequently during bench press. The rupture occurs when the humerus is extending at the beginning of the lift. In this position, the sternoclavicular head is under maximum stretch and is also exerting maximum force. In more chronic tears, patients often complain of cramping of the chest wall during heavy lifting and weakness of the affected arm.

Examination in the acute setting reveals a hematoma in either the proximal medial arm or the chest wall. Musculotendinous ruptures tend to produce a hematoma along the chest wall; tendinous avulsions from the humeral shaft produce a small area of ecchymosis near the insertion on the proximal humerus. The defect in the anterior axillary fold can be visualized by having the patient simultaneously abduct both shoulders to 90° and forward flex to approximately 45°, thus extending the anterior axillary folds. Side-to-side comparisons readily demonstrate the defect in the anterior axillary folds. Palpation of the anterior axillary fold and pectoralis muscle may be deceiving. A readily recognizable defect is revealed in a majority of patients. However, many patients have remaining fascial attachments that extend from the muscle onto the humeral shaft; these can mislead the examiner to the incorrect diagnosis of partial tendon rupture. In addition, the intact clavicular head of the pectoralis major may deceive the inexperienced examiner. Finally, on physical examination, the patient may demonstrate weak internal rotation.

DIAGNOSTIC IMAGING

X-rays are routinely performed, although in the majority of cases they fail to reveal any bone abnormality. MRI is useful for establishing the diagnosis when it is in question (Fig. 48–1) but is not usually required for assessment of the acute rupture.

NONOPERATIVE MANAGEMENT

Partial ruptures of the pectoralis major can be managed with a conservative program of rest and initial icing, followed by heat and a progressive stretching and strengthening program. If the status of the tendon is in question, it is highly recommended to confirm a partial rupture with MRI, because complete rupture should be managed surgically. After 6 weeks of a conservative program, progressive strengthening exercises can be initiated. Bench pressing of heavy weights should be delayed for at least 3 months.

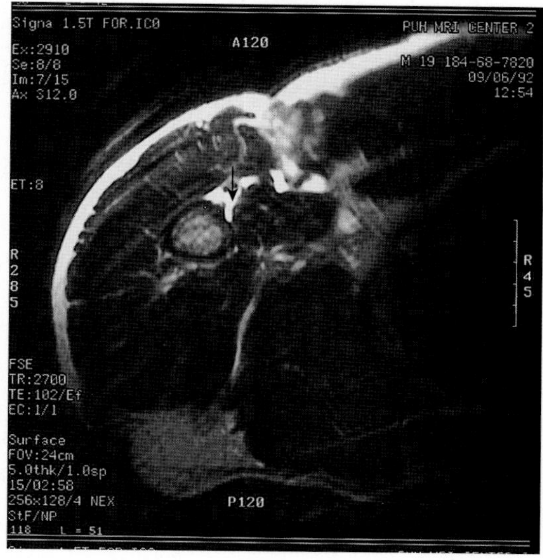

FIGURE 48–1. MRI shows avulsion of the pectoralis tendon *(arrow)*.

RELEVANT ANATOMY

The pectoralis major tendon is a broad, bilaminar tendon that inserts into the lateral lip of the bicipital groove. Two heads—a sternocostal head and a clavicular head—form the tendon. The upper clavicular head forms the anterior tendon insertion, and the sternocostal head forms the posterior tendon insertion. The sternocostal head spirals on itself to produce the rounded appearance of the anterior axillary fold such that the most inferior fibers of the sternocostal head insert superiorly and the superior fibers insert inferiorly (Fig. 48–2). This layered effect of the tendon can be deceiving on palpatory examination of a complete rupture. In the vast majority of cases, the clavicular head remains intact and the sternocostal head avulses.

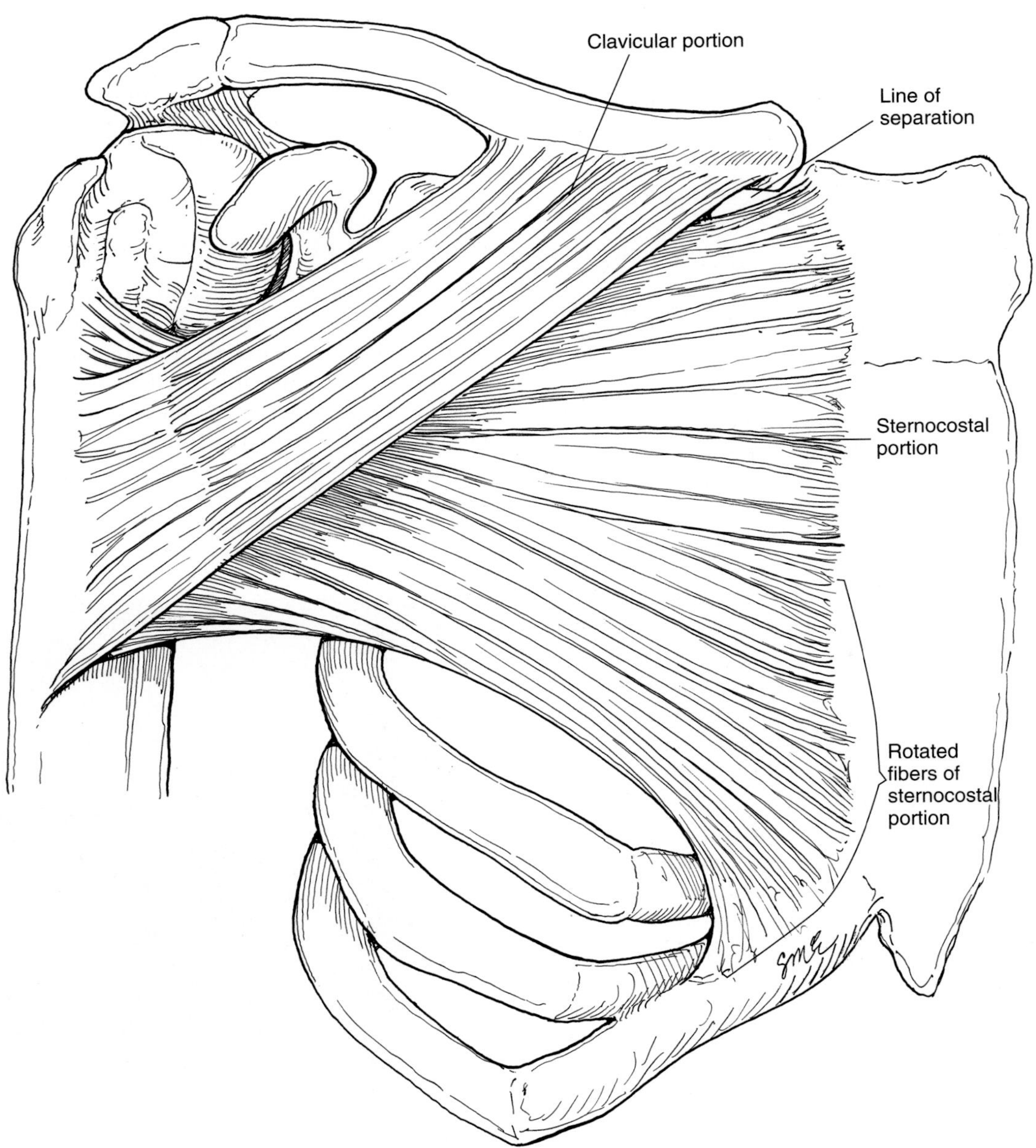

FIGURE 48–2. The clavicular and sternal heads of the pectoralis major. The tendon insertion onto the humerus is in two layers. The deeper sternal head spirals toward its insertion so that the inferior fibers insert superiorly and the superior fibers insert inferiorly.

SURGICAL *TECHNIQUE*

Indications

Complete rupture of the pectoralis major tendon is an indication for repair. This injury occurs in young, active people in whom, without repair, significant weakness persists. In addition, chronic rupture should be given consideration for repair. Repairs have been successfully performed as late as 6 years after injury in symptomatic athletes.

Technique

1. Positioning: The patient is placed in a supine position on the operating table with a rolled towel placed under the affected scapula to elevate the shoulder off the table surface for prepping and draping. The shoulder region is prepped and draped such that the arm is free for unrestricted manipulation.
2. Incision: A 5-cm incision is made in the inferior aspect of the deltopectoral groove centered over the biceps tendon.
3. Procedure: The intact clavicular head is palpable near its insertion onto the humeral shaft, lateral to the biceps tendon. Exposure immediately deep to this tendon reveals the avulsion site at the sternal head (Fig. 48–3). Long dissection can be carried out along the inferior margin of the clavicular head until the avulsed stump tendon is encountered. The

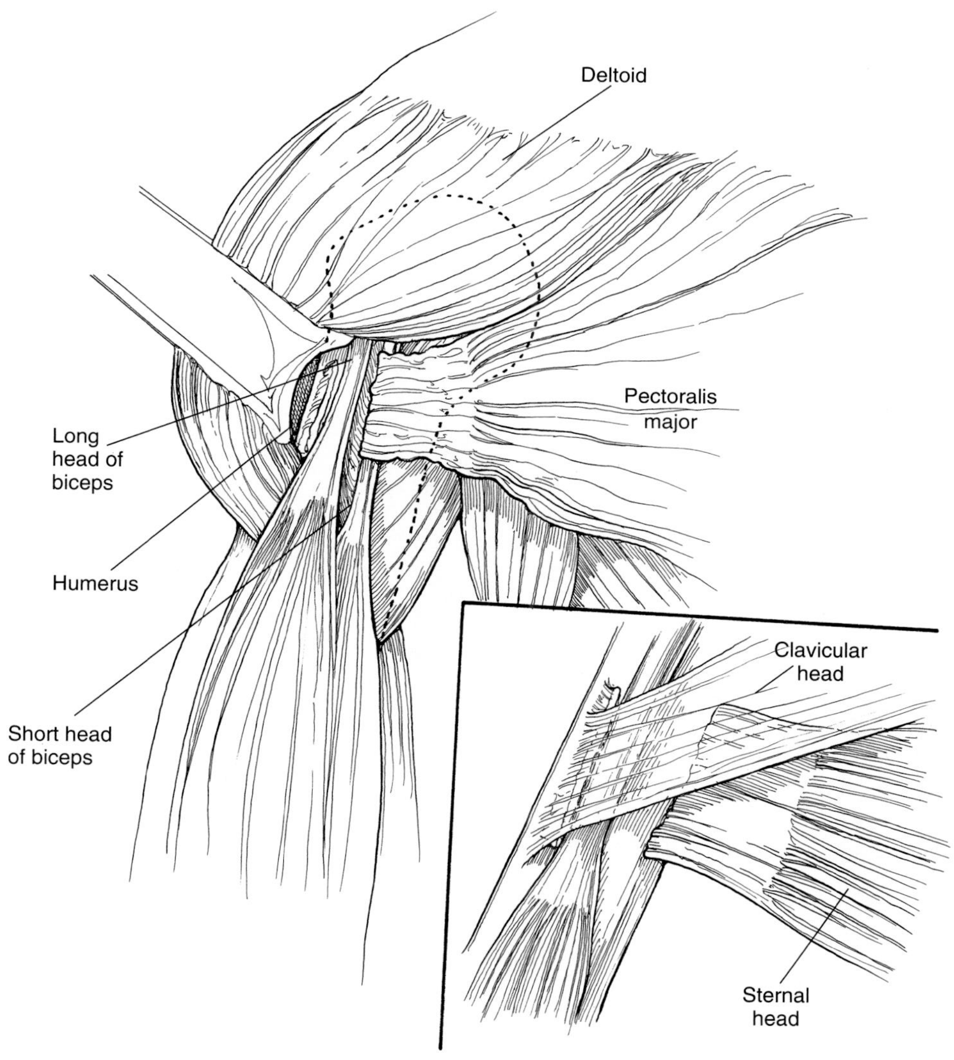

FIGURE 48–3. The clavicular head of the pectoralis major usually is found intact. The sternal head usually avulses near its insertion. With the arm adducted, the clavicular head is retracted superiorly to expose the insertion of the sternal head.

tendon stump is grasped with a Kocher and is delivered into the surgical wound. The tendon stump is sutured with three or four No. 2 braided nonabsorbable sutures, using a Mason-Allen suture technique (Fig. 48–4). Attention is directed to the humeral shaft, and a retractor is placed on the intact clavicular head tendon to retract it superiorly. The arm is brought into adduction to relax the tendon and into some rotation to expose the shaft of the humerus. A 4-mm Acorn burr is used to a cut a longitudinal slot in the anterior humeral shaft. The arm is internally rotated, and the humeral shaft lateral to the clavicular head insertion is exposed. Holes are drilled through the cortex toward the base of the previously cut bone trough. Looped 28-gauge stainless steel wire is passed through the drill holes into the trough. The sutures on the tendon stump are passed through the loops of wire; then the wire loops are retracted to deliver the sutures through the drill holes. The arm is brought into adduction and the sutures are pulled taut, delivering the tendon stump into the bone trough. Sutures are tied over the cortex. The wound is closed in layers and a light dressing is applied. A standard arm sling is applied.

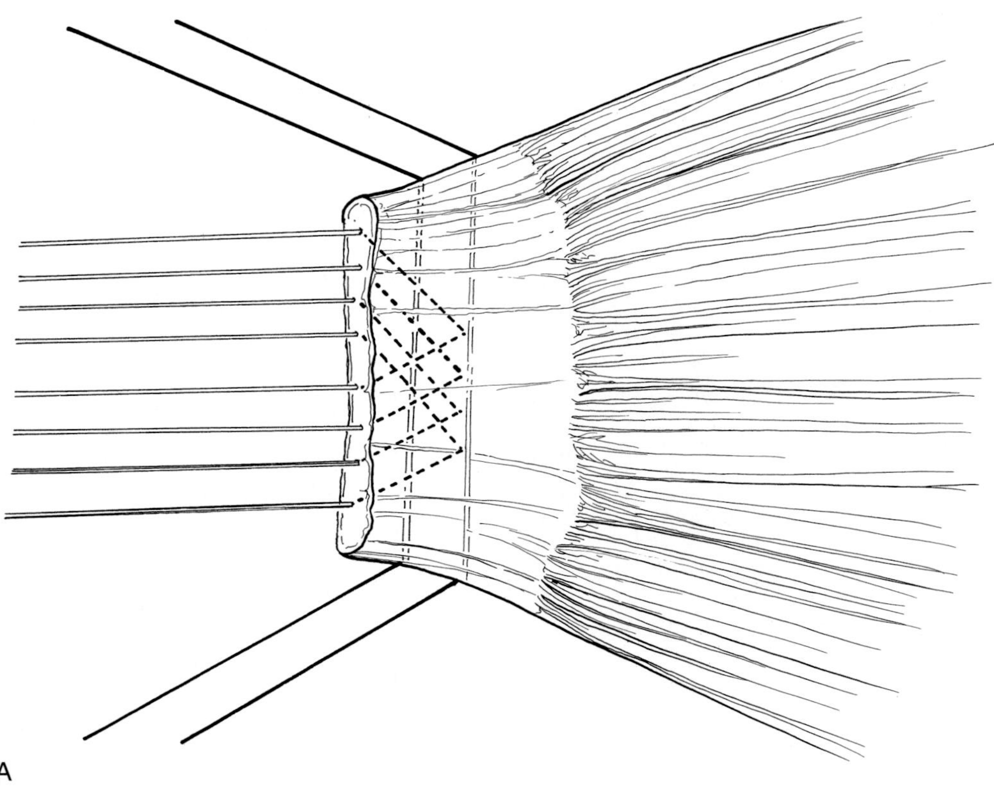

FIGURE 48–4. *A*, Number 2 braided nonabsorbable sutures are placed in the tendon stump using a Mason-Allen suture technique.

FIGURE 48–4 *Continued. B,* Suture anchors can be used to repair the tendon, as shown here, or the tendon can be repaired similar to a traditional rotator cuff repair, as shown in *C* and *D. C,* A slot is cut in the anterior cortex of the humerus at the tendon insertion using a 4-mm burr; 2-mm drill holes are placed through the cortex, lateral to the clavicular head insertion and angled toward the slot. Looped surgical wires are passed through the drill holes to act as suture passers. *D,* The sutures are put under tension to deliver the tendon into the slot. The sutures are tied over the cortex.

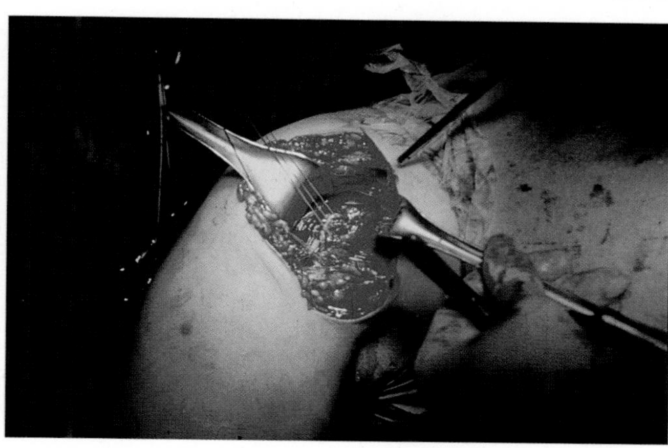
B

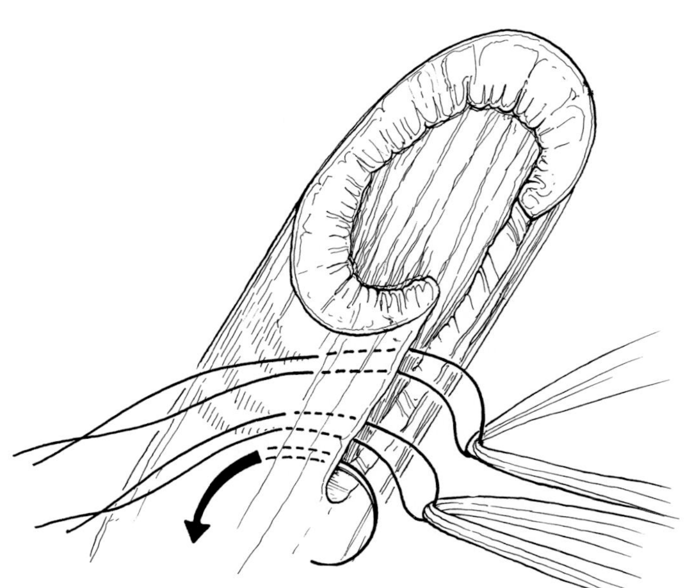
C

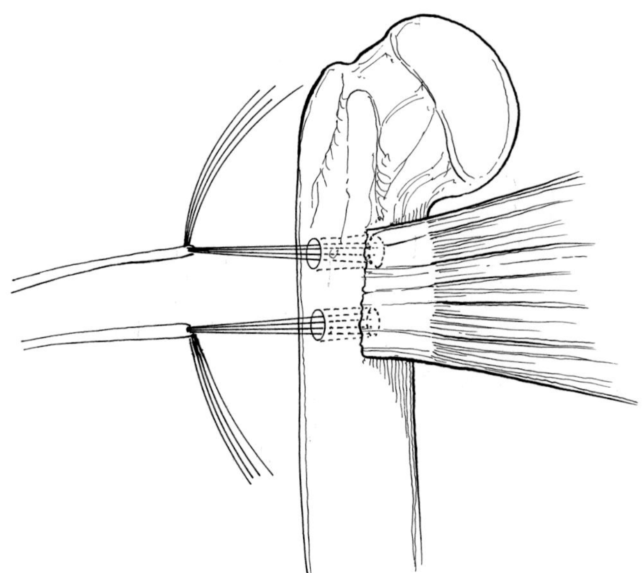
D

POSTOPERATIVE MANAGEMENT

The light dressing is removed after 5 to 7 days, and the patient is instructed to perform pendulum exercises and frequent range-of-motion exercises of the elbow and wrist. An arm sling is used to encourage the patient to rest the arm. The sling is discontinued at 4 weeks. Patients then begin a gentle active range-of-motion program. At 6 weeks after surgery, an active and passive motion program is initiated. Once full range of motion is restored, progressive resistive exercises are begun; these use of different resistance (thickness) elastic bands. Heavy lifting is avoided for 3 months, and return to full lifting, including bench presses, is restricted until 6 months. At 6 months, patients are released to full activity.

COMPLICATIONS

Because of the limited reporting of this injury in the literature, no large series have detailed the complications. Complications can include hematoma with pseudocyst formation, infection, and ruptured repair. Rupture of the repair is most likely to occur with tendinous repairs at the musculotendinous junction. Re-repair of these ruptures has been successful, especially if the repair is delayed until some mature scar has formed in the avulsed tendon stump, thus allowing improved suture purchase.

RESULTS

In 1970, Park and Espiniella reviewed 31 patients reported in the literature. They reported that surgical treatment produced excellent results in 80% of these patients, and an additional 10% had good results. In contrast, good results were reported in only 58% of the patients who were treated nonoperatively. Zeman and colleagues described nine athletes with pectoralis major ruptures. Four patients were treated surgically, and all had excellent results. The five nonoperatively treated patients had residual weakness and residual symptoms in all cases. Kretzler and Richardson reported on the repair of 16 of 19 patients with pectoralis major rupture. Thirteen of these patients reported full return of function without symptoms. In addition, this study included two patients who underwent repair 5½ years after injury. Delayed repair did not achieve full return of strength; however, significant improvement in function was attained.

These results indicate that operative treatment for pectoralis major ruptures is the treatment of choice in the active population. Consideration of repair is generally recommended, even in those patients who present several years after injury.

REFERENCES

Connell DA, Potter HG, Sherman MF, Wickiewicz TL: Injuries of the pectoralis major muscle: Evaluation with MR imaging. Radiology 210:785–791, 1999.

Jones MW, Matthews JP: Rupture of pectoralis major in weight lifters: A case report and review of the literature [review]. Injury 19:219, 1988.

Kretzler HH Jr, Richardson AB: Rupture of the pectoralis major muscle. Am J Sports Med 17:453–458, 1989.

Park JY, Espiniella JL: Rupture of pectoralis major muscle. A case report and review of literature. J Bone Joint Surg [Am] 52:577–581, 1970.

Wirth MA, Rockwood CA Jr: Operative treatment of irreparable rupture of the subscapularis. J Bone Joint Surg [Am] 79:722–731, 1997.

Wolfe SW, Wickiewicz TL, Cavanaugh JT: Ruptures of the pectoralis major muscle. An anatomic and clinical analysis. Am J Sports Med 20:587–593, 1992.

Zeman SC, Rosenfeld RT, Lipscomb PR: Tears of the pectoralis major muscle. Am J Sports Med 7:343–347, 1979.

CHAPTER 49

Treatment of Suprascapular Nerve Entrapment

INTRODUCTION

Entrapment neuropathy occurs uncommonly around the shoulder. Suprascapular nerve entrapment is the most common nerve compression lesion around the shoulder. Patients with suprascapular nerve lesions can be divided into two general groups. One group includes patients with acute onset of nerve palsy symptoms after violent activity or injury. The other group includes those with the gradual onset of vague shoulder pain and eventual supraspinatus or infraspinatus muscle atrophy. Patients with acute onset of symptoms can be expected to recover with conservative treatment. In contrast, patients with gradual, progressive compromise of function and progression of muscle atrophy constitute most of the candidates for surgical decompression.

HISTORY AND PHYSICAL EXAMINATION

Patients with suprascapular nerve disease tend to complain of posterolateral shoulder pain that is vague and poorly localized. Although the suprascapular nerve may contain sensory fibers that supply the skin of the posterior shoulder, paresthesias are usually not observed in this syndrome. Patients have weakness in external rotation of the shoulder and weakness in activities requiring overhead use of the hand.

Physical examination reveals weakness in external rotation of the shoulder. Careful examination may demonstrate atrophy of the supraspinatus or infraspinatus muscles. Nerve entrapment occurs in one of two locations—in the suprascapular notch or in the spinoglenoid notch. Thus, tenderness may be localized to either of these areas. Isolated atrophy of the infraspinatus muscle suggests entrapment at the spinoglenoid notch. Spinoglenoid notch entrapment occurs most often secondary to a ganglion from the glenohumeral joint. Recent studies suggest a high association between glenoid labrum tears and shoulder ganglions.

DIAGNOSTIC IMAGING

Standard anteroposterior and lateral views of the scapula should be performed to rule out obvious skeletal lesions or tumors. In cases demonstrating isolated atrophy of the infraspinatus, we have routinely obtained MRI scans of the shoulder to rule out ganglions of the spinoglenoid notch. Recent experience has suggested a high association between labral disease and spinoglenoid notch ganglions. Electromyography and nerve conduction velocities may be helpful in confirming the diagnosis and further delineating the exact location of compression.

NONOPERATIVE MANAGEMENT

Nonoperative management of suprascapular nerve lesions consists of activity modification to avoid further stretching of the nerve. In addition, a gentle resistance exercise program to strengthen the external rotators is emphasized to assist in reducing muscle weakness. Patients are seen on a regular basis and are observed closely for evidence of progressive atrophy or weakness.

RELEVANT ANATOMY

The suprascapular nerve is derived from the upper trunk of the brachial plexus. The nerve enters the supraspinatus fossa through the suprascapular notch, then passes down the floor of the supraspinatus fossa and enters the infraspinatus fossa through the spinoglenoid notch (Fig. 49–1). In the region of the spinoglenoid notch, the nerve passes through this hiatus, the lateral margin of which is a fibrous band called the spinoglenoid ligament. The nerve is relatively immobile in this area; thus, ganglions frequently compress the nerve.

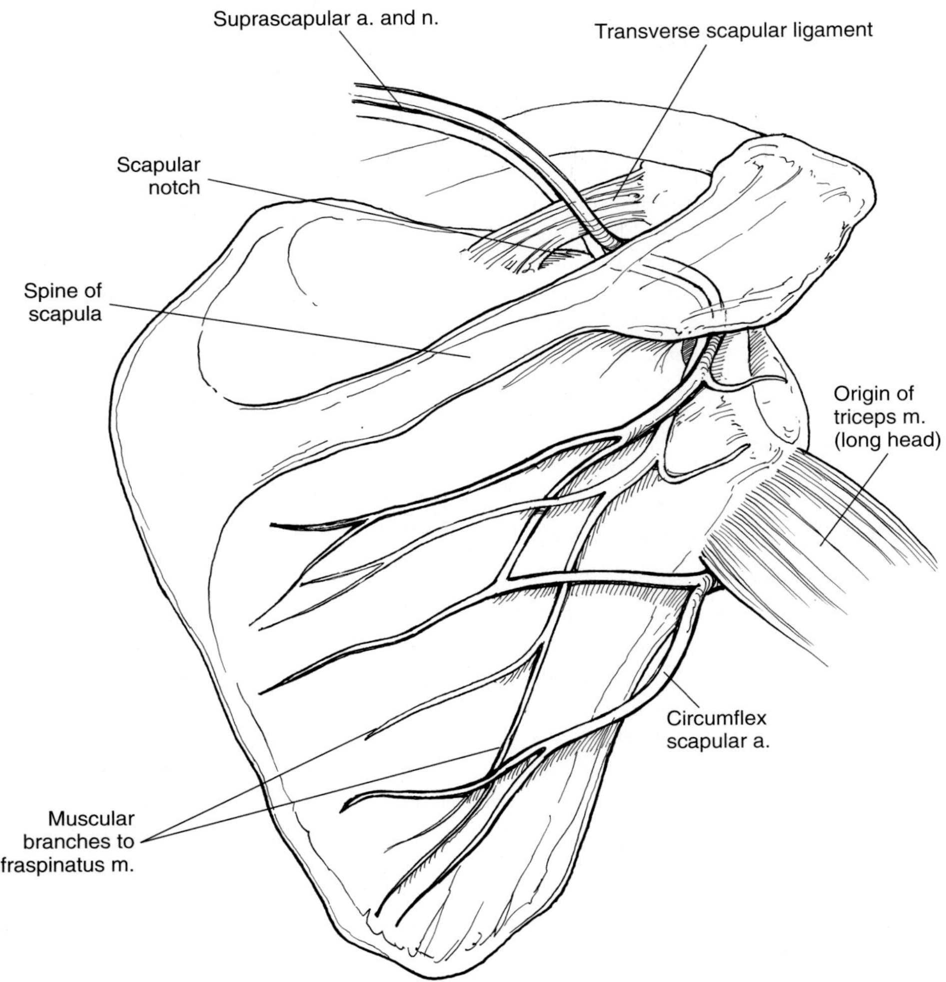

FIGURE 49–1. The suprascapular nerve accompanied by the suprascapular artery enters the supraspinatus fossa through the scapular notch passing deep to the transverse scapular ligament. The nerve enters the infraspinatus fossa by passing lateral to the spinoglenoid notch.

SURGICAL TECHNIQUE

Indications

Patients with evidence of progressive neuropathy are candidates for surgical decompression. In addition, patients who fail to show significant improvement after 2 to 3 months of close observation should be considered for nerve decompression. Spinoglenoid notch ganglions should be managed with surgical decompression. Recent reports have shown success with arthroscopic decompression of the cysts and management of associated labral disease. We have had success with this approach in a small series of cases, but we continue to favor direct decompression of the ganglion until long-term studies demonstrate the superiority of arthroscopic cyst decompression.

Technique

Two approaches to the nerve are used, depending on the area of compression. The superior approach is used to decompress the suprascapular notch. The posterior approach is used to access the spinoglenoid notch. Both approaches are reviewed here.

Superior Approach

1. Position: The patient is placed in a lateral position on a beanbag, and an axillary roll is placed. The arm is draped free so there is free access to the entire scapula and shoulder girdle. The table is positioned in approximately 30° reverse Trendelenburg position to allow gravity retraction of the shoulder girdle.
2. Incision: The superior edge of the scapula is palpated as the skin incision is made over the midsuperior aspect of the scapula along Langer's lines (Fig. 49–2). The fibers of the trapezius muscle are split longitudinally in line with the fibers that expose the supraspinatus muscle. The supraspinatus is then retracted posteriorly, and dissection is carried down its anterior border to expose the superior edge of the scapula (Fig. 49–3).

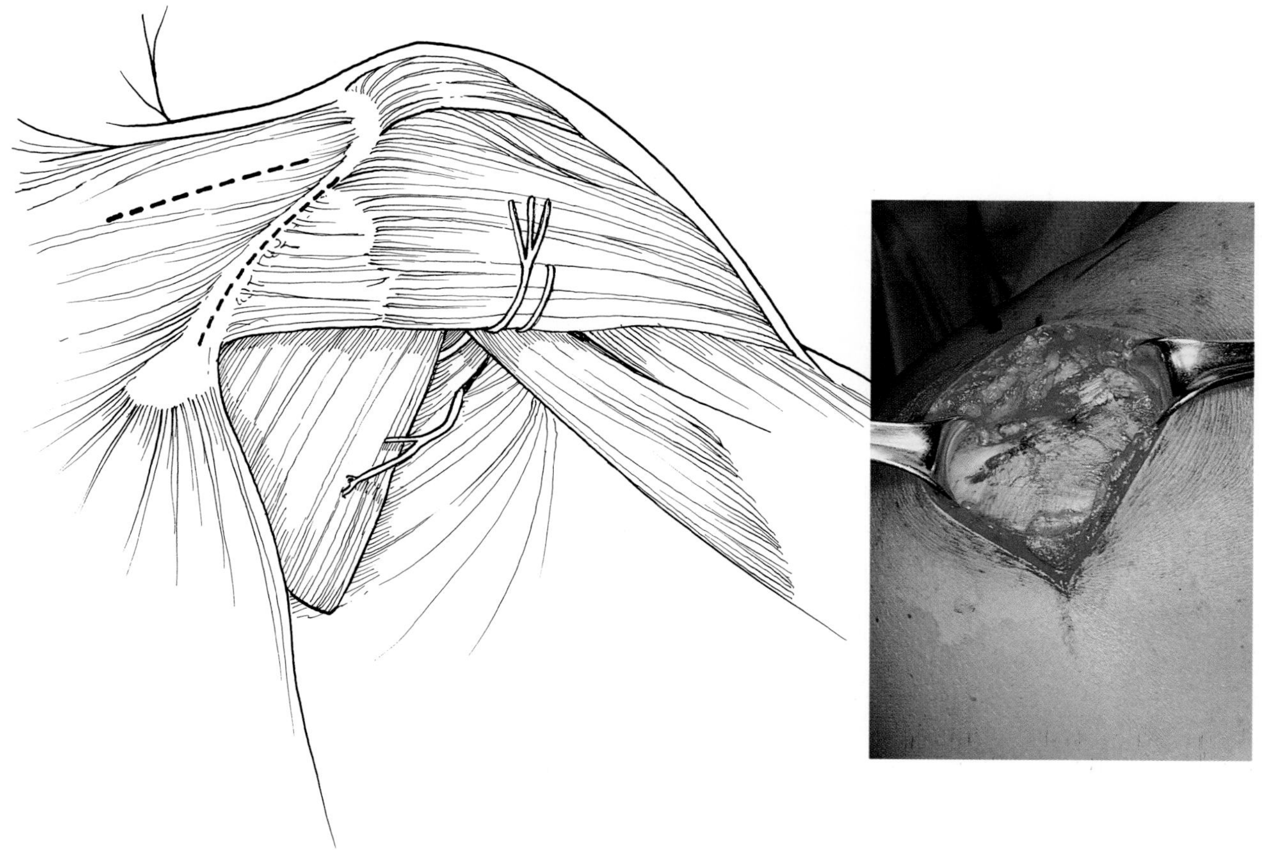

FIGURE 49–2. The solid line indicates the incision for the superior exposure of the scapular notch. The dashed line indicates the incision for exposure of the spinoglenoid notch.

3. Nerve decompression: Palpation along the superior margin of the scapula reveals the suprascapular notch. The superior transverse scapular ligament is identified and resected. A right-angle clamp placed deep to the ligament during resection can assist in avoiding injury to the suprascapular artery and venae comitantes. Following complete release of the ligament, the nerve is elevated from the notch and inspected, with care taken to avoid injury to the associated vascular structures. The nerve should be inspected proximally and distally to ensure that there are no other areas of entrapment or local ganglions. The wound is closed in layers in standard fashion.

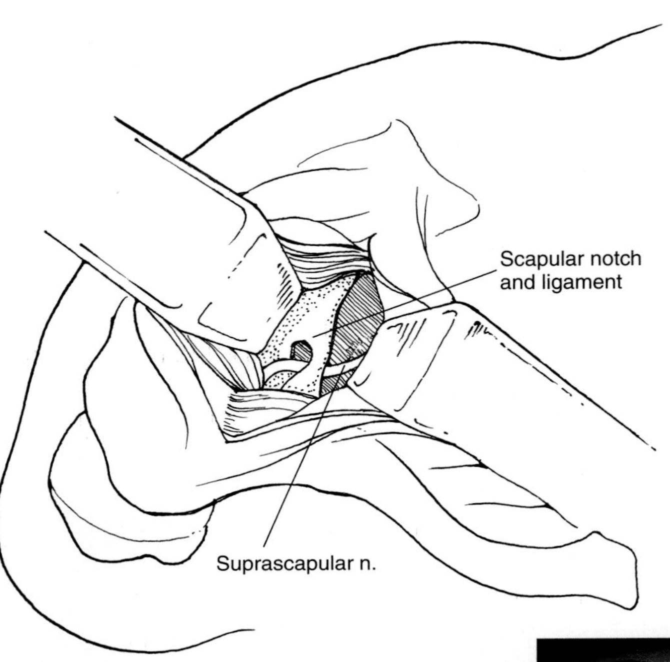

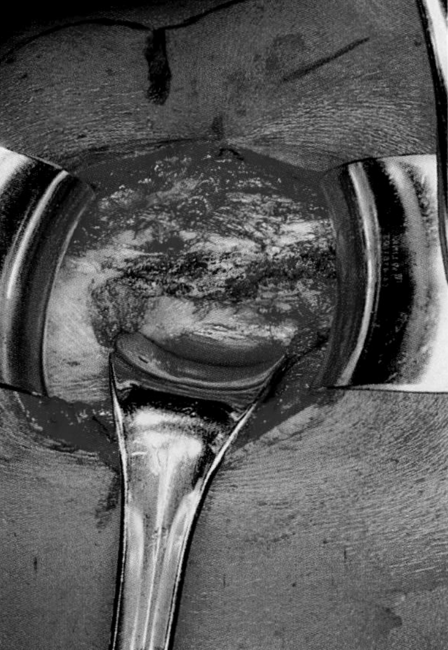

FIGURE 49–3. Superior exposure of the suprascapular nerve. The trapezius is split in line with its fibers, and the supraspinatus is retracted posteriorly to expose the scapular notch.

Posterior Approach

1. Skin incision: A skin incision is placed along Langer's lines. Skin flaps are elevated, and the spine of the scapula is exposed.
2. Deep dissection: The deltoid is sharply released from the spine, preserving the tendon and periosteum for later repair. With the deltoid reflected off the spine, the transverse fibers of the infraspinatus come into view. The infraspinatus can then be retracted inferiorly, and the spinoglenoid notch is visualized (Fig. 49–4). If access to the supraspinatus fossa is required, the trapezius insertion can be reflected off superiorly and the supraspinatus muscle can be retracted gently. Care must be taken to avoid applying traction to the nerve if both the superior and inferior exposures are used. With the nerve exposed, the spinoglenoid ligament is resected; any associated ganglion is resected and the wound is closed in layers.

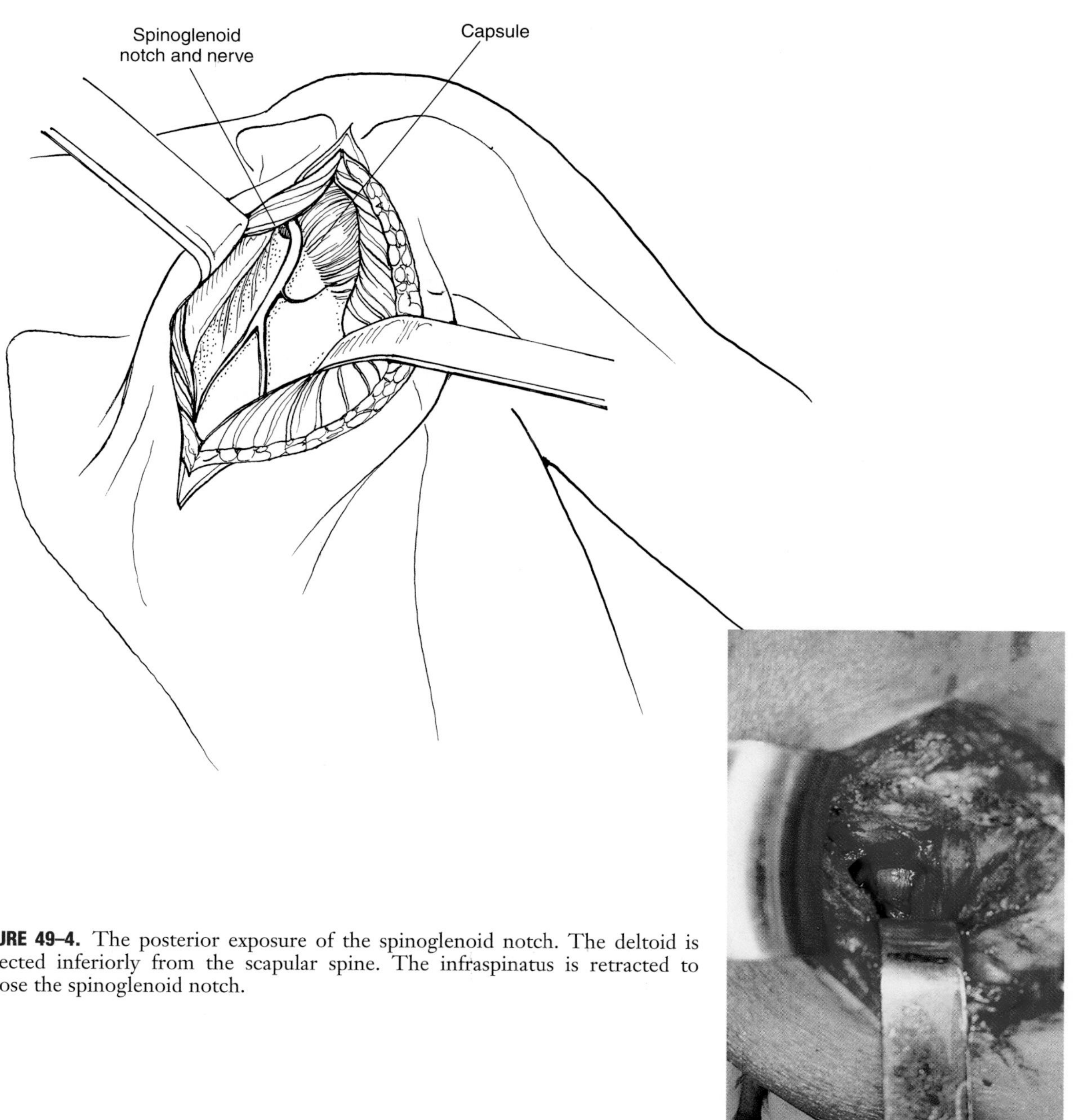

FIGURE 49–4. The posterior exposure of the spinoglenoid notch. The deltoid is reflected inferiorly from the scapular spine. The infraspinatus is retracted to expose the spinoglenoid notch.

POSTOPERATIVE CARE

Patients are placed in a sling for comfort and are given a light dressing approximately 1 week after surgery. Gentle active range of motion is initiated as tolerated. In patients who have had a superior exposure of the suprascapular notch, activity can be progressed as tolerated. However, patients who have had a posterior exposure require activity restriction to allow the deltoid and/or trapezius insertions to heal. After the posterior exposure, abduction of the arm and overhead use of the hand are restricted for the first 4 weeks; then a gentle progressive program is initiated for the following 2 weeks. Full, unrestricted activities can be initiated after 6 weeks.

RESULTS

The largest study on suprascapular nerve entrapment was published in 1993 by Vastamaki and Goransson, in the journal *Clinical Orthopedics and Related Research*. In their review of 56 operations, 81% of patients were improved. However, some patients remained significantly symptomatic. Patients who have had severe atrophy and compression for longer than 6 months are far more likely to have poor outcomes.

COMPLICATIONS

No large series have reviewed the complications of this infrequent operation. The most frequent problem is failure to improve. Injury to the suprascapular vessels can be problematic, resulting in hematoma and subsequent infection. When the region of the spinoglenoid notch is repaired, great care is taken to avoid excessive retraction of the supraspinatus or infraspinatus muscles, which could result in injury to the nerve.

REFERENCES

Callahan JD, Scully TB, Shapiro SA, Worth RM: Suprascapular nerve entrapment. A series of 27 cases [see comments]. J Neurosurg 74:893–896, 1991.
Chochole MH, Senker W, Meznik C, Breitenseher MJ: Glenoid-labral cyst entrapping the suprascapular nerve: Dissolution after arthroscopic debridement of an extended SLAP lesion. Arthroscopy 13:753–755, 1997.
Drez D Jr: Suprascapular neuropathy in the differential diagnosis of rotator cuff injuries. Am J Sports Med 4:43–45, 1976.
Ferretti A, DeCarli A, Fontana M: Injury of the suprascapular nerve at the spinoglenoid notch. The natural history of infraspinatus atrophy in volleyball players. Am J Sports Med 26:759–763, 1998.
Martin SD, Warren RF, Martin TL, et al: Suprascapular neuropathy. Results of non-operative treatment. J Bone Joint Surg [Am] 79:1159–1165, 1997.
Post M, Mayer J: Suprascapular nerve entrapment. Diagnosis and treatment. Clin Orthop (223):126–136, 1987.
Ticker JB, Djurasovic M, Strauch RJ, et al: The incidence of ganglion cysts and other variations in anatomy along the course of the suprascapular nerve. J Shoulder Elbow Surg 7:472–478, 1998.
Vastamaki M, Goransson H: Suprascapular nerve entrapment. Clin Orthop (297):135–143, 1993.

CHAPTER 50

Treatment of Acromioclavicular Injuries

INTRODUCTION

Acromioclavicular (AC) injuries are common. They range from separations that result from direct trauma to distal clavicle osteolysis, an overuse injury common in weight lifters. Nonoperative management is successful in treating a number of these disorders, and treatment options must be individualized based on the patient's needs.

HISTORY AND PHYSICAL EXAMINATION

A direct fall onto the shoulder can result in a distal clavicle fracture or an AC separation. Based on the degree of injury, patients may complain of pain, loss of motion, or a deformity. AC abnormalities not associated with an injury may present with insidious onset of pain in the joint. This is commonly seen in weight lifters. In addition to notation of any deformities and crepitus in or around the joint, the standard shoulder examination should be completed.

DIAGNOSTIC IMAGING

Standard anteroposterior (AP) and axillary lateral radiographs usually characterize AC injuries (Fig. 50–1). The axillary lateral radiograph is essential in documenting type IV AC injuries (discussed later) because the deformity usually is not obvious with an AP radiograph alone. Stress radiographs (bilateral AC views with 10 to 15 pounds of weight *hanging* from both wrists) may occasionally be useful in distinguishing a subtle type II from

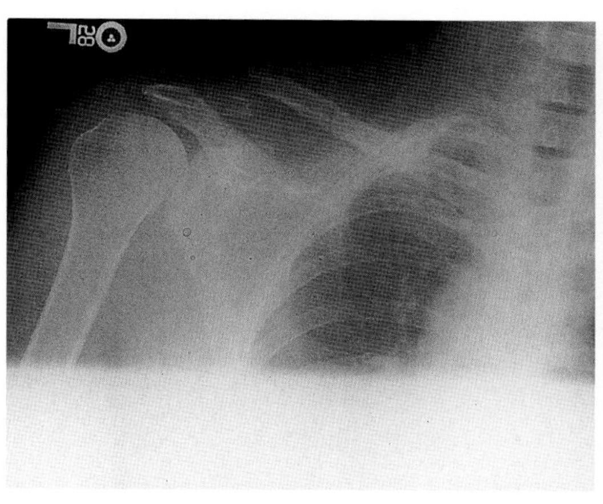

A

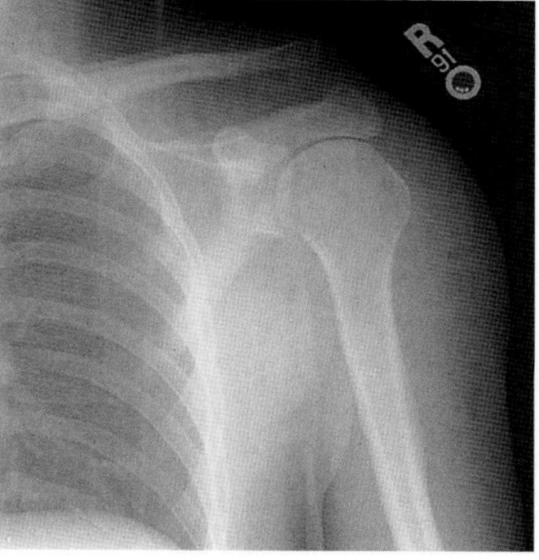

B

FIGURE 50–1. Acromioclavicular injuries. *A*, Type II fracture of the distal clavicle. *B*, Anteroposterior radiograph of a type V acromioclavicular separation. Note the increased coracoclavicular distance. *C*, Axillary lateral radiograph of a type IV acromioclavicular separation. *Arrowheads* indicate the anterior edge of the acromion. *Arrow* indicates posterior displacement of the clavicle. *D*, Anteroposterior radiograph of distal clavicle osteolysis *(arrow)*. (*D* from Pitchford KR, Cahill BR: Osteolysis of the distal clavicle in the overhead athlete. Op Tech Sports Med 5:72–77, 1997.)

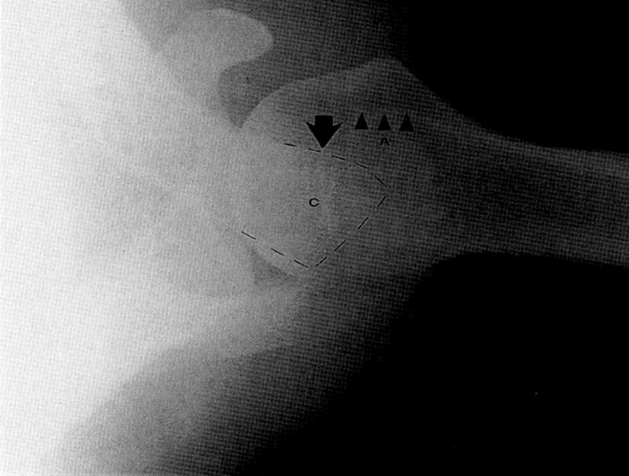

C

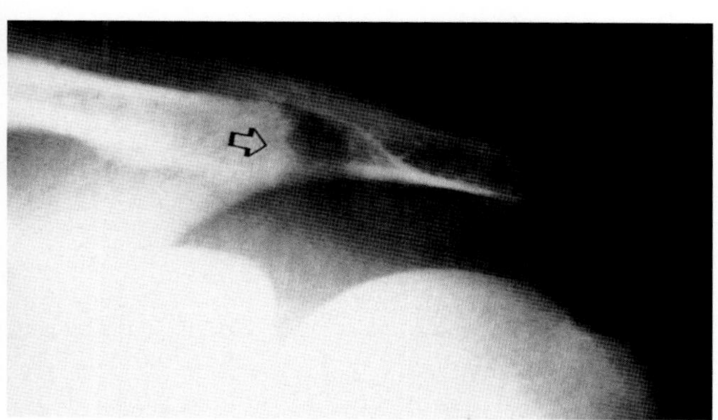

D

a type III injury, but they usually are not necessary. The coracoclavicular distance (measured vertically from the superior aspect of the coracoid to the inferior surface of the clavicle) is helpful in classification of these injuries (see later). A 10° cephalic tilt view with soft tissue technique (Zanca) can be helpful in the diagnosis of distal clavicle osteolysis.

NONOPERATIVE MANAGEMENT

Most authors agree that nonoperative management is indicated for types I and II and most type III AC separations. Closed reduction should be considered in some type IV separations (i.e., those without significant displacement through the trapezius muscle). Following reduction or the initial injury period, a brief period of immobilization should be followed by range-of-motion and a rotator cuff–strengthening program. Most fractures (especially types I, III, and IV) can be managed similarly. Distal clavicle osteolysis can be managed by activity modification (abstaining from weight training for a period), technique modification, a limited number of injections, and physical therapy.

RELEVANT ANATOMY

An understanding of the anatomy of the AC joint is essential for the classification of injuries of this joint (Fig. 50–2). The distal clavicle is stabilized in the anteroposterior direction by the AC ligament, which is actually a capsule that is reinforced with thickenings (ligaments). The distal clavicle is stabilized in the vertical direction by the coracoclavicular (CC) ligaments (which are actually two distinct structures—a cone-shaped ligament and a broad trapezoid ligament). The coracoacromial (CA) ligament's function is widely debated; it has been implicated as a source of impingement, and it may have a role in restraining superior migration of the humeral head. Its utility in the management of AC injuries, however, is as a ligament substitute; when transferred to the end of a recessed distal clavicle, it functions as a CC ligament.

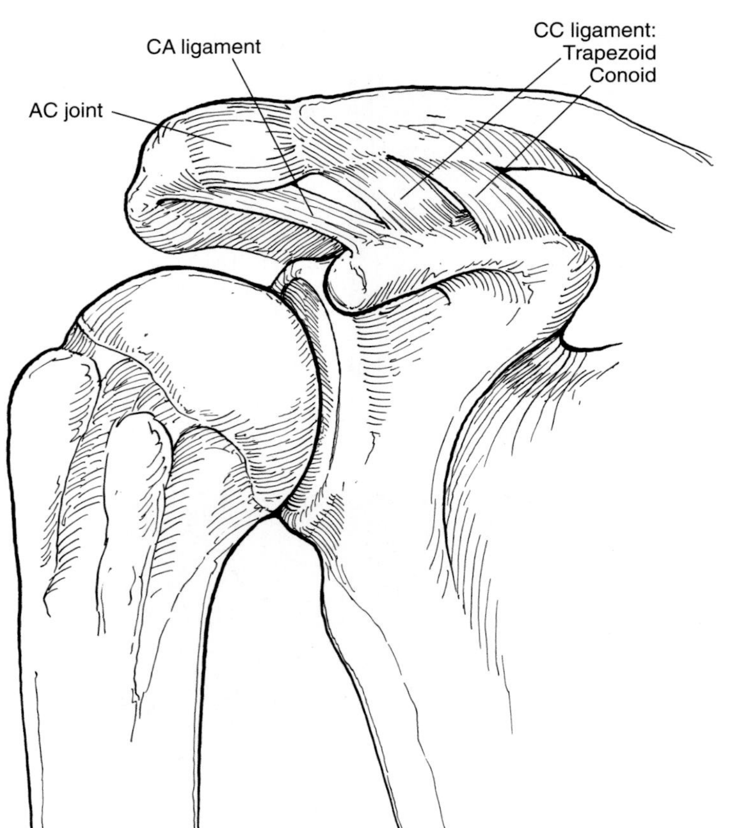

FIGURE 50–2. Normal anatomy of the acromioclavicular joint. AC, acromioclavicular; CA, coracoacromial; CC, coracoclavicular.

CLASSIFICATION OF ACROMIOCLAVICULAR INJURIES

Distal Clavicle Fractures

Distal clavicle fractures have been classified into five types, based on the location of the fracture(s) in relation to the coracoclavicular ligaments (Fig. 50–3). Typically, types II and V require operative intervention.

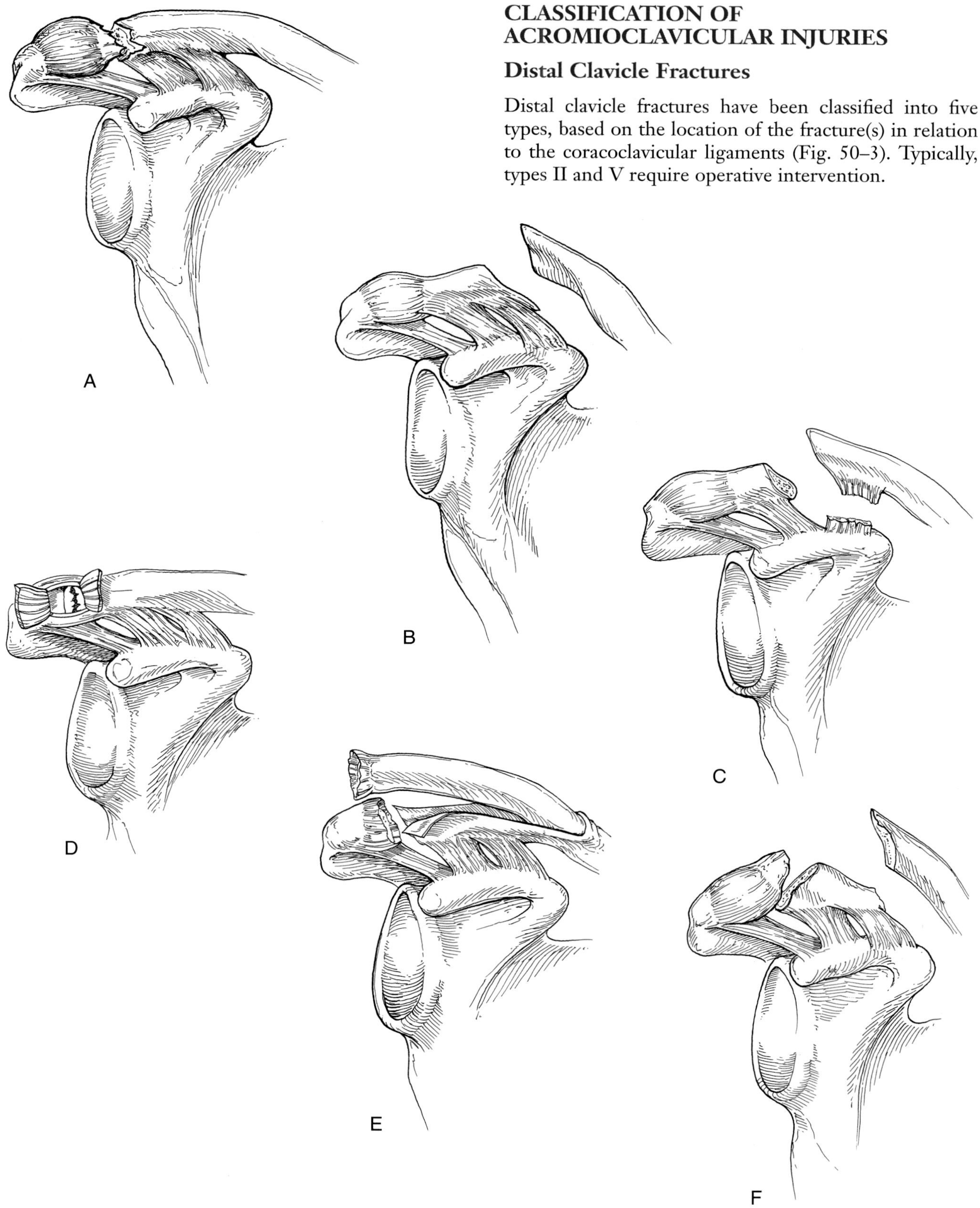

FIGURE 50–3. Classification of distal clavicle fractures. *A*, Type I, lateral to the coracoclavicular ligaments. *B*, Type IIA, medial to coracoclavicular ligaments. *C*, Type IIB, between the coracoclavicular ligaments. *D*, Type III, lateral to the coracoclavicular ligaments and extra-articular. *E*, Type IV, periosteal sleeve fracture (also can occur in young adults). *F*, Type V, segmental fracture with intact coracoclavicular ligaments but displaced medial and lateral fragments.

Acromioclavicular Separations

AC separations have been classified into six different types, based on the degree of displacement and the location of the distal clavicle (Fig. 50–4). The difference between a type III injury and a type V separation is based on the CC distance as compared with the opposite side. Type V separations are displaced by more than 100% on the opposite side. Again, type IV injuries are best visualized on an axillary lateral radiograph. Type IV injuries are so unusual that some authors question their existence.

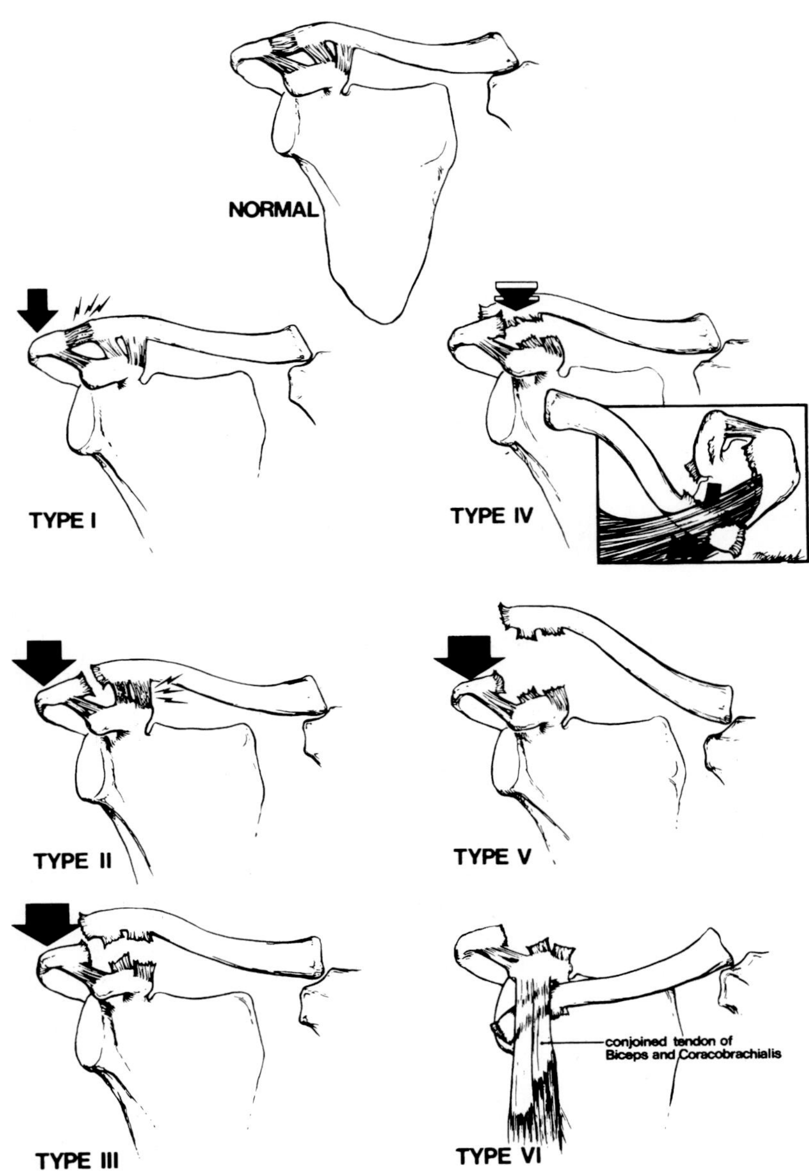

FIGURE 50–4. Classification of acromioclavicular separations. (From Rockwood CA Jr, Williams GR Jr, Young DC: Disorders of the acromioclavicular joint. In Rockwood CA Jr, Matsen FA III [eds]: The Shoulder. Philadelphia, WB Saunders, 1998, p 495.)

SURGICAL *TECHNIQUE*

Indications

Distal clavicle fractures: Although no consensus has been reached, most authors recommend operative stabilization for acute type II and V injuries and for chronic, painful type III fractures.

Acromioclavicular separations: Again, there is some controversy regarding the treatment of both type III and type IV AC separations. Most authors recommend initial nonoperative treatment of type III injuries, then consider late reconstruction (Weaver-Dunn procedure) if these become symptomatic later. Recent evidence suggests that at least some type IV separations can be reduced closed (with anterior to posterior traction applied to the acromion of both shoulders). Types V and VI separations, as well as those type IV injuries that cannot be reduced, should be treated operatively.

Distal clavicle osteolysis: Operative treatment (open or arthroscopic distal clavicle resection) should be considered for patients who have failed extended nonoperative management.

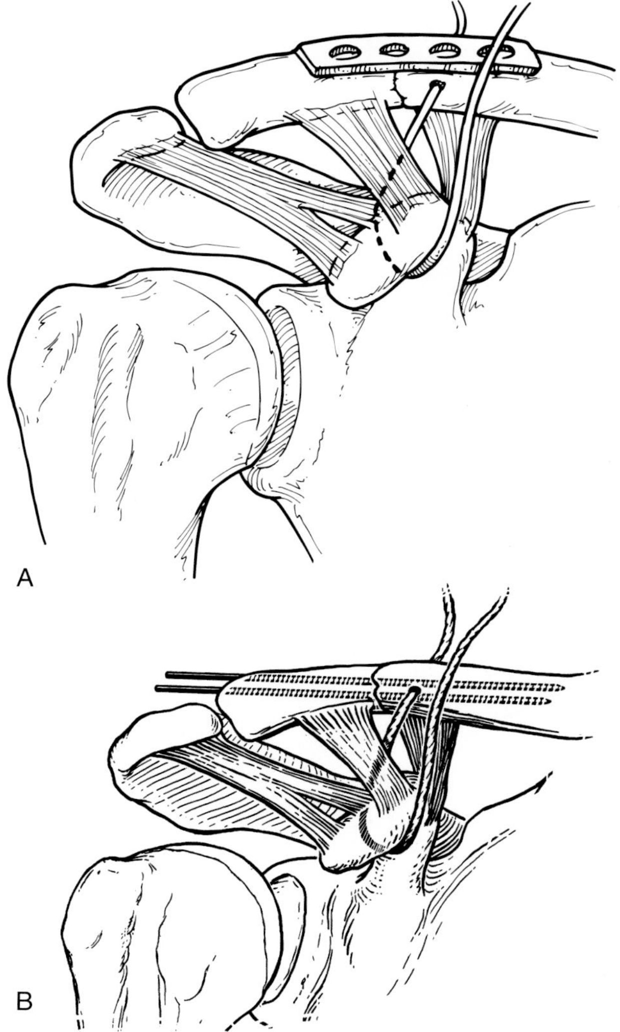

Technique

Open Reduction and Internal Fixation of Distal Clavicle Fracture

1. Positioning: Following successful administration of anesthesia, the patient is placed in a beach-chair position, and the shoulder is prepped and draped. Special care should be taken to ensure that medial exposure is possible.
2. Incision: A 5- to 7-cm incision is made directly over the fracture in Langer's line. If additional exposure is required, the incision can be made directly over the clavicle.
3. Exposure: The deltotrapezial fascia is carefully dissected off the clavicle subperiostally. The ends of the fracture are exposed and débrided.
4. Reduction: The fracture is reduced and stabilized. A variety of internal fixation approaches are possible. Interfragmentary screws, plates, intramedullary pins (from the acromion to the clavicle), and various coracoclavicular stabilization techniques should be considered, based on the character of the injury (Fig. 50–5).
5. Closure: The deltotrapezial fracture is carefully reapproximated with heavy nonabsorbable sutures. Subcutaneous tissues and skin are closed in the standard fashion.

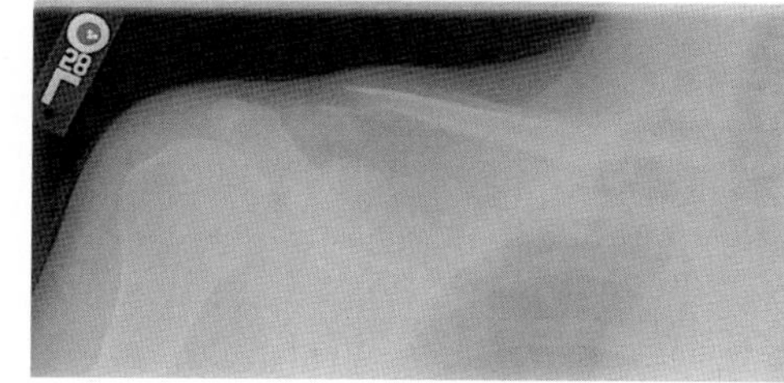

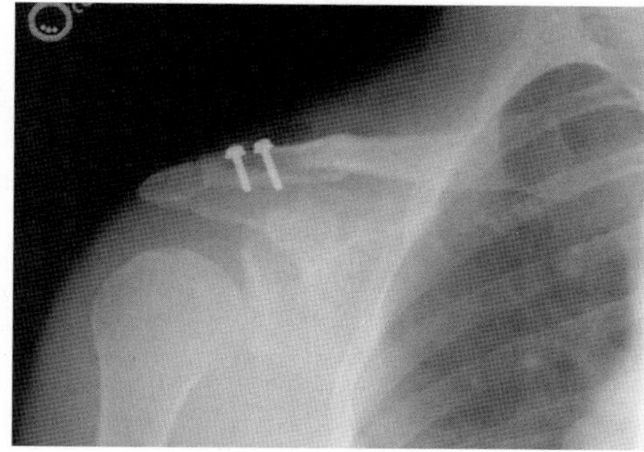

FIGURE 50–5. *A*, Fixation of a distal clavicle fracture using a plate and cable. *B*, Fixation of a distal clavicle fracture using K-wires and a cable. *C* and *D*, Radiographs of primary open reduction and internal fixation of a distal clavicle fracture *(C)* with interfragmentary screws and a cable *(D)*. (*A* redrawn from and *B* from Schlegel TF, Hawkins RJ: Management of distal clavicle fractures. Op Tech Sports Med 5:93–99, 1997.)

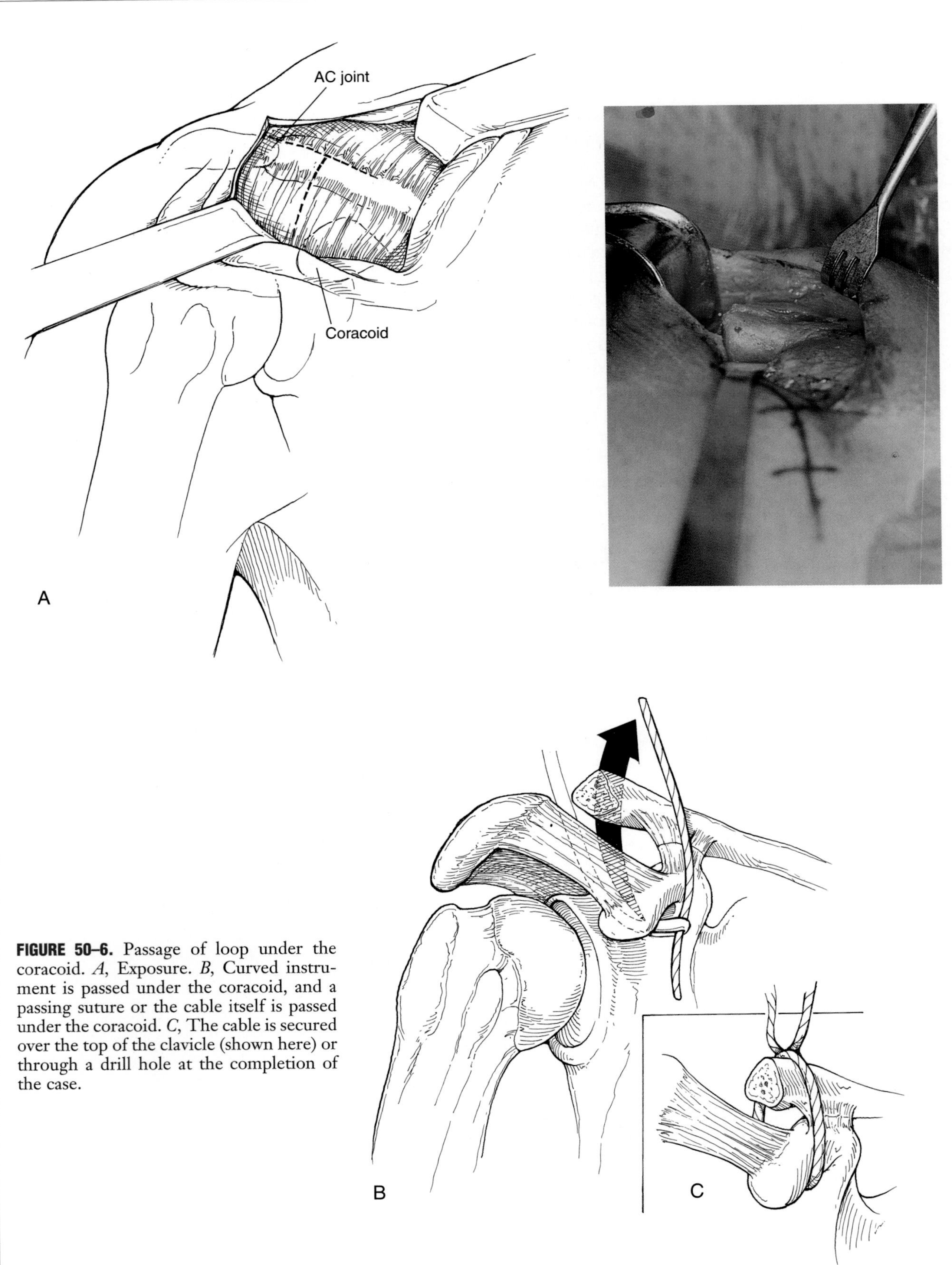

FIGURE 50–6. Passage of loop under the coracoid. *A*, Exposure. *B*, Curved instrument is passed under the coracoid, and a passing suture or the cable itself is passed under the coracoid. *C*, The cable is secured over the top of the clavicle (shown here) or through a drill hole at the completion of the case.

Acute Repair of Acromioclavicular Separation

1. Positioning/incision/exposure—similar to above: If CC fixation is planned, the coracoid is exposed by blunt dissection; then a loop is placed under the coracoid with any of a variety of curved instruments (Fig. 50–6).
2. CC ligament repair: Although it may be difficult to anatomically restore these ligaments, the torn ends are reapproximated with the use of heavy suture (Fig. 50–7).

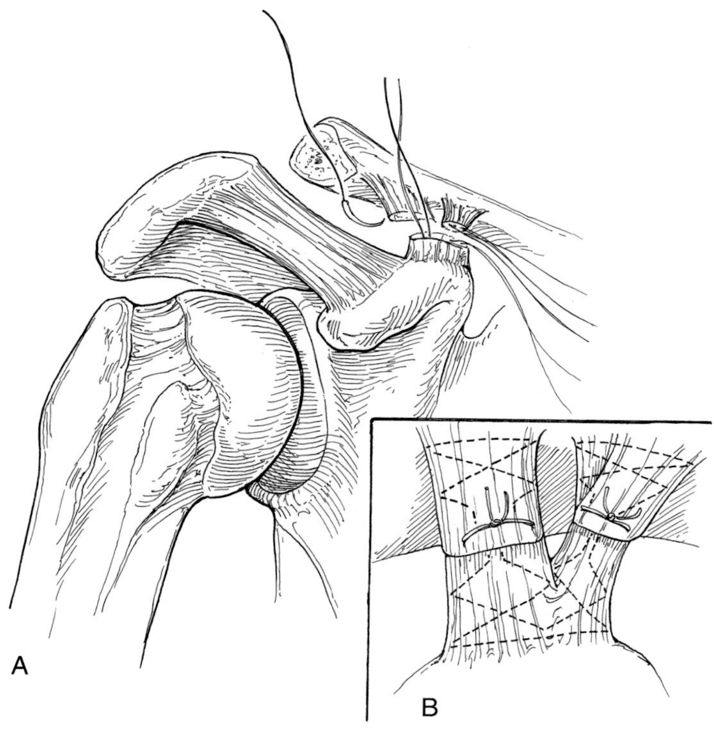

FIGURE 50–7. Repair of coracoclavicular ligament. *A*, Exposure. *B*, Repair.

3. Temporary CC stabilization: The clavicle is reduced in its anatomic position (the AC joint can easily be palpated) and is secured with a variety of fixation devices. A coracoclavicular (modified Bosworth) screw, popularized by Rockwood, can be used; however, it must be removed at some later date. Alternatively, a loop of braided absorbable suture provides excellent fixation, and no removal is required. The fixation "cable" (as described separately by Warren, Hawkins, and Warner) is prepared on the back table using nine strands of No. 1 polydioxanone (PDS) suture braided into three groups of three sutures each, which in turn are braided into one cable (Fig. 50–8). The cable is passed under the coracoid, then around or through a drill hole in the clavicle; it is then secured with several knots (Fig. 50–9).
4. Closure: The wound is irrigated and closed as described earlier, with meticulous regard for reapproximation of the deltotrapezial fascia. Several nonabsorbable sutures are used to repair the AC ligaments/capsule.

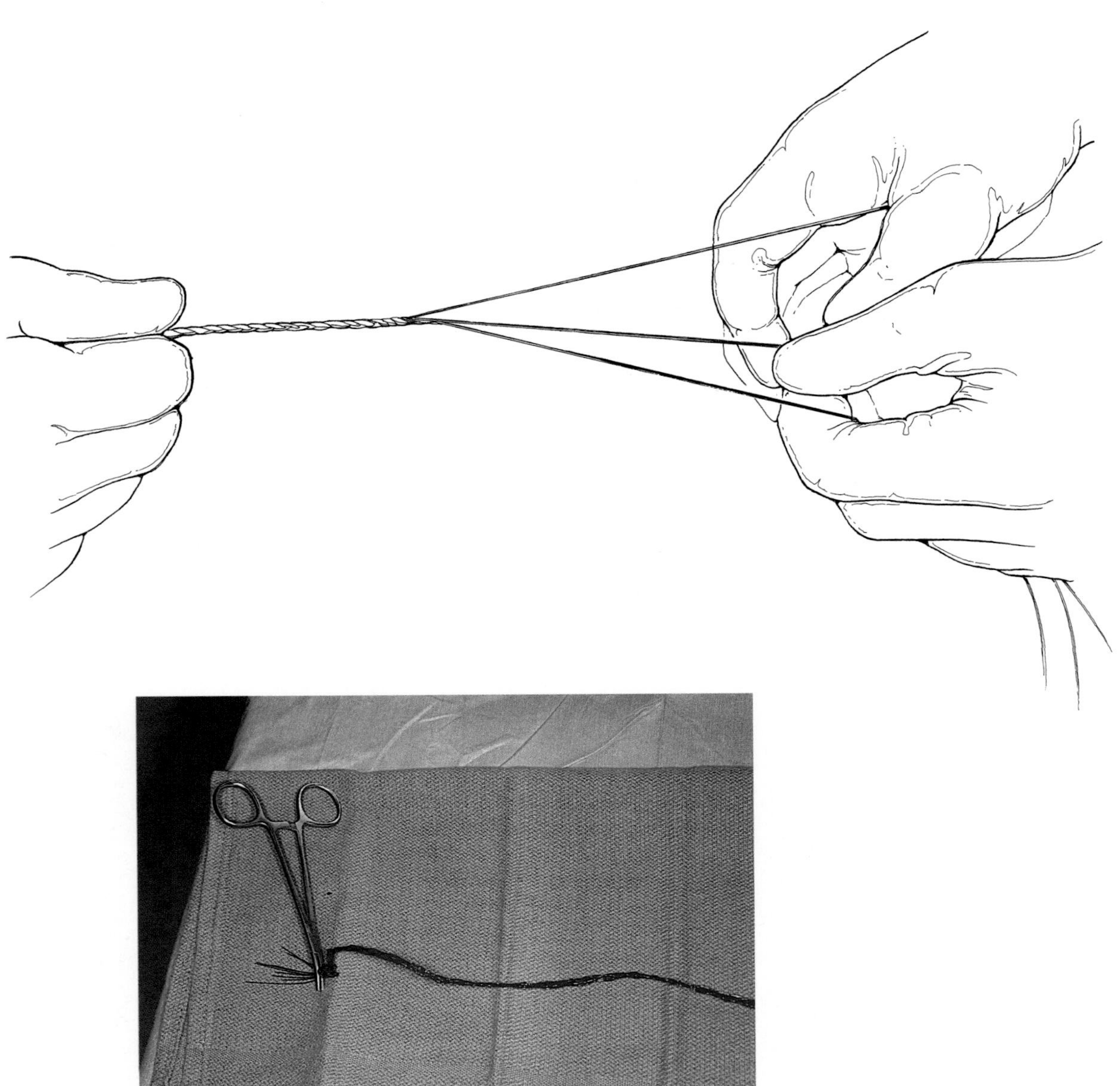

FIGURE 50–8. Fixation cable is made using nine strands of number 1 PDS suture (shown here) or Panacryl suture (which we now prefer). Three groups of three braided sutures are braided together to make the cable *(inset)*.

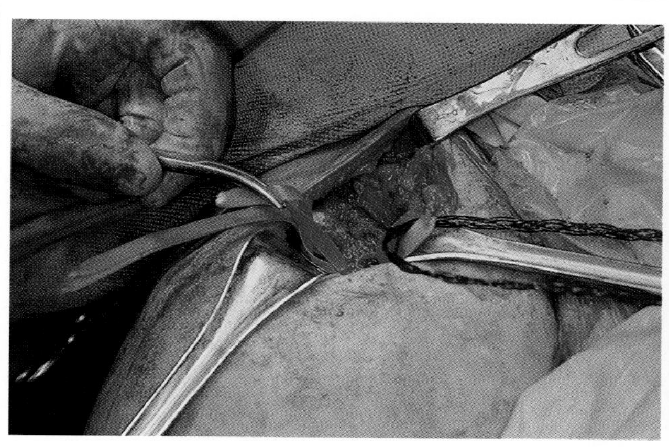
A

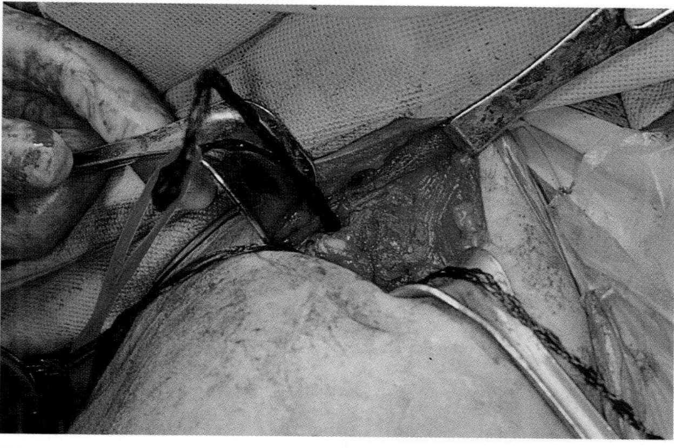
B

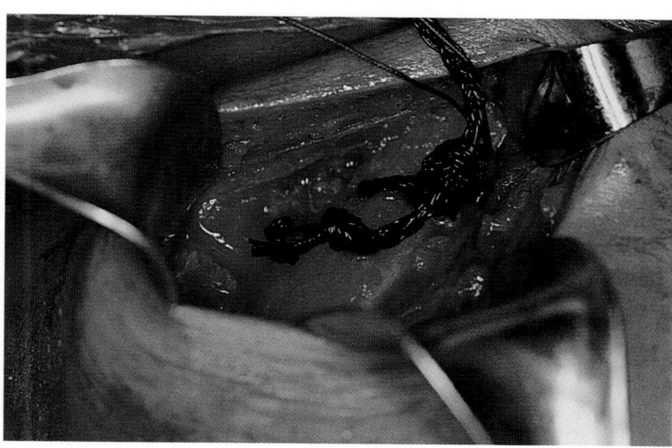
C

FIGURE 50–9. Securing of the cable. Cable is passed under the coracoid *(A)*, retrieved *(B)*, and secured on top of the clavicle *(C)* or through a drill hole.

Long-term Reconstruction of Acromioclavicular Separations (Modified Weaver-Dunn Procedure)

1. Positioning/incision/exposure—discussed earlier: It is also necessary that the CA ligament be exposed. The deep deltoid muscle fibers are bluntly dissected off the ligament, a Bunnell-type suture is placed into it, and it is mobilized for transfer.
2. Distal clavicle resection: Approximately 1 cm of the distal clavicle is excised with an oscillating saw or an osteotome (Fig. 50–10). Holes are drilled from the superior surface of the clavicle into the intramedullary canal so that the sutures can be accepted from the CA ligament.
3. Temporary CA stabilization: The clavicle is reduced in its anatomic position (an intraoperative radiograph is sometimes useful to determine the ideal height), and it is secured as described earlier.
4. CA ligament transfer: The mobilized CA ligament is transferred into the end of the clavicle with a suture passer or looped 24-gauge wire. The sutures are secured on the superior surface of the clavicle, thus restoring tension to the ligament (Fig. 50–11).
5. Closure: The wound is irrigated and closed as described earlier, with meticulous regard for reapproximation of the deltotrapezial fascia.

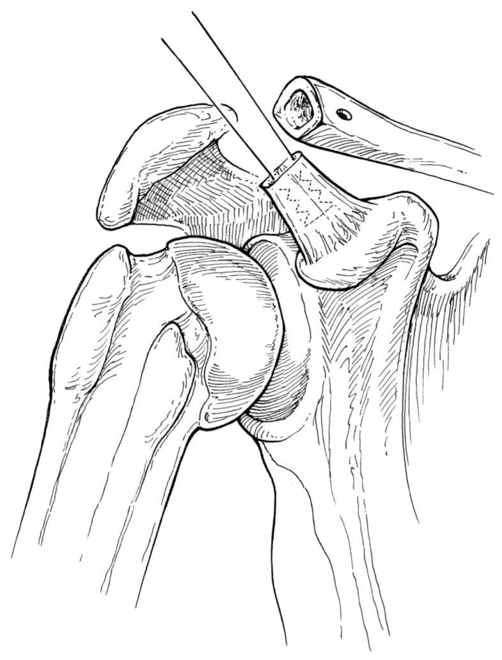

FIGURE 50–10. Mobilization of the coracoacromial ligament and distal clavicle resection.

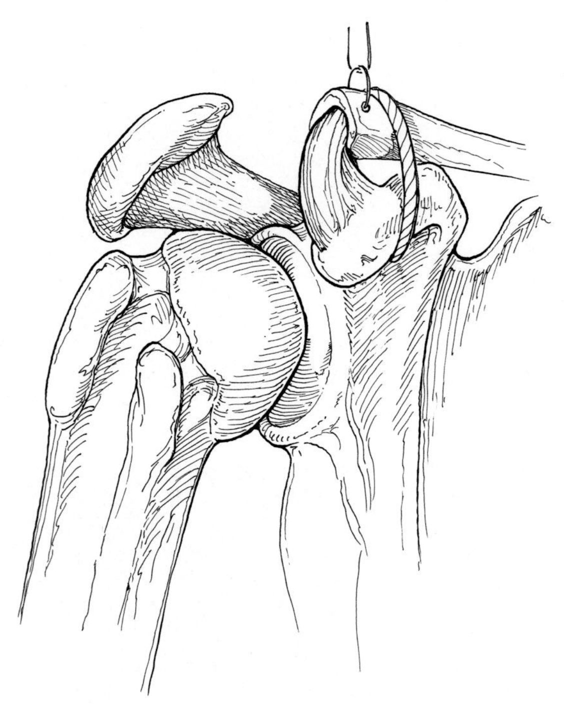

FIGURE 50–11. The coracoacromial ligament is transferred into the intramedullary canal of the clavicle, and sutures are tied over the superior cortex. A cable is used for reinforcement.

Open Distal Clavicle Resection (Mumford)

1. Positioning: The patient is placed in a beach-chair position and is prepped and draped.
2. Incision: A 3-cm incision is made just medial to the AC joint. If an arthroscopic portal was used, this can be extended posteriorly.
3. Exposure: The deltotrapezial fascia is subperiostally dissected, thereby exposing the distal clavicle. The dissection is carried all the way around the clavicle, and the AC joint is exposed.
4. Distal clavicle resection: With the use of a saw, osteotome, or burr, approximately 1 cm of distal clavicle is excised. The exposed surface is palpated for any remaining osteophytes, sharp edges, or spurs, which are removed with a burr or rasp.
5. Closure: The wound is closed, as described earlier.

Arthroscopic Distal Clavicle Resection

1. Positioning/prepping/diagnostic arthroscopy: This is accomplished as described in Chapter 46. An acromioplasty is often accomplished concurrently.
2. Distal clavicle resection: With the use of an arthroscopic burr and a variety of portals, the distal clavicle is resected, beginning at the acromioclavicular joint. Electrocautery is used liberally to control hemostasis. The arthroscope is placed in the lateral portal; it can be placed in the anterior portal periodically to assess the amount of resection (Fig. 50–12).

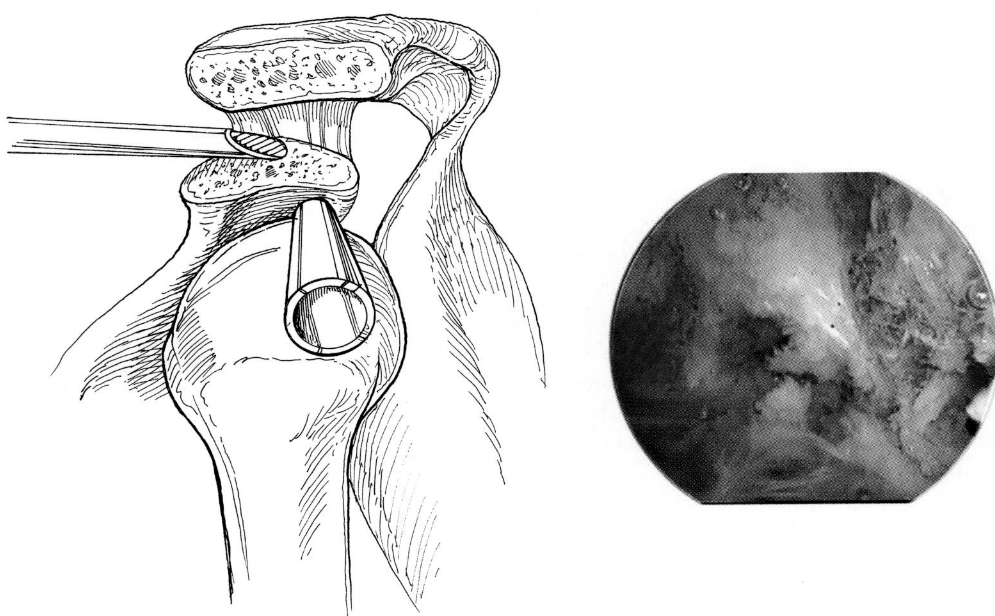

FIGURE 50–12. Arthroscopic distal clavicle resection. *A*, Arthroscope is placed in the lateral portal, and a burr is used for distal clavicle resection from the anterior portal. *B*, Arthroscopic view from anterior portal shows distal clavicle resection. (*B* courtesy of Brian J. Cole, MD.)

POSTOPERATIVE MANAGEMENT

Depending on the stability of the fixation, early motion should be encouraged. A brief period in a sling or immobilizer is followed by several weeks of passive motion. Active motion and strengthening should then be initiated until strength and function are regained.

COMPLICATIONS

In addition to complications that can occur with any procedure (e.g., bleeding, infection), perhaps the biggest concern with the management of AC injuries is recurrent instability. Treatment of this problem must be individualized.

RESULTS

In several series, surgical results are very encouraging. Restoration of normal anatomy results in successful outcomes.

REFERENCES

Lemos MJ: Current concepts. The evaluation and treatment of the injured acromioclavicular joint in athletes. Am J Sports Med 26:145–149, 1998.

Nuberg W, Bowen MK: Acromioclavicular joint injuries and distal clavicle fractures. J Am Acad Orthop Surg 5:11–18, 1997.

Richards RR: Acromioclavicular joint injuries. Instr Course Lect 42:259–269, 1993.

Rockwood CA Jr, Williams GR, Young DC: Injuries to the acromioclavicular joint. In Rockwood CA Jr, Green DP, Bucholz RW (eds): Rockwood and Green's Fractures in Adults, 3rd ed. Philadelphia, JB Lippincott, 1991, pp 1181–1251.

Slawski DP, Cahill BR: Atraumatic osteolysis of the distal clavicle: Results of open surgical excision. Am J Sports Med 22:267–271, 1994.

Snyder SJ, Banas MP, Karzel RP: The arthroscopic Mumford procedure: An analysis of results. Arthroscopy 11:157–164, 1995.

Weaver JK, Dunn HK: Treatment of acromioclavicular injuries; especially complete acromioclavicular separation. J Bone Joint Surg [Am] 54:1187–1197, 1972.

CHAPTER 51

Treatment of Sternoclavicular Injuries

INTRODUCTION

Sternoclavicular injuries are rare, and sternoclavicular injuries that require surgery are even rarer. It is for good reason that most surgeons consider surgery for sternoclavicular injuries with much trepidation. Sternoclavicular instability accounts for less than 3% of all shoulder instabilities, with anterior instability much more common than posterior instability. Instability can be classified based on its cause (e.g., traumatic vs nontraumatic), direction, degree, and chronicity.

HISTORY AND PHYSICAL EXAMINATION

Anterior instability may result from a direct blow or, more commonly, from an anterior blow to the clavicle. Posterior instability is usually the result of a direct blow, most commonly from motor vehicle accidents. Acutely, patients may present with the arm held closely to the side. Patients with anterior dislocation may note a prominence over the joint. Posterior dislocation is less obvious on inspection because swelling obscures any depression. Patients with posterior dislocation are at serious risk for vascular or tracheal injuries, and any signs of these necessitate emergent treatment.

DIAGNOSTIC IMAGING

Plain radiographs usually are not helpful. Special views, including the Hobbs and serendipity views, have been described, but the diagnosis, especially with posterior dislocations, is best made with computed tomography (Fig. 51–1).

NONOPERATIVE MANAGEMENT

Most anterior dislocations can be treated with simple observation. Severe anterior dislocations can be treated with closed reduction. The patient is placed supine with a sandbag between the scapulae; traction is placed on the affected abducted arm, and direct pressure is applied over the medial clavicle. Usually, the patient is then placed into a figure-eight brace for 4 weeks. Posterior dislocations can have disastrous consequences and may require emergent reduction. This can be accomplished with longitudinal arm traction that attempts to elevate the clavicle medially; a sterile towel clip may be needed to grasp and reduce the medial clavicle. Following reduction, recurrent posterior instability is unusual.

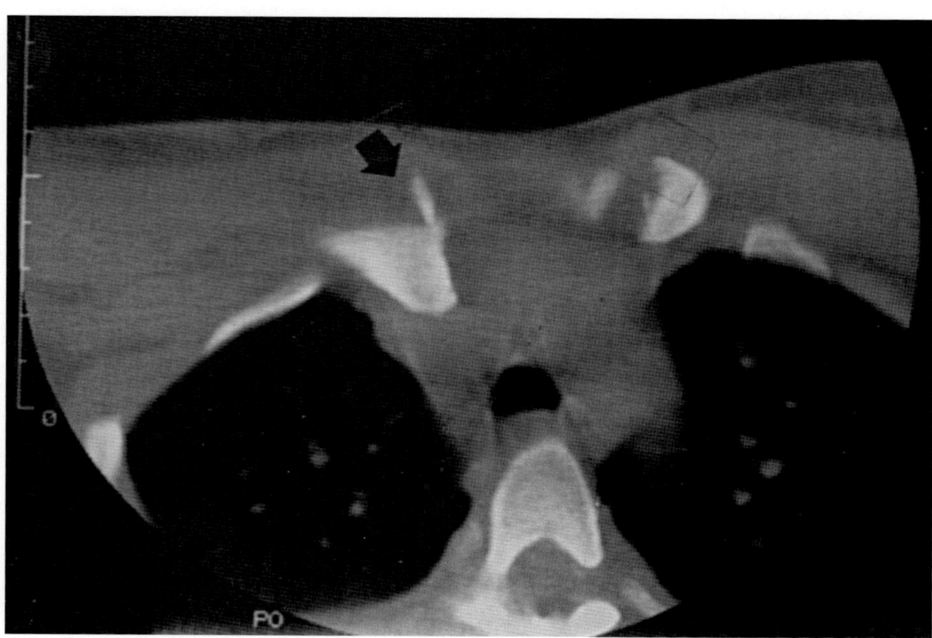

FIGURE 51–1. CT scan of patient with posterior dislocation of the left sternoclavicular joint *(arrow)*. Note normal sternoclavicular joint on the opposite side. (From Miller ME, Ada JR: Injuries to the shoulder girdle: Fractures of the scapula, clavicle, and glenoid. In Browner BD, Jupiter JB, Levine AM, Trafton PG [eds]: Skeletal Trauma, 2nd ed. Philadelphia, WB Saunders, 1998, pp 1657–1670.)

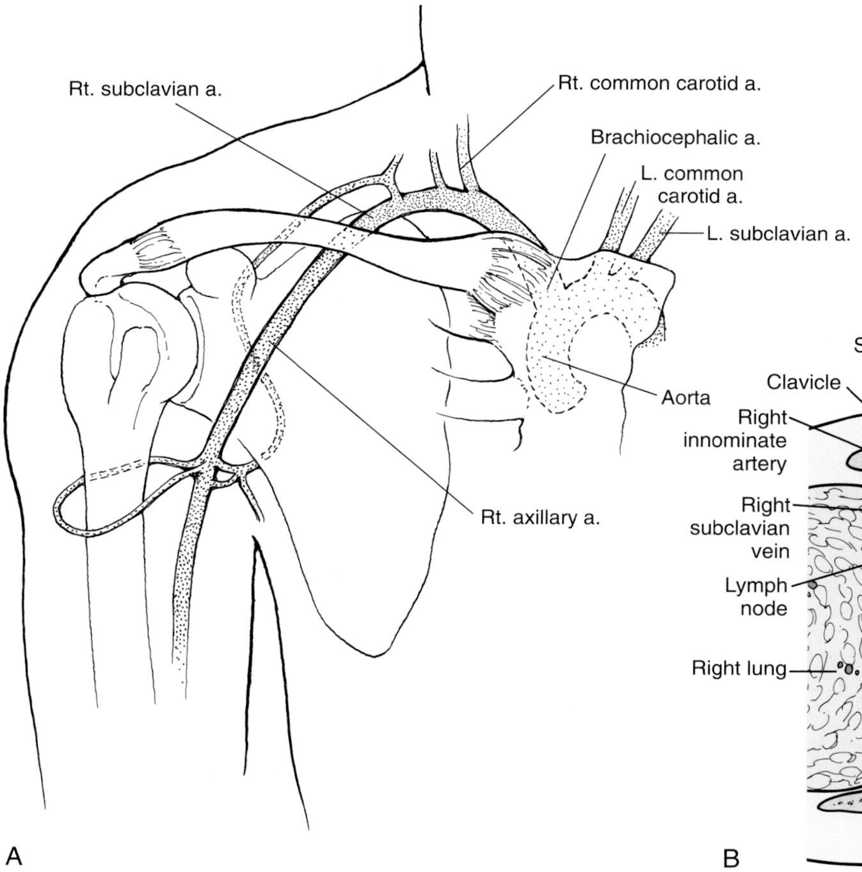

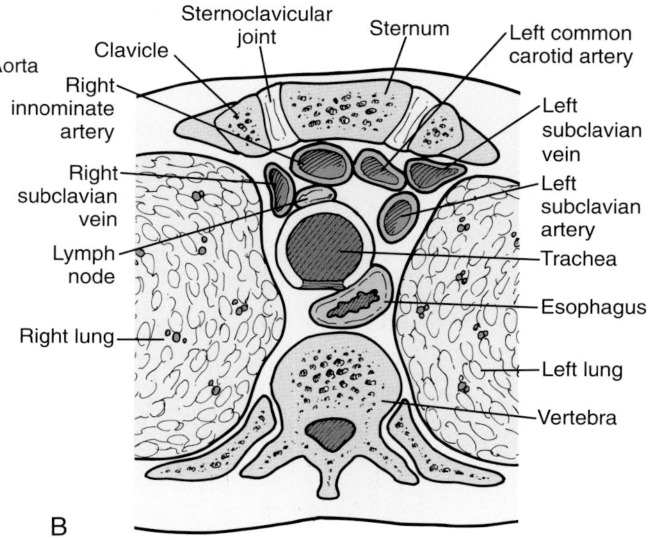

FIGURE 51–2. Relationship of the sternoclavicular joints to the underlying great vessels and other vital structures. *A*, Frontal view. *B*, Cross-sectional view. (*B* Redrawn from Rockwood CA Jr, Wirth MA: Disorders of the sternoclavicular joint. In Rockwood CA Jr, Matsen FA III [eds]: The Shoulder, 2nd ed. Philadelphia, WB Saunders, 1998, pp 555–609.)

RELEVANT ANATOMY

The great vessels lie directly behind the sternoclavicular joint (Fig. 51–2). Additionally, a great deal of rotational motion occurs at the sternoclavicular joint. This has been implicated as a factor in hardware migration and its disastrous consequences during attempted stabilization of the joint. The joint is composed of capsular ligaments, costoclavicular ligaments (like the coracoclavicular ligament, these are thought to be the most important stabilizing structures), and an intervening interarticular disk (Fig. 51–3). Finally, the medial clavicle is one of the last physes to fuse, and physeal injuries can occur in patients up to 25 years old. Injuries in these younger patients can often be treated less aggressively because of the tremendous remodeling potential.

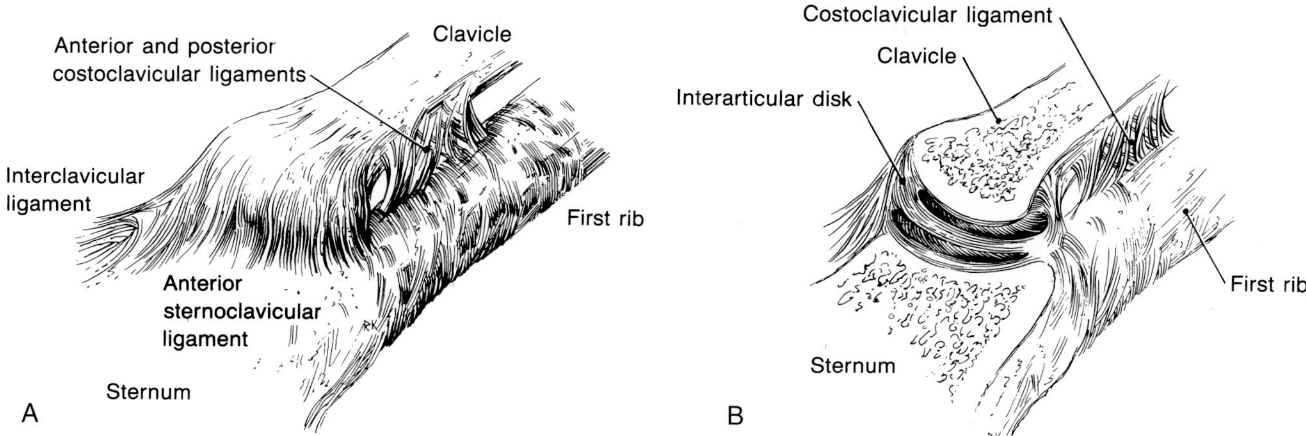

FIGURE 51–3. Ligaments and structures of the sternoclavicular joint. *A*, Ligaments. Note the location and structure of the costoclavicular ligaments, thought to be the main stabilizer of the joint. *B*, Cross-sectional view shows the presence of an interarticular disk. (From Jobe CM: Gross anatomy of the shoulder. In Rockwood CA Jr, Matsen FA III [eds]: The Shoulder, 2nd ed. Philadelphia, WB Saunders, 1998, pp 34–97.)

SURGICAL *TECHNIQUE*

Indications

Although there is some controversy, most authors do not recommend open treatment for acute anterior sternoclavicular injuries. Posterior dislocations that cannot be reduced closed may require open reduction. Open management for recurrent or chronic anterior dislocations should be considered only in patients with intractable pain or loss of function.

Technique

Although a variety of reconstructive procedures have been described, most authors recommend simple open reduction for acute posterior dislocations (without hardware), as well as excision of the medial clavicle with or without reconstruction of the costoclavicular ligament for both anterior and posterior chronic or recurrent dislocations.

Excision of the Medial Clavicle (Fig. 51–4)

1. Incision: A 5-cm transverse incision is made over the affected joint.
2. Exposure: The joint is exposed, and the costoclavicular ligaments are identified. The joint is dissected, and retractors are carefully placed to protect the posterior structures.

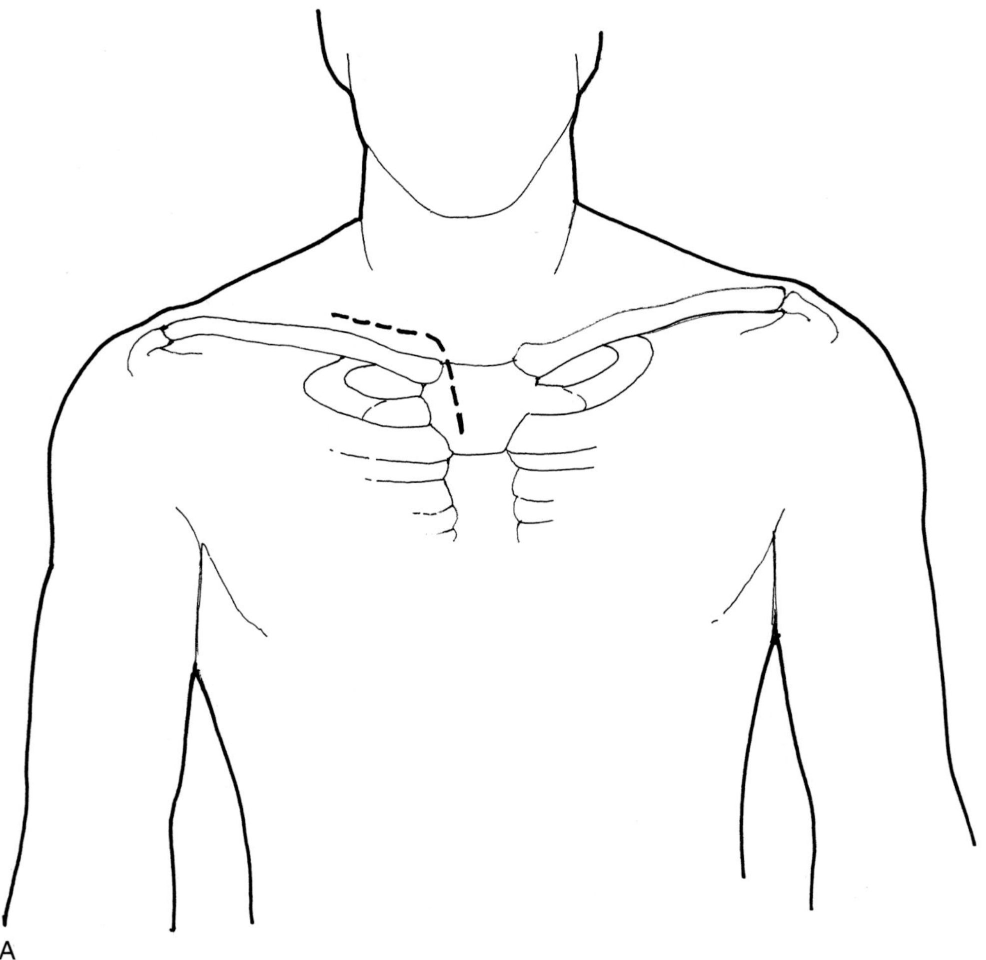

FIGURE 51–4. Resection of the medial clavicle. *A*, A 5-cm incision is made over the sternoclavicular joint.

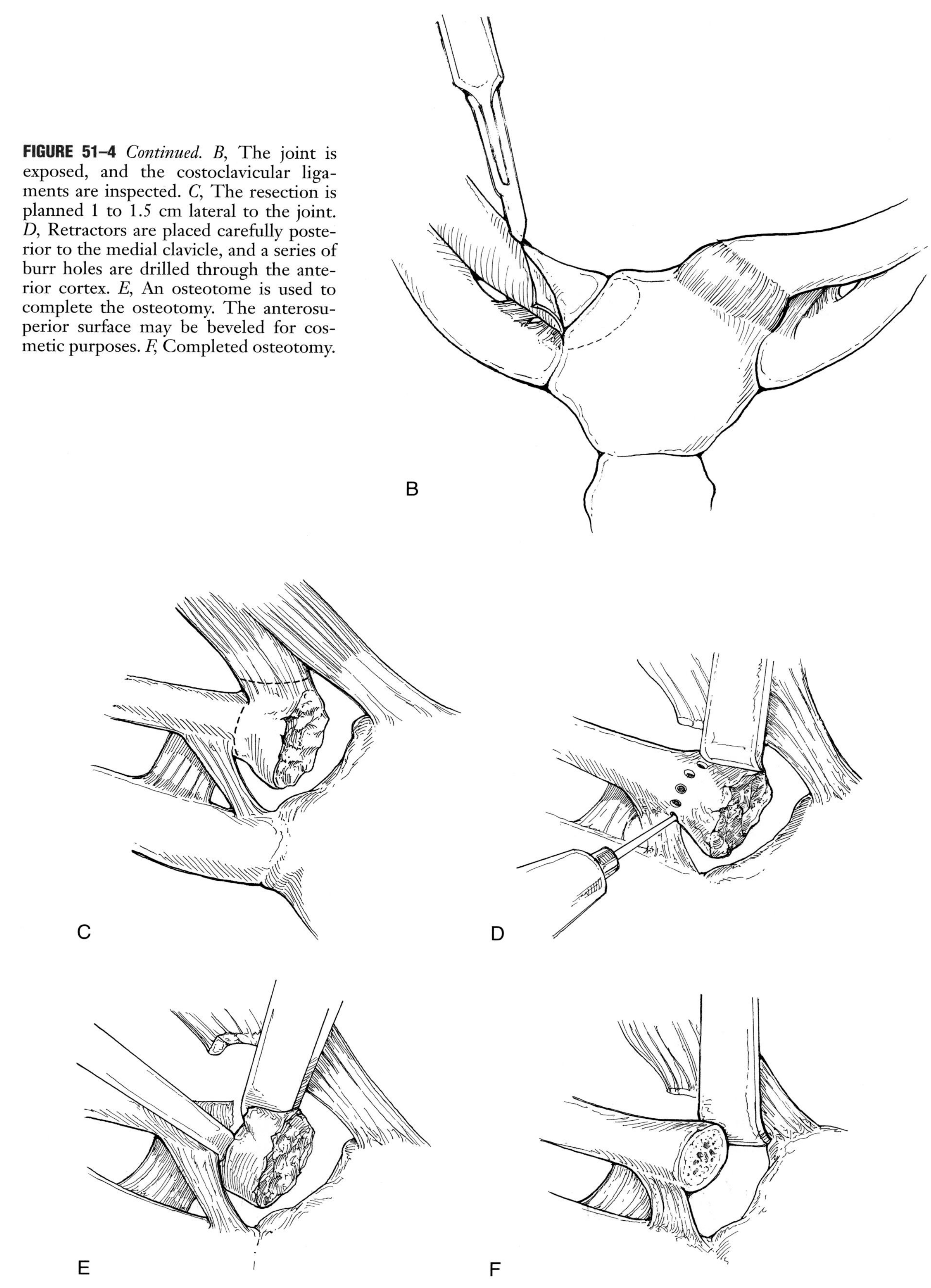

FIGURE 51–4 *Continued. B*, The joint is exposed, and the costoclavicular ligaments are inspected. *C*, The resection is planned 1 to 1.5 cm lateral to the joint. *D*, Retractors are placed carefully posterior to the medial clavicle, and a series of burr holes are drilled through the anterior cortex. *E*, An osteotome is used to complete the osteotomy. The anterosuperior surface may be beveled for cosmetic purposes. *F*, Completed osteotomy.

3. Osteotomy: One to 1½ cm of the medial clavicle is osteotomized. Some surgeons recommend burring several holes in the anterior cortex to outline the resection before using an osteotome.

Costoclavicular Ligament Reconstruction (Fig. 51–5)

If the costoclavicular ligaments are torn and irreparable, they can be reconstructed with the use of the subclavius tendon or a strip of fascia or tendon.

4. Wounds are closed in standard fashion: The periosteum is carefully reapproximated over the joint, especially in younger patients.

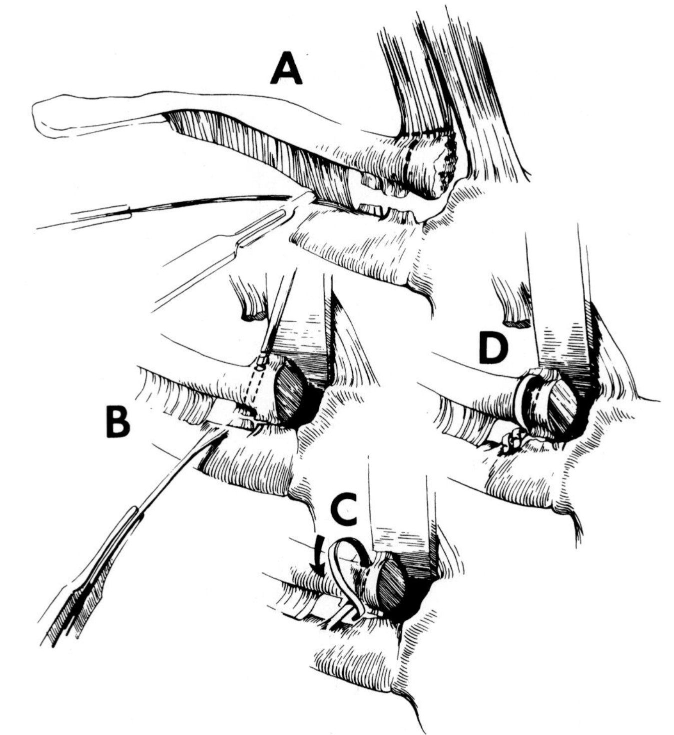

FIGURE 51–5. Technique described by Burrows for reconstruction of the costoclavicular ligaments. A, The subclavius tendon is freed from its muscle fibers that insert superiorly. B, A drill hole is placed from superior to inferior approximately 1 cm lateral to the resected clavicle. C, The tendon is woven through the drill holes. D, Completed reconstruction. (From Rockwood CA Jr, Wirth MA: Disorders of the sternoclavicular joint. In Rockwood CA Jr, Matsen FA III [eds]: The Shoulder, 2nd ed. Philadelphia, WB Saunders, 1998, pp 555–609.)

POSTOPERATIVE MANAGEMENT

A sling is used for 2 to 3 weeks. Passive motion is quickly instituted, followed by active motion and strengthening.

COMPLICATIONS

The most disastrous complication that occurs with treatment of these injuries is vascular injury or injury to other midline structures such as the trachea and esophagus. The use of pins and hardware is strongly discouraged around the sternoclavicular joint. Most authors recommend that a cardiothoracic surgeon be involved in the operative management of these cases.

RESULTS

As was indicated earlier, most patients do well with nonoperative treatment. Surgical treatment that consists of medial clavicle resection with or without costoclavicular stabilization has been successful in several series.

REFERENCES

Burrows HJ: Tenodesis of subclavius in treatment of recurrent dislocation of the sternoclavicular joint. J Bone Joint Surg [Br] 33:240, 1951.

Rockwood CA Jr, Wirth MA: Disorders of the sternoclavicular joint. In Rockwood CA Jr, Matsen FA III (eds): The Shoulder, 2nd ed. Philadelphia, WB Saunders, 1998, pp 555–609.

Warren RF: The acromioclavicular and sternoclavicular joints. In Evarts CM (ed): Surgery of the Musculoskeletal System, 2nd ed. New York, Churchill Livingstone, 1990, p 1519.

Wirth MA, Rockwood CA Jr: Acute and chronic traumatic injuries of the sternoclavicular joint. J Am Acad Orthop Surg 4:268–278, 1996.

CHAPTER 52

Treatment of Malunion and Nonunion of Clavicle Fractures

INTRODUCTION

Most clavicle fractures, with the exception of some distal clavicle fractures discussed in Chapter 50, heal with no sequelae. Occasionally, however, this is not the case, and these fractures require open reduction and internal fixation with bone grafting.

HISTORY AND PHYSICAL EXAMINATION

The acute presentation of clavicular fractures is fairly obvious. Patients relate a history of trauma (direct or indirect—a fall onto outstretched hand), pain, and usually a deformity. Most of these fractures are successfully treated closed. Occasionally (less than 5% of the time), nonunion can occur. Up to 75% of these patients develop symptoms—pain, crepitation, posture-related problems, or neurovascular symptoms. Physical examination may reveal crepitus, restricted motion, or neurovascular findings.

DIAGNOSTIC IMAGING

Standard anteroposterior (AP) views can be supplemented with a 45° cephalic tilt view (Fig. 52–1). In cases of nonunion, CT scans can be helpful.

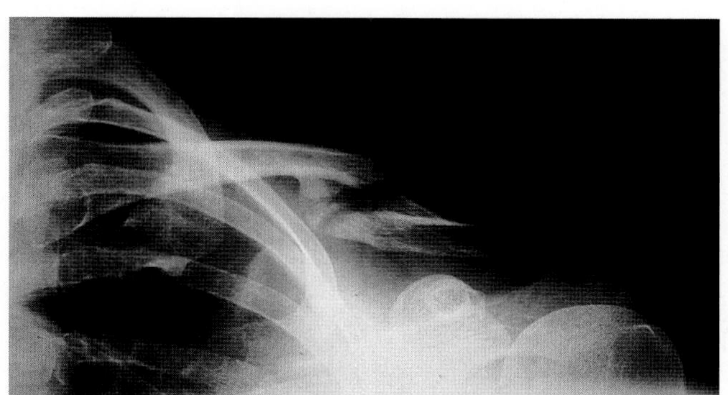

FIGURE 52–1. A 45° cephalic tilt view of a clavicle nonunion.

NONOPERATIVE MANAGEMENT

For acute injuries, unless the fracture is open, is a type II distal fracture, or is associated with other injuries (e.g., "floating shoulder"), treatment of most clavicle fractures is nonoperative. Asymptomatic nonunions should also be treated nonoperatively.

RELEVANT ANATOMY

The clavicle forms an S-shaped double curve when viewed superiorly, and its cross section is variable (Fig. 52–2). It has secure fixation laterally (acromioclavicular joint) and medially (sternoclavicular joint). The brachial plexus and the great vessels are immediately posterior to the medial clavicle. The clavicle is subcutaneous and serves as an attachment for the deltoid and trapezius muscles.

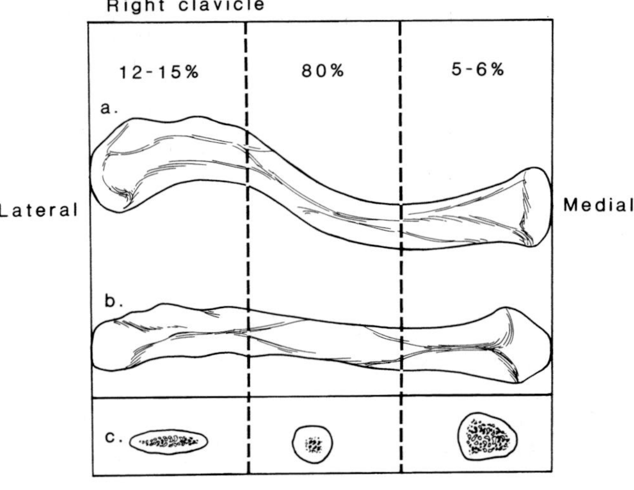

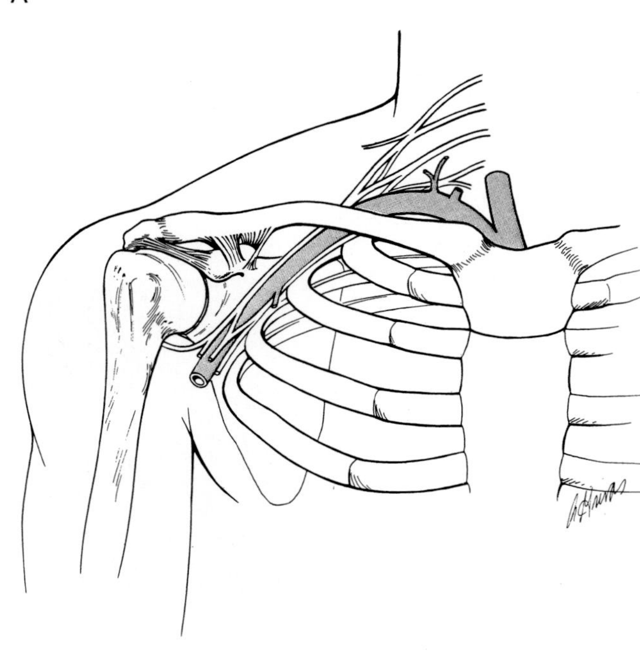

FIGURE 52–2. Anatomy of the clavicle. *A*, Viewed from superiorly, the clavicle makes a double S curve. Viewed from the front, it appears straight. Cross sections vary throughout the clavicle. *B*, The clavicle is anchored by the acromioclavicular joint laterally and the sternoclavicular joint medially. The brachial plexus and greater vessels are just inferior to the medial clavicle. (From Craig EV: Fractures of the clavicle. In Rockwood CA Jr, Matsen FA III [eds]: The Shoulder, 2nd ed. Philadelphia, WB Saunders, 1998, pp 428–482.)

SURGICAL *TECHNIQUE*

Indications

Surgery is recommended for symptomatic nonunion or malunion that has failed nonoperative management.

Technique

1. Positioning: The patient is placed in a low beach-chair position and is prepped and draped in the standard fashion. It is critical that the entire clavicle can be accessed; therefore, the preparation must extend past the midline.
2. Incision: A horizontal incision is made along the superior border of the clavicle. The deltotrapezial interval is identified and the clavicle is exposed subperiosteally (Fig. 52–3).

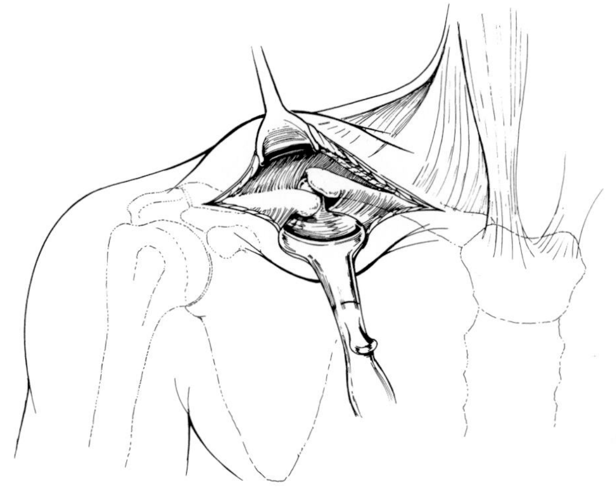

A

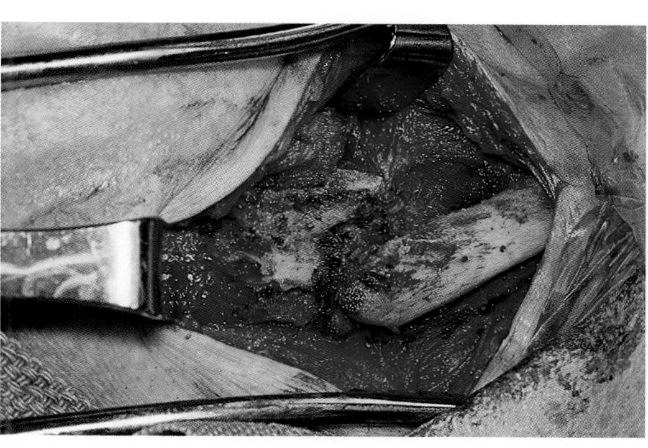

B

FIGURE 52–3. Approach to the clavicle. *A*, Artist's depiction. *B*, Operative approach. (*A* from Craig EV: Fractures of the clavicle. In Rockwood CA Jr, Matsen FA III [eds]: The Shoulder, 2nd ed. Philadelphia, WB Saunders, 1998, pp 428–482.)

3. Exposure: The scleroric ends are resected, and fixation is planned. Intercalary bone grafts must often be used (Fig. 52–4).
4. Fixation: A 6- or 7-hole 3.5-DCP (dynamic compression plate) or pelvic reconstruction plate is fashioned according to the shape of the clavicle, and the bone graft is secured to the plate. The

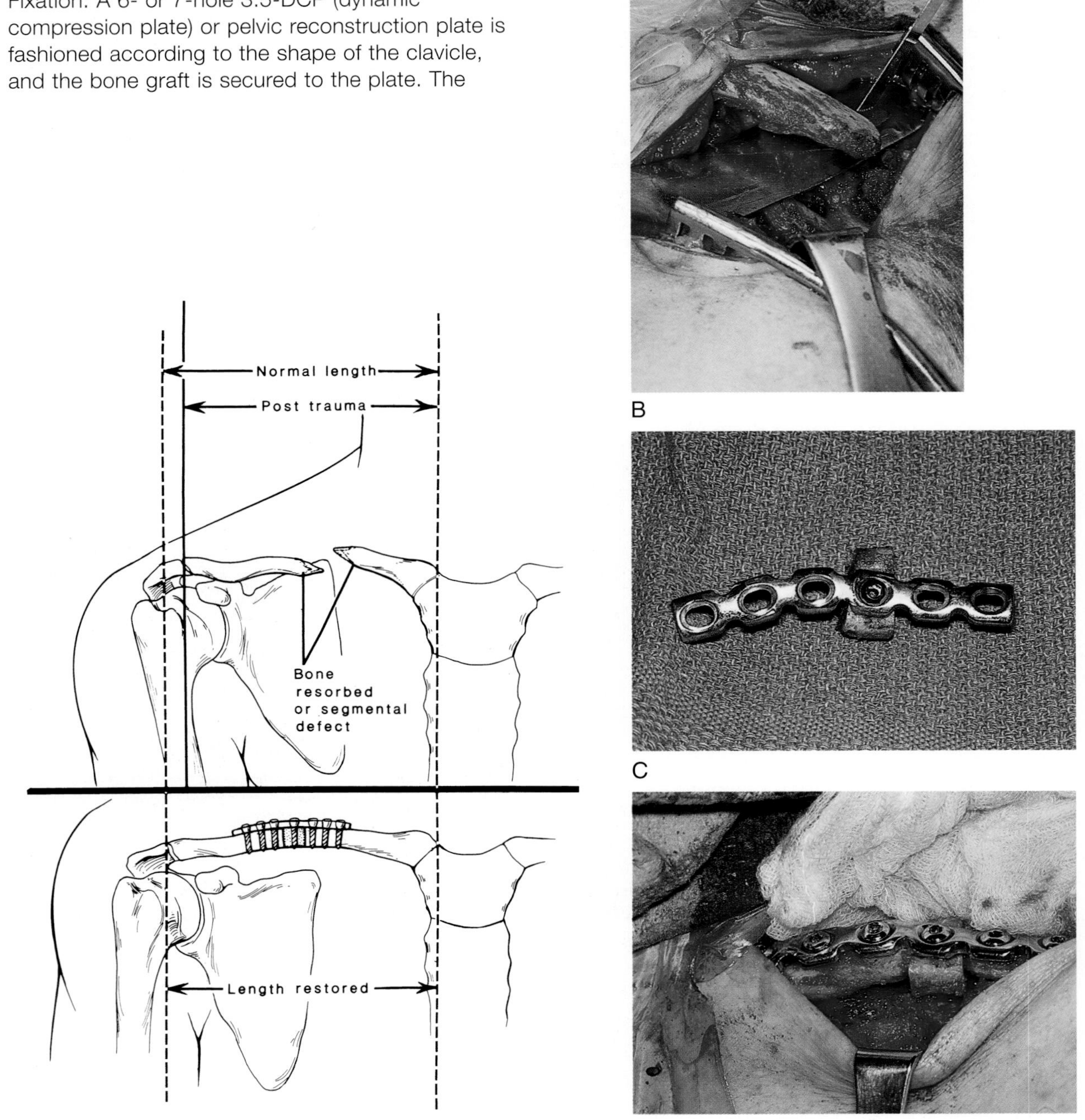

FIGURE 52–4. Planning for restoration of the length of the clavicle using an intercalary graft. *A*, Plan based on restoring the length (as measured from opposite side). *B*, After exposure and débridement, the width of the fracture gap is determined. *C*, A tricortical iliac crest graft that matches the size of the gap is harvested and secured in the middle of the plane. *D*, Final fixation. (*A* from Craig EV: Fractures of the clavicle. In Rockwood CA Jr, Matsen FA III [eds]: The Shoulder, 2nd ed. Philadelphia, WB Saunders, 1998, pp 428–482.)

plate is then used to stabilize the fracture and the graft.

5. Closure: The deltotrapezial fascia is secured over the plate, and the subcutaneous tissue and skin are closed.

Primary Clavicle Fracture Fixation

In unusual circumstances, primary fixation of clavicle fractures may be indicated. These indications include open fractures or those tenting the skin, as well as fractures associated with vascular injuries. Relative indications include significant displacement and shortening of 2 cm or more. Fixation can be performed with screws and plates, or intramedullary fixation can be used (Fig. 52–5).

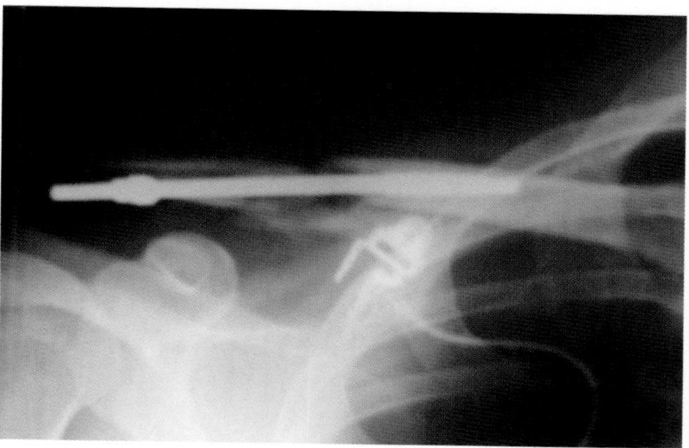

FIGURE 52–5. Radiograph shows primary fixation of clavicle fracture using modified Hage pin.

POSTOPERATIVE MANAGEMENT

The patient is placed in an immobilizer, and limited motion is allowed until there are early signs of union (at least 1 month postoperatively). Isometric exercises and limited pendulum exercises are allowed during this period. Following radiographic union, full motion and rehabilitative exercises are initiated. Prolonged immobilization does not have the same adverse effects as do other procedures involving the shoulder, because the glenohumeral joint is not disrupted.

COMPLICATIONS

As with all nonunions, the risk of infection is great; in fact, the nonunion may have been caused by an infection (especially in cases of revision surgery). Other risks include persistent nonunion, malunion, and devastating neurovascular injury. Late removal of hardware is not advised because of the risk of refracture.

RESULTS

With appropriate indications and meticulous technique, excellent results can be expected.

REFERENCES

Boyer MI, Axelrod TS: Atrophic nonunion of the clavicle: Treatment by compression plate, lag-screw fixation and bone graft. J Bone Joint Surg [Br] 79:301–303, 1997.

Craig EV: Fractures of the clavicle. In Rockwood CA Jr, Matsen FA III (eds): The Shoulder, 2nd ed. Philadelphia, WB Saunders, 1998, pp 428–482.

Simpson NS, Jupiter JB: Clavicular nonunion and malunion: Evaluation and surgical management. J Am Acad Orthop Surg 4:1–8, 1996.

SECTION V
ELBOW

CHAPTER 53
Elbow Arthroscopy

INTRODUCTION

Whereas the role of arthroscopy in the management of elbow disorders is evolving, the technique of diagnostic arthroscopy has become standardized. This chapter addresses basic diagnostic arthroscopic technique and its application for removal of loose bodies and for joint débridement in degenerative arthritis. Advanced techniques are not discussed.

ANATOMY

A thorough understanding of elbow anatomy is essential for the safe placement of arthroscopic portals. Because neurovascular structures lie near the elbow capsule, attention to detail is paramount during this procedure. The ulnar nerve lies in direct contact with the posteromedial aspect of the joint; therefore, there are no posteromedial arthroscopy portals. The radial nerve is most at risk for injury during elbow arthroscopy (Fig. 53–1). It lies anteromedially in the interval between the brachialis and brachioradialis muscles. The nerve is 6 mm from the elbow capsule, and the capsule-to-nerve distance does not change significantly with joint distention. However, joint distention can significantly displace the capsule from the joint surface, thereby increasing the margin of safety (Fig. 53–2). In contrast, arthroscopy of the stiff elbow poses inherently greater risk of nerve injury owing to the loss of capsular compliance. The clinician must recognize that the margin of safety is eliminated with elbow extension. Therefore, anterior portals are made with the elbow flexed. The median nerve lies in the interval between the brachialis and pronator teres muscles, and it is located 12 mm from the elbow capsule. Because of the greater distance of the median nerve from the capsule, as compared with the radial nerve, the superomedial portal is the preferred initial portal.

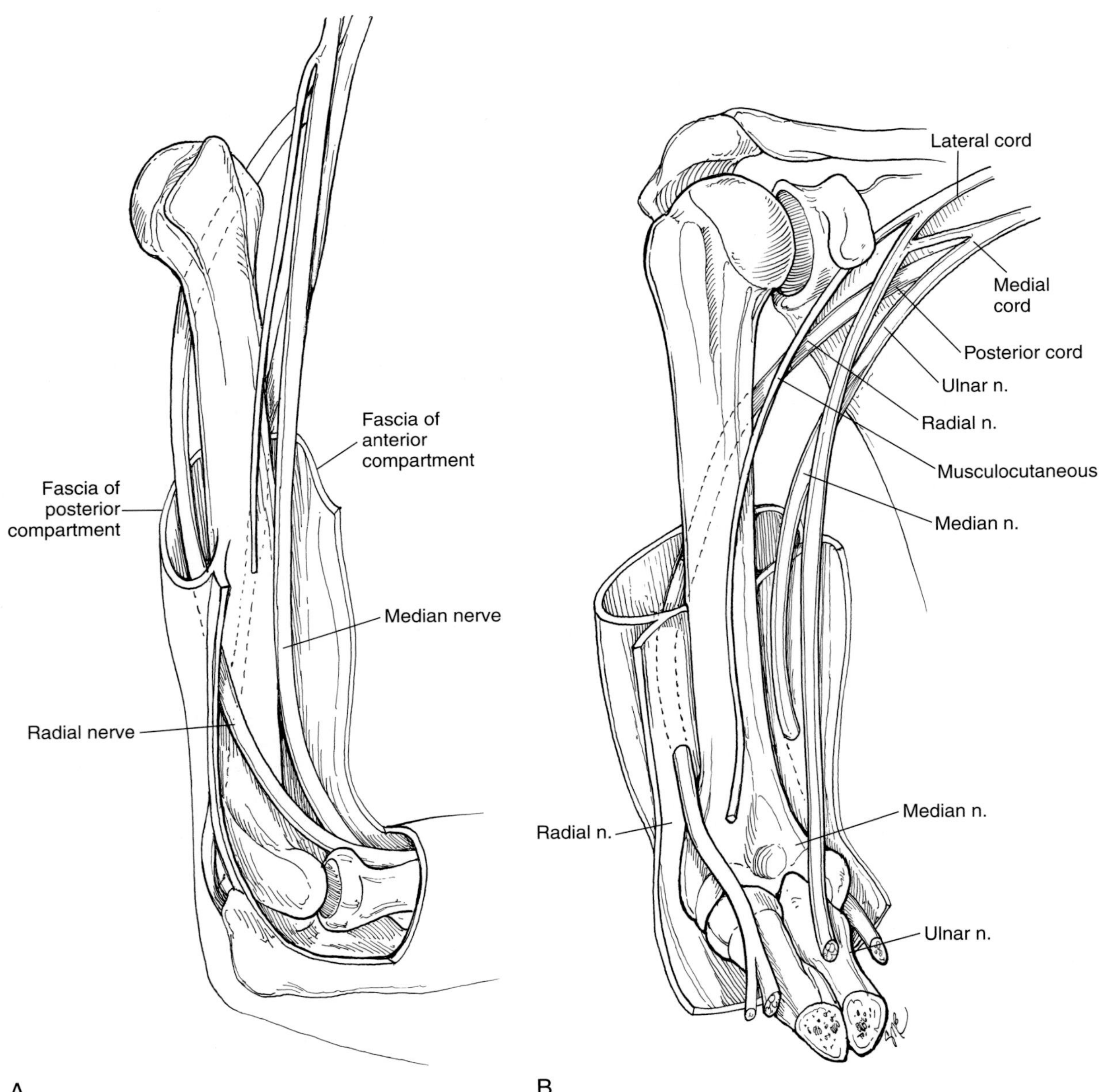

FIGURE 53–1. *A*, The lateral view illustrates the close proximity of the radial nerve to the joint capsule. *B*, On anterior view, the relative position of the median and radial nerves can be appreciated.

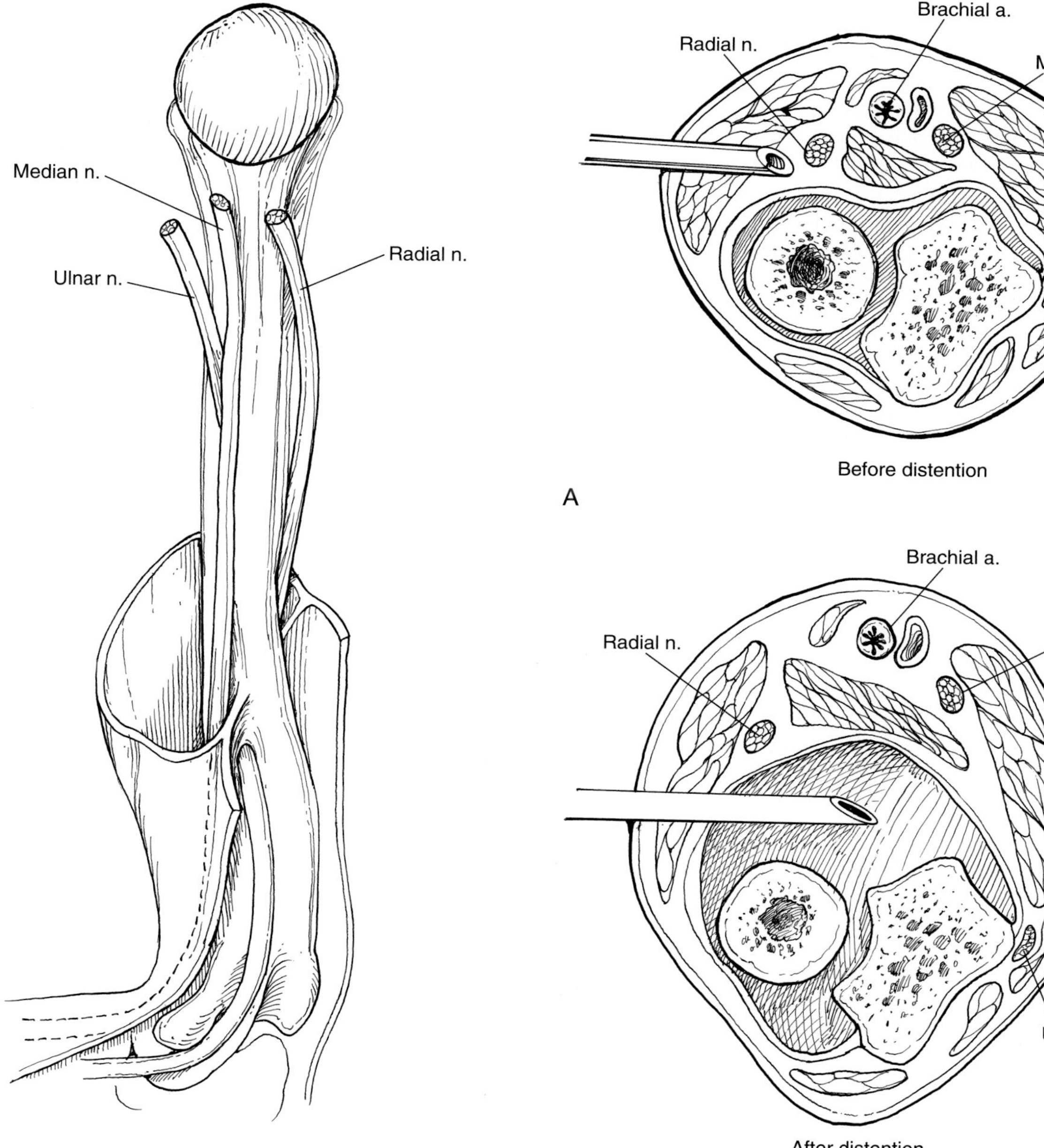

FIGURE 53–1 *Continued. C,* The medial view illustrates the relation of the median nerves to the capsule; this position provides a greater zone of safe passage of trocars as compared with the lateral side.

FIGURE 53–2. Distention of the elbow capsule increases the margin of safe trocar passage past the radial nerve from 4 mm to 11 mm. *A,* Before distention; *B,* after distention.

SURGICAL *TECHNIQUE*

Indications

Arthroscopy of the elbow, as of other joints, can be both diagnostic and therapeutic. Arthroscopy can help the physician determine the cause of chronic elbow pain in patients who gain relief from intra-articular injection of local anesthetic but whose cause of pain is unclear from the history and physical examination. Therapeutic indications include the removal of loose bodies and foreign bodies, the removal of osteophytes, synovectomy, and the assessment and treatment of osteochondritis dissecans of the capitellum.

Technique

Diagnostic Arthroscopy

1. Equipment: A standard 30°, 4.0-mm arthroscope can accomplish the tasks required in the vast majority of procedures. Similarly, a variety of grasping and biting forceps, as used in knee arthroscopy, function well in the elbow. Small joint instruments offer no particular advantages.
2. Examination under anesthesia (EUA): Before the patient is positioned for arthroscopy, EUA is performed with the patient in the supine position. If medial instability is suspected, the valgus stress test is assessed with fluoroscopy. Posterolateral rotary instability is also assessed.
3. Positioning: The patient is positioned laterally on a deflatable beanbag with the affected arm superior. Most surgeons prefer the lateral position, which offers the same advantages as the prone position without its inherent difficulties in positioning the patient; the lateral position also allows easy conversion to an open procedure when indicated. An axillary roll is placed under the contralateral chest wall. The arm is flexed to 90° over a padded support with the forearm hanging free (Fig. 53–3).

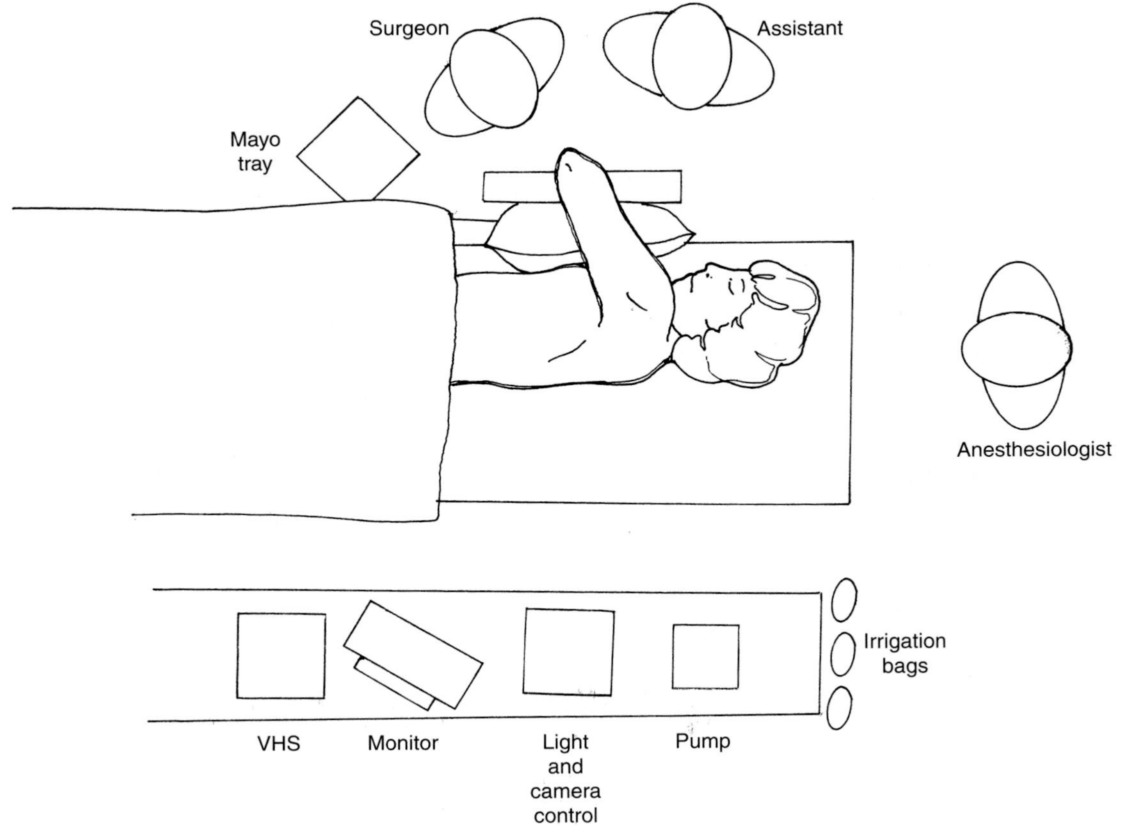

FIGURE 53–3. Operating room setup for elbow arthroscopy. A deflatable beanbag provides support to the chest. The well-padded arm support is positioned at the midshaft of the humerus to facilitate free access to the entire elbow. Monitors are positioned behind the patient for comfortable viewing by the surgeon.

The chest must be well supported to prevent trunk rotation toward or away from the support arm. The neck is maintained in neutral alignment, and the hips and knees are flexed.

4. After the patient has been sterilely prepped and draped, a sterile tourniquet is applied as proximally as possible on the arm. The forearm is wrapped with an elastic compression wrap (Coban 3M Wrap 3M, St. Paul, MN) from the fingertips to just below the operative field. This elastic wrap limits the diffusion of fluid into the soft tissues of the forearm. The elbow joint is insufflated with normal sterile saline via an 18-gauge needle puncture through the *midlateral portal,* which is located in the center of a triangle formed by the lateral epicondyle, the radial head, and the olecranon process (Fig. 53–4).
5. Portal selection is determined by the anticipated disease. There are four anterior and four posterior portals. The posterior portals are inherently the safest. The midlateral portal is placed first. If anterior disease is anticipated, this portal serves as an inflow for capsule distention during anterior portal placement. The additional posterior portals are the accessory lateral, posterolateral, and posterior.

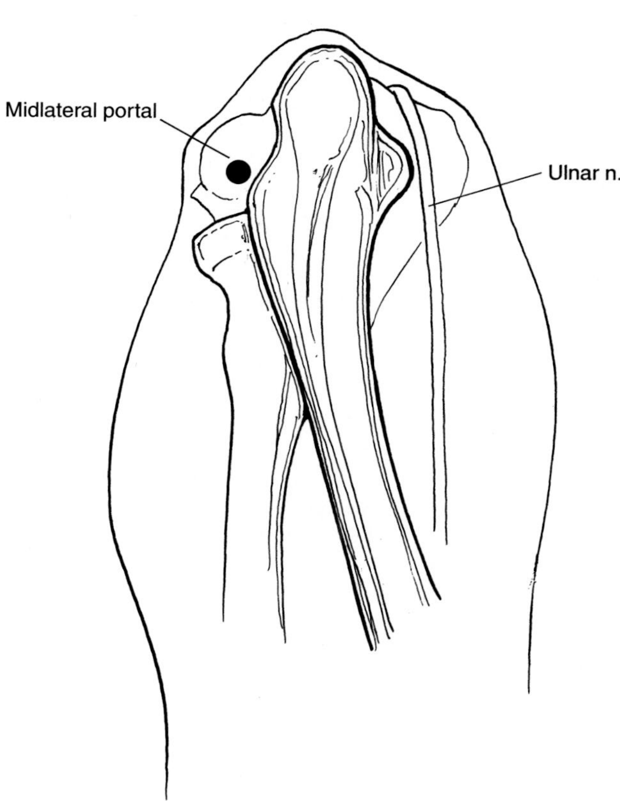

FIGURE 53–4. From the direct posterior view, the midlateral portal lies at the center of a triangle formed by the lateral epicondyle, the radial head, and the olecranon process.

6. Anterior portals are near cutaneous nerves. Therefore, care is taken to incise only the skin and to bluntly dissect down to the capsule before trocar insertion. The four anterior portals are the anterolateral, anteromedial, superomedial, and superolateral. The anteromedial and anterolateral portals are located at the joint line and can be joined by a switching stick (Fig. 53–5). The superior, or high, anterior portals increase the safe margin for nearby nerves. The radial nerve is at greatest risk of injury during anterior elbow arthroscopy. Thus, the *superomedial portal* is created first. This portal is 2 cm proximal to the medial epicondyle and just anterior to the medial intramuscular septum (Fig. 53–6). It is critical to the safe placement of the portal that the medial intramuscular septum remain posterior to the introduced sheath and blunt trocar.

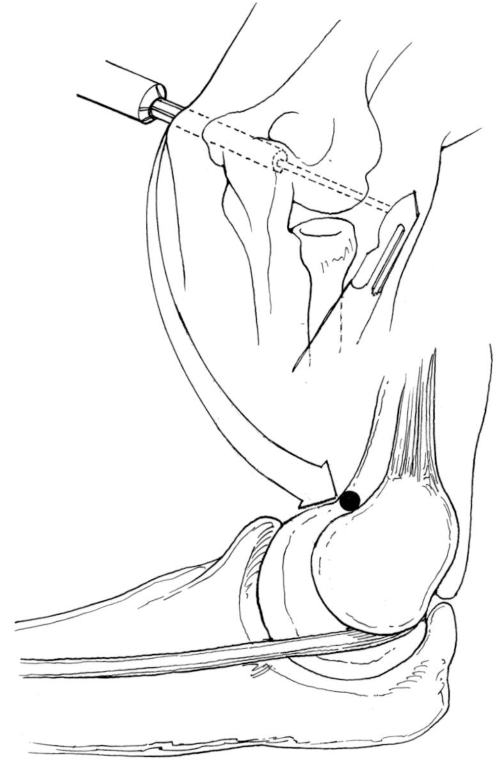

FIGURE 53–5. The anterolateral portal is established by passing a switching stick from the medial side toward the capsule at the juncture of the radial head and the capitellum.

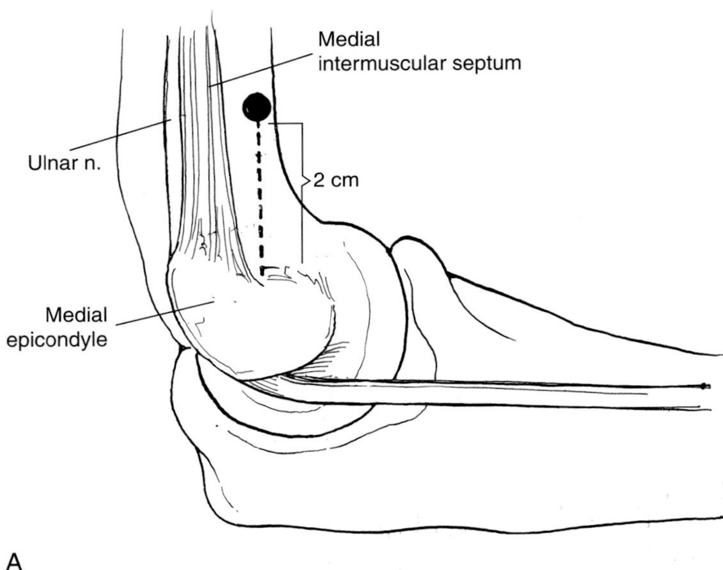

FIGURE 53–6. *A*, Landmarks for the superior medial portal. The portal is 1 to 2 cm proximal to the medial epicondyle.

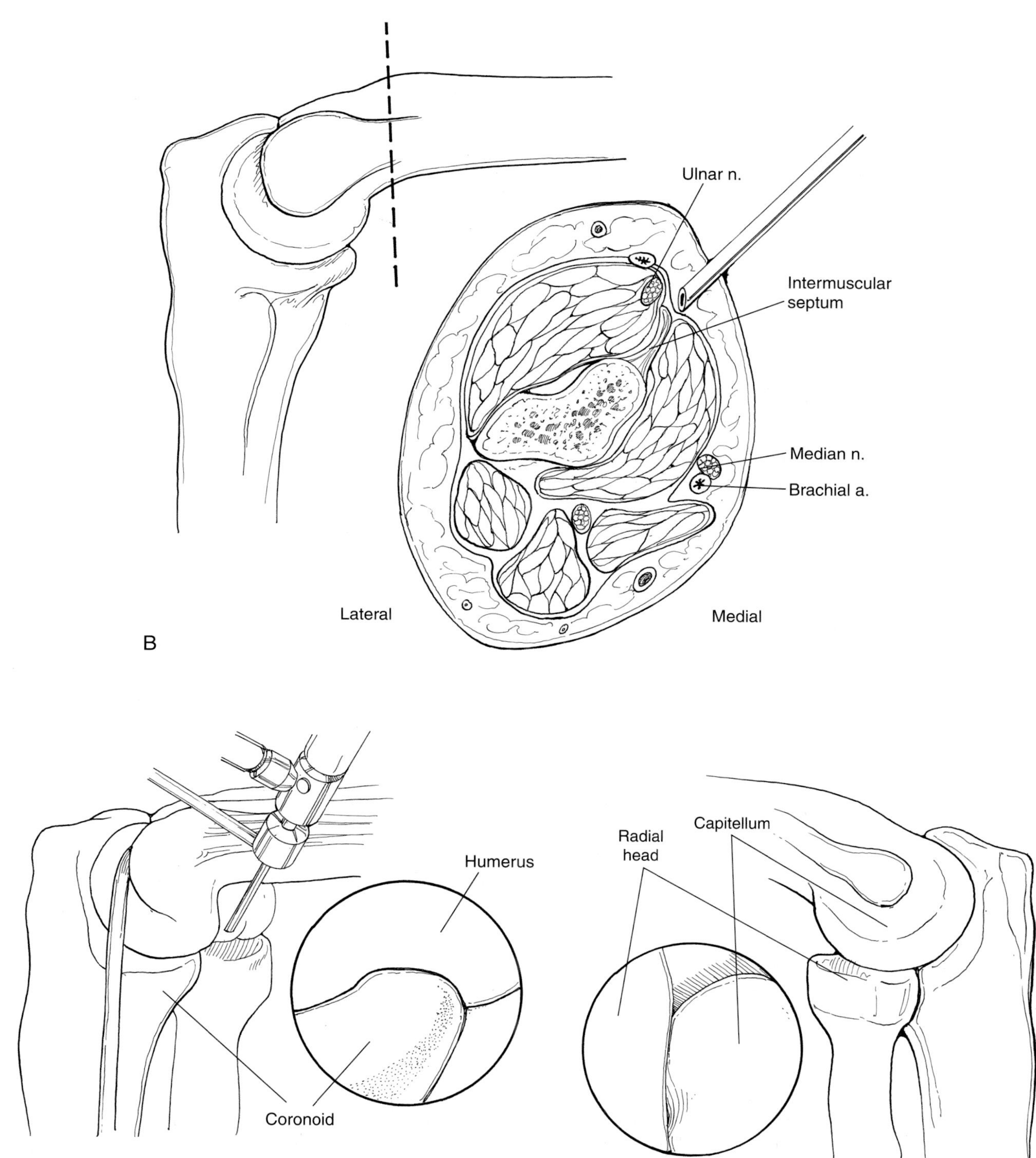

FIGURE 53–6 *Continued. B,* The trocar passes just anterior to the lateral intermuscular septum. *C,* This view illustrates the positioning of the scope and provides views of the joint looking toward the medial side *(C1)* and the lateral side *(C2)*.

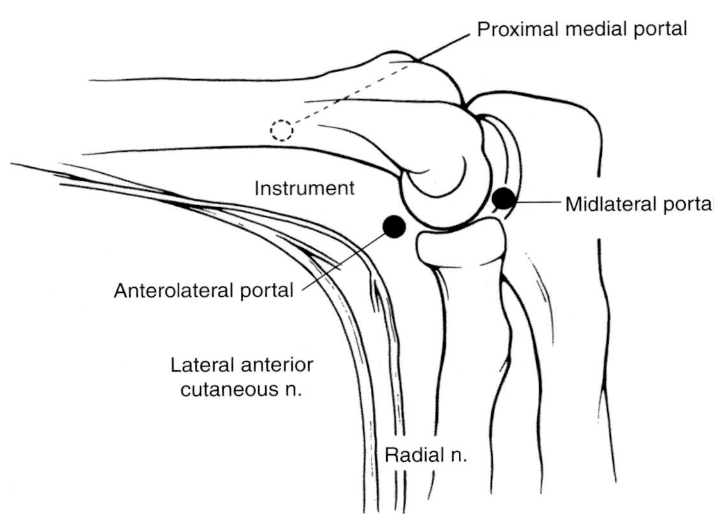

FIGURE 53–7. The relation of the radial head to the anterolateral portal is appreciated in the lateral view. The proximity of the radial nerve is demonstrated. (From Ekman EF, Poehling GG: Arthroscopy of the elbow. Hand Clin 10:453–460, 1994.)

7. The *anterolateral portal* is 1 cm inferior and 1 cm anterior to the lateral epicondyle (Fig. 53–7). The inside-out technique offers the lowest risk of radial nerve injury. Although many surgeons familiar with elbow arthroscopy prefer to establish this portal first, failure to flex the elbow leaves the radial nerve perilously close to this portal. With the elbow flexed to 90°, the anterolateral portal is established by positioning the scope at the intersection of the radial head and the capitellum. Elbow capsular distention with saline is maintained to maximize displacement of the radial nerve. The scope is pushed up against the capsule, and the arthroscope is withdrawn with the sheath held in place. Then, a 4-mm Steinmann pin or switching stick is passed through the lateral capsule until it tents the skin. A small incision is made over the pin; then a disposable, threaded, dammed cannula is placed over the pin and screwed into the elbow.

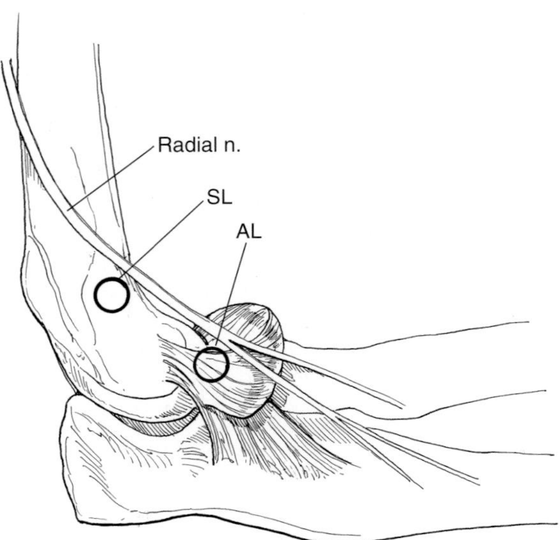

FIGURE 53–8. The superolateral (SL) portal allows increased distance from the radial nerve as compared with the anterolateral (AL) portal.

8. The *superolateral portal*, as described by Stothers, Day, and Regan, is located 1 to 2 cm superior to the lateral epicondyle and lies directly on the anterior surface of the humerus. Compared with the anterolateral portal, this portal provides an additional margin of safety with regard to the risk of radial nerve injury (Fig. 53–8). This portal can be created by using either the inside-out technique with a switching stick or a direct technique, as described for the superomedial portal.
9. The posterior portals are the posterior, posterolateral, and midlateral (Fig. 53–9). The posteromedial portal is described in the literature; however, we do not advocate its use because of the inherent risk of ulnar nerve injury. For diagnostic arthroscopy, we prefer the posterior and posterolateral portals. The *posterior portal* is 1 to 2 cm superior to the tip of the olecranon in midline posteriorly. The *posterolateral portal* is midway between the midlateral and posterior portals and 1 to 2 cm from the olecranon tip. The surgeon should be especially careful to avoid fluid extravasation into

the subcutaneous tissues posteriorly because the resulting "mass effect" prevents effective visualization. In the degenerative elbow, arthroscopy of the posterior elbow can be challenging. The posterior compartment of the inflamed elbow may provide the same poor visualization initially experienced by arthroscopists performing subacromial decompression of the shoulder. Visualization is enhanced by flexing the joint to 45° and maintaining fluid pressure within the joint. Standard technique is used to create these portals.

10. After completion of the procedure, all saline is drained from the joint and the tourniquet is released. Any excessive bleeding from portal sites is addressed at this time. This minimizes the incidence of postoperative wound hematomas. Portals are then sutured or closed with skin tape according to the surgeon's preference. We prefer to leave the wounds open to allow free drainage of saline and blood, and we see no cosmetic difference when compared with sutured wounds. However, if the portal is enlarged beyond 5 mm, the portal is sutured. In most cases, a light dressing is applied to allow uninhibited range of motion during the early postoperative period.

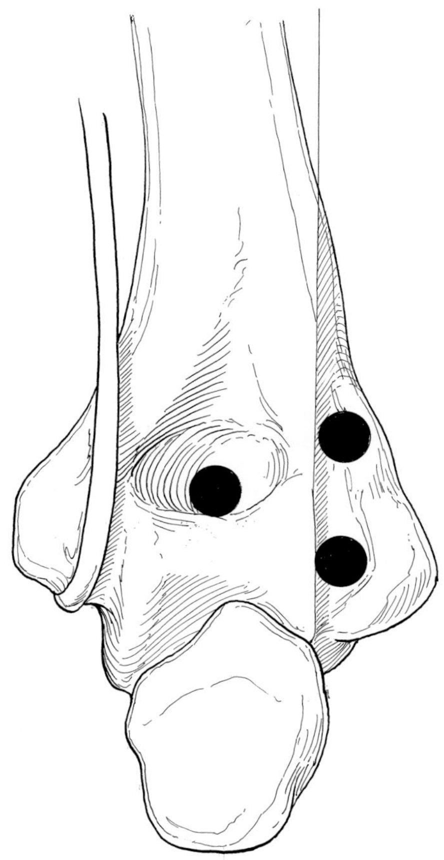

FIGURE 53–9. Posterior view of the elbow. As can be seen here, the posterior portals include those positioned posteriorly, posterolaterally, and midlaterally.

Removal of Loose Bodies

Removal of loose bodies from the elbow is one of the primary indications for elbow arthroscopy. The initial sequence of steps in the procedure is outlined in the diagnostic arthroscopy section.

1. Loose fragments are removed in sequence according to their size. The smallest fragments to pass through the arthroscope sheath or cannulas are removed first. Larger fragments may require enlargement of the portal, which can result in loss of joint distention. This loss of joint distention may increase the difficulty of locating and removing additional loose bodies.
2. To remove fragments through the scope cannula, the surgeon attaches the outflow to the arthroscope cannula and partially withdraws the scope, while visualizing the fragment as it passes up the cannula. The scope is fully withdrawn, and the fragments are captured in a basin. Larger fragments that pass through a 6-mm disposable cannula are removed by attaching the outflow to the sideport of the cannula. The cannula, like a vacuum cleaner, is then used to remove loose bodies.
3. Loose bodies larger than available cannulas are removed with an arthroscopic grasper that is passed through the portal without the aid of a cannula, or they are cut into smaller fragments and removed. The surgeon orients the fragment such that the smallest cross-sectional area will pass through the soft tissues. A stout grasper is in invaluable for this technique. The loose body is visualized as it exits the joint capsule, and it is carefully inspected after removal to ensure that the entire fragment was removed from the joint, and that it did not fragment in the subcutaneous tissues. An alternative technique for large fragments is to pass the grasper through a smooth 6-mm cannula. The loose body is withdrawn into the cannula until it wedges in the opening. The arthroscope is pushed up against the loose body, and the scope is uncoupled from the scope sheath. The sheath is used to push the loose body out as the grasper withdraws it. The large cannula can be reinserted into the joint by passing it over the scope sheath. Next, the scope sheath is withdrawn into the joint, and the scope is recoupled to the sheath.

Degenerative Elbow Débridement

Several words of caution are in order on this topic. First, the capsular compliance of the degenerative elbow is restricted. As a result, the margin for safe passage of cannulas past neurovascular structures is decreased.

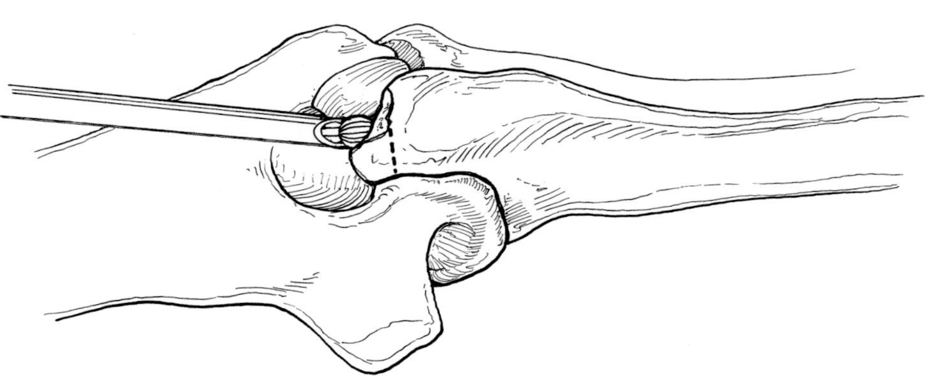

FIGURE 53–10. The olecranon osteophytes are resected, and approximately one third of the olecranon tip is removed.

Consequently, the degenerative elbow can present a formidable challenge to the inexperienced elbow arthroscopist. These procedures may be safer in the hands of more experienced colleagues. Furthermore, there is a role for open débridement of the degenerative joint. Whereas arthroscopic débridement provides many of the usual advantages over the open procedure, in severe cases with involvement of both anterior and posterior compartments, an open approach may be more expedient and technically less demanding. In our opinion, the best candidates for arthroscopic débridement are those with posterior compartment impingement and minimal anterior compartment degeneration.

1. The posterior and posterolateral portals are established, as described previously. A 4.5-mm round burr is introduced from the posterior portal while the surgeon views the procedure from the posterolateral portal. Attention is first directed at the osteophytes along the tip and the medial aspect of the olecranon. After the osteophytes are removed with the burr, the tip of the olecranon is resected, thereby removing approximately one third of the tip (Fig. 53–10).
2. Attention is directed to the olecranon fossa. The osteophytes are located primarily on the medial margin of the fossa. Special attention to detail is required to avoid injury to the ulnar nerve (Fig. 53–11).

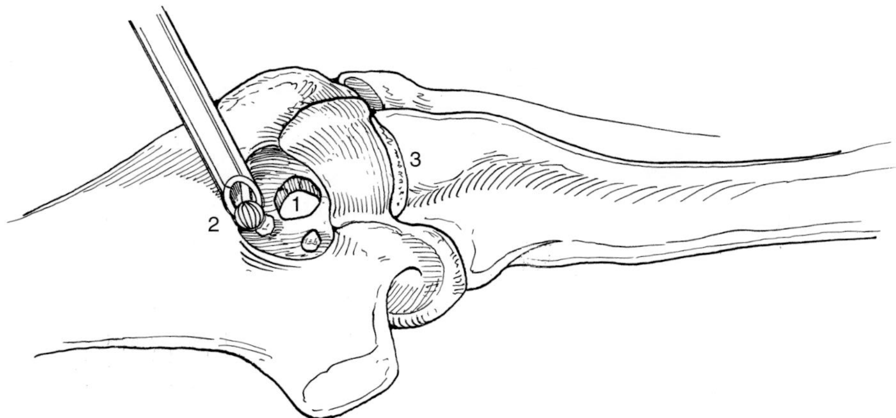

FIGURE 53–11. Bone is removed from the olecranon fossa (1). Fenestration of the fossa floor occurs in most cases, but this is not required for adequate decompression. Osteophytes are removed from the rim of the olecranon fossa with the burr (2). The tip of the olecranon is removed with a small osteotome (3).

POSTOPERATIVE MANAGEMENT

The dressings are removed 4 to 5 days after surgery. At this time, the portals are usually dry and healing. A light dressing is applied, if needed, and the patient is encouraged to initiate active range of motion. Patients with low pain tolerance, moderate to severe edema, or postdegenerative elbow débridement may require formal physical therapy. The goal is to restore full motion within 3 weeks after surgery. The patient is evaluated 2 weeks after surgery to ensure that satisfactory progress toward this goal has been made.

COMPLICATIONS

Complications from elbow arthroscopy, which are infrequent and usually minor, include persistent portal drainage, transient nerve palsies secondary to local anesthetic extravasation, and loss of motion secondary to capsular contracture. The most significant complication is injury to a major peripheral nerve. We have not experienced this problem, but we have consulted on cases in which the radial nerve or the ulnar nerve has been transected. This devastating complication is avoided when the surgeon provides careful attention to detail. In our experience, radial nerve injury seems to occur when the portal is placed too far anteriorly, or the trocars are passed through the tissue with the elbow extended. The cases of ulnar nerve transection referred to here occurred during posterior compartment débridement, thus illustrating the extreme caution required when the posterior medial elbow is débrided.

RESULTS

O'Driscoll and Morrey reviewed the benefits of elbow arthroscopy from their experience with 71 arthroscopies. In their series, 75% of patients benefited from the procedure. The benefits were categorized into three groups: diagnostic benefit in 31%, therapeutic benefit in 17%, and both diagnostic and therapeutic benefit in 24%. Patients undergoing treatment for posterior elbow impingement with degenerative arthritis were reviewed by Ogilvie-Harris and associates. They reported 14 excellent and 7 good results in their series of 21. However, the dissatisfaction of two of their patients, despite improvement, illustrates the potential difficulties associated with management of the degenerative elbow in a physically active patient. The ideal indication for elbow arthroscopy is the removal of loose bodies.

REFERENCES

Andrews JR, Carson WG: Arthroscopy of the elbow. Arthroscopy 1:97–107, 1985.

Ekman EF, Poehling GG: Arthroscopy of the elbow. Hand Clin 10:453–460, 1994.

Lindenfeld TN: Medial approach in elbow arthroscopy. Am J Sports Med 18:413–417, 1990.

Miller CD, Jobe CM, Wright MH: Neuroanatomy in elbow arthroscopy. J Shoulder Elbow Surg 4:168–174, 1995.

O'Driscoll SW, Morrey BF: Arthroscopy of the elbow. Diagnostic and therapeutic benefits and hazards. J Bone Joint Surg [Am] 74:84–94, 1992.

Ogilvie-Harris DJ, Gordon R, MacKay M: Arthroscopic treatment for posterior impingement in degenerative arthritis of the elbow. Arthroscopy 11:437–443, 1995.

Poehling GG, Ekman EF: Arthroscopy of the elbow. Instr Course Lect 44:217–223, 1995.

Stothers K, Day B, Regan WR: Arthroscopy of the elbow: Anatomy, portal sites, and a description of the proximal lateral portal. Arthroscopy 11:449–457, 1995.

CHAPTER 54

Treatment of Osteochondritis

INTRODUCTION

A review of the literature on this topic can leave one confused because of the variety of names used to describe it. Terms such as *osteochondritis dissecans (OCD), Panner's disease, Little Leaguer's elbow, osteochondrosis,* and *osteochondral fracture* have all been used to describe the same condition. Osteochondrosis occurs in children between the ages of 4 and 8 years and affects the entire capitellum. It is a self-limiting process without long-term sequelae, and it is not the focus of this section. The majority of patients with OCD of the capitellum are adolescents or young adults participating in gymnastics or throwing sports.

The surgeon must understand the natural history to appropriately manage these difficult problems. Surgical treatment of osteochondritis of the capitellum can improve function and decrease pain; however, it is important that the young athlete be counseled and accept that this is not a benign diagnosis and that it signals the end of hard, painless throwing. Similarly, in Jackson's series of ten high-level gymnasts with OCD of the capitellum, only one returned to competition after treatment. The majority of the literature on this subject addresses techniques that use elbow arthrotomy. More recent experience has demonstrated equal or superior results with the use of elbow arthroscopy techniques. For this reason, this chapter does not address arthrotomy techniques

HISTORY AND PHYSICAL EXAMINATION

The pain of OCD on the lateral aspect of the elbow is insidious and progressive. The pain is usually aggravated by elbow valgus loading activity and is relieved by rest. Loss of motion is a frequent complaint, with limited extension being most common. Some patients may be predisposed to the disorder if they have a history of osteochondritis in other parts of the body. Complaints of catching, grinding, or clicking in the joint may signal more advanced stages of disease with loose articular fragments in the joint.

Physical examination often shows tenderness around the lateral elbow, along with a mild elbow extension deficit. The radiocapitellar compression test consists of active pronation and supination with the elbow held in extension, which often aggravates the pain of OCD. The contralateral elbow is carefully examined because the disease can be present bilaterally.

DIAGNOSTIC IMAGING

Standard anteroposterior and lateral x-rays usually allow visualization of the lesion in the capitellum. The radiographic appearance is radiolucency with irregularity and flattening of the capitellum. There may be a sclerotic rim in the central or lateral aspect of the capitellum. If the fragment separates, loose bodies may be seen. The radial head view is helpful because it enables greater appreciation of the anatomy of the capitellum.

Treatment of OCD is determined by the status of the involved fragment and articular surface. Lesions are characterized as intact, separated and attached, or loose. Computed tomography (CT) or CT arthrogram (CTA) of the elbow is helpful for the clinician in defining these lesions. Specifically, CTA gives detailed information about the condition of the articular cartilage around the OCD lesion. Lesions that are loose or that have separated from the bone require operative intervention; CTA can facilitate decision making regarding whether to operate.

Magnetic resonance imaging (MRI) and magnetic resonance arthrography (MRA) provide information beyond that provided by CTA. MRI allows earlier detection of disease before x-ray changes are visible. MRA can accurately assess the integrity of the articular surface. MRA is our preferred assessment tool when articular surface integrity is in question (Fig. 54–1).

NONOPERATIVE MANAGEMENT

When the articular surface around the OCD lesion is intact, conservative treatment is indicated. However, nonsurgical treatment is not indicated when the fragment is partially or completely detached, or when the patient complains of mechanical symptoms such as locking or catching.

To manage conservatively, elbow valgus and axial loading activities are discontinued. A hinge elbow brace is useful for restricting activity and encouraging elbow rest. This brace can be locked temporarily if pain is severe. Splinting and rest continue until the pain resolves. After 3 to 6 weeks, the pain has usually subsided, and a progressive therapy program is begun. Initial therapy focuses on the goal of restoring full range of motion with stretching exercises. As elbow motion returns, the therapy program focuses on strengthening. The patient is closely monitored during this program for

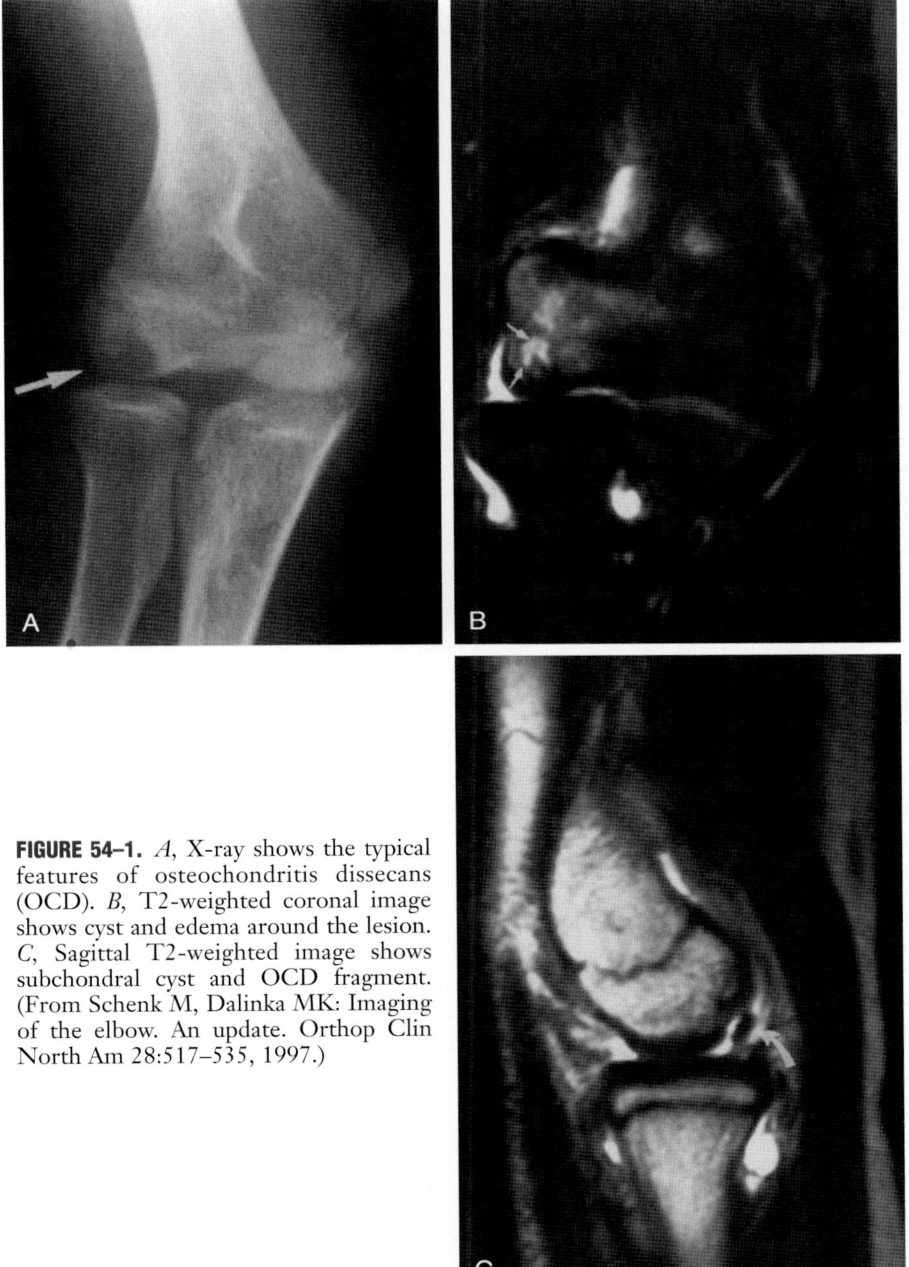

FIGURE 54–1. *A*, X-ray shows the typical features of osteochondritis dissecans (OCD). *B*, T2-weighted coronal image shows cyst and edema around the lesion. *C*, Sagittal T2-weighted image shows subchondral cyst and OCD fragment. (From Schenk M, Dalinka MK: Imaging of the elbow. An update. Orthop Clin North Am 28:517–535, 1997.)

development of mechanical symptoms. Catching, locking, or elbow effusions are indications for further evaluation with MRA or arthroscopy. X-ray cannot be reliably used to monitor progress because changes occur over several years. Patients progressing through therapy may return to activity 3 to 6 months after initiation of therapy.

A word of caution: Failure of the lesion to heal with conservative treatment signals the end of strenuous competition for most athletes. Thus, return to activity must be delayed long enough to allow full healing of the lesion; both the parent and the athlete should be counseled regarding the potential long-term sequelae.

RELEVANT ANATOMY

The distal articular surface of the humerus consists of the trochlea, which articulates with the ulna, and the capitellum, which articulates with the radial head. The convex surface of the capitellum articulates with the concave surface of the radial head through the entire arc of elbow motion. The capitellum has a hemispheric articular surface. On the lateral view, the center of the hemisphere rests on a line defined by the anterior humeral cortex (Fig. 54–2). The articular surface terminates inferiorly near the coronal plane of the humerus. Thus, fixation of the capitellum is possible from the entire posterolateral surface of the lateral condyle. When the elbow is axially loaded in extension, 60% of the load is carried on the radiocapitellar articulation; the remaining 40% is carried on the ulnotrochlear articulation. Maximal radiocapitellar loading occurs in pronation.

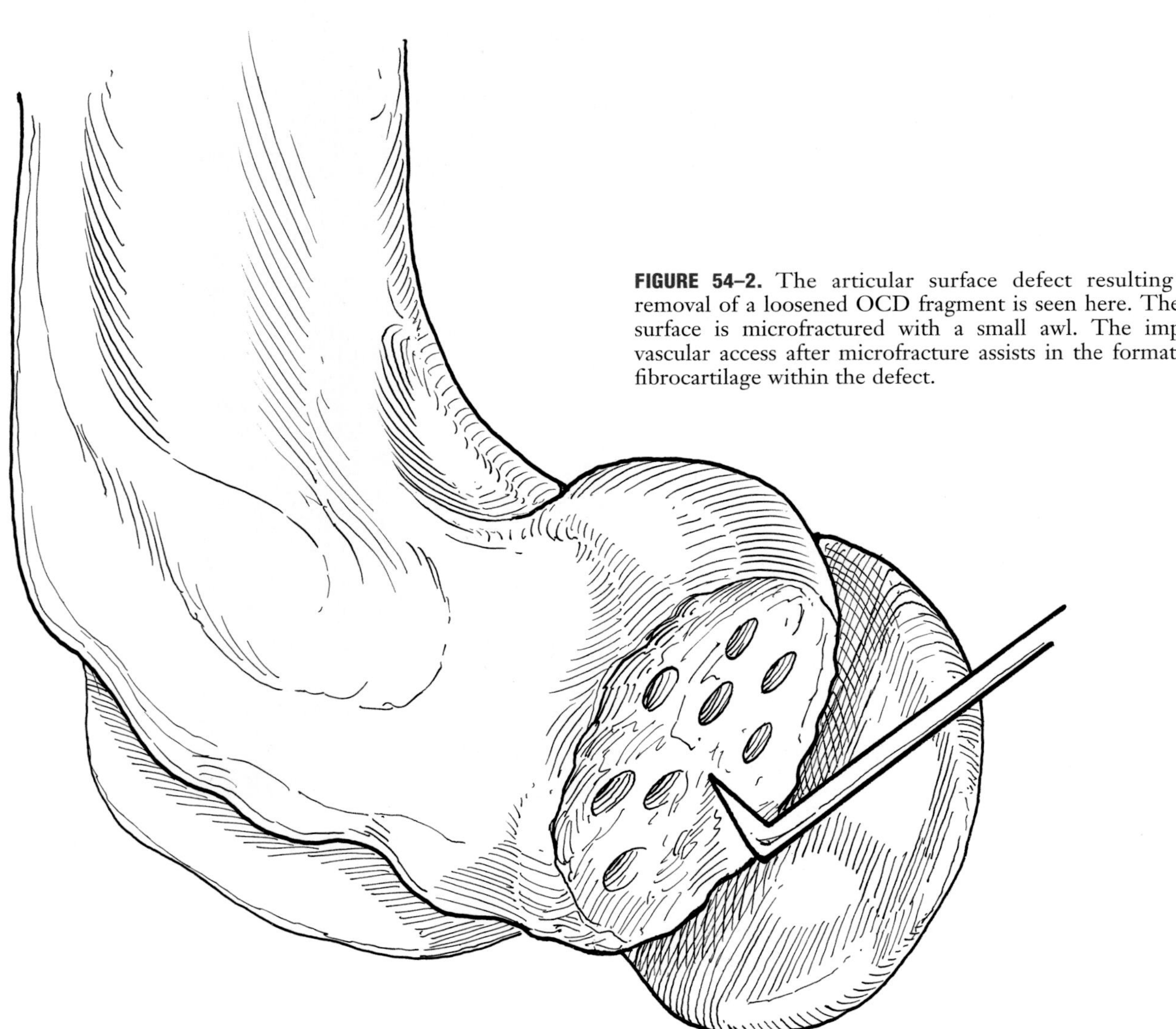

FIGURE 54–2. The articular surface defect resulting from removal of a loosened OCD fragment is seen here. The bone surface is microfractured with a small awl. The improved vascular access after microfracture assists in the formation of fibrocartilage within the defect.

SURGICAL *TECHNIQUE*

Surgical treatment consists of one of two choices. The first includes excision of the loose fragment and abrasion, drilling, or microfracture of the resulting articular deficit to stimulate fibrocartilage ingrowth. The second involves reduction and fixation of the loose fragment. Fragment fixation can be performed with Kirschner wires, Herbert screws, or absorbable pins. There is controversy regarding which approach is superior. The literature to date fails to demonstrate superiority of any technique; the surgeon must therefore use his or her own judgment to determine which approach to use. We have been discouraged by the need to reoperate on patients who failed to heal after fragment fixation was attempted. In addition, the lack of clear evidence of superiority of any technique leads us to favor fragment excision in most cases.

Indications

The primary indication for operative treatment is a loose fragment that causes mechanical symptoms in the elbow. In addition, if conservative treatment for 6 to 12 weeks has failed to relieve pain, or if imaging studies show a detached or loose fragment, surgical intervention is indicated.

Technique

1. Positioning: The procedure is performed arthroscopically; see Chapter 53 on elbow arthroscopy and removal of loose bodies. The lateral position allows easy conversion to elbow arthrotomy, if needed; therefore, the prone position is not recommended.
2. Arthroscopy: The midlateral, anterolateral, and superomedial portals are used for this procedure. Visualization from the superomedial portal with instruments that enter the lateral portals allows good access to the fragment. Following removal of the loose fragment, the resulting defect is microfractured with a 45° awl. The awl technique is preferred because of its relative ease as compared with drilling. The tourniquet is released at the completion of the microfracturing to ensure that the bone defect bleeds.

POSTOPERATIVE MANAGEMENT

Postoperative management for this procedure is similar to the nonoperative treatment of this disorder. The immediate postsurgical rehabilitation plan is outlined in Chapter 53.

COMPLICATIONS

The complications of elbow arthroscopy for OCD are the same as those discussed in Chapter 53. A majority of problems are minor. The major complications involve peripheral nerve injuries. The radial nerve is at greatest risk during this procedure; careful review of the technical details of portal placement is key if this problem is to be avoided.

RESULTS

No long-term follow-up studies on arthroscopic treatment of OCD of the elbow have been undertaken. However, short-term studies show more rapid recovery when compared with open treatment. In general, the prognosis for improvement in pain is good, although the potential for the athlete to return to high-level competitive throwing or gymnastics is limited. The longest average follow-up in the literature is 23 years. Half of these patients had degenerative changes noted on x-rays; in two thirds, enlargement of the radial head occurred. In spite of these findings, patients had little functional limitation.

REFERENCES

Bauer M, Jonsson K, Josefsson PO, Linden B: Osteochondritis dissecans of the elbow. A long-term follow-up study. Clin Orthop 284:156–160, 1992.

Baumgarten TE, Andrews JR, Satterwhite YE: The arthroscopic classification and treatment of osteochondritis dissecans of the capitellum. Am J Sports Med 26:520–523, 1998.

Brown R, Blazina ME, Kerlan RK, et al: Osteochondritis of the capitellum. J Sports Med 2:27–46, 1974.

Jackson DW, Silvino N, Reiman P: Osteochondritis in the female gymnast's elbow. Arthroscopy 5:129–136, 1989.

Ruch DS, Cory JW, Poehling GG: The arthroscopic management of osteochondritis dissecans of the adolescent elbow. Arthroscopy 14:797–803, 1998.

Takahara M, Shundo M, Kondo M, et al: Early detection of osteochondritis dissecans of the capitellum in young baseball players. Report of three cases. J Bone Joint Surg [Am] 80:892–897, 1998.

CHAPTER 55

Treatment of Epicondylitis

INTRODUCTION

Epicondylitis, either medial or lateral, results from repetitive overloading of the involved tendon insertion. However, this syndrome can also result from a single traumatic event. A great majority of patients with this common disorder recover with conservative treatment. In Nirschl's review of his experience with more than 1200 cases of lateral epicondylitis, only 7% eventually required surgical treatment. Thus, the need to proceed to surgical treatment should be uncommon in most practices.

HISTORY AND PHYSICAL EXAMINATION

The pain from epicondylitis is usually well localized by the patient to the affected area with radiation down the forearm into the associated muscle group. Some patients can clearly identify the precipitating event; however, many with repetitive strain are unaware of the cause of their pain.

Lateral epicondylitis causes tenderness to palpation over the insertion of the conjoined tendon slightly distal to the lateral epicondyle. In contrast, tenderness more distally over the arcade of Frohse is suggestive of radial tunnel syndrome. Some authors believe that lateral epicondylitis that is recalcitrant to conservative treatment is suggestive of radial tunnel syndrome, which should be considered in the differential diagnosis. The pain that results from lateral epicondylitis is typically aggravated by resisted wrist extension and passive wrist flexion with the elbow fully extended.

Medial epicondylitis results in point tenderness in the conjoined tendon of the flexor-pronator muscles at the medial epicondyle. The diagnosis of medial epicondylitis can be confused with ulnar neuropathy or medial collateral ligament instability. Pain is aggravated by resisted pronation and wrist flexion, and by passive wrist extension, elbow extension, and forearm supination. In more severe cases, elbow extension may be limited.

DIAGNOSTIC IMAGING

Standard views of the elbow are usually normal in epicondylitis; however, up to 25% of patients have calcification within the involved tendon. Calcification within the conjoined tendon laterally has little significance. In contrast, calcification within the medial collateral ligament may indicate insufficiency of the ligament.

NONOPERATIVE MANAGEMENT

Initial treatment focuses on eliminating the aggravating activities and controlling inflammation. Activities are modified to reduce symptoms. A careful analysis of sport techniques or work ergonomics may identify potential areas for technique modification. Nonsteroidal anti-inflammatory medications (NSAIDs) assist in pain management during this phase of treatment. If NSAIDs, rest, and counterforce bracing fail to produce adequate symptom reduction, local injection with a corticosteroid is indicated. Approximately 60% of patients have significant relief of symptoms, but in 54%, symptoms recur. Furthermore, whereas steroid injection provides short-term benefit for some patients, it does not appear to affect the long-term natural history of this disorder. No carefully controlled studies have evaluated the efficacy of various steroid preparations. Thus, the choice of steroid preparation remains arbitrary. Every effort is made to avoid depositing steroid into the subcutaneous tissues. Counterforce bracing can provide significant relief of symptoms by reducing extensor muscle activity.

After symptoms are brought under control, the focus of rehabilitation changes to stretching and strengthening of the involved muscles. Up to 15% of patients have a relapse of symptoms. A majority of those who relapse have failed to complete the appropriate second phase of rehabilitation.

RELEVANT ANATOMY

The lateral epicondyle is the origin for the extensor carpi radialis brevis, the extensor digitorum communis, and the extensor carpi ulnaris muscles. Innervation of the dorsal compartment of the forearm is provided by the posterior interosseous branch of the radial nerve (PIN). The radial nerve branches into the PIN and the superficial branch (SBRN) anterior to the elbow. The PIN passes deep to the mobile wad (brachioradialis, extensor carpi radialis longus, and extensor carpi radialis brevis [ECRB]) as it enters the dorsal compartment of the forearm. Deep to the extensor carpi radialis brevis, the PIN enters the supinator, passing through the arcade of Frohse (Fig. 55–1). Compression of the PIN in this region may produce symptoms of radial tunnel syndrome, which

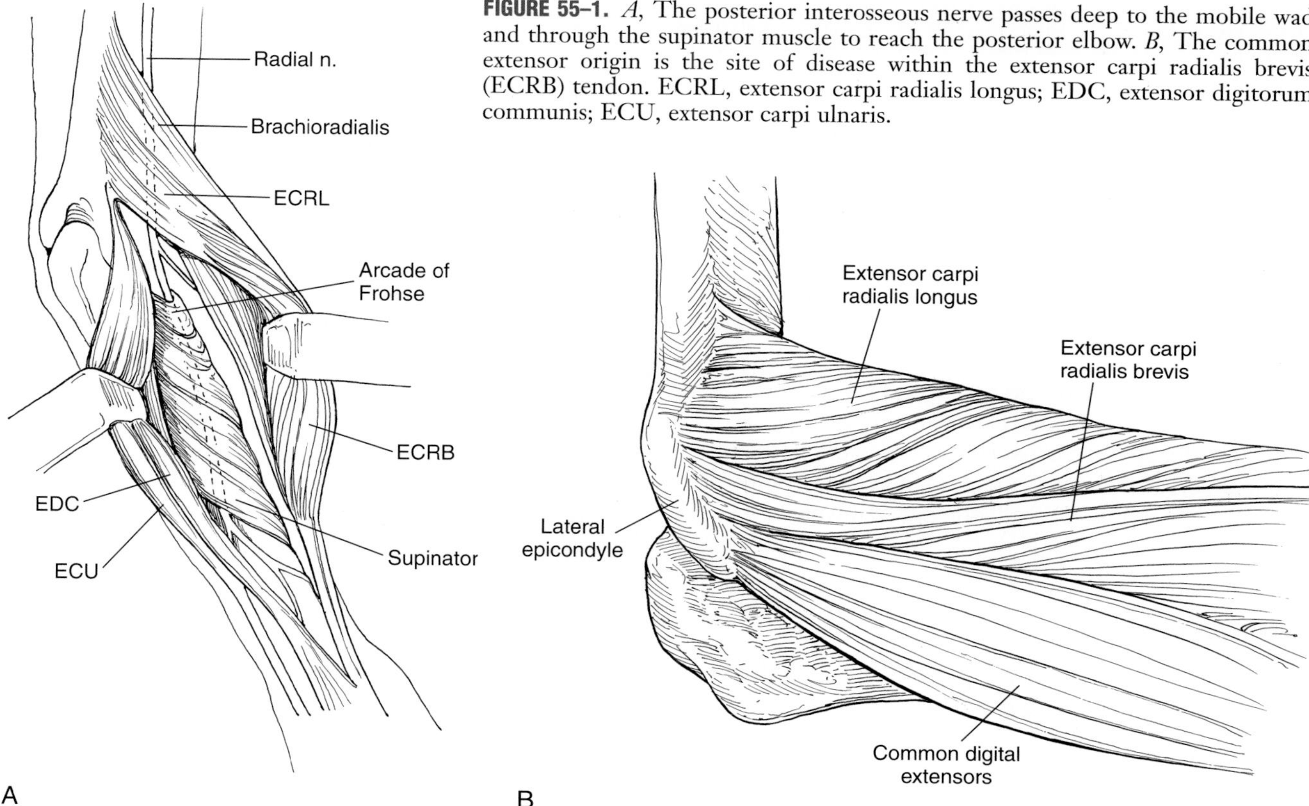

FIGURE 55–1. *A*, The posterior interosseous nerve passes deep to the mobile wad and through the supinator muscle to reach the posterior elbow. *B*, The common extensor origin is the site of disease within the extensor carpi radialis brevis (ECRB) tendon. ECRL, extensor carpi radialis longus; EDC, extensor digitorum communis; ECU, extensor carpi ulnaris.

must be considered in the differential diagnosis of lateral epicondylitis.

The medial epicondyle is the origin for the pronator teres, flexor carpi radialis, flexor digitorum superficialis, palmaris longus, and flexor carpi ulnaris. The soft tissue lesion from medial epicondylitis typically lies in the interval between the pronator teres and the extensor carpi radialis (Fig. 55–2). The skin overlying the medial epicondyle is innervated by branches of the medial antebrachial cutaneous nerve (MACN). A majority of patients have a medial epicondylar branch from the MACN passing directly over the medial epicondyle. Subcutaneous dissection near the medial epicondyle may injure this nerve.

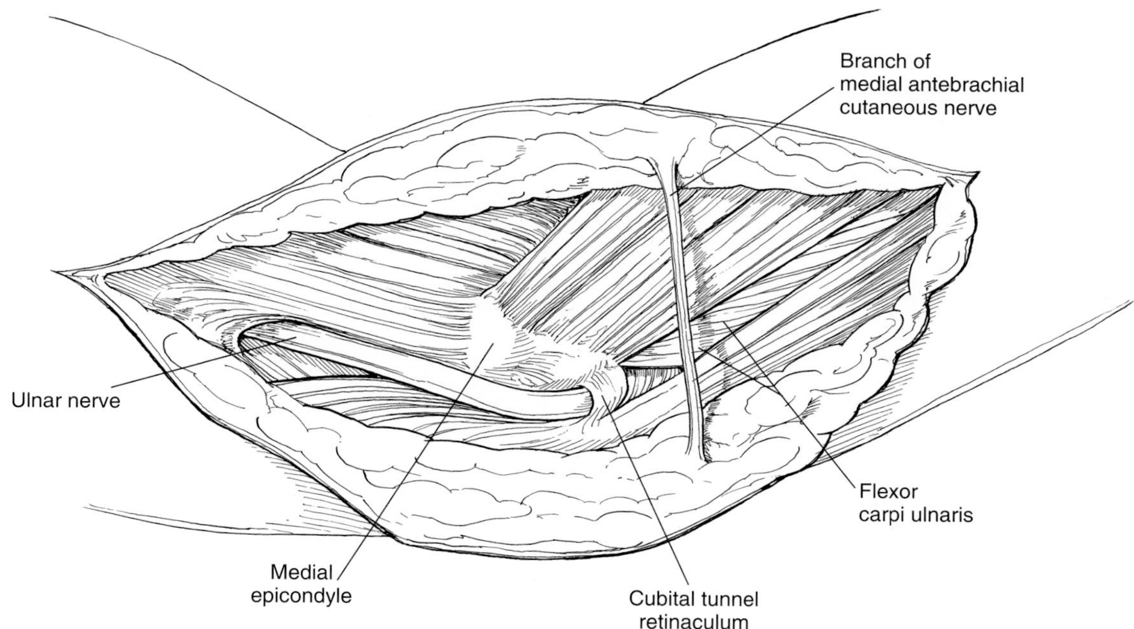

FIGURE 55–2. Conjoined tendons insert on the medial condyle. Note the close proximity of the ulnar nerve.

SURGICAL TECHNIQUE

Indications

Indications for surgical treatment include (1) failure of conservative treatment to adequately control symptoms, (2) symptoms that persist beyond 6 months during appropriate conservative treatment, and (3) exclusion of other potential diagnoses.

Technique

A variety of techniques are advocated for the surgical treatment of epicondylitis. However, most surgeons agree on these three essential principles of treatment: (1) excision of the diseased tissue, (2) closure of the tendon defect, and (3) reattachment of the elevated tendon to the bone.

Lateral Epicondylitis

1. Positioning: The patient is placed supine on the operating table with the affected arm extended on a hand table. A standard upper arm tourniquet is used. General or regional anesthesia is recommended for this procedure.
2. Incision: A longitudinal incision extends from just posterior to the lateral epicondyle and distally in the axis of the ECRB tendon for a distance of 5 to 7 cm. Dissection down to the deep fascia reveals the longitudinal fibers of the ECRB originating from the anterior aspect of the lateral epicondyle. The ECRB is incised in line with the fibers in its midsubstance for 3 to 4 cm (Fig. 55–3).
3. Débridement: The intratendinous lesion is identified by its amorphous appearance against the background of longitudinally oriented tendon fibers. This lesion is sharply excised in its entirety. The adjacent surface of the epicondyle is rongeured back to bleeding bone (Fig. 55–4).
4. Repair: Any elevated tendon insertion is reattached to the bone with nonabsorbable 2–0 sutures passed through drill holes in the bone. The defect in the ECRB is closed with interrupted sutures (Fig. 55–5).

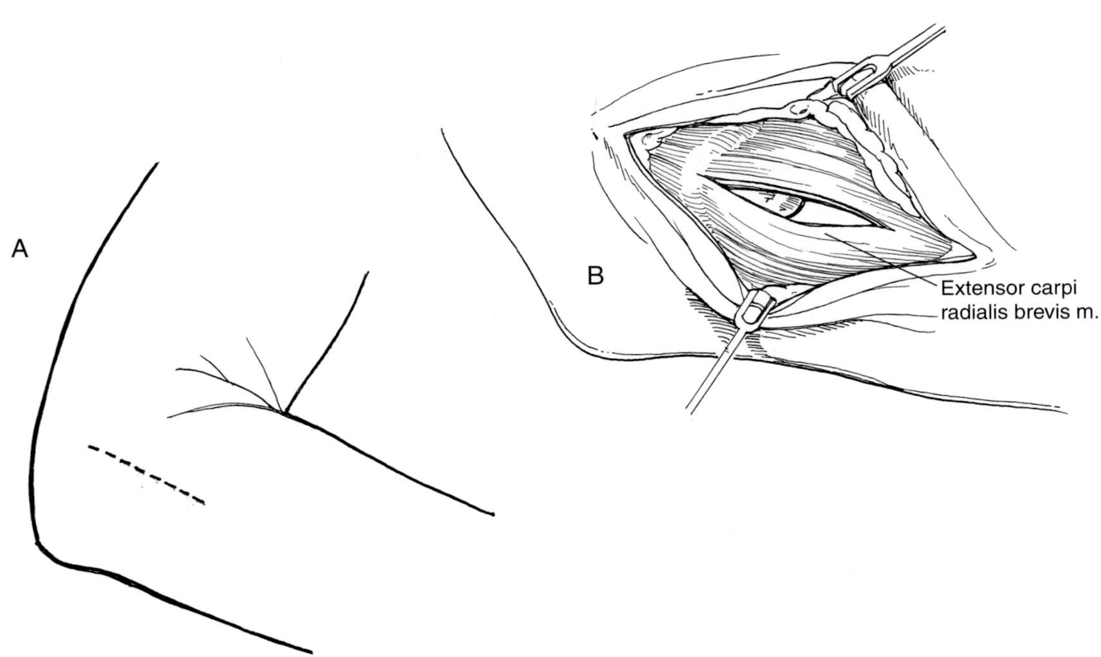

FIGURE 55–3. The extensor carpi radialis brevis tendon is longitudinally incised. *A*, Incision placement over the lateral epicondyle extending 5 cm distal to the epicondyle. *B*, ECRB tendon split along its anterior margin.

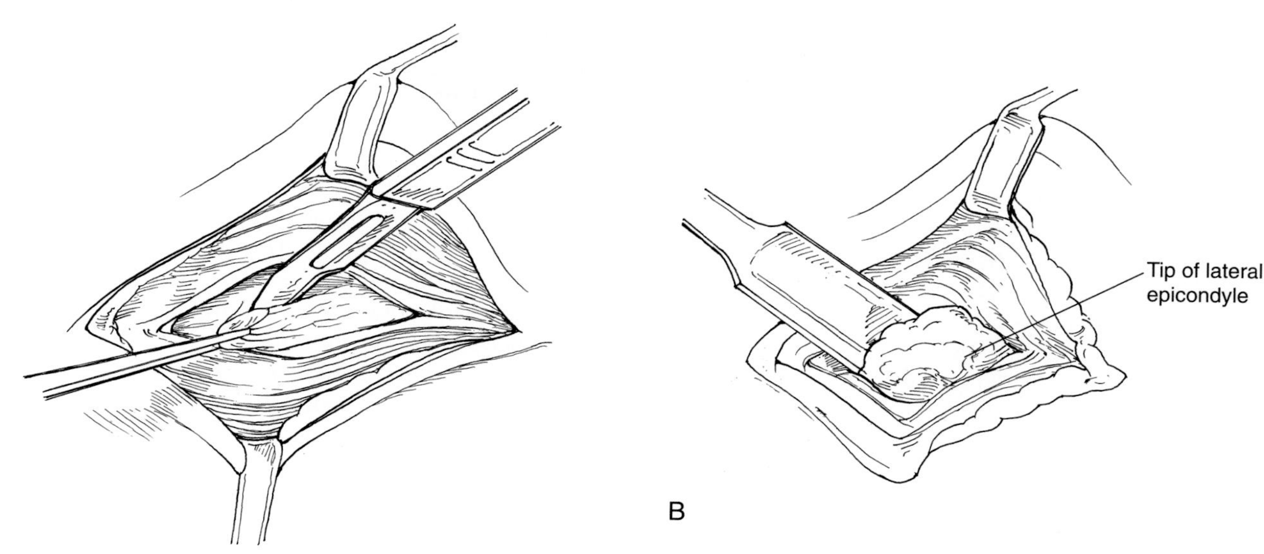

FIGURE 55–4. *A*, Amorphous-appearing tissue is excised from the tendon until healthy, longitudinally oriented fibers are visualized. *B*, The tip of the lateral epicondyle is removed.

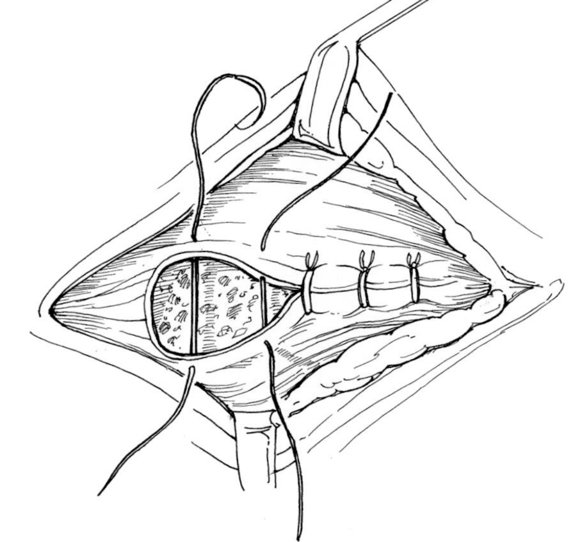

FIGURE 55–5. The tendon is repaired with interrupted sutures.

Medial Epicondylitis

1. Positioniong: The setup and positioning are the same as in lateral epicondylitis, but the arm is maximally externally rotated to expose the medial elbow to the surgeon seated in the axilla.
2. Incision: A 5- to 7-cm incision is placed obliquely from just anterior to the medial epicondyle apex in line with the flexor-pronator muscles. Care is taken during subcutaneous dissection to identify and protect the branches of the medial antebrachial cutaneous nerve (Fig. 55–6).
3. Débridement: The common flexor-pronator tendon is incised in line with its fibers in the interval between the pronator teres and the flexor carpi radialis. The intratendinous lesion is identified by its amorphous appearance against the background of longitudinally oriented tendon fibers. The lesion is sharply excised in its entirety. The exposed medial epicondyle is rongeured back to bleeding bone. The medial collateral ligament and the ulnar nerve can be inspected as indicated for coexistent disease, although this is not routinely required or recommended.
4. Repair: Any tendon elevated from the bone is reattached through drill holes with the use of 2–0 nonabsorbable sutures. The defect in the flexor-pronator conjoined tendon is repaired side to side with simple absorbable sutures.

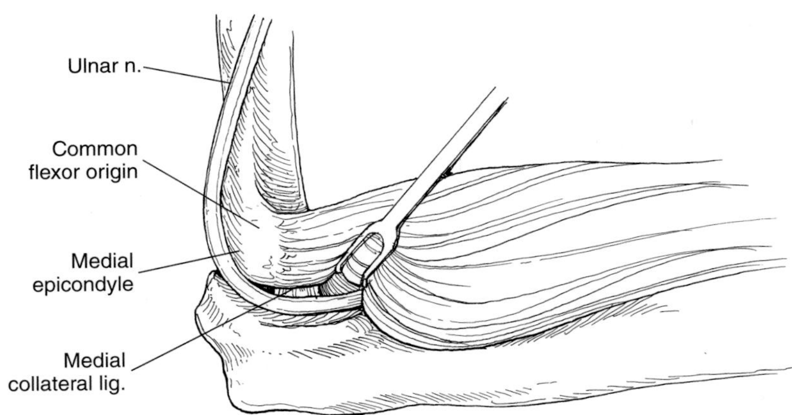

FIGURE 55–6. The common flexor origin is the site of tendon disease. This area is resected along with the tip of the epicondyle.

POSTOPERATIVE MANAGEMENT

Patients are encouraged to resume full active range of motion of the elbow and wrist as soon as tolerable after surgery. A period of splinting, not to exceed 14 days, may be required for control of postoperative pain. At 4 weeks after surgery, gentle strengthening exercises are initiated. Strengthening exercises may advance to full effort after 6 weeks. Return to full sports participation is permitted after 4 months.

COMPLICATIONS

Complications from surgical treatment of epicondylitis are infrequent. The most frequent problem is failure of the procedure to resolve symptoms, which may result from incomplete resection of the diseased tissue.

Surgical treatment of medial epicondylitis is inherently perilous because of the local anatomy. Injury of the MACN is a significant cause of patient dissatisfaction with any procedure on the medial side of the elbow.

Injury to the ulnar nerve may result from overzealous dissection around the medial epicondyle. Unrecognized coexistent ulnar neuropathy and medial epicondylitis can be successfully managed with débridement and nerve transposition. Failure to recognize and treat the neuropathy is a potential pitfall in management.

RESULTS

The surgical treatment of lateral epicondylitis results in return to full activity without pain for 85% to 90% of patients. For treatment after failed lateral epicondyle débridement, some authors have advocated wide resection of the conjoined tendon and rotation flap coverage with the anconeus muscle. The results of medial epicondyle débridement are similar. However, the coexistence of ulnar neuropathy may compromise the results.

REFERENCES

Almquist EE, Necking L, Bach AW: Epicondylar resection with anconeus muscle transfer for chronic lateral epicondylitis. J Hand Surg [Am] 23:723–731, 1998.

Ciccotti M: Epicondylitis in the athlete. Instr Course Lect 48:375–381, 1999.

Gellman H: Tennis elbow (lateral epicondylitis) [review]. Orthop Clin North Am 23:75–82, 1992.

Leach RE, Miller JK: Lateral and medial epicondylitis of the elbow [review]. Clin Sports Med 6:259–272, 1987.

Nirschl R, Pettrone F: The surgical treatment of lateral epicondylitis. J Bone Joint Surg [Am] 61:832–839, 1979.

Plancher KD, Halbrecht J, Lourie GM: Medial and lateral epicondylitis in the athlete [review]. Clin Sports Med 15:283–305, 1996.

Stahl S, Kaufman T: The efficacy of an injection of steroids for medial epicondylitis. A prospective study of sixty elbows. J Bone Joint Surg [Am] 79:1648–1652, 1997.

CHAPTER 56

Treatment of Cubital Tunnel Syndrome

INTRODUCTION

Cubital tunnel syndrome may result from compression, traction, friction, or direct trauma to the ulnar nerve. Compression is thought to be the most frequent cause. Ulnar nerve entrapment at the elbow is the second most common compressive neuropathy in the upper extremity. Surgical decompression of cubital tunnel syndrome has been the focus of much contentious debate. Numerous procedures and modifications addressing the underlying disease are described in the literature, and it is beyond the scope of this chapter to address all the issues related to procedure selection. The most widely employed procedures are in situ decompression, medial epicondylectomy, subcutaneous transposition, and submuscular transposition. The technical aspects of these procedures are the focus of this chapter.

HISTORY AND PHYSICAL EXAMINATION

The hallmark complaints of the patient with cubital tunnel syndrome are numbness and tingling in the ring and small fingers and medial forearm pain. The absence of paresthesias in this distribution should raise suspicion of another diagnosis. Patients with cubital tunnel syndrome frequently suffer from nocturnal symptoms. Inquiring as to the distribution of nocturnal paresthesias can assist in the differential diagnosis. In addition, complaints of vague ulnar forearm pain, tenderness on the medial aspect of the elbow, and hand clumsiness frequently are reported. A history of previous trauma may indicate the presence of scarring around the nerve, which contributes to local compression or limited excursion, resulting in nerve traction. Throwing athletes may suffer from chronic traction injury to the ulnar nerve. Studies have shown a threefold increase in ulnar nerve pressure with elbow flexion and wrist extension; when the arm is placed in the cocking position of the throw, the pressure increases to six times resting pressure (Fig. 56–1). Prolonged periods of elbow flexion often provoke symptoms, and such information should be sought in the history. Radiculopathy of the C7 root, thoracic outlet syndrome, ulnar tunnel syndrome, and ulnar artery thrombosis may manifest with similar symptoms. Patients with radiculopathy more frequently complain of neck and shoulder pain. Nerve compression in the ulnar tunnel causes symptoms similar to cubital tunnel syndrome; however, the diagnosis is readily distinguished on physical examination. Ulnar artery thrombosis usually has an acute onset, and Allen's test is positive. Thoracic outlet syndrome is a diagnosis of exclusion.

Initial observation of the elbow should reveal the presence of cubitus valgus or cubitus varus; either may contribute to cubital tunnel compression. Active elbow range of motion is observed during inspection and palpation of the ulnar nerve in search of evidence of subluxation. The hands are inspected for evidence of intrinsic atrophy. Cervical spine examination is included in the evaluation. Patients with radiculopathy may have a positive Spurling's sign, triceps muscle weakness or diminished reflex, and decreased sensation in the middle finger. Patients with cubital tunnel syndrome often have a Tinel's sign at or just distal to the elbow. The elbow flexion test frequently reproduces the characteristic paresthesia and dysesthesia. Similar to Phalen's test in carpal tunnel syndrome, the elbow flexion test is a timed test, and posture should be maintained for at least 1 minute. Measuring two-point discrimination in the fingertips assesses sensation, and special attention is directed to the dorsal ulnar hand. Decreased sensation on the dorsal ulnar aspect of the hand indicates a lesion of the ulnar nerve proximal to the dorsal cutaneous branch. Motor examination may identify diminished strength in the abductor digiti minimi and the ulnar-innervated flexor digitorum profundus muscles. Allen's test is performed to assess ulnar arterial inflow to the hand. Ulnar artery thrombosis will result in a positive test and may be misconstrued as cubital tunnel syndrome. Physical examination in ulnar tunnel syndrome frequently reveals a positive Tinel's sign at Guyon's tunnel. A volar wrist ganglion causes ulnar tunnel syndrome in 80% of cases.

DIAGNOSTIC IMAGING

Standard anteroposterior and lateral radiographs adequately evaluate bone disease. The cubital tunnel view is useful for evaluation if heterotopic ossification or osteophytes are present in the cubital tunnel. The humerus should lie in the plane of the film cassette for this view. Calcification or avulsion fractures of the medial collateral ligament (MCL) may be visible on the cubital tunnel view.

Nerve conduction velocity (NCV) testing and electromyography (EMG) of the ulnar-innervated muscles,

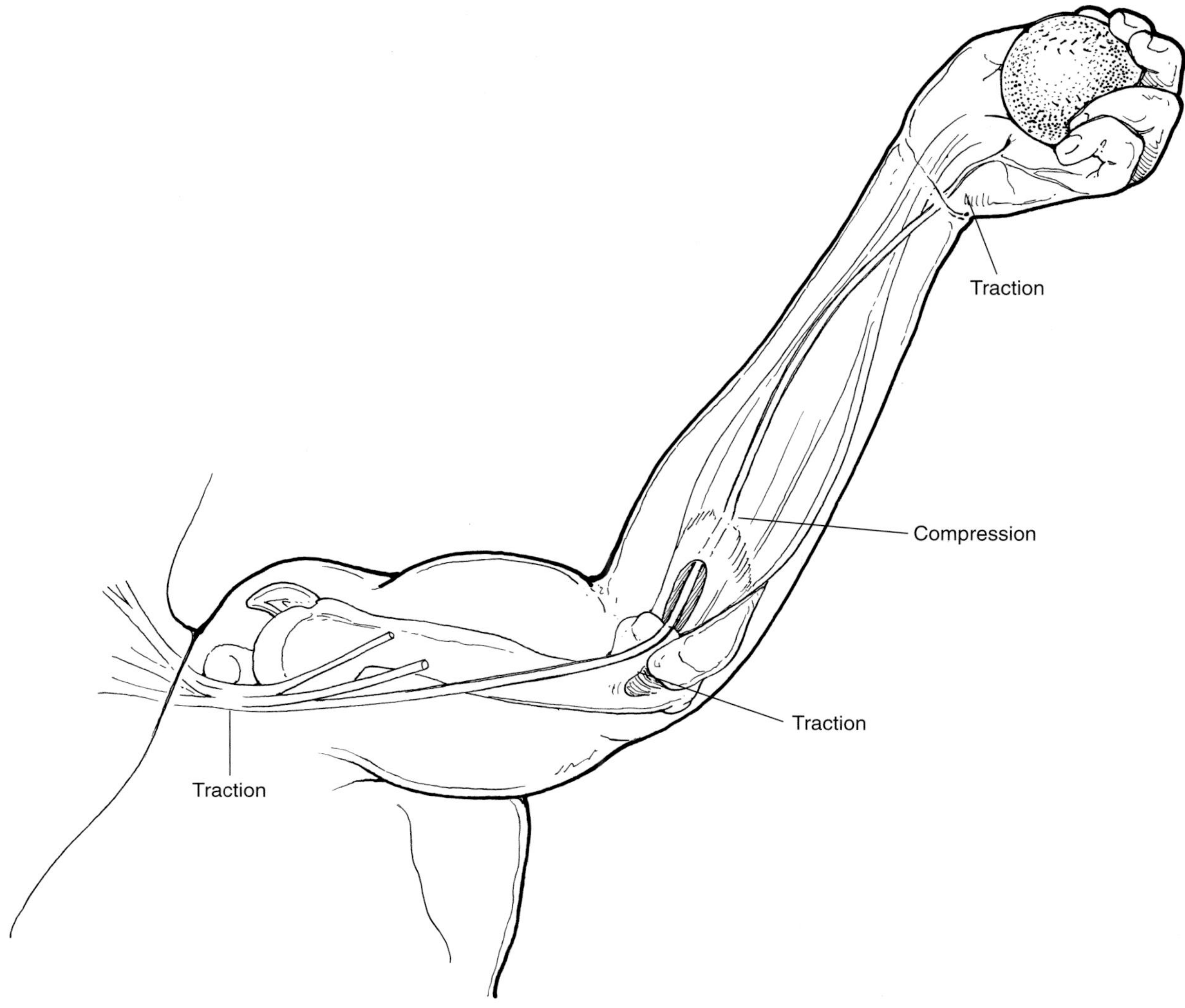

FIGURE 56–1. In the cocking position, the pressure in the cubital tunnel is six times greater than the resting pressure. The pressure elevation is the result of forces of traction from the shoulder, elbow, and wrist. The flexor carpi ulnaris generates compressive force.

when they are positive, are helpful for diagnosis of ulnar nerve entrapment at the elbow. Normal nerve studies do not exclude the diagnosis of cubital tunnel syndrome. When the history and clinical examination are consistent with cubital tunnel syndrome and NCV and EMG studies are normal, the neuropathy is considered mild. Electrical studies may not become positive until late in the process. The staging system of McGowan is helpful in classifying the disease and predicting patient response to treatment. Patients with McGowan stage I neuropathy have paresthesias and hypesthesias without sensory or motor loss. Stage II is characterized by weakness of the interosseous muscles. Finally, stage III patients have atrophy of the interossei and may have ulnar clawhand. These patients also have irreversible nerve damage and demonstrate less predictable improvement after surgical decompression.

NONOPERATIVE MANAGEMENT

Nonoperative management of cubital tunnel syndrome is frequently successful. Prolonged periods of elbow flexion are often the source of nerve irritation. A careful history of work and lifestyle habits often reveals obvious sources of nerve irritation. Patients should be educated to avoid prolonged periods of elbow flexion and to limit resting the elbow on hard surfaces. An elbow pad assists in protecting the nerve and serves as a constant reminder to avoid pressure on the nerve. Patients with nocturnal symptoms often benefit from night splints. The elbow pad worn backward at night may provide sufficient deterrence to elbow flexion at night. Greater limitation to elbow flexion can be achieved with towel splints, which are made by wrapping the elbow with a bath towel. The free end of the towel is pinned or taped. The towel can be slid off the arm in the morning. Many patients prefer the comfort of this homemade splint to conventional splints. If more rigid immobilization is required, a custom anterior elbow splint that maintains the joint at 45° is well tolerated. We do not recommend the injection of corticosteroids into the cubital tunnel. Fat atrophy is a significant risk in this area and may compromise wound healing with later surgery.

RELEVANT ANATOMY

The ulnar nerve lies in the anterior compartment of the proximal arm along the medial intermuscular septum. This nerve enters the posterior compartment near the midhumerus, passing through the medial intermuscular septum at the arcade of Struthers. The nerve passes distally along the posterior aspect of the medial intermuscular septum, passing deep to Osborne's fascia as it enters the cubital tunnel. Immediately distal to the cubital tunnel, the ulnar nerve passes between the two heads of the flexor carpi ulnaris (FCU) muscle. The most frequent site of compression of the nerve is between the two heads of the FCU. The cubital tunnel is bordered anteriorly by the medial epicondyle of the humerus; laterally, by the olecranon process of the ulna; and posteriorly, by Osborne's fascia. The ulnar nerve is accompanied by the superior ulnar recurrent artery proximally and by the posterior ulnar collateral artery distally. The arteries segmentally supply branches to the ulnar nerve.

Studies of the ulnar nerve's vascularity have demonstrated that up to 15 cm of nerve can be mobilized from the cubital tunnel without resultant nerve ischemia. However, cases of ischemic injury of the ulnar nerve have occurred after transposition procedures. Thus, it is prudent to preserve as many segmental branches as possible when transposing the nerve. As the nerve passes through the cubital tunnel, the first branch is the articular branch to the elbow. The articular branch can be sacrificed. The next branches are the motor branches to the FCU, which arise from the nerve as it passes between the heads of the FCU. The surgeon should preserve all FCU motor branches. If the nerve is being transposed and the motor branch limits transposition, the branch can be safely dissected away from the main nerve trunk for a distance of 5 to 8 cm. The medial antebrachial cutaneous nerve supplies the skin over the medial elbow. Anatomic studies demonstrate a consistent branch of this nerve that passes directly over the medial epicondyle. Medial elbow incisions risk injury to the medial antebrachial cutaneous nerve. Risk of cutaneous nerve injury is minimized by careful attention during subcutaneous dissection and by placing the incision farther posteriorly.

SURGICAL *TECHNIQUE*

Indications

Surgical release of the cubital tunnel has significant potential for debilitating complications, and the surgeon must scrutinize the decision to operate on the ulnar nerve. Indications are considered in two categories—relative and absolute. Indications for nerve decompression are considered *absolute* when failure to perform the procedure will likely result in progressive, permanent nerve deficit. *Relative* indications refer to situations in which nonoperative treatment has failed to relieve the symptoms, and the patient agrees that the surgical risks are worth an attempt to relieve the symptoms. Absolute indications for ulnar nerve decompression are a history consistent with the diagnosis and physical examination findings of atrophy or loss of static two-point discrimination, and nerve conduction studies consistent with ulnar nerve compression at the elbow. In addition, electromyography demonstrating axonal loss, a moderate to severe neuropathy, is an absolute indication. Relative indications include a history consistent with the diagnosis, positive provocative maneuvers, and failure to improve with a reasonable duration of conservative treatment. In our clinic, we prefer to provide 6 months of conservative care in patients with normal nerve conduction studies, and 3 to 6 months in patients with positive studies.

The selection of surgical technique is controversial, and a detailed discussion of procedure selection is beyond the scope of this chapter. Some general concepts are important. First, Dellon's review of the literature on this subject suggests that results of operative treatment for mild to moderate cubital tunnel are independent of the surgical technique. Second, in severe neuropathy, results of submuscular transposition are better than those for other decompression techniques. Recent reports have indicated success with subcutaneous transposition in severe and in recurrent neuropathy. Finally, the surgeon should be familiar with a variety of decompression techniques from which to choose so that various clinical situations can be addressed optimally.

Our preferences are based on a balance of potential risks and ease of surgical technique. We prefer in situ release for mild neuropathy not caused by nerve subluxation. In the case of moderate neuropathy or ulnar nerve subluxation, subcutaneous transposition is preferred. Medial epicondylectomy is reserved for cases of cubital tunnel syndrome associated with medial epicondylitis. Subcutaneous transposition with a fascial sling is employed in traumatic or elbow reconstructive cases, such as open reduction and internal fixation of supracondylar fractures, or total elbow arthroplasties. Submuscular transposition is reserved for severe neuropathy (McGowan III) or revision cases.

Technique

In Situ Decompression

1. Positioning: The patient is positioned in one of two ways. The first option, and our preference, is placing the patient supine with the arm extended on a hand table. The shoulder is maximally externally rotated and the elbow is flexed to 90°. The surgeon sits on the side of the hand table facing the axilla. This position provides a comfortable, stable position for dissection of the nerve; however, this position cannot be used in patients with stiff shoulders. The second option is to place the patient supine with arms across the chest. This position is used in patients with stiff shoulders. The surgeon stands on the affected side, and the arm is adducted across the chest wall in approximately 90° of forward flexion (Fig. 56–2). A sterile tourniquet is recommended to allow maximum access to the nerve. The surgical draping is done such that the tourniquet is placed as proximally on the arm as possible.

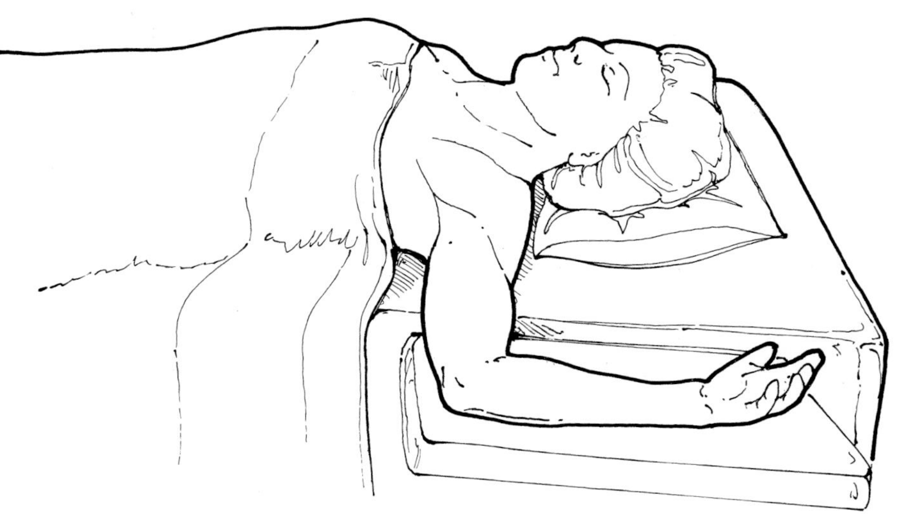

FIGURE 56–2. Positioning for cubital tunnel release. *A*, The supine position provides excellent arm support for the surgeon, but it requires maximum external rotation of the patient's shoulder. *B*, The across-chest position is useful in patients with stiff shoulders, but it offers less support for the wrists and forearms of the surgeon.

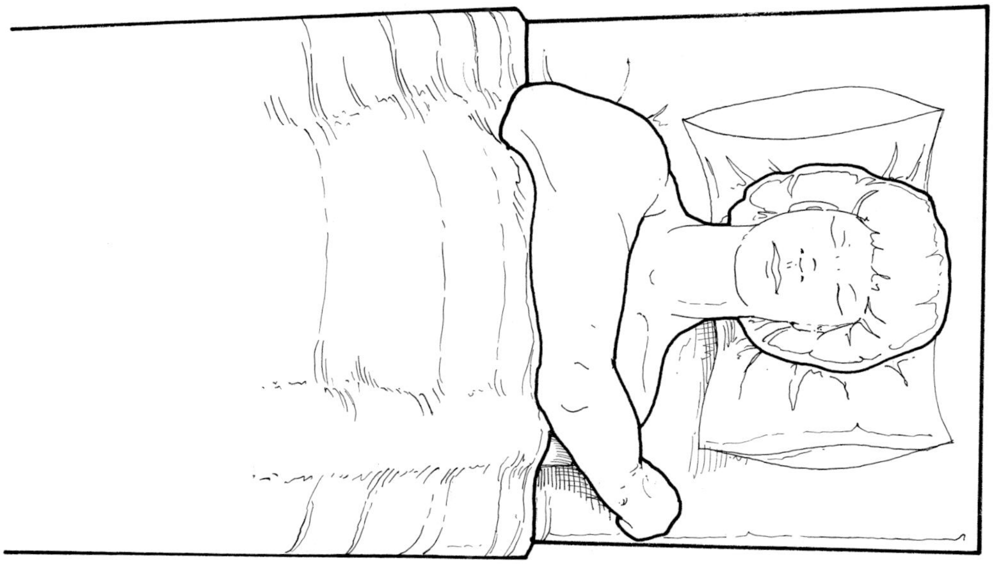

B

2. Incision: The incision is placed medial to the posterior midline of the elbow, just off the olecranon and subcutaneous boarder of the ulna. Because this incision is not placed directly over the nerve, risk of injury to the medial antebrachial cutaneous nerve branches is minimized (Fig. 56–3).
3. Deep exposure: Next, to further minimize risk of injury to the medial antebrachial cutaneous nerve, blunt scissors dissection is recommended to gain exposure of the deep fascial plane. The nerve is identified proximal to the arcuate ligament and posterior to the medial intermuscular septum.
4. Nerve decompression: During dissection from proximal to distal, the arcuate ligament and fascia of the FCU are released to a point sufficient for decompressing the nerve. In most cases, the nerve is visibly compressed at the fascial arcade between the two heads of the FCU (Fig. 56–4). It is not necessary for the proximal dissection to extend beyond the arcuate ligament in primary cases. Careful blunt scissors dissection just distal to the FCU heads ensures that no deep fascial bands entrap the nerve. Great care is exercised in this area to ensure that the scissors are in direct vision at all times; gentle spreading of the scissors is used to prevent injury to the numerous small motor branches from the ulnar nerve in this region.
5. Closure: Finally, the tourniquet is released and meticulous hemostasis is achieved. The wound is closed in standard fashion, and a light dressing is applied to allow early elbow motion postoperatively.

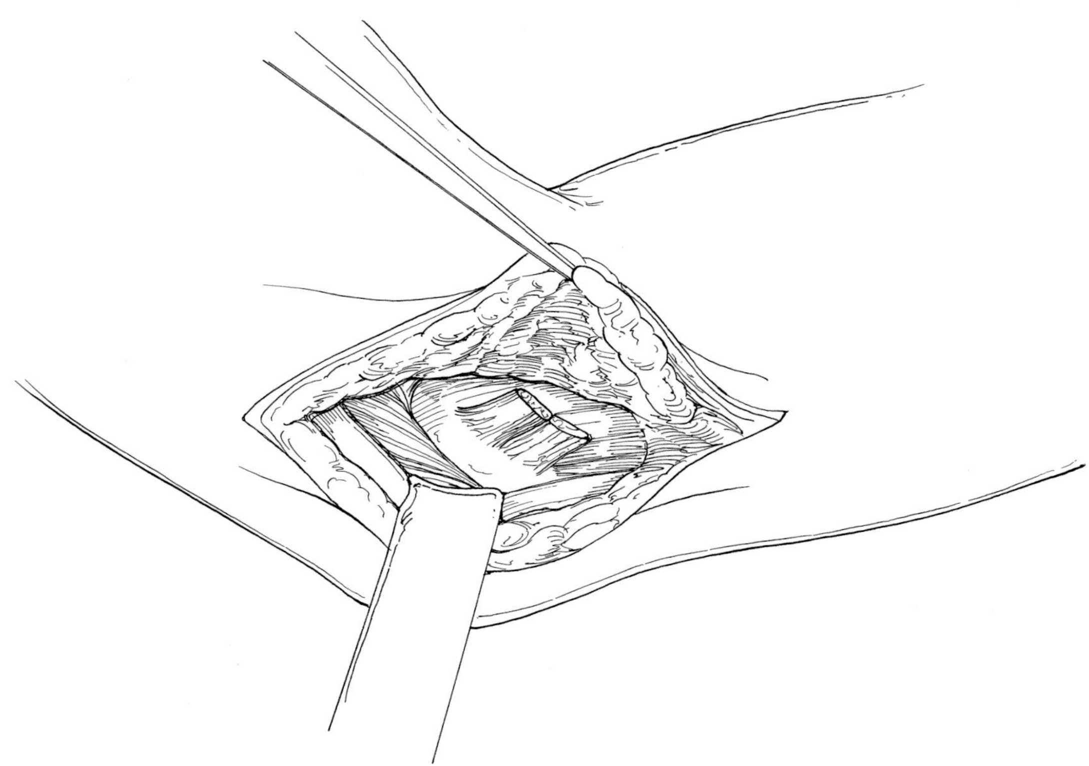

FIGURE 56–3. The incision for in situ release. A more posterior incision placement minimizes the risk of cutaneous nerve injury.

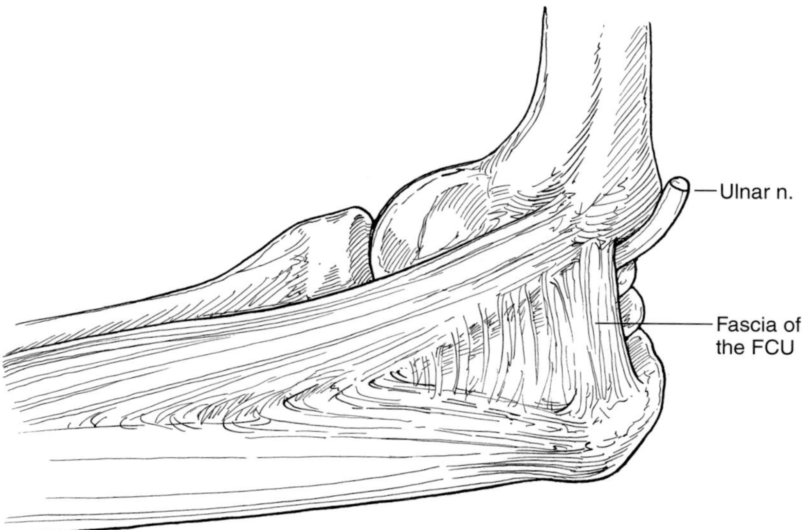

FIGURE 56–4. The flexor carpi ulnaris (FCU) fascia is the most frequent site of compression. Fascial bands within the muscle may be secondary sites of compression.

Medial Epicondylectomy

1. Positioning: Positioning and setup are as described for in situ release.
2. Incision: The skin incision extends from 5 cm distal and 8 cm proximal to the medial epicondyle (Fig. 56–5).
3. Epicondylectomy: Medial epicondylectomy is performed after completion of in situ release. The ulnar nerve is mobilized enough to allow retraction away from the medial epicondyle while the segmental blood supply is preserved. The distal 3 to 4 cm of the medial intermuscular septum is exposed and

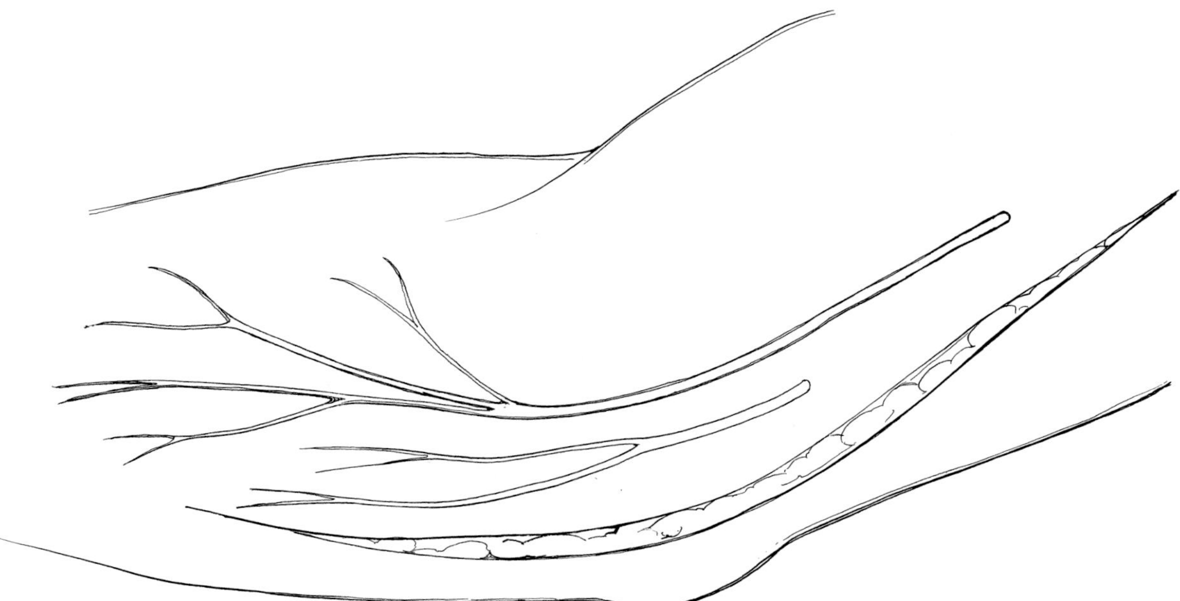

FIGURE 56–5. The incision for medial epicondylectomy or anterior transposition of the ulnar nerve extends from 8 cm proximal to the medial epicondyle to 5 cm distal to the epicondyle. The incision is placed posterior to the ulnar nerve and anteromedial to the posterior midline of the arm.

resected. An incision is carried from the medial epicondylar ridge to the inferior aspect of the medial epicondyle. Subperiosteal dissection is used to raise the soft tissues to the base of the epicondyle posteriorly, and to the middle of the epicondyle anteriorly. Special care is taken to preserve the thin tissue posteriorly; this serves as a gliding surface for the nerve and covers the cancellous bone exposed by the osteotomy. In addition, the MCL insertion is preserved. Next, the epicondyle is scored with an osteotome along the intended plane of resection (Fig. 56–6). The osteotomy is done from distal to proximal in a plane that is 45° posteriorly oblique from the coronal plane, such that the entire posterior surface and 50% of the anterior surface of the medial epicondyle are resected. This plane of resection does not significantly weaken the MCL.

4. Closure: The cancellous bone surface is covered with bone wax, and the periosteal envelope is closed with absorbable sutures. The elbow is taken through its range of motion to ensure that the nerve freely glides anteriorly. Any areas of nerve kinking with elbow flexion are resolved with further nerve mobilization.

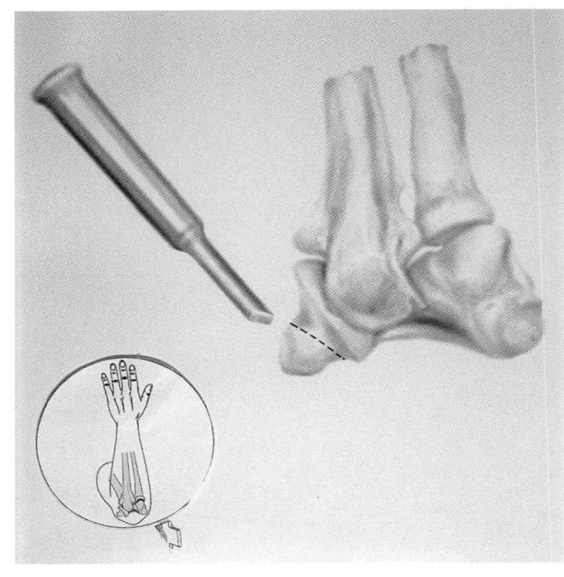

FIGURE 56–6. The plane of medial epicondyle resection is 45° oblique to the coronal plane of the humerus. The anteromedial surface of the epicondyle is preserved, along with the attachment of the anterior band of the medial collateral ligament. (Courtesy of William B. Kleinman, MD, The Indiana Hand Center, Indianapolis, IN.)

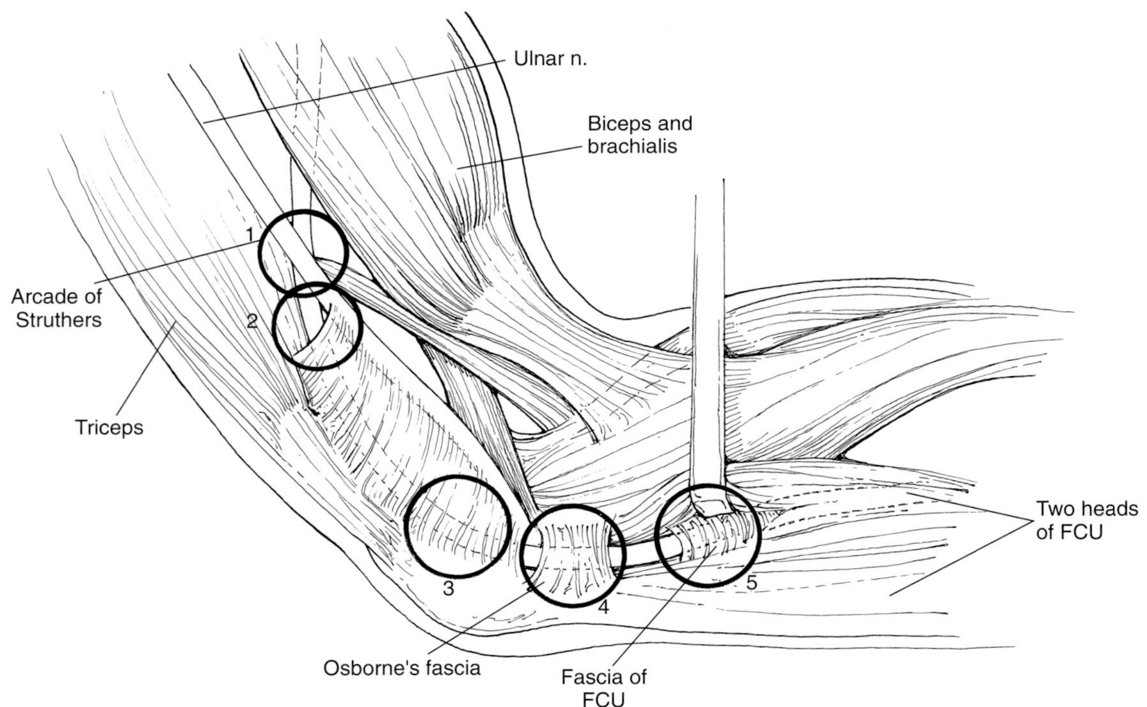

FIGURE 56–7. The ulnar nerve may be entrapped by (1) the arcade of Struthers, (2) the medial intermuscular septum, (3) the distal transverse fibers of the arcade of Struthers, (4) Osborne's ligament, and (5) the fascia of the flexor carpi ulnaris (FCU) heads and deeper fascial origins of the FCU.

Subcutaneous Transposition

1. Positioning: Positioning and setup are performed as described in the section on in situ release.
2. Incision: The skin incision is made as described for medial epicondylectomy.
3. Nerve decomression: The nerve is then mobilized from the arcade of Struthers to the proximal aspect of the FCU. All potential sites of compression are released (Fig. 56–7). The nerve is mobilized such that there is no kinking of the nerve proximally or distally after anterior transposition. Thus, the amount of mobilization required varies among patients.
4. A fascial sling is created by elevating a fascial flap from the superficial surface of the flexor-pronator mass based anterior to the medial epicondyle (Fig. 56–8). The nerve is transposed anteriorly. Transposition may require gentle dissection of the more proximal FCU motor branches from the ulnar nerve. The fascia is sutured to the subdermal tissue anterior to the medial epicondyle with interrupted absorbable sutures. The elbow is taken through a full range of motion while the ulnar nerve is inspected for evidence of kinking. The nerve should remain lax through the range of motion.

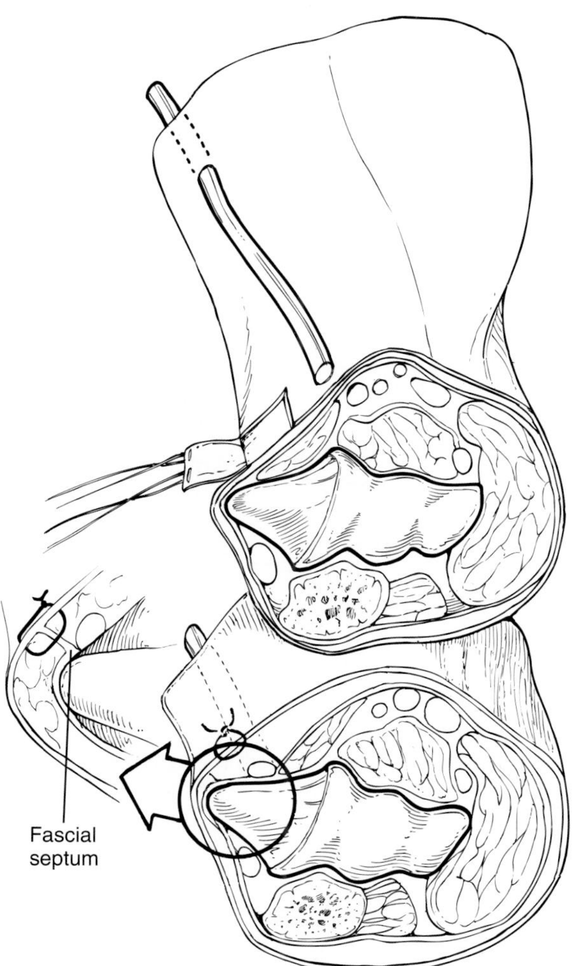

FIGURE 56–8. A flap of fascia is raised from the surface of the flexor-pronator insertion *(top)*. The flap is left attached anterior to the medial epicondyle *(bottom)*. The end of the flap is sutured to the subcutaneous tissue to form a septum that blocks posterior subluxation of the nerve.

Submuscular Transposition

1. Positioning and nerve decompression: Positioning and nerve decompression are the same as for in situ release, although the proximal mobilization of the nerve extends up to the arcade of Struthers. The nerve is mobilized as described for subcutaneous transposition. The medial intermuscular septum is excised (Fig. 56–9).
2. The flexor-pronator mass is elevated from the medial epicondyle distally enough to allow the ulnar nerve a straight path to the proximal one third of the FCU. The tendinous origin of the muscle mass is incised while the MCL is preserved (Fig. 56–10). Care is exercised in developing the plane between the MCL and the flexor-pronator mass. Beginning the dissection anteromedially and passing a clamp between the visualized edge of the MCL and the muscle mass can facilitate the procedure. The intermuscular septum of the FCU arising from the anteromedial edge of the ulnar shaft must be released distally enough to prevent it from entrapping or kinking the nerve. Similarly, the fascia inserting on the posteromedial aspect of the ulnar shaft must be released distally enough to prevent nerve kinking.
3. The nerve is transposed deep to the FCU. Then, the flexor-pronator tendon mass is approximated with interrupted sutures. The tourniquet is released and hemostasis is obtained. The wound is closed in standard fashion.

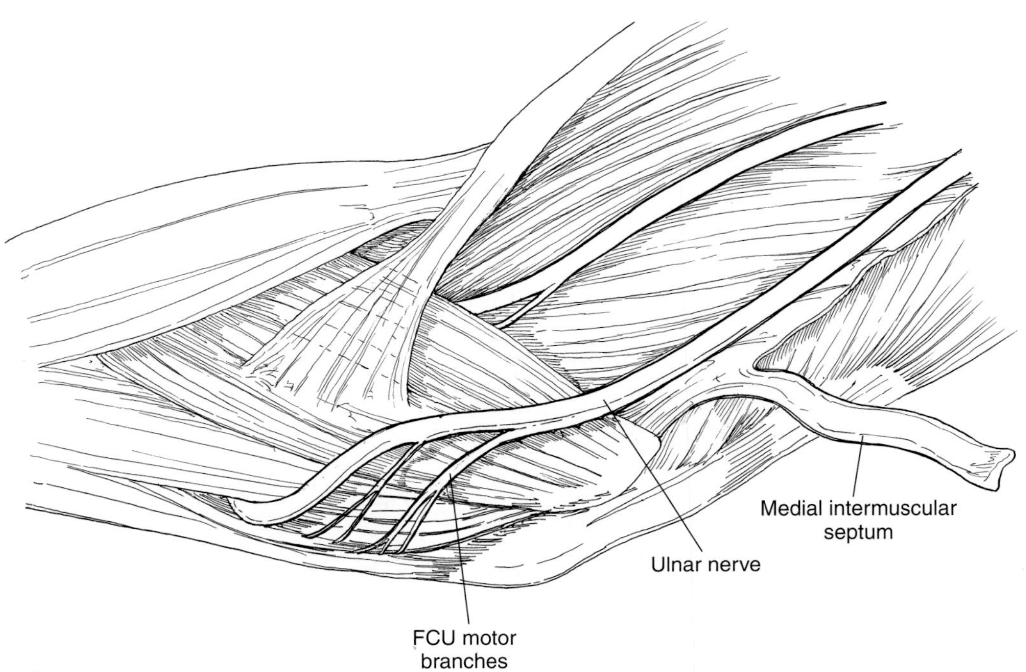

FIGURE 56–9. The medial intermuscular septum is excised. FCU, flexor carpi ulnaris.

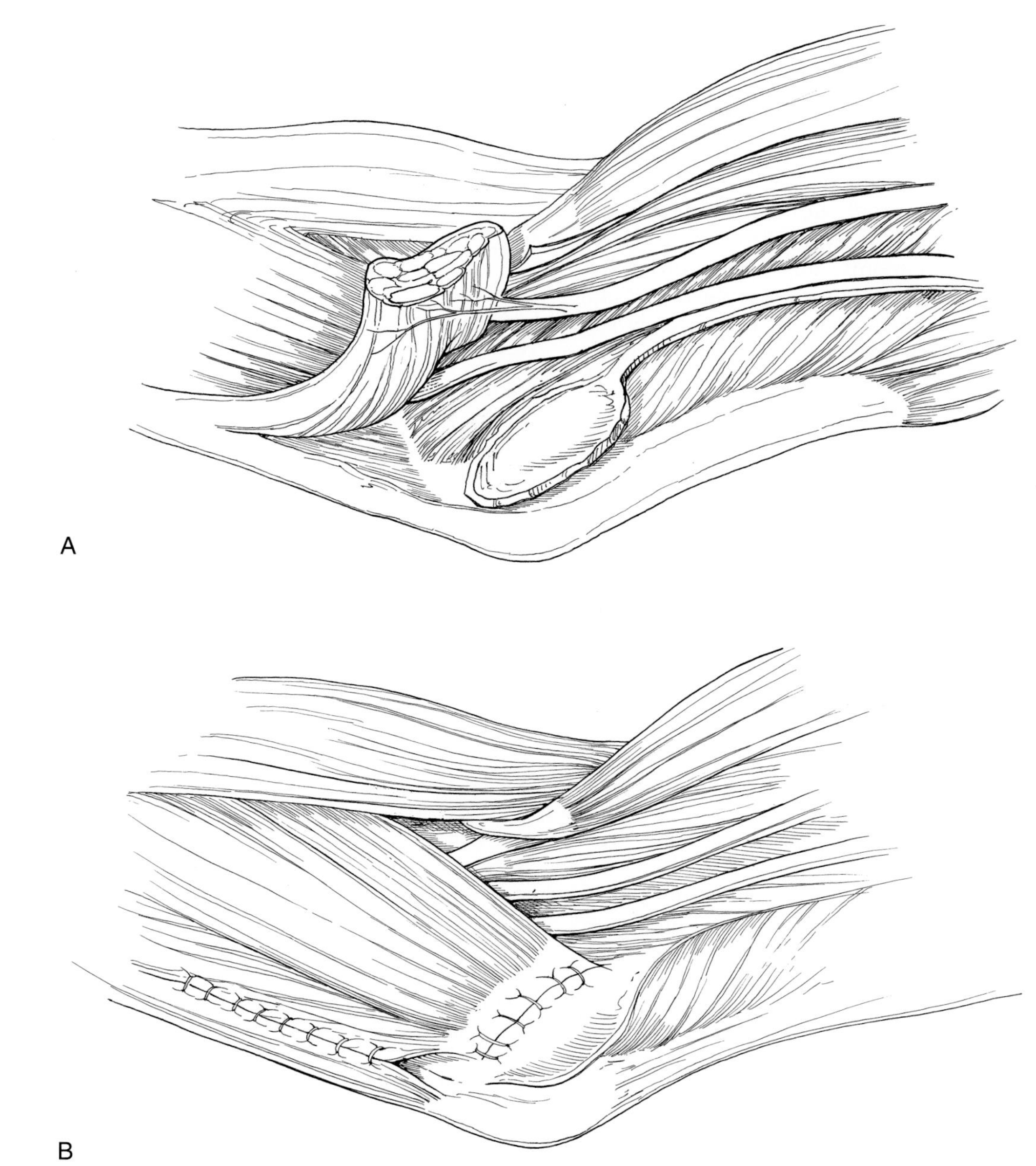

FIGURE 56–10. *A*, The flexor-pronator mass is elevated from the elbow capsule and the medial collateral ligament. The ulnar nerve is transposed adjacent to the median nerve. *B*, The flexor-pronator mass is sutured back to the medial epicondyle, ensuring that the nerve glides freely deep to the muscle.

POSTOPERATIVE MANAGEMENT

Early motion is important if the patient is to regain elbow range of motion with minimal difficulty, and it fosters gliding of the transposed nerve. Postoperative splinting is avoided. If splinting is required for pain control, it is limited to a few days. Minimal restrictions are applied in cases of in situ release and subcutaneous transposition. In cases treated with medial epicondylectomy or submuscular transposition, lifting is limited to light activity only for 1 month, followed by progressive strengthening activity. Patients are encouraged to resume daily activities and regain full elbow motion within the first 2 weeks. Beginning at 3 weeks, regardless of procedure, patients are taught scar massage to mobilize the subcutaneous scar and to decrease scar sensitivity.

COMPLICATIONS

The complications of ulnar nerve decompression vary according to the surgical procedure selected. However, complications seen in all these procedures include failure to resolve symptoms, scar tenderness, and sensory loss over the olecranon and proximal ulna. Scar tenderness, which most frequently results from injury to the medial antebrachial cutaneous nerves, is the most frequent complication of all these procedures. Injury to the cutaneous nerves is minimized by careful attention and blunt scissors dissection during the superficial wound exposure. In addition, a more posterior incision, as suggested by Saldana and Race, has greatly reduced the incidence of this problem in our experience.

The complications resulting from in situ decompression include failure to resolve symptoms and ulnar nerve subluxation. Although this is inherently the safest option in terms of risk of complication, the potential for persistent symptoms is significant in McGowan stage II and stage III neuropathy. Thus, this problem is avoided by careful patient selection. Limiting the proximal release of the nerve to where the nerve intersects a line from the medial epicondyle to the olecranon minimizes the risk of nerve subluxation. This area is not usually a source of compression; however, if it appears tight, it should be released and nerve transposition should be performed.

Complications of medial epicondylectomy include inadequate bone resection, excess bone resection with resulting compromise of the MCL, and bone tenderness at the osteotomy site. Underresection can significantly increase the risk of persistent symptoms. Overresection and underresection are avoided by attention to detail during the osteotomy. Bone tenderness is fortunately uncommon, but it can be a great source of dissatisfaction. This problem is beyond the control of the surgeon and is the primary reason we limit the use of this procedure.

Anterior subcutaneous transposition is associated with an increased risk of injury to the cutaneous nerves. In addition, nerve subluxation and new sites of compression are significant risks. Nerve subluxation can be eliminated with a fasciodermal sling, as suggested by Eaton. New sites of compression result most frequently from failure to address the arcade of Struthers, the medial intermuscular septum, and unresected deep flexor pronator aponeurosis.

Anterior submuscular transposition may result in the same problems seen in subcutaneous transposition. In addition, approximately 5% to 10% of patients develop elbow flexion contractures.

RESULTS

Dellon in 1989 reported on his review of the literature with regard to the operative treatment of ulnar nerve entrapment at the elbow. His review suggests that all these procedures have similar results when used to treat McGowan stage I or II ulnar neuropathy. In general, 80% or more of patients can expect good to excellent results. However, in McGowan stage III, the results are less predictable, and submuscular transposition appears to yield results superior to those of the other techniques. With severe neuropathy, less than 50% of patients recover their sensory innervation, and only 35% experience motor recovery; however, in most cases of severe neuropathy, submuscular transposition halts the progression of motor and sensory loss.

REFERENCES

Broudy AS, Leffert RD, Smith RJ: Technical problems with ulnar nerve transposition at the elbow: Findings and results of reoperation. J Hand Surg [Am] 3:85–89, 1978.

Dellon AL: Review of the treatment results for ulnar nerve entrapment at the elbow. J Hand Surg [Am] 14:688–700, 1989.

Dellon AL, Hament W, Gittelshon A: Nonoperative management of cubital tunnel syndrome: An 8-year prospective study. Neurology 43:1673–1677, 1993.

Dellon AL, MacKinnon SE: Injury to the medial antebrachial cutaneous nerve during cubital tunnel surgery. J Hand Surg [Br] 10:33–36, 1985.

Eaton RG, Crowe JF, Parkes JCI: Anterior transposition of the ulnar nerve with a non-compressing fasciodermal sling. J Bone Joint Surg [Am] 62A:820–825, 1980.

Gellman H, Campion DS: Modified in situ decompression of the ulnar nerve at the elbow. Hand Clin 12:405–410, 1996.

Heitoff SJ, Millender LH: Medial epicondylectomy for treatment of ulnar nerve compression at the elbow. Clin Orthop 139:174, 1979.

Jackson LC, Hotchkiss RN: Cubital tunnel surgery. Complications and treatment of failures. Hand Clin 12:449–456, 1996.

Race M, Saldana M: Anatomic course of the medial cutaneous nerves of the arm. J Hand Surg [Am] 16:48–52, 1991.

Rettig AC, Ebben JR: Anterior subcutaneous transfer of the ulnar nerve in the athlete. Am J Sports Med 21:836–840, 1993.

CHAPTER 57

Posterior Interosseous Nerve Release

INTRODUCTION

Two syndromes are associated with compression of the posterior interosseous nerve (PIN). First, posterior interosseous nerve syndrome refers to the clinical situation characterized by loss of motor function to some or all of the muscles innervated by the PIN. Second, radial tunnel syndrome (RTS) refers to vague forearm pain without associated motor function loss. RTS is frequently associated with lateral epicondylitis recalcitrant to conservative treatment. The diagnosis of RTS is based on subjective symptoms and limited objective findings, and electrophysiologic studies are not usually helpful in making the diagnosis. In contrast, in PIN syndrome, electrophysiologic studies are often diagnostic.

HISTORY AND PHYSICAL EXAMINATION

Patients with PIN syndrome describe vague, poorly localized dorsal forearm pain, and they often report associated extensor weakness. Some patients may present with complete PIN palsy, manifesting as complete loss of finger and thumb extensor function. Patients with RTS complain of vague, poorly localized forearm pain. They may have paresthesias in the radial nerve distribution, but more often they do not. Such paresthesias are more likely associated with C6 radiculopathy, which should be considered in the differential diagnosis. Commonly, patients have undergone unsuccessful treatment for lateral epicondylitis. Vague forearm pain that awakens the patient from sleep is particularly helpful in the diagnosis of RTS, especially if it occurs with associated positive provocative tests on physical examination.

Examination includes a careful neurologic assessment of the arm to rule out the presence of nerve compression syndromes. The presence of Tinel's sign over the radial nerve is suggestive of compression proximal to the radial tunnel. A positive Spurling's sign suggests the presence of the more common C6 radiculopathy. Physical examination may reveal pain reproduction with resisted supination from the positions of elbow extension, wrist flexion, and full pronation. The radial tunnel compression test is positive when compression of the area of the radial tunnel with the examiner's thumb reproduces the symptoms of vague forearm pain. Careful evaluation of the extensor muscles may reveal subtle weakness in selected extensors because PIN syndrome often manifests as an incomplete palsy.

DIAGNOSTIC IMAGING

Imaging is not usually helpful in establishing this diagnosis. However, standard anteroposterior and lateral radiographs of the elbow and proximal forearm are obtained to evaluate the bone for deformity or lesions. Lipomas or ganglions may produce soft tissue shadows on radiographs. If physical examination demonstrates a palpable mass in the region of the radial tunnel, MRI is indicated.

NONOPERATIVE MANAGEMENT

Literature on the nonoperative management of PIN compression is scarce. In PIN syndrome, a period of observation and limited activity is warranted. However, progression of neurologic deficit is an indication for decompression of the nerve. In contrast, RTS has limited objective findings, and a long period of rest and observation is recommended. The use of splinting and avoidance of pronation and supination may help alleviate symptoms. Surgery should not be considered in the treatment of RTS before the patient has experienced symptoms for 6 months.

RELEVANT ANATOMY

The radial nerve lies in the interval between the brachialis and the brachioradialis muscles as the nerve enters the cubital fossa. Within the area of the elbow, the nerve divides into the superficial and PIN branches. Just proximal to the radiocapitellar joint, the PIN enters the radial tunnel. As described by Roles and Maudsley, this is not a true anatomic tunnel, but its definition aids in our understanding of the potential sites of nerve compression (Fig. 57–1). A fascia lies superficial to the PIN as it passes anterior to the radiocapitellar joint. The next potential compression site is the radial recurrent artery and its venae comitantes, as described by Henry (consequently, it bears the name "leash of Henry"). Next, the nerve passes deep to the fibrous edge of the extensor carpi radialis brevis (ECRB). The PIN then passes through the arcade of Frohse. Dissection studies of this anatomic region by Spinner demonstrated that 30% of patients have a fibrous edge, which may compress the PIN. When a mass arises in this region, it is usually this fascia that becomes the point of nerve compression. Finally, the nerve can be compressed by fascial bands that lie at the exit from the supinator distally.

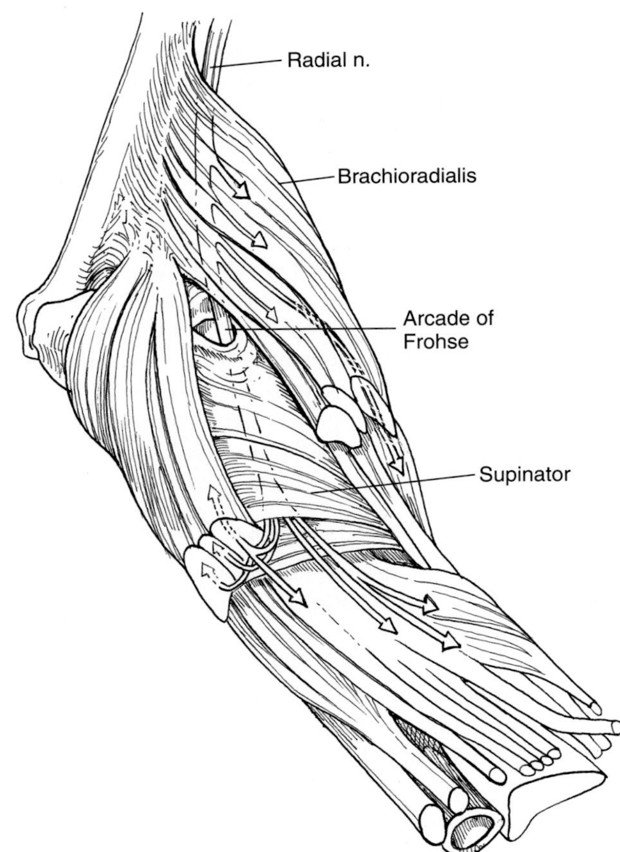

FIGURE 57–1. The posterior interosseous nerve enters the supinator through the fibrous arcade of Frohse. Immediately proximal to the arcade, the nerve may be compressed by fibrous bands or by the radial recurrent branches of the radial artery. Compression can also occur at the distal edge of the supinator.

SURGICAL TECHNIQUE

Indications

Progressive PIN palsy from compression and nerve palsy secondary to a compressing mass are clear indications for nerve decompression. In addition, iatrogenic PIN palsy after a surgical procedure around the elbow should be explored surgically immediately. The adage "to look is to know" applies. Although iatrogenic injuries are more likely secondary to traction injury from retractors, the best chance of identifying and resolving an incarcerated or lacerated nerve occurs during the immediate postsurgical period. Nonprogressive PIN syndrome should be observed for 4 to 12 weeks from the onset of symptoms. Failure of the patient to improve during this time is an indication for decompression of the nerve.

The indications for operative treatment of RTS are controversial. These recommendations are based on the literature and on our experience with this difficult diagnosis. Patients are treated conservatively for a minimum of 6 months. Serial examination should eliminate all potential differential diagnoses. Furthermore, examinations should consistently show pain with the radial tunnel compression test. Night pain, when present, foretells a good candidate for operative decompression.

Technique

Three popular approaches to decompression of this nerve have been used, and there are well-respected proponents of each. These approaches include brachioradialis splitting, the brachioradialis–extensor carpi radialis longus interval, and the posterior or Thompson approach in the extensor digitorum communis–extensor carpi radialis brevis interval. In our experience, the Thompson approach provides an extensile view of the nerve and all potential sites of compression. In addition, more proximal exposure of the nerve can be obtained through the same skin incision by exploiting the interval between the brachioradialis and the extensor carpi radialis longus.

1. Positioning: The patient is placed supine on the table with the affected limb on a hand table, the elbow flexed to 90°, and the shoulder internally rotated. The pneumatic tourniquet is placed as proximally on the arm as possible. In patients with short arms, it may be beneficial to use a sterile tourniquet.
2. Incision: The incision is a straight line from the lateral epicondyle toward the "bare area" of the midradius shaft. This "bare area" is located between the distal end of the radial wrist extensor muscle bellies and the outcropping muscles. The incision is marked with a sterile pen with the arm in neutral rotation. The surgeon must look for branches of the posterior antebrachial cutaneous nerve and protect them from injury during superficial dissection (Fig. 57–2).
3. Procedure: After the deep fascia is exposed, a fascial septum is visible between the extensor digitorum communis (EDC) and the extensor carpi radialis brevis (ECRB). This fascia is part of the ECRB, and it is longitudinally incised just ulnar to the

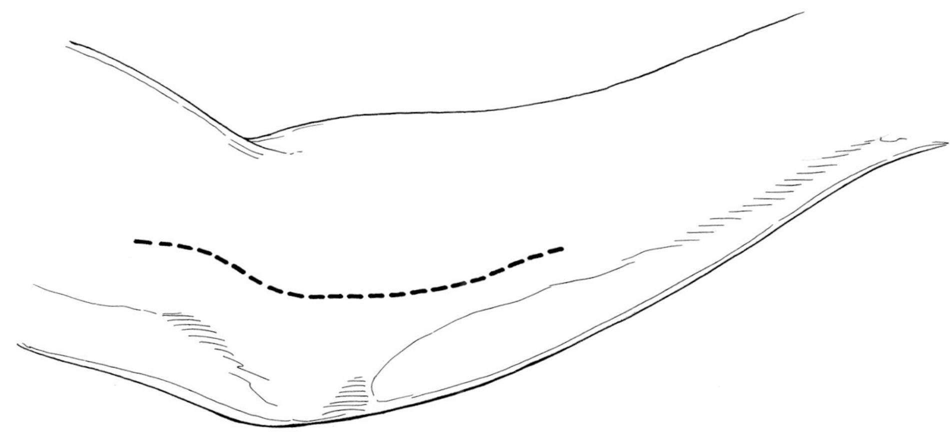

FIGURE 57–2. Superficial and deep incisions. *A*, The line of incision is from the lateral epicondyle toward the bare area of the radius distally.

Illustration continued on following page

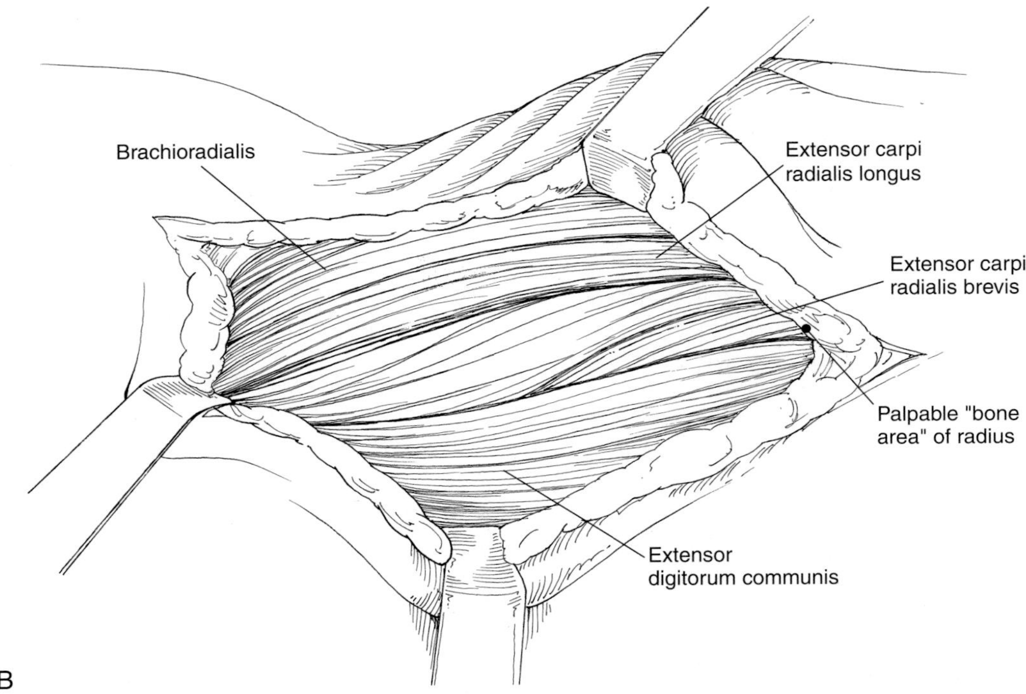

FIGURE 57–2 *Continued. B,* The deep exposure is between the extensor carpi radialis brevis and the extensor digitorum communis. The dissection is carried deep on the ulnar side of the fascial plane between the muscles.

fascial septum. Attempting the approach from the radial side of the septum leads the surgeon into the substance of the ECRB muscle belly. As the deep plane of dissection develops, fibers of the EDC inserting into the fascial septum are easily swept free with a Freer elevator or knife in a distal-to-proximal direction. A double skin hook placed in the midsubstance of the septum and lifted away from the radius facilitates the dissection. As the plane develops, the fibers of the supinator are visible as they course obliquely to the plane of the septum. With the supinator in view, the plane between the supinator and the ECRB is developed proximally and distally (Fig. 57–3). Care is taken in the distal aspect of the wound to avoid injury to small delicate branches of the PIN that exit the distal aspect of the supinator.

4. An Army-Navy retractor is placed under the ECRB to elevate it from the supinator. The PIN is visualized as it enters the arcade of Frohse. The view of the PIN is limited by the noncompliance of the fascial septum and fascia on the deep surface of the ECRB. These two fascial planes are completely incised perpendicular to the axis of the forearm superior to the arcade of Frohse (Fig. 57–4). This maneuver eliminates this potential cause of compression and dramatically increases the exposure of the PIN. It is important to note that the exposure depicted in Figure 57–4 is not possible until the fascia of the ECRB is incised. Before the fascial incision is made, the view of the PIN is limited.
5. The arcade of Frohse and the surrounding supinator muscle fibers are released. The nerve is followed to its exit from the supinator distally. Finally, the proximal aspect of the PIN is explored. This is facilitated by elbow flexion while an Army-Navy retractor elevates the ECRB. The proximal PIN is explored for compression by either the fascia or the radial recurrent vessels. Gentle scissors dissection around the leash of Henry is recommended because these vessels are often tortuous and friable. Bleeding from the venae comitantes can be difficult to identify and control.
6. If more proximal exposure of the nerve is required, the proximal aspect of the incision is extended and the interval between the brachioradialis (BR) and the

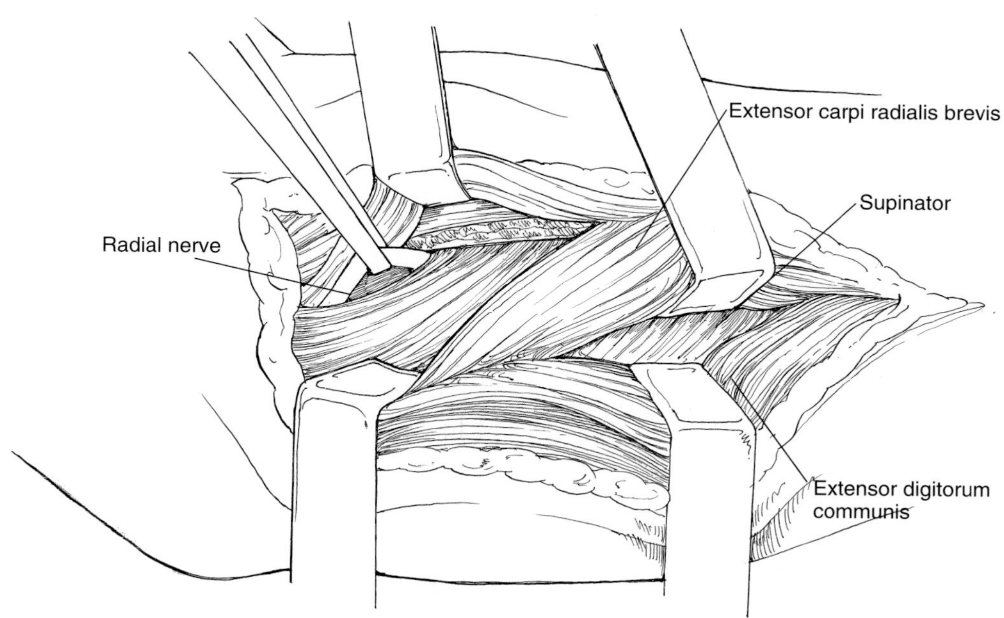

FIGURE 57–3. Supinator exposure. The supinator fibers are recognized by their oblique orientation to the extensor carpi radialis brevis and the extensor digitorum communis as the deep plane is exposed.

extensor carpi radialis longus (ECRL) is used. This is accomplished by elevating the anterior skin flap, carefully protecting the branches of the lateral antebrachial cutanous nerve, and identifying the interval between the BR and the ECRL.

7. The tourniquet is released and meticulous hemostasis is obtained. The deep fascia is loosely reapproximated to avoid a cosmetic defect, and the wound is closed in standard fashion. Drains are not usually required.

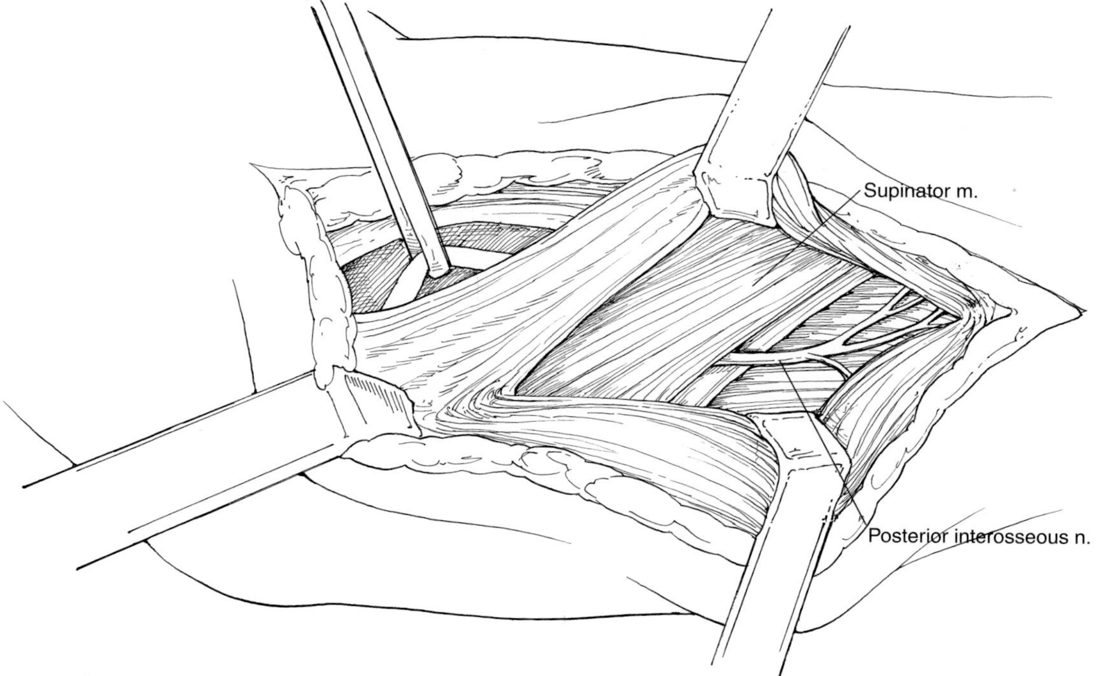

FIGURE 57–4. Release of the fascia on the deep surface of the extensor carpi radialis brevis allows the muscle to be retracted and substantially improves the nerve exposure.

POSTOPERATIVE MANAGEMENT

A light dressing is applied postoperatively so as not to inhibit elbow range of motion. Patients are encouraged to resume daily activities as pain permits. Forearm rotation and wrist extension cause the greatest discomfort postoperatively owing to the release of the ECRB fascia and the supinator muscle. Consequently, the wrist is supported with a cock-up wrist splint during the first week for comfort.

COMPLICATIONS

Complications include failure to relieve symptoms, injury to the PIN, hematoma, and injury to the posterior antebrachial cutaneous nerve. All of these problems are averted by careful attention to the details of the procedure and avoidance of vigorous retraction of the nerves.

RESULTS

This discussion of results must emphasize the difference between RTS and PIN syndrome. PIN syndrome has clear objective criteria for establishing the diagnosis; diagnosis of RTS is based on subjective complaints and limited physical findings. Consequently, surgical treatment of PIN syndrome is much more reliable than that of RTS.

PIN decompression for RTS has been reported to result in approximately 70% good and excellent results. However, other authors caution that results are less predictable, and they suggest that surgeons take a cautious approach to indicating this operation. Our unpublished experience in 22 cases of RTS parallels the experience recorded in the literature—30% of patients improve but are dissatisfied with the relief of pain. This experience is the result of a very conservative approach to RTS that includes a minimum of 6 months (in most cases, 12 months) of nonoperative treatment.

The results of decompression of PIN syndrome are directly related to the severity of the neuropathy. Denervated muscles have little chance of recovery if the condition continues for longer than 18 months. In the case of acute onset with gradual progression of symptoms followed by prompt decompression, complete recovery is anticipated.

REFERENCES

Atroshi I, Johnsson R, Ornstein E: Radial tunnel release. Unpredictable outcome in 37 consecutive cases with a 1–5 year follow-up. Acta Orthop Scand 66:255–257, 1995.

Fardin P, Negrin P, Sparta S, et al: Posterior interosseous nerve neuropathy. Clinical and electromyographical aspects. Electromyogr Clin Neurophysiol 32:229–234, 1992.

Jebson PJ, Engber WD: Radial tunnel syndrome: Long-term results of surgical decompression. J Hand Surg [Am] 22:889–896, 1997.

Lawrence T, Mobbs P, Fortems Y, Stanley JK: Radial tunnel syndrome. A retrospective review of 30 decompressions of the radial nerve [see comments]. J Hand Surg [Br] 20:454–459, 1995.

Ritts GD, Wood MB, Linscheid RL: Radial tunnel syndrome. A ten-year surgical experience. Clin Orthop 219:201–205, 1987.

Roles NC, Maudsley RH: Radial tunnel syndrome: Resistant tennis elbow as a nerve entrapment. J Bone Joint Surg [Br] 54:499–508, 1972.

Spinner RJ, Berger RA, Carmichael SW, et al: Isolated paralysis of the extensor digitorum communis associated with the posterior (Thompson) approach to the proximal radius. J Hand Surg [Am] 23:135–141, 1998.

CHAPTER 58

Lateral Collateral Ligament Repair

INTRODUCTION

Recognition of lateral collateral ligament (LCL) insufficiency of the elbow is increasing among orthopaedic surgeons. The instability that results from LCL rupture is rotational. This rotation results in widening of the lateral joint line and rotation of the radial head posterior to the capitellum, which is referred to as *posterior lateral rotary instability (PLRI) of the elbow* (Fig. 58–1). Although the mechanism of LCL injury is quite different from that of medial collateral ligament instability, the surgical technique of LCL reconstruction is remarkably similar to that for the medial collateral ligament.

HISTORY AND PHYSICAL EXAMINATION

Most patients with LCL rupture sustained a traumatic injury. Josefsson and associates demonstrated in open treatment of elbow dislocations that both medial and lateral collateral ligaments are ruptured. In addition, they showed that in the majority of cases, the ligaments heal without residual instability, and surgical repair of the acute ligament injury does not improve outcome.

By far the most common cause of PLRI is elbow dislocation. In addition, iatrogenic injury during lateral elbow exposures is not uncommon. These issues should be evaluated in the patient history. Patients may report pain or discomfort with elbow extension and supination. Popping or catching in the joint may occur during flexion and pronation from the extended position. This catching sensation occurs with reduction of the posteriorly subluxed radial head onto the capitellum.

The physical examination usually shows normal motion, although pain and apprehension may occur with supination and extension, especially when combined with axial loading. The posterior lateral rotary instability test (lateral pivot shift test), as described by O'Driscoll and colleagues, is the most reliable maneuver for confirming

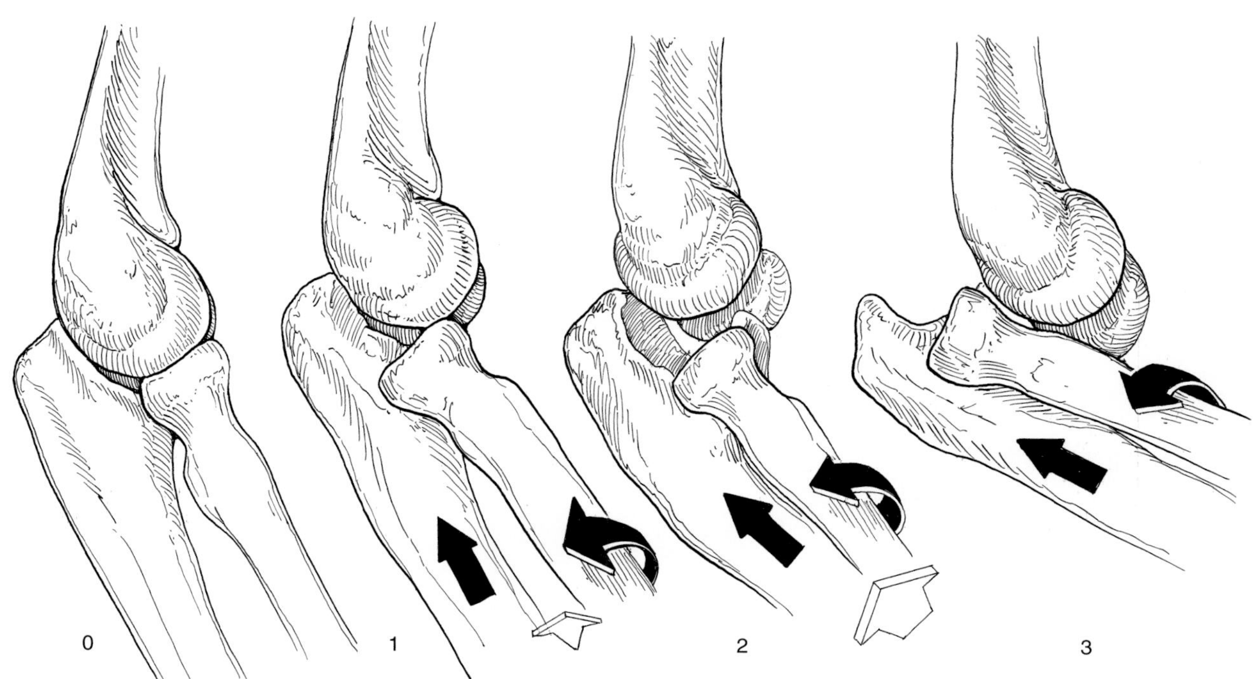

FIGURE 58–1. Posterolateral elbow instability is progressive from subluxation (0) to dislocation. The three stages are illustrated here: (1) posterior lateral rotary instability; (2) perched; and (3) dislocated.

the diagnosis (Fig. 58–2), causing pain and apprehension. In most cases, actual subluxation of the radiocapitellar joint with the resulting "dimple sign" occurs only during examination under anesthesia, or after injection of the joint with local anesthetic. If examination under anesthesia is unclear, diagnostic arthroscopy may assist the clinician in visualizing the instability.

DIAGNOSTIC IMAGING

Standard anteroposterior and lateral radiographs of the elbow are usually unremarkable. Recent advances in MRI have increased our ability to visualize the collateral ligaments. Fluoroscopy is useful for visualizing radial head displacement during the PLRI test.

NONOPERATIVE MANAGEMENT

In the acute elbow injury, rupture of the LCL can be managed with a brief period of immobilization with the forearm in pronation. After 10 to 14 days, a progressive motion program is initiated, as in the treatment of elbow dislocations. In the setting of a chronic injury, symptoms are unlikely to improve with nonsurgical treatment. Patients wishing to avoid surgery may benefit from braces that limit elbow extension. In contrast, patients wishing to return to full activity do best with ligament reconstruction.

RELEVANT ANATOMY

Morrey and An in 1985 described the detailed anatomy of the LCL. The ligament has an oblique orientation as it originates from the anterior inferior aspect of the lateral epicondyle, then passes medially and inferiorly to insert on the supinator tubercle of the ulna inferior to the radial neck. The fibers of the annular ligament blend with the ligament near its insertion (Fig. 58–3). The isometric point on the lateral epicondyle is located on a line that extends down the anterior cortex of the humeral shaft.

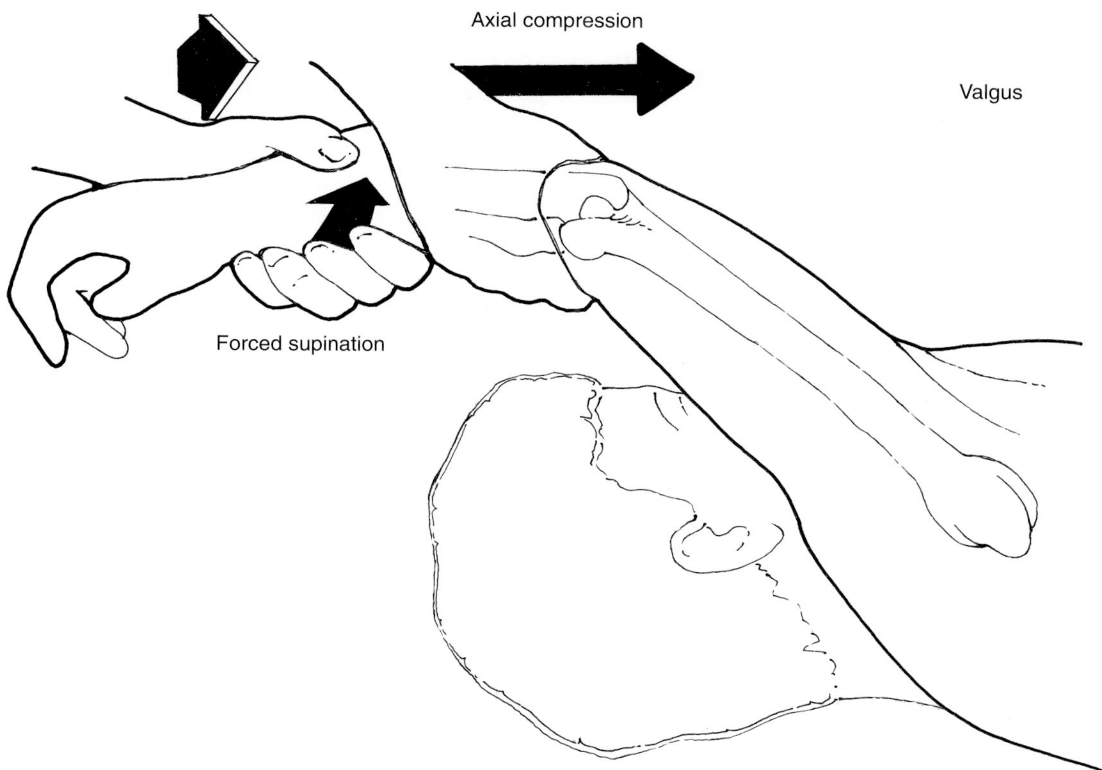

FIGURE 58–2. The posterior lateral rotary instability (PLRI) test is performed by applying supination, valgus, and axial compression while flexing and extending the elbow. Reduction of the radial head is palpable, and a dimple occurs posteriorly as the radial head subluxes. A "dimple sign" is most often seen on examination with the patient under anesthesia.

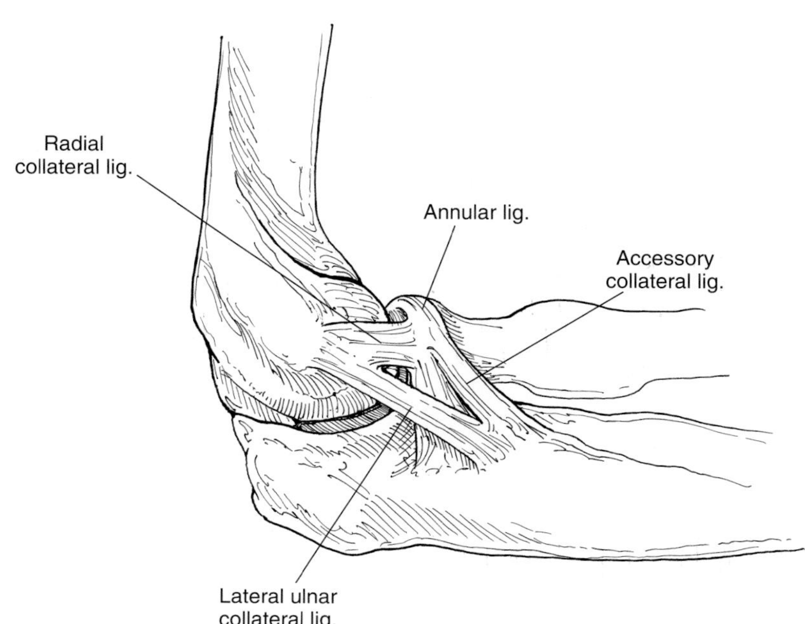

FIGURE 58–3. The lateral collateral ligament passes distal, posterior, and medial to the radial head in the insert on the supinator tubercle of the ulna. The oblique orientation allows it to act as both a lateral and a posterior stabilizer of the elbow.

SURGICAL *TECHNIQUE*

Indications

Active patients with PLRI are candidates for LCL reconstruction. Most patients are not satisfied with bracing and activity limitation. Because of the difficulty in demonstrating PLRI on physical examination, the decision to proceed to ligament reconstruction is often made after the examination under anesthesia is performed.

Technique

1. Positioning: The patient is placed supine on the operating table with the affected arm extended on an arm table. If the patient does not have a palmaris longus tendon, preparation for harvest of plantaris or semitendinosus tendon is made. The arm tourniquet is placed high to allow maximum access to the elbow.
2. Incision: A 10- to 12-cm Kocher incision is used. The deep exposure is carried through the interval between the anconeus and extensor carpi ulnaris muscles. The muscles are elevated off the capsuloligamentous structures (Fig. 58–4). With the capsule exposed, the PLRI is demonstrated under direct visualization. The lateral epicondylar origin of the LCL is exposed by incising the capsule vertically, proximal to the annular ligament (Fig. 58–5).

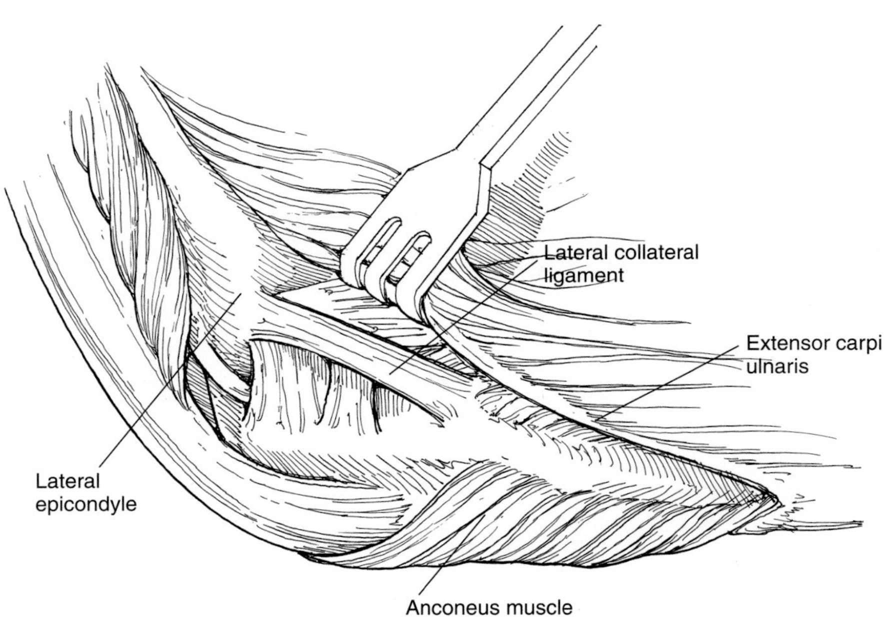

FIGURE 58–4. Kocher exposure preserves the elbow capsule integrity.

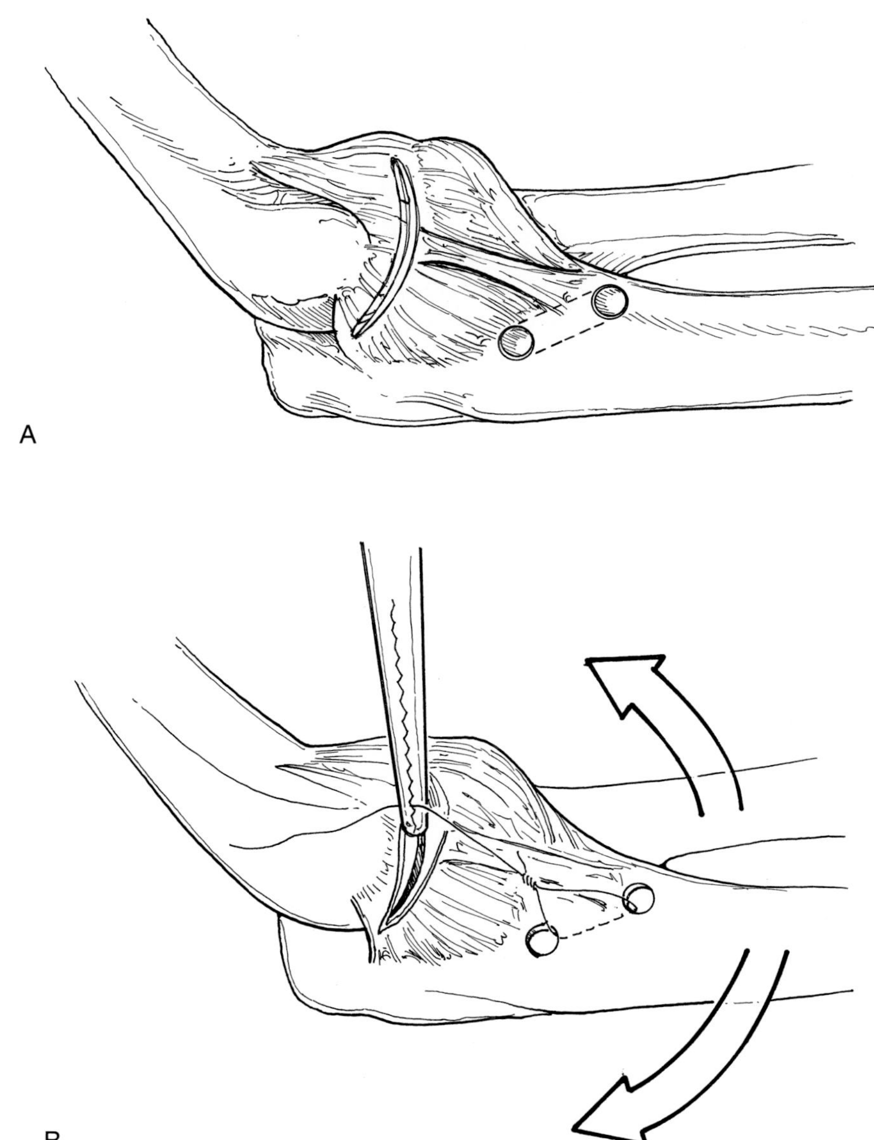

FIGURE 58–5. *A*, The capsule is incised transversely to expose the lateral epicondyle. These flaps are used to reinforce the repair at the capsular closure. *B*, A suture placed through the drill holes is used to identify the isometric point on the lateral epicondyle. The elbow is flexed and extended *(arrows)* while a clamp holds the suture over the isometric point of the epicondyle.

3. Graft harvest: A 2-cm transverse incision is made at the volar wrist crease centered over the palmaris longus tendon. The palmaris longus tendon insertion is grasped with a hemostat and transected distally. A 1–0 nonabsorbable braided suture is passed through the tendon stump several times. The suture is then passed through a tendon stripper of appropriate size. Note that the suture is required to pass the tendon into the tendon stripper because the tendon stripper that is the correct size is too small to allow a clamp to pass through. Traction is applied to the tendon stump by pulling firmly with a hemostat on the end of the tendon. The tendon stripper is then rotated back and forth while it is advanced up the forearm (Fig. 58–6). As the tendon stripper engages the musculotendinous junction, some increased resistance to advancement will be felt. Shortly after the tendon stripper has been advanced past the point of resistance, the tendon will pull loose from the muscle and can be withdrawn with the tendon stripper. If difficulty is encountered, a second incision is placed proximally to expose and release the tendon.
4. Ligament reconstruction: Two 3.2-mm holes are drilled on the supinator tubercle 1 cm apart. A suture is passed through the holes and is held to the lateral epicondyle near the anticipated isometric point (Fig. 58–7). The isometry is checked by flexing and extending the elbow. Two divergent 3.2-mm holes are drilled just posterior and superior to the isometric point such that they exit the posterior cortex of the lateral epicondyle at least 1 cm apart (Fig. 58–8). A 28-gauge wire loop is used as a ligament passer to thread the graft through the tunnels. The graft is passed through the ulnar drill holes first and then is sutured to itself with No. 1 nonabsorbable braided sutures (Fig. 58–9). The graft is then passed through the isometric humeral drill hole and out the back of the epicondyle, then back into the other posterior drill hole and out the isometric hole. The graft is tensioned with the elbow flexed to 90° and the forearm fully pronated. The free end of the graft is sutured to itself and to the annular ligament and capsule. Sutures are not placed directly over the joint line where they may cause crepitus with motion of the elbow.
5. Closure: The capsular flap is closed over the graft with absorbable No. 1 or No. 0 sutures. The musculotendinous interval between the anconeus and the extensor carpi ulnaris is closed with absorbable sutures.

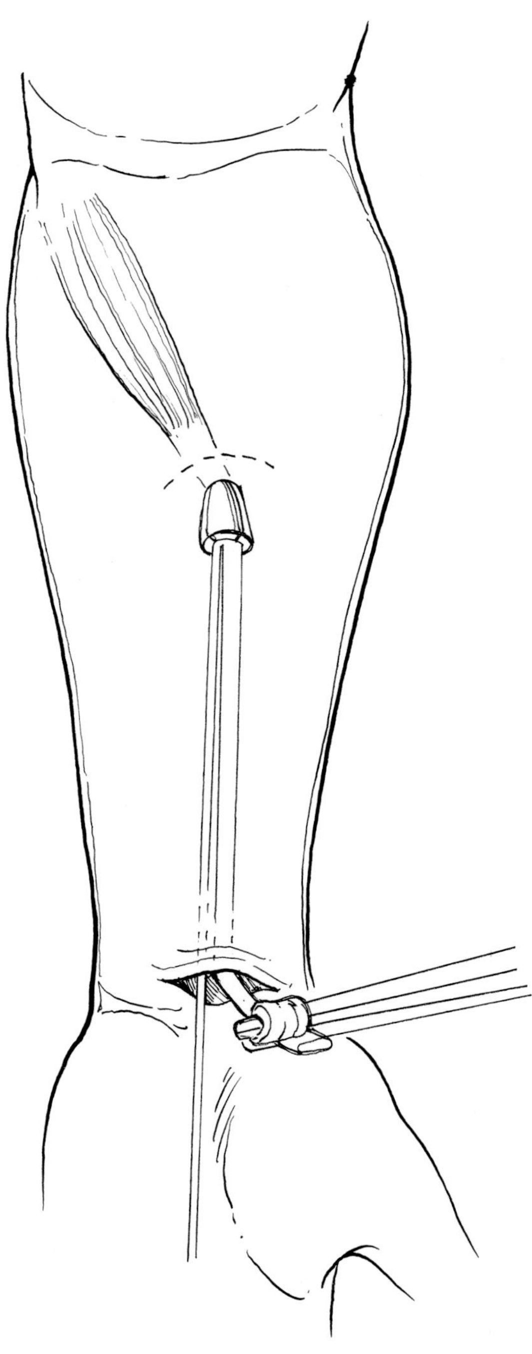

FIGURE 58–6. An incision in the wrist flexion crease exposes the palmaris longus. The tendon stripper harvests the palmaris longus by passing over the tendon from distal to proximal. A second incision can be made proximally, but it is not usually required.

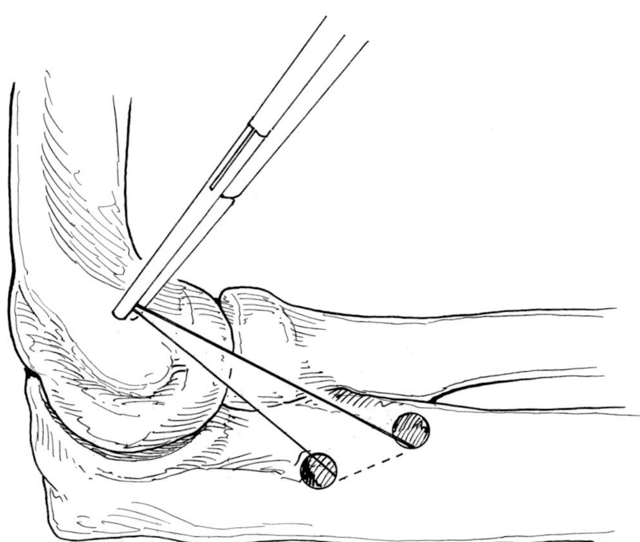

FIGURE 58–7. Isometry is checked with a large suture held by a clamp.

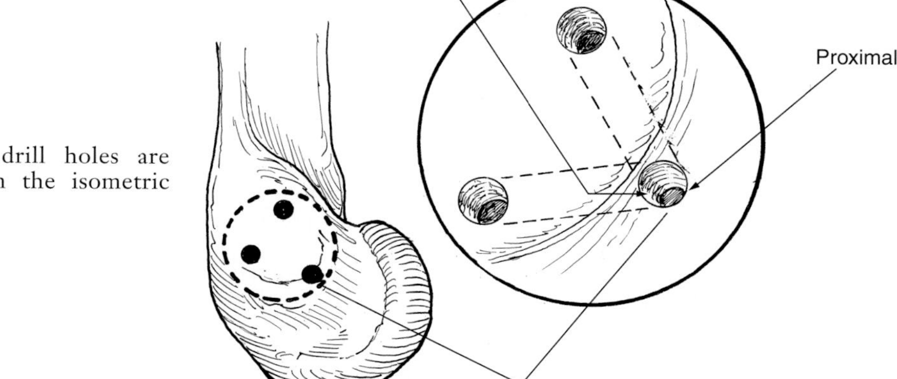

FIGURE 58–8. Divergent drill holes are created, originating from the isometric point.

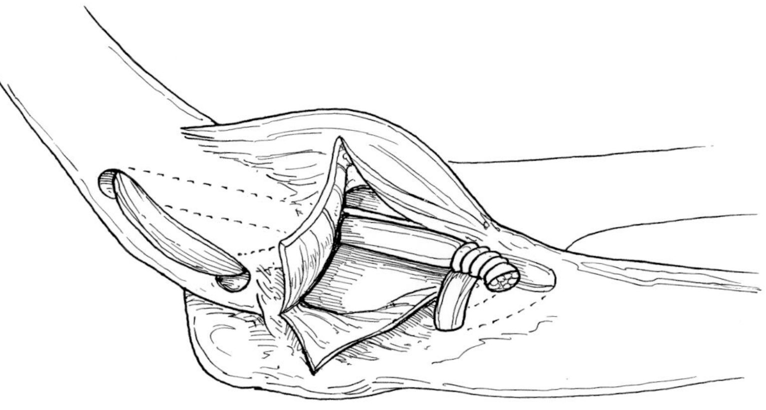

FIGURE 58–9. The palmaris graft is weaved through the drill holes as shown and is sutured to itself with multiple interrupted nonabsorbable sutures.

POSTOPERATIVE MANAGEMENT

Postoperatively, the limb is immobilized in full pronation with the elbow in 90° of flexion until a brace is applied. The brace that we use consists of a custom-molded orthoplast arm cuff and forearm clamshell connected with a hinge from a Bledsoe brace (Bledsoe Brace Systems, Medical Technology, Inc., Grand Prairie, TX) that is riveted to the orthoplast. The hinge is set to a 30° extension block for 4 weeks. Full motion in the brace is permitted from 4 to 6 weeks. The brace is discontinued at 6 weeks. Individuals with ligamentous laxity and no evidence of capsular contracture may be braced for a longer period of time. From 6 weeks to 12 weeks, patients are allowed unrestricted daily activities, but they should avoid elbow loading in extension and supination. At 3 months, a graduated progressive strengthening program is initiated with the goal of achieving full extensor power by 6 to 9 months. However, restrictions on varus stress and heavy loading in extension and supination are continued until 9 months. Sport-specific training begins at 9 months with the goal of returning to unrestricted activity at 12 months.

COMPLICATIONS

Potential problems include elbow stiffness, posterior interosseous nerve injury, and rupture of the graft. Elbow stiffness is best avoided by isometric graft placement and attention to detail during the postoperative rehabilitation. Similarly, attention to detail during surgical exposure will prevent injury to the posterior interosseous nerve. We have, however, seen one case of radial tunnel syndrome that occurred 1 year after reconstruction secondary to scar near the nerve. The symptoms resolved with nerve decompression.

RESULTS

Owing to the relatively recent description of this disorder, large numbers of long-term results are not available. Morrey and O'Driscoll reported their early experience with 10 cases, of which 6 outcomes were rated as excellent, 1 good, and 3 fair. This included 1 case of recurrent instability.

REFERENCES

Clarke RP: Symptomatic, lateral synovial fringe (plica) of the elbow joint. Arthroscopy 4:112–116, 1988.

Cohen MS, Hastings H: Rotatory instability of the elbow. The anatomy and role of the lateral stabilizers. J Bone Joint Surg [Am] 79:225–233, 1997.

Jobe FW, Elattrache NS: Diagnosis and treatment of ulnar collateral ligament injuries in athletes. In Morrey BF (ed): The Elbow and Its Disorders, 2nd ed. Philadelphia, WB Saunders, 1993, pp 566–572.

Josefsson PO, Gentz CF, Johnell O, Wendeberg B: Surgical versus non-surgical treatment of ligamentous injuries following dislocation of the elbow joint. A prospective randomized study. J Bone Joint Surg [Am] 69:605–608, 1987.

Morrey BF, An KN: Functional anatomy of the ligaments of the elbow. Clin Orthop 201:84–90, 1985.

Morrey BF, O'Driscoll SW: Lateral collateral ligament injury. In Morrey BF (ed): The Elbow and Its Disorders, 2nd ed. Philadelphia, WB Saunders, 1993, pp 573–595.

O'Driscoll SW: Elbow instability. Hand Clin 10:405–415, 1994.

O'Driscoll SW, Bell DF, Morrey BF: Posterolateral rotatory instability of the elbow. J Bone Joint Surg [Am] 73:440–446, 1991.

Potter HG, Weiland AJ, Schatz JA, et al: Posterolateral rotatory instability of the elbow: Usefulness of MR imaging in diagnosis. Radiology 204:185–189, 1997.

CHAPTER 59

Medial Collateral Ligament Repair

INTRODUCTION

The anterior band of the medial collateral ligament (MCL) is the primary soft tissue restraint to valgus stress. However, the stability of the elbow comes primarily from the osseous anatomy. Thus, the majority of patients with laxity of the MCL of the elbow are asymptomatic. Patients who apply extreme valgus loads to the elbow, such as throwing athletes, may develop symptoms. This chapter addresses this unique group of patients.

HISTORY AND PHYSICAL EXAMINATION

Patients often have a long history of overhand throwing. Approximately 40% have symptoms of ulnar neuropathy, which may be the primary complaint. Most report medial elbow pain, especially under valgus loading. Some recall a specific injury associated with an acute "pop" in the elbow, after which they could not throw at full velocity.

Examination often shows limited elbow extension. Crepitus may occur with range of motion. A careful neurologic examination is performed to evaluate the ulnar nerve. Tenderness along the cubital tunnel or Tinel's sign at the cubital tunnel is often present with ulnar neuropathy secondary to valgus instability of the elbow. Palpatory examination attempts to differentiate tenderness in the flexor-pronator musculotendinous origin from that in the MCL. An acute tear of flexor-pronator origin may result in a clinical picture similar to acute MCL rupture. Pain primarily with resisted wrist pronation and supination is indicative of injury to the musculotendinous unit.

The valgus stress test of the elbow assesses the competence of the MCL. This test is performed with the elbow flexed past 25° to minimize the effect of bone stability on valgus stress. The MCL is palpated while valgus stress is applied. A positive test is characterized by pain, tenderness, and end point laxity of the MCL. Performing it under fluoroscopy facilitates the examination (Fig. 59–1). The intact MCL prevents widening of the medial joint space. In some cases, examination under anesthesia may be required to establish the diagnosis. In addition, diagnostic arthroscopy can identify the persistently painful partial tear on the articular side of the ligament.

DIAGNOSTIC IMAGING

Standard anteroposterior and lateral views of the elbow may show calcification within the MCL, loose bodies, osteophytes, and degenerative changes of the radiocapitellar joint. These findings are helpful, but their absence does not eliminate the diagnosis of MCL rupture. In addition, stress radiographs may confirm the diagnosis by demonstrating medial joint widening with valgus stress. Recently, we have used MRI with gadolinium arthrography for evaluation of the collateral ligaments. This imaging technique is investigational; however, we are impressed with its diagnostic accuracy when interpreted by a musculoskeletal radiologist.

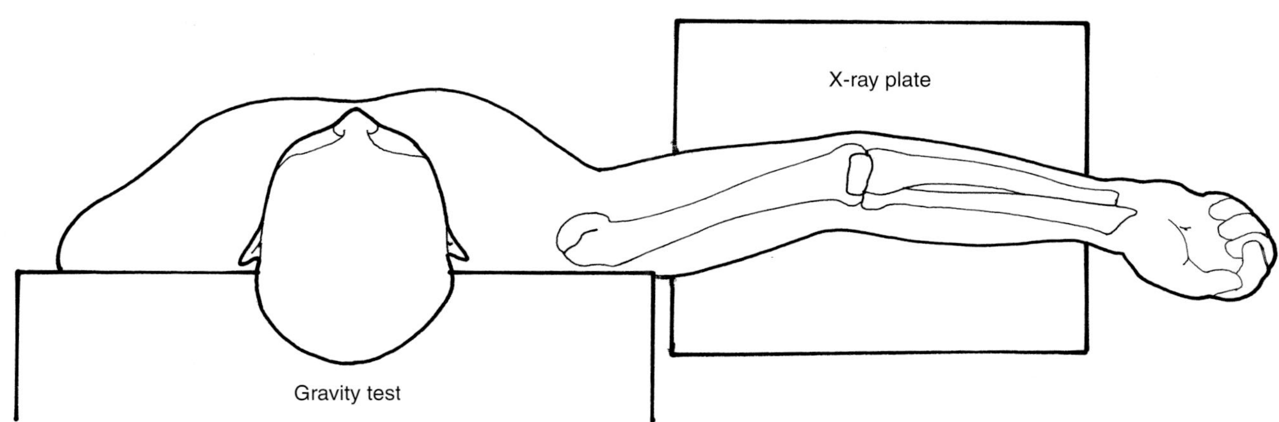

FIGURE 59–1. Valgus stress test.

NONOPERATIVE MANAGEMENT

Initial treatment consists of rest and anti-inflammatory medication. After the acute inflammatory period has passed, a progressive strengthening and endurance rehabilitation program is initiated. For many noncompetitive athletes, this approach often resolves their symptoms, allowing return to play in 6 to 12 weeks. The highly competitive overhand throwing athlete is unlikely to respond to this program when the MCL has ruptured.

RELEVANT ANATOMY

The MCL is composed of 3 bundles—the anterior bundle, the posterior bundle, and the transverse ligament (Fig. 59–2). The anterior bundle originates from the anterior inferior medial two thirds of the medial epicondyle and inserts on the coronoid tubercle. The posterior bundle is a thickening in the posterior capsule that inserts along the margin of the semilunar notch. The transverse ligament plays no role in elbow stability and is often not identified in gross dissection. Biomechanically, the anterior bundle is the key soft tissue stabilizer and is the focus of clinical attention in surgical reconstruction.

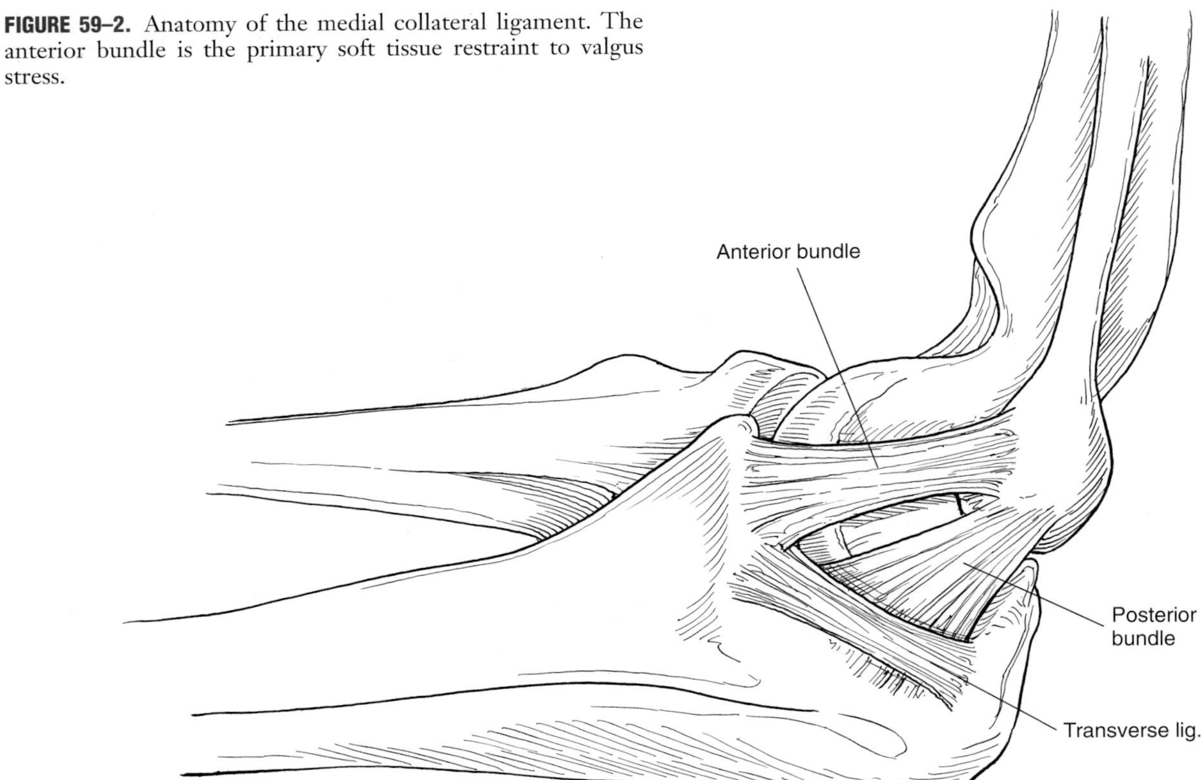

FIGURE 59–2. Anatomy of the medial collateral ligament. The anterior bundle is the primary soft tissue restraint to valgus stress.

SURGICAL *TECHNIQUE*

Indications

Symptomatic MCL laxity in the high-performance patient is the primary indication for MCL reconstruction. Infrequently, acute traumatic avulsion of the MCL can be managed with ligament repair. However, the repairable ligament is a rare finding. In cases in which the ligament is avulsed, intraoperative findings often show attenuation or calcification of the ligament. When this occurs, reconstruction with tendon graft is preferred over ligament repair.

Technique

1. Positioning: The patient is placed supine on the operating table with the affected arm extended on a hand table. The arm is surgically prepped to the axilla, and a sterile tourniquet is used to allow maximum access to the ulnar nerve and elbow. If the patient does not have a palmaris longus tendon, the lower extremity is prepped for harvest of the plantaris tendon.
2. Incision: A 10- to 12-cm incision is created on the posteromedial aspect of the elbow, centering on the joint line. The more posterior placement minimizes the dissection around branches of the medial antebrachial cutaneous nerves (Fig. 59–3).
3. Ulnar nerve mobilization: The ulnar nerve is mobilized from its bed, preserving as many vascular attachments as possible. A ½-inch Penrose drain is passed around the nerve to aid in atraumatic manipulation of the nerve. A clamp is not placed on the Penrose drain because of the risk of traction injury to the nerve when the clamp catches in the drapes. If ulnar neuropathy is present, the ulnar nerve is mobilized and transposed anteriorly and subcutaneously with the aid of a fasciodermal sling. The details of this technique are outlined in Chapter 56. We prefer subcutaneous transposition because it does not require release of the flexor-pronator origin and the resulting disruption of the neural elements within the conjoined tendon of the flexor-pronator muscle mass. However, surgeons who prefer submuscular transposition can elevate the muscle mass as described in Chapter 56.

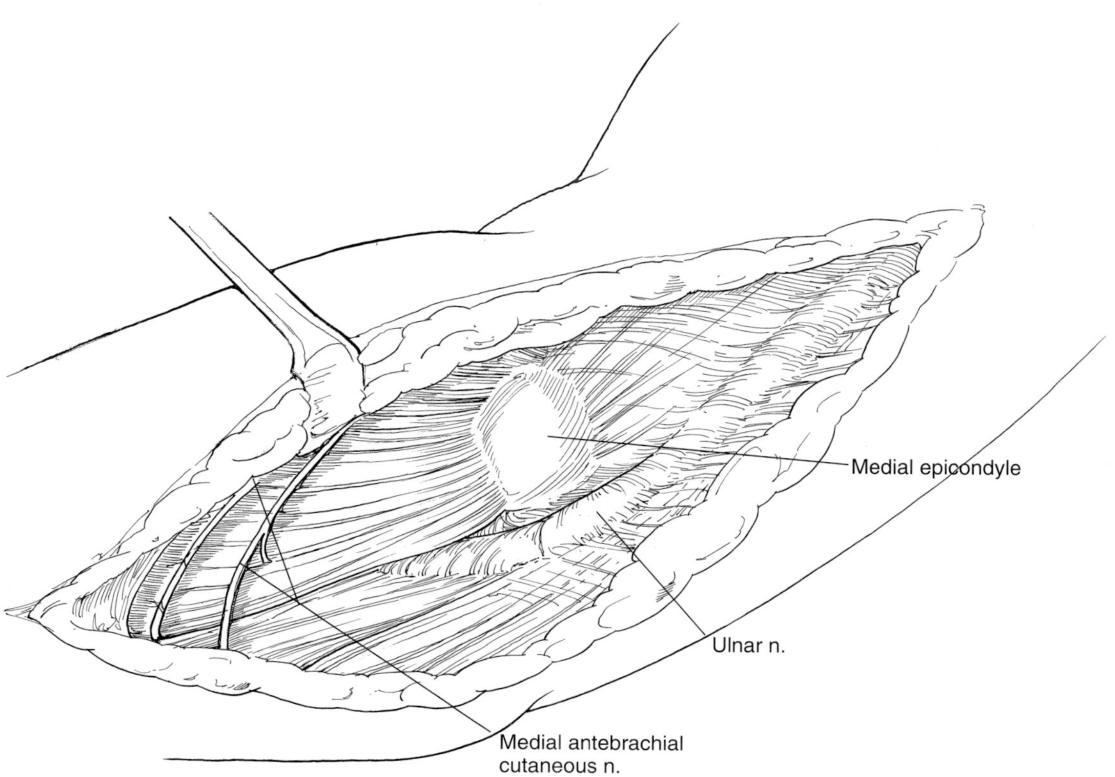

FIGURE 59–3. Posteromedial elbow incision. The anterior flap is elevated while it protects the cutaneous nerves.

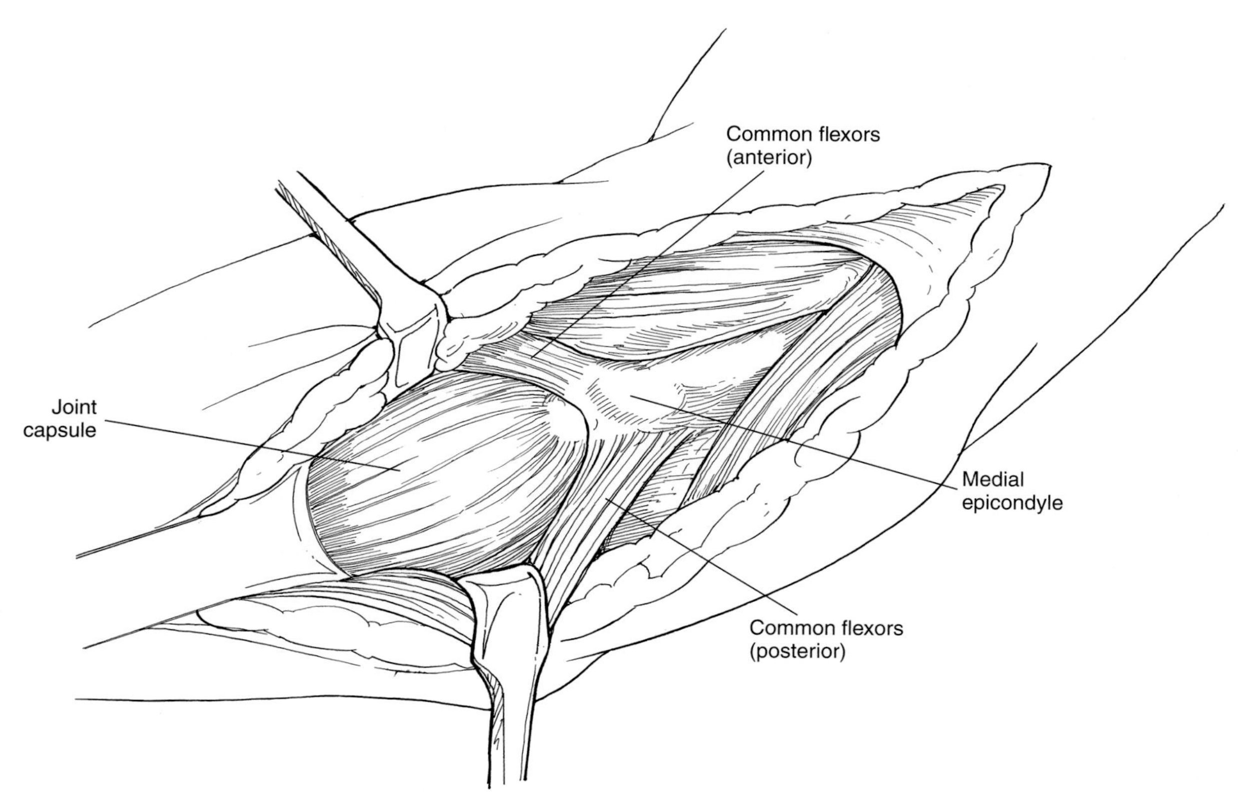

FIGURE 59–4. The medial collateral ligament is exposed when the flexor-pronator mass is split on a line between the anterior and middle thirds.

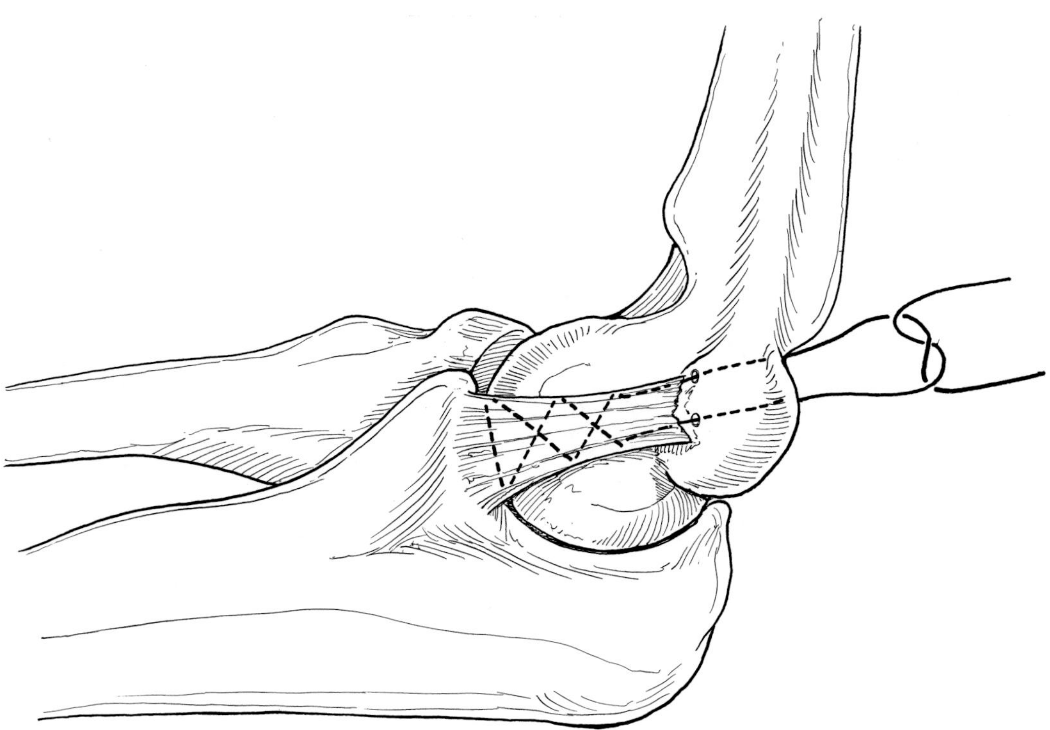

FIGURE 59–5. Bunnell suture technique is used to reattach the avulsed ligament.

4. Deep exposure: The flexor-pronator tendon is split longitudinally from the medial epicondyle distally for approximately 5 cm on a line between the anterior and middle thirds (Fig. 59–4). A small Weitlaner retractor maintains the exposure while an elevator sweeps away any additional muscle fibers. In traumatic ruptures, the ligament may appear avulsed from the medial epicondyle. In this case, the ligament is repaired with No. 2 nonabsorbable sutures using a Bunnell technique and passing the sutures through drill holes in the medial epicondyle (Fig. 59–5). If the MCL is intact, the ligament is split longitudinally and inspected. If preservation of the ligament is desired, it can be tightened by placing a longitudinally oriented figure-eight nonabsorbable suture within it. If reconstruction is planned, the split ligament is elevated to expose the medial epicondyle and coronoid process.
5. Graft harvest: A 2-cm transverse incision is made at the volar wrist crease centered over the palmaris longus tendon. The palmaris longus tendon insertion is grasped with a hemostat and transected distally. A 1–0 nonabsorbable braided suture is passed through the tendon stump several times. The suture is then passed through a tendon stripper of appropriate size. Note that the suture is required to pass the tendon into the tendon stripper because the tendon stripper that is the correct size is too small to allow a clamp to pass through. Traction is applied to the tendon stump by pulling firmly with a hemostat on the end of the tendon. The tendon stripper is then rotated back and forth while it is advanced up the forearm (Fig. 59–6). As the tendon stripper engages the musculotendinous junction, some increased resistance to advancement will be felt. Shortly after the tendon stripper has been advanced past the point of resistance, the tendon will pull loose from the muscle and can be withdrawn with the tendon stripper.

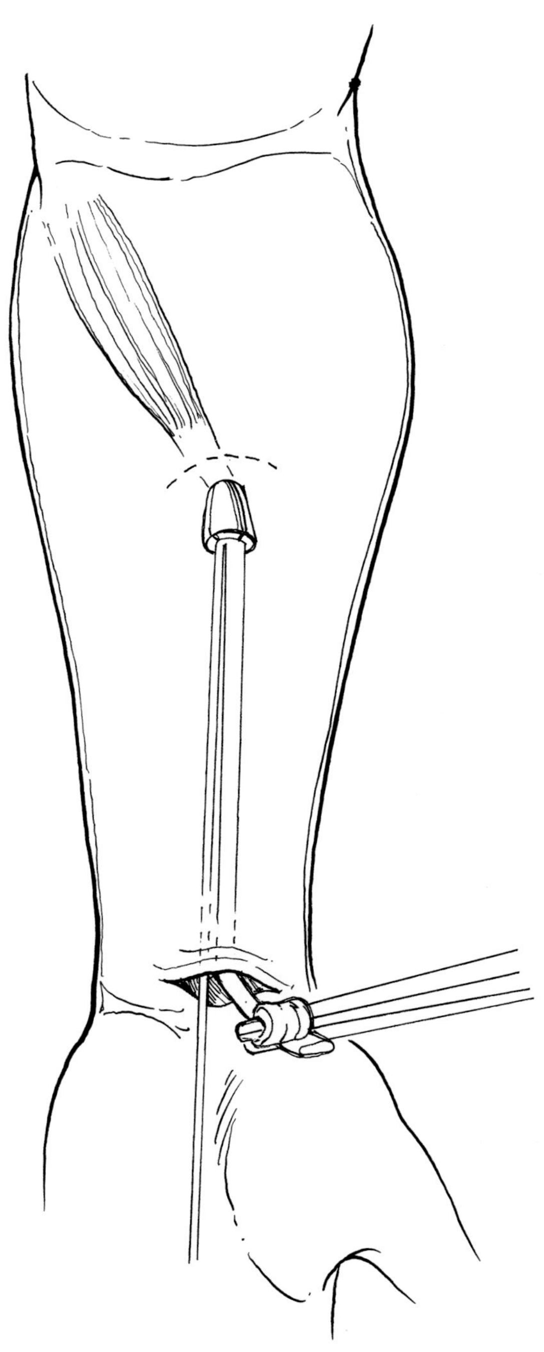

FIGURE 59–6. An incision in the wrist flexion crease exposes the palmaris longus. The tendon stripper harvests the palmaris longus by passing over the tendon from distal to proximal. A second incision can be made proximally, but it is not usually required.

6. Graft placement: Convergently drilled 3.2-mm holes are placed in the coronoid process 1 cm apart and centered on the tubercle. Divergent 3.2-mm drill holes are placed in the medial epicondyle. The drill holes start at the origin of the MCL and exit the posterior epicondyle such that they are at least 1 cm apart where they exit (Fig. 59–7). A loop of 28-gauge surgical wire is passed through the bone tunnels to facilitate passage of the tendon graft. The tendon is weaved through the tunnels in a figure-eight pattern (Fig. 59–8). The elbow is held in 45° of flexion and neutral varus-valgus while the graft is tensioned. The graft is sutured to itself and to remnants of the MCL with nonabsorbable braided suture on a tapered needle.
7. Closure: The graft is inspected for isometry by placing the elbow through a full range of motion and gentle valgus stress. The tourniquet is released and hemostasis achieved. A drain is placed when indicated. The flexor-pronator mass is approximated with interrupted sutures. The wound is closed in standard fashion. The elbow is immobilized at 90° in a splint with the hand and wrist free.

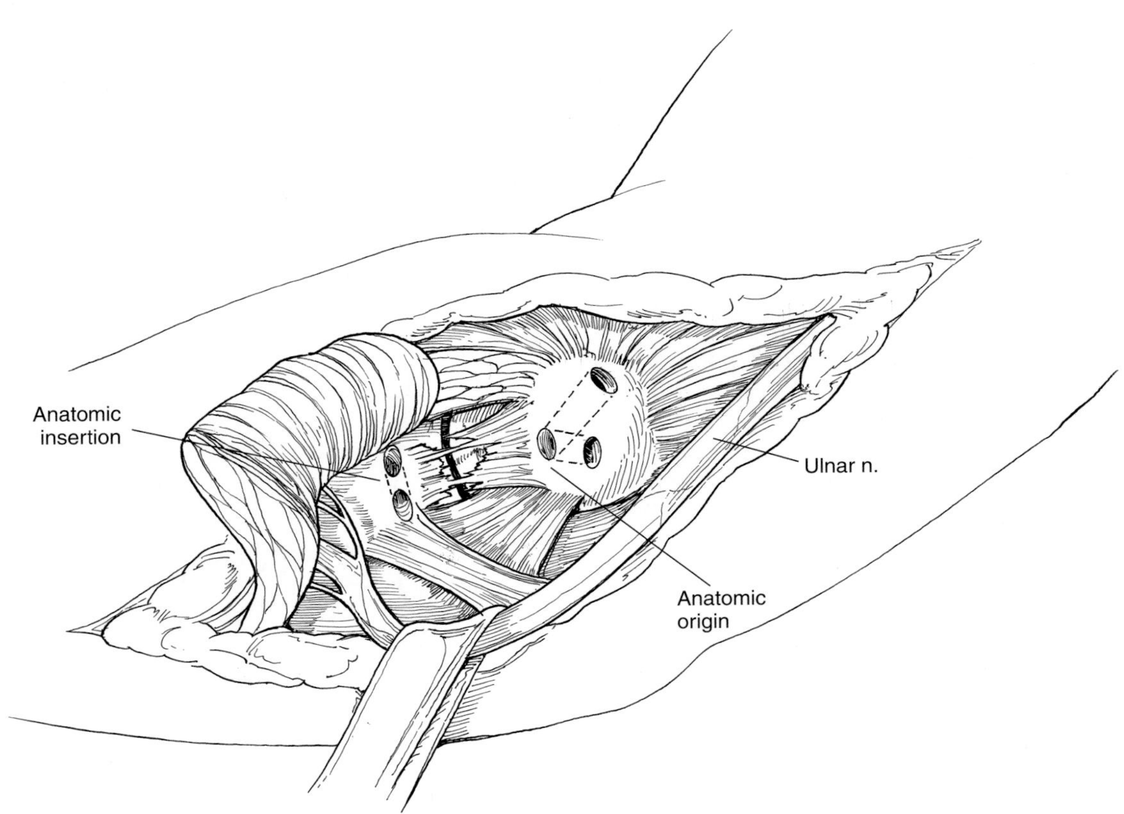

FIGURE 59–7. On the coronoid process, 3.2-mm drill holes are 1 cm apart. Divergent 3.2-mm drill holes in the medial epicondyle originate from the isometric point of the medial collateral ligament.

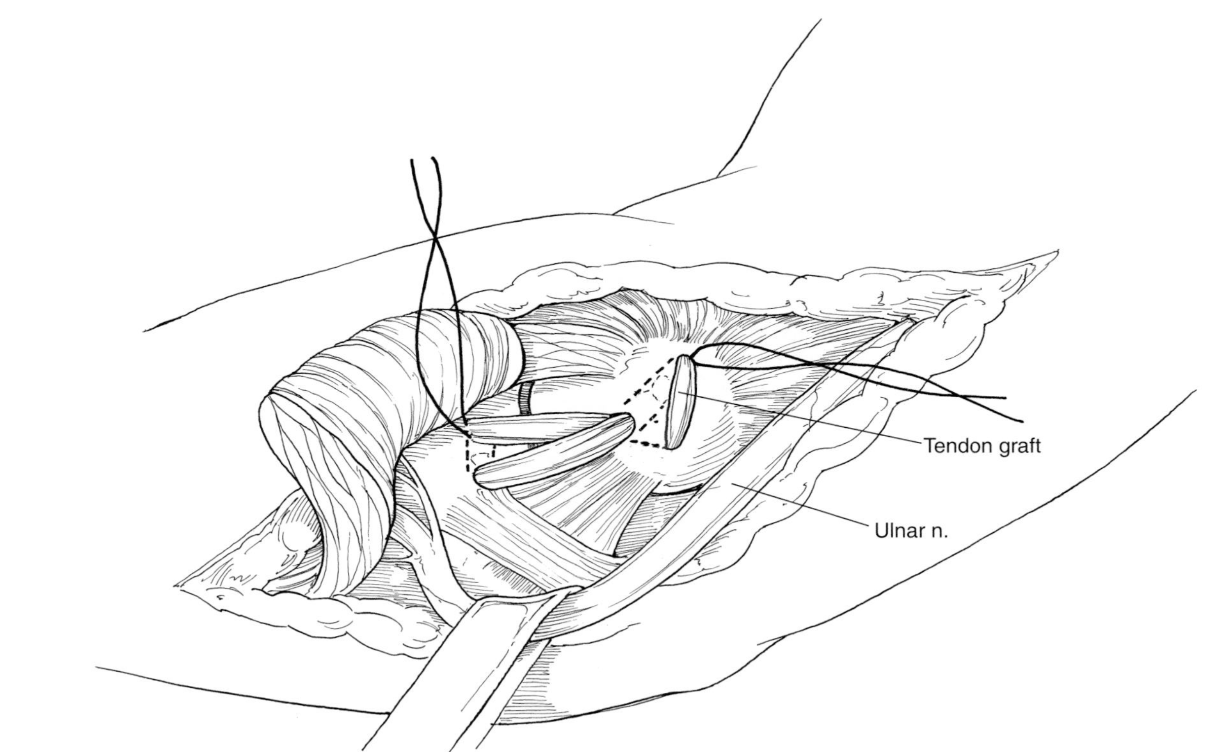

FIGURE 59–8. Palmaris longus tendon is weaved through the drill hole in a figure-eight pattern. The weave results in three strands of graft over the medial joint. Note that sutures are placed away from the joint line where the knot may cause late crepitus.

POSTOPERATIVE MANAGEMENT

Immediate active range of motion of the shoulder and wrist is encouraged. After 10 days, immobilization is discontinued and active elbow motion is initiated. In addition, a grip-strengthening program is started. When submuscular transposition of the ulnar nerve has been performed, grip strengthening is delayed for 1 month to allow healing of the flexor mass insertion. Full elbow motion should be achieved by 4 weeks. At 6 weeks, any residual motion loss is managed with dynamic and static splints. At 6 weeks, elbow strengthening exercises begin, yet no valgus loading of the elbow is permitted until 4 months. After 4 months, the patient may toss a ball up to 60 feet without a windup. At 6 months, a graduated progressive throwing program is initiated with the goal of reaching 100% velocity by the end of the eighth month. This graduated program emphasizes proper throwing mechanics. It may take as long as 12 to 18 months for the athlete to regain previous throwing ability.

COMPLICATIONS

A majority of the problems associated with this procedure involve the nerves. Injury to the medial antebrachial cutaneous nerve branches or the ulnar nerve can occur in up to 25% of cases. Careful attention to detail during the exposure is key to the prevention of nerve injury. Gentle handling of the ulnar nerve and preservation of blood supply to the nerve can minimize trauma to the nerve. Injury to the ulnar nerve can be minimized by leaving the nerve minimally disturbed and performing transposition only when preoperative symptoms indicate that the procedure is needed. Failure of reconstruction is possible but occurs rarely if the postsurgical program is followed. Failure of ligament repairs should be followed by ligament reconstruction.

RESULTS

In a series of 70 operations on 68 patients at the Kerlan-Jobe Orthopaedic Clinic, with an average followup of

6.2 years, 68% of the 56 patients who underwent ligament reconstruction returned to their previous level of participation. Of the 14 patients who underwent direct repair, 50% returned to their previous level of play. The average time to return to competition was 9 months in the repair groups and 12 months in the reconstruction group.

REFERENCES

Conway JE, Jobe FW, Glousman RE, Pink M: Medial instability of the elbow in throwing athletes: Surgical treatment by ulnar collateral ligament reconstruction. J Bone Joint Surg [Am] 74:67–83, 1992.

Field LD, Callaway GH, O'Brien SJ, Altchek DW: Arthroscopic assessment of the medial collateral ligament complex of the elbow. Am J Sports Med 23:396–400, 1995.

Jobe FW, Kvitne RS: Elbow instability in the athlete. Instr Course Lect XX:17–23, 1991.

Morrey BF, Tanaka S, An KN: Valgus stability of the elbow. A definition of primary and secondary constraints. Clin Orthop 265:187–195, 1991.

O'Driscoll SW, Jaloszynski R, Morrey BF, An KN: Origin of the medial ulnar collateral ligament. J Hand Surg [Am] 17:164–168, 1992.

Regan WD, Korinek SL, Morrey BF, An KN: Biomechanical study of ligaments around the elbow joint. Clin Orthop 271:170–179, 1991.

Rijke AM, Goitz HT, McCue FC, et al: Stress radiography of the medial elbow ligaments. Radiology 191:213–216, 1994.

CHAPTER 60

Treatment of Biceps Tendon Rupture

INTRODUCTION

Biceps tendon rupture is uncommon, but it is the most common tendon rupture that occurs in the elbow region. Repair of the acute ruptured biceps tendon often produces excellent results. Recently, the introduction of suture anchors has facilitated distal biceps repair through a single incision. Although we prefer to use a two-incision technique, both techniques are presented here.

HISTORY AND PHYSICAL EXAMINATION

Patients with biceps tendon rupture often present with a history of acute onset of pain in the antecubital fossa during lifting. The typical patient is 50 years old but may be between 21 and 70 years of age; a majority of cases occur in weight lifters. Patients report ecchymosis anterior to the elbow and a period of limited elbow motion secondary to acute inflammation and swelling in the region. If care is sought after the acute inflammation has resolved, patients may present with complaints of weak elbow flexion and supination.

Palpation of the antecubital fossa reveals absence of the biceps tendon; however, if the tendon is palpable, a partial rupture has likely occurred. Partial rupture often demonstrates palpable crepitus with pronation and supination. With complete rupture, many patients are left with deformity of the arm.

DIAGNOSTIC IMAGING

Plain radiographs of the elbow are performed routinely, but they are not usually helpful in establishing the diagnosis. Radiographic changes in the radial tuberosity are suggestive of a chronic lesion. MRI can assist in confirming the diagnosis, although it is not necessary in most cases. However, MRI may be useful in confirming the diagnosis of partial rupture when the diagnosis remains uncertain despite a careful history and physical examination.

RELEVANT ANATOMY

The biceps tendon inserts on the tuberosity of the radius. The tuberosity is oriented such that the biceps has maximum efficiency in its primary function as a forearm supinator. Thus, the tuberosity lies opposite the radial bow so that it is lateral in full pronation and medial in full supination. This "crankshaft" effect is important when repair of the tendon is considered (Fig. 60–1). The tendon must be inserted to the apex of the tuberosity to give it maximum mechanical efficiency. We find this most easily accomplished with a two-incision technique. The posterior interosseous nerve (PIN) is the primary structure at risk for injury during biceps tendon repair. The nerve branches from the radial nerve within millimeters of the radiocapitellar joint. The PIN passes deep to the mobile wad and enters the supinator at the arcade of Frohse. The nerve then continues distally as it spirals around the neck of the radius (Fig. 60–2).

NONOPERATIVE MANAGEMENT

A review of operative and nonoperative treatment of distal biceps tendon rupture clearly demonstrates superior results with operative repair. In the biomechanical analysis of distal biceps rupture by Morrey and associates, patients with unrepaired tendons lost an average of 40% of elbow supination strength and 30% of elbow flexion strength. An important additional finding was that flexion strength returned to normal with attachment of the biceps to the brachialis tendon. This alternative to anatomic repair should be considered in selected cases when anatomic repair is not possible and loss of elbow flexion strength is a problem.

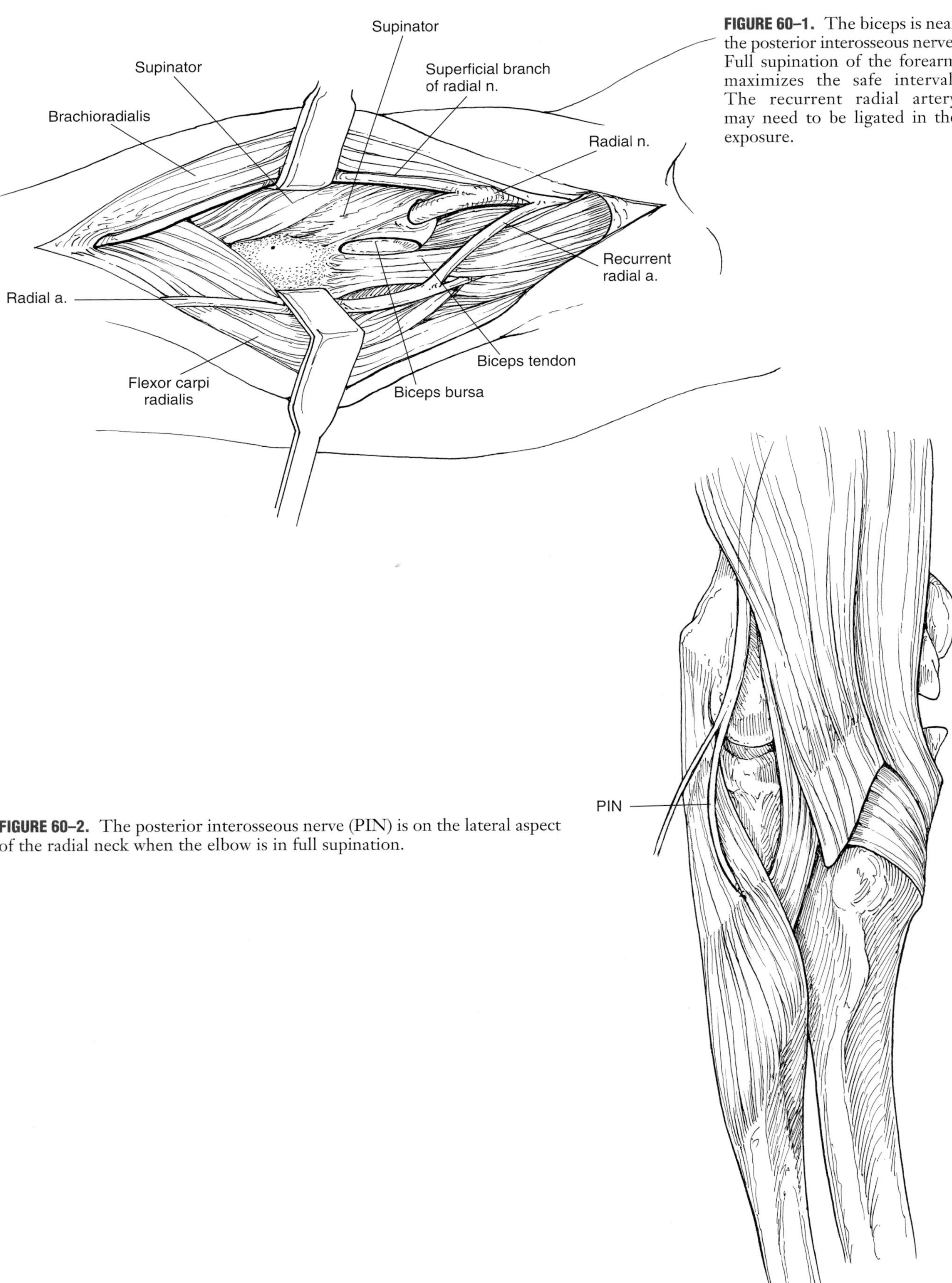

FIGURE 60–1. The biceps is near the posterior interosseous nerve. Full supination of the forearm maximizes the safe interval. The recurrent radial artery may need to be ligated in the exposure.

FIGURE 60–2. The posterior interosseous nerve (PIN) is on the lateral aspect of the radial neck when the elbow is in full supination.

SURGICAL *TECHNIQUE*

Indications

Surgical repair is recommended in all acute cases unless advanced age or poor medical condition circumscribes operative treatment. In cases of chronic rupture in which improved elbow flexion strength is needed, the tendon can be attached to the brachialis tendon.

Technique

We prefer the two-incision technique, modified from Boyd and Anderson's original description (Mayo modification). Single-incision techniques report similar results; however, we find that the two-incision approach facilitates easy, accurate placement and secure approximation of the tendon stump to the radial tuberosity. In our estimation, the force required to approximate the tendon to the bone in some cases would be difficult to apply with the one-incision technique. Both techniques are reviewed in this section.

Two-Incision Technique

1. Positioning: The patient is placed supine on the table with the affected arm extended on an arm table. A sterile pneumatic tourniquet is used to facilitate maximal access to the proximal arm in the event that difficulty is encountered in delivering the tendon stump into the wound.
2. Incision: An incision is placed from the lateral aspect of the distal biceps muscle, extending distally (approximately 5 cm) to the elbow flexion crease, then medially (Fig. 60–3). The incision is easily extended to a more extensile exposure if difficulty is encountered delivering the tendon stump into the wound. Surgeons more experienced with this procedure may prefer the more cosmetic transverse incision as described by Morrey.

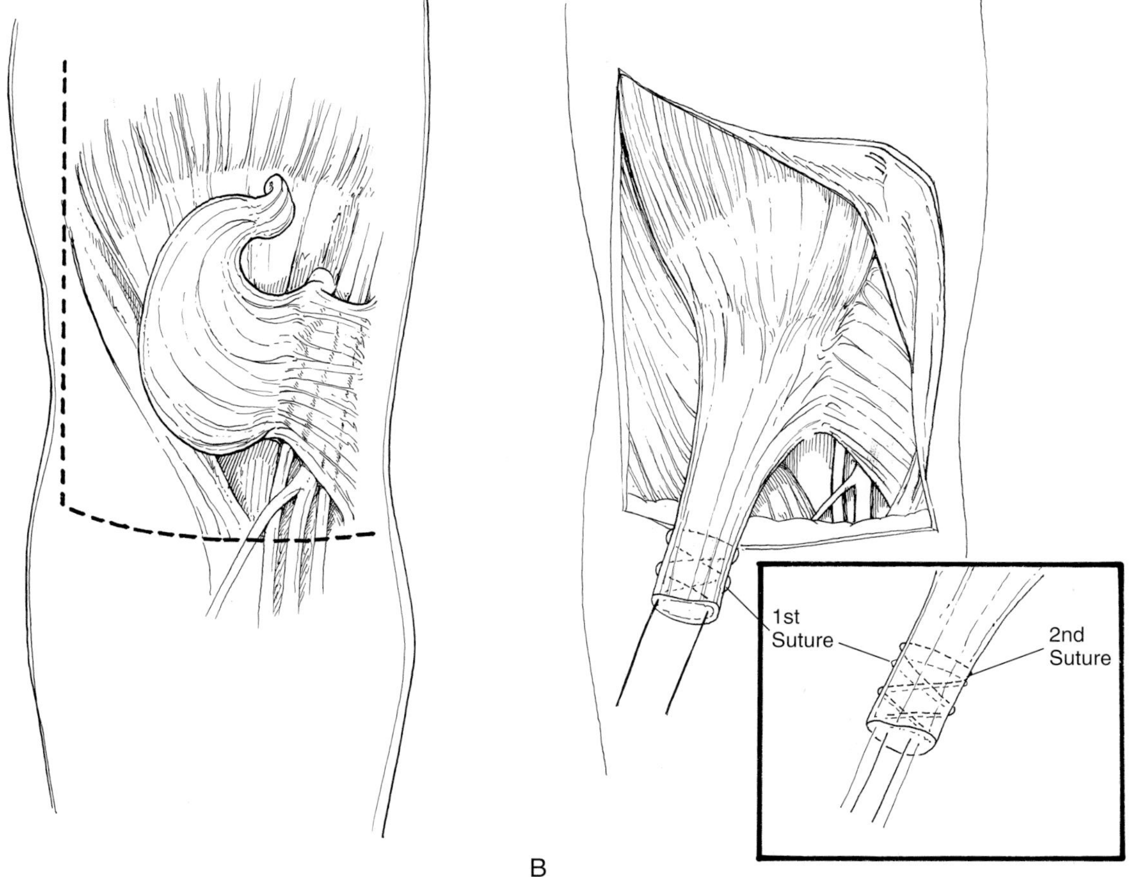

FIGURE 60–3. *A*, The incision depicted here provides adequate exposure in most cases. The tendon stump is usually proximal to the elbow, but further retraction is prevented by the lacertus fibrosus. *B*, No. 2 nonabsorbable braided suture is placed in the tendon using the Bunnell technique.

3. The biceps tendon is delivered into the wound and is sutured with a Bunnell technique using two No. 2 Ethibond sutures. In cases of acute rupture, a finger is easily passed through the soft tissue interval to the tuberosity of the radius. With the forearm in maximum supination, a Kelly clamp is used to palpate the tuberosity. The clamp is then passed beyond the radius in the radioulnar interval through the posterior muscles until it tents the skin posteriorly (Fig. 60–4). The skin is incised posteriorly and blunt dissection is carried down to the radius. Hohmann retractors are placed on each side of the radius. The periosteum of the ulna is not disturbed.
4. The forearm is pronated to bring the biceps tuberosity into view from the posterior incision. A 4-mm round burr is used to create a hole in the tuberosity of sufficient size to accept the tendon stump. Holes are drilled though the cortex adjacent to the burr hole. These drill holes should be staggered such that the cortex will not fracture. The sutures from the biceps tendon are passed from the burr hole out the drill hole. Next, a clamp holds the tip of the tendon within the burr hole while the sutures are tied (Fig. 60–5).

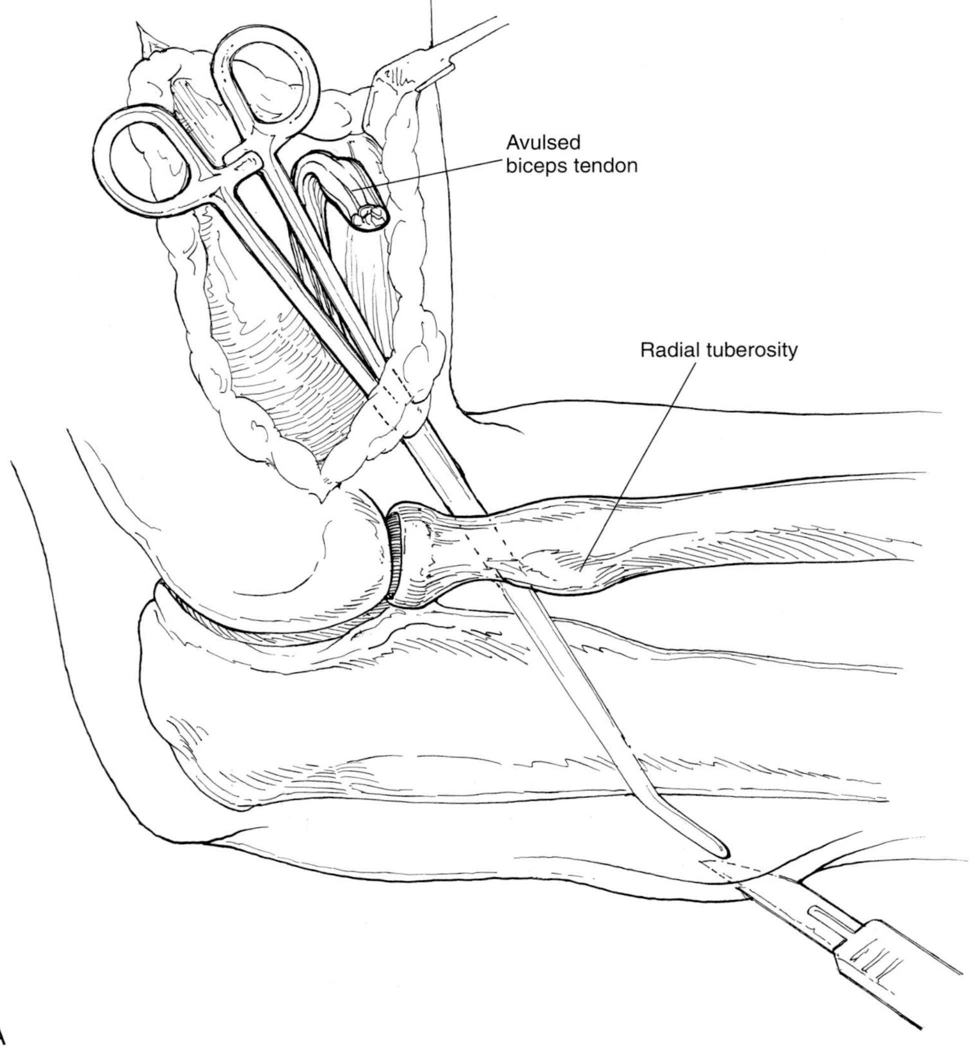

FIGURE 60–4. *A*, A Kelly clamp is passed around the radius and out posteriorly until it reaches the skin.

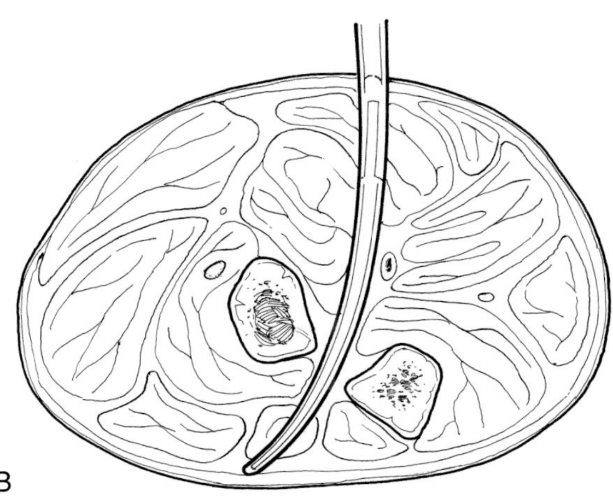

FIGURE 60–4 *Continued. B*, The curve of the clamp is passed such that the ulna is not disturbed. Note the relatively posterior exit point of the clamp.

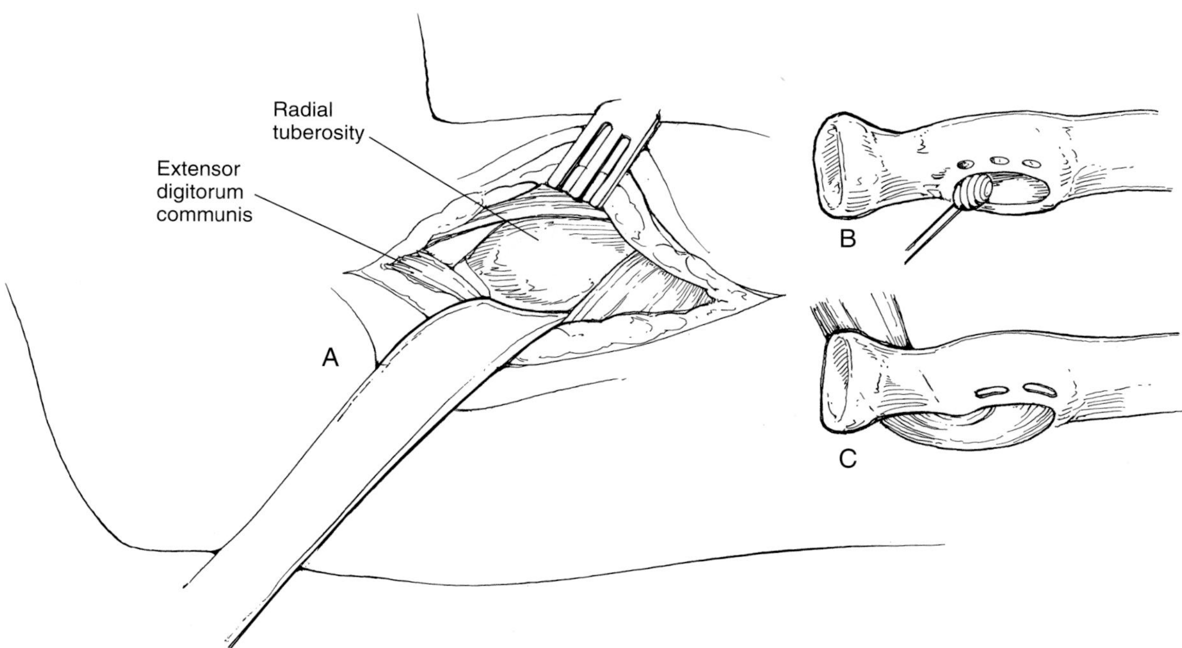

FIGURE 60–5. *A*, Dissection down over the clamp to the radius with the arm in full pronation exposes the tuberosity. *B*, The tuberosity is excavated to accept the tendon stumps. Holes are drilled through the cortical bone for passage of the No. 2 sutures in the tendon stump. *C*, The tendon is sutured into the burr hole with No. 2 nonabsorbable suture.

Suture Anchor Technique (One-Incision Technique)

1. Positioning and incision: The positioning and incision are identical to those used in the open technique, excluding the posterior incision. A narrow Hohmann retractor placed on each side of the radius facilitates the exposure. The arm is maintained in full supination during the entire procedure. The biceps tuberosity is roughened with a rongeur or burr. The cortex of the radius is not penetrated (Fig. 60–6).
2. Traction is maintained on the tendon stump while the tuberosity exposure is performed. This important step reduces the force required to approximate the repair during suture tying.
3. Next, two screw-in suture anchors are placed in the biceps tuberosity. Each anchor is loaded with No. 2 nonabsorbable suture. The tendon is sutured with the use of the Kessler technique. The end of the tendon is grasped with a Kocher clamp and held in position on the tuberosity while the sutures are tied (Fig. 60–7). The wound is closed in standard fashion.

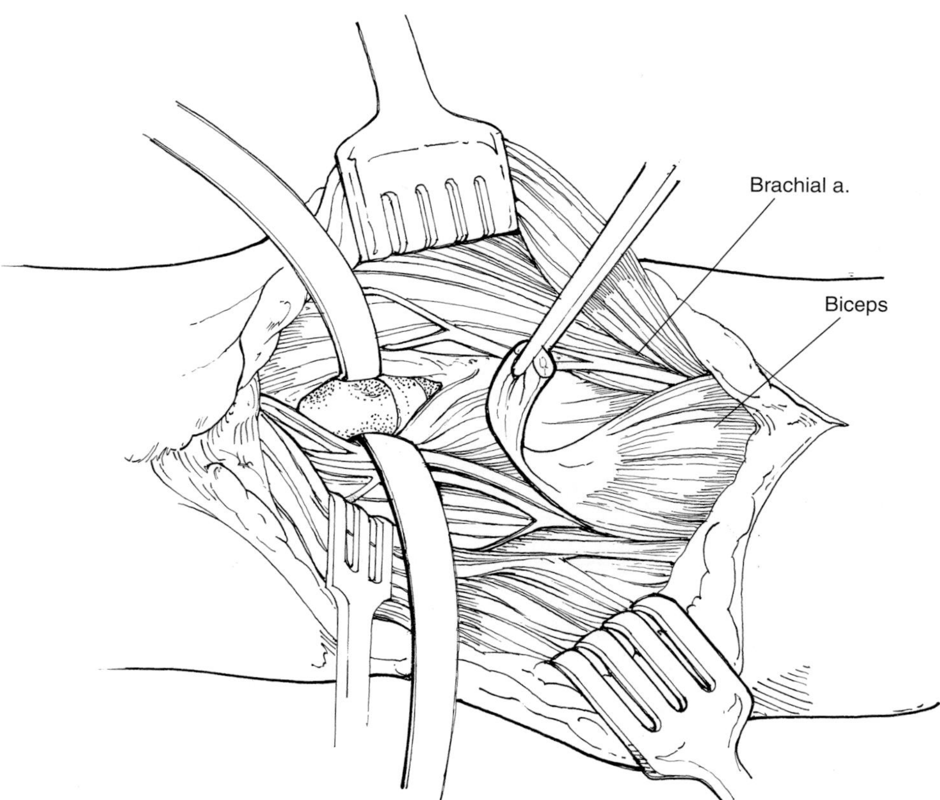

FIGURE 60–6. The exposure for the single-incision technique is identical to the anterior incision used in the two-incision technique. Full supination brings the radial tuberosity into view from the anterior exposure.

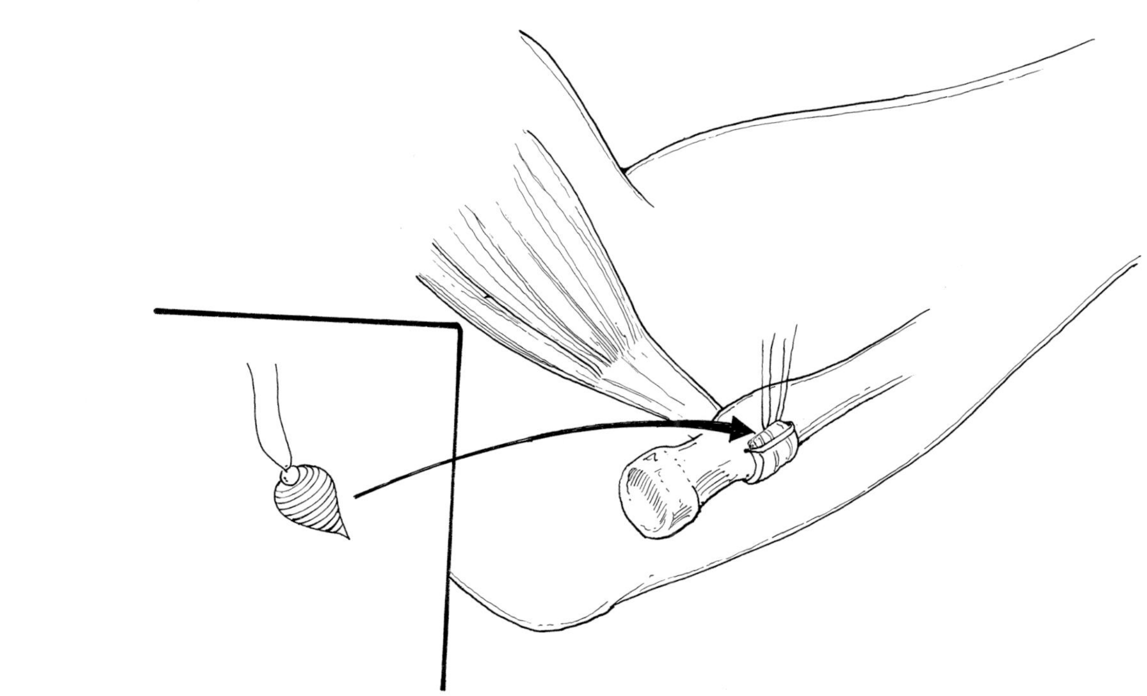

FIGURE 60–7. A clamp holds the tendon reduced while the sutures are tied. Two anchors in the tuberosity provide excellent fixation. Note the correct insertion of the tendon when the arm is pronated. The repair must be performed with the arm supinated. *Arrow* indicates proper placement of the screw in the suture anchors *(inset)*.

POSTOPERATIVE MANAGEMENT

Postoperative splints are discontinued within the first week, and gentle passive elbow extension and forearm supination are begun. Active elbow flexion and forearm rotation are initiated at 10 to 14 days without resistance. The goal is full active range of motion by 3 to 4 weeks. At 6 weeks, progressive resistance exercises begin, with the goal of release to full activity by 3 months.

COMPLICATIONS

Complications include radial nerve palsy, posterior interosseous nerve palsy, heterotopic ossification, radioulnar synostosis, and elbow flexion contracture. Nerve palsy is best avoided by careful attention to placement and force applied to soft tissue retractors. Heterotopic ossification is beyond the surgeon's control, although it has not been a major problem in our experience if the ulna is not disturbed. Radioulnar synostosis can result with the two-incision technique; however, the Mayo modification of the Boyd-Anderson technique eliminates this problem. Elbow flexion contracture can occur after repair of subacute or chronic distal biceps tendon rupture, and it is a direct result of shortening of the musculotendinous unit. This is best avoided by attention to passive range of motion after repair and by graft reconstruction in patients significantly lacking passive extension after repair.

RESULTS

Full range of motion and restoration of normal strength are expected in acute cases. Restoration of full flexion and extension is expected, although some patients lose up to 30° of pronation and supination. Because most of these patients are weight lifters, they must be cautioned to delay heavy lifting until 9 to 12 months after repair. Rerupture is a potential problem, and treatment is less likely to have a good result.

REFERENCES

Boyd HB, Anderson LD: A method for reinsertion of the distal biceps brachi tendon. J Bone Joint Surg [Am] 43:1041–1043, 1961.

Davison BL, Engber WD, Tigert LJ: Long term evaluation of repaired distal biceps brachii tendon ruptures. Clin Orthop 333:186–191, 1996.

Lintner S, Fischer T: Repair of the distal biceps tendon using suture anchors and an anterior approach. Clin Orthop 322:116–119, 1996.

Morrey BF, Askew LJ, An KN, Dobyns JH: Rupture of the distal tendon of the biceps brachii. A biomechanical study. J Bone Joint Surg [Am] 67:418–421, 1985.

Strauch RJ, Michelson H, Rosenwasser MP: Repair of rupture of the distal tendon of the biceps brachii. Review of the literature and report of three cases treated with a single anterior incision and suture anchors. Am J Orthop 26:151–156, 1997.

CHAPTER 61

Treatment of Degenerative Arthritis

INTRODUCTION

Arthritis in the elbow has many causes; this chapter focuses on post-traumatic degenerative arthritis and valgus extension overload injury of the elbow. Arthrotomy and joint débridement can produce gratifying results in properly selected patients. Moreover, recent advances in arthroscopy of the elbow have expanded the theraputic armamentarium available to treat these disorders.

HISTORY AND PHYSICAL EXAMINATION

Patients with elbow arthritis have symptoms similar to those reported in other joints, such as morning stiffness, night pain, aggravation with activity, and improvement with rest. These patients can be categorized into two broad groups by history. One group includes patients who have a chronic history of throwing or other valgus extension overload activity. The other group includes those patients with a history of elbow trauma or primary osteoarthritis.

The patient with chronic posterior elbow impingement from valgus extension overload often complains of insidious and progressive posterior elbow pain and limited elbow extension. These patients tend to be younger than those with post-traumatic arthritis. Many have coexistent ulnar neuropathy and report numbness or tingling in the ring and small fingers. The ulnar nerve is carefully evaluated. Physical examination shows limited elbow extension and full forearm rotation. Pain in the posterior elbow is intensified at the end point of extension. The presence of posterior fossa impingement can be confirmed by an injection test. Pain should be completely relieved by posterior fossa injection with local anesthetic. Furthermore, full elbow extension may be achieved in some patients after the injection test has been completed. This group is further subdivided based on the integrity of the ulnar collateral ligament. Physical examination of the ulnar collateral may reveal laxity of the ligament. In chronic ulnar collateral ligament laxity, radiocapitellar arthritis is manifest as lateral elbow pain and tenderness aggravated by valgus load and forearm rotation.

Patients with primary osteoarthritis or post-traumatic elbow arthritis are almost exclusively men in the fourth to sixth decades of life. Signs and symptoms of ulnar neuropathy are seen infrequently in this group. Arthritic changes in the joint are more global, with osteophytes noted in the anterior and posterior compartments of the elbow. Motion may be limited in both flexion and extension. Limitation of forearm rotation suggests that radial head osteophytes are present.

DIAGNOSTIC IMAGING

Standard anteroposterior and lateral x-rays are routinely recommended. The lateral view shows the olecranon and coronoid processes clearly and often shows osteophytic deformity. Visualization of the radiocapitellar joint is best attained with the radial head view when disease in this area is suspected. A majority of degenerative changes occur on the radial side of the joint. Valgus stress views are used when ulnar collateral ligament laxity is suspected. Both CT and MRI provide additional information about loose bodies and osteophytes filling the olecranon and coronoid fossa. We prefer CT because of its lower cost and better bone imaging detail; however, it is rarely needed in the evaluation of the degenerative elbow.

NONOPERATIVE MANAGEMENT

The goals of treatment are pain relief and restoration of function. Patient education is the cornerstone of management. Patients should understand the cause of the pain and the need for rest and activity modification. Many patients come to the physician only after an acute event has resulted in severe exacerbation of long-standing symptoms. A period of rest and a short course of nonsteroidal anti-inflammatory medication may return them to their preinjury status. A gentle stretching and strengthening program is initiated after the acute pain has subsided. The patient and therapists are advised to avoid aggressive stretching, which will likely aggravate the pain. Achieving a preinjury level of pain and function often satisfies the low-demand patient with primary or post-traumatic arthritis.

Throwing atheletes require a more organized rehabilitation program. Following the resolution of acute symptoms, a progressive rehabilitative program that emphasizes improvement in strength is begun.

RELEVANT ANATOMY

A comprehensive understanding of elbow anatomy is essential to the successful execution of these procedures. It is beyond the scope of this chapter to review this anatomy in detail. The surgeon should be familiar with the relationship of the elbow capsule to the surrounding neurovascular structures. These relationships are outlined in the chapter on elbow arthroscopy (Chapter 53).

SURGICAL *TECHNIQUE*

Arthroscopy of the degenerative elbow can be technically challenging. Similar results are reported from both open and arthroscopic techniques. Because of the limited margin of safety around neurovascular structures during elbow arthroscopy, the surgeon should not hesitate to convert to an open procedure when arthroscopic visualization is suboptimal. Surgeons unfamiliar with elbow arthroscopy should consider the open technique first. We find the arthroscopic technique most useful in patients with extension overload secondary to throwing in whom the disease is confined to the posterior elbow. However, in patients with both anterior and posterior osteophytes, the open technique is expedient and allows thorough assessment and débridement of the joint.

Indications

The primary indication for elbow débridement is pain at terminal extension or flexion secondary to impinging osteophytes. Pain through the arc of motion is a contraindication because it suggests advanced degenerative changes that are likely to remain symptomatic after débridement. Catching and locking of the elbow are indications that loose bodies are present; patients must understand that similar symptoms may continue after surgery owing to the underlying joint deformity. Limited motion may be a relative indication if the elbow lacks a functional arc (30° to 130°); osteophytes and capsular contracture are contributing factors.

Technique

1. Positioning: The patient is placed supine on the operating table with a rolled towel placed under the scapula. The unsupported arm should rest across the patient's chest. A pneumatic tourniquet is placed high on the arm. If the patient's arm is short, a sterile tourniquet may be needed to maximize access to the elbow region.
2. Incision: If the disease is found to be posterior only, a direct posterior trans-triceps tendon approach can be used, as described by Morrey (Fig. 61–1). In cases

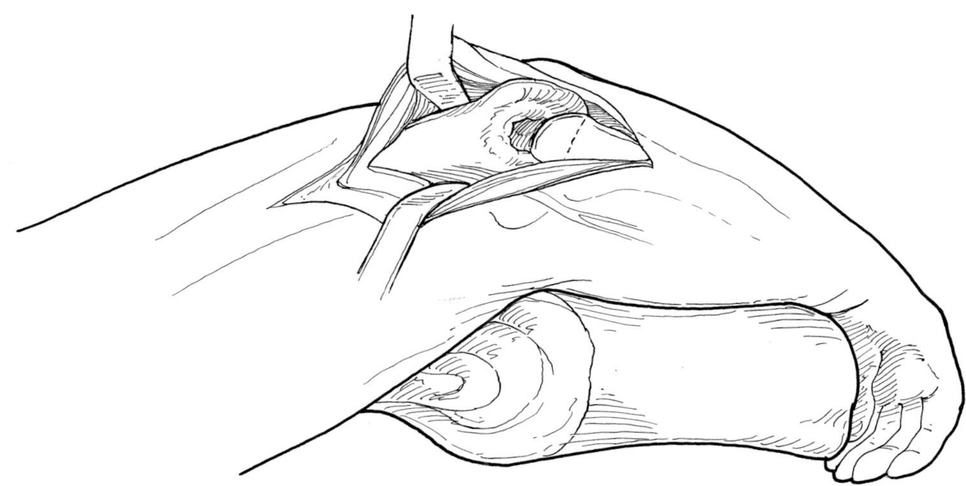

FIGURE 61–1. The triceps-splitting approach provides excellent exposure of the posterior compartment.

requiring access to the anterior and posterior compartments, a standard Kocher approach is used. The interval between the anconeus and extensor carpi ulnaris muscles is used to access the joint. Care is taken to preserve the lateral collateral ligament complex. The extensor muscle origins are reflected off the humerus in the subperiosteal plane as needed for the exposure (Fig. 61–2).

3. Débridement: The osteophytes are resected with a rongeur (Fig. 61–3). The olecranon and coronoid fossa are débrided with a 6-mm round power burr. The floor of the fossa is removed with the burr (Fig. 61–4). The elbow is taken through a range of motion and is inspected for other areas of impingement. If capsular contracture is a problem,

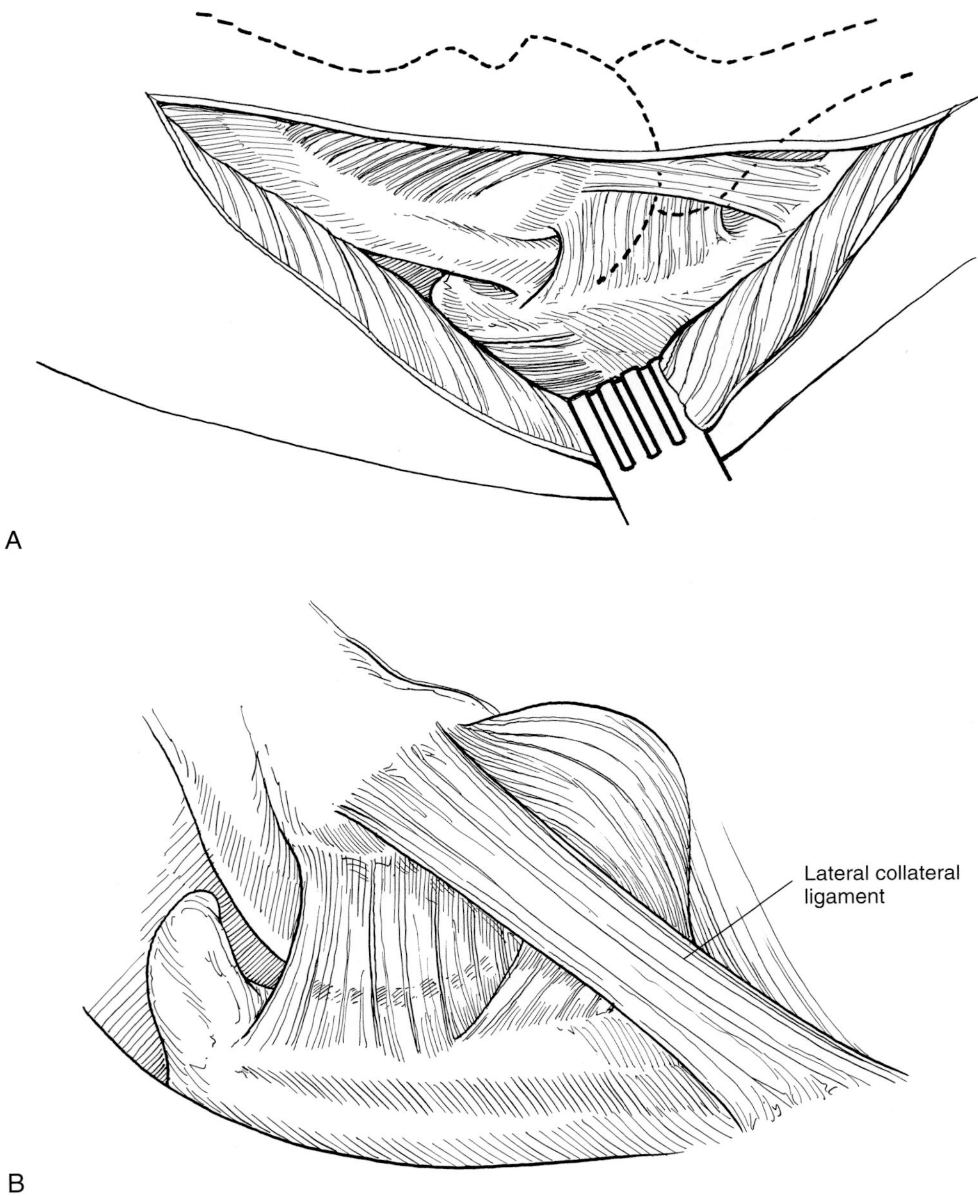

FIGURE 61–2. The Kocher approach provides an extensile view anteriorly and posteriorly. The muscle envelope is elevated off the capsule to preserve the lateral collateral ligament complex. *A*, A retractor on the anconeous exposes the posterolateral elbow capsule. *B*, Preservation of the lateral collateral ligament maintains elbow stability. The capsule anterior and posterior to the ligament can be excised.

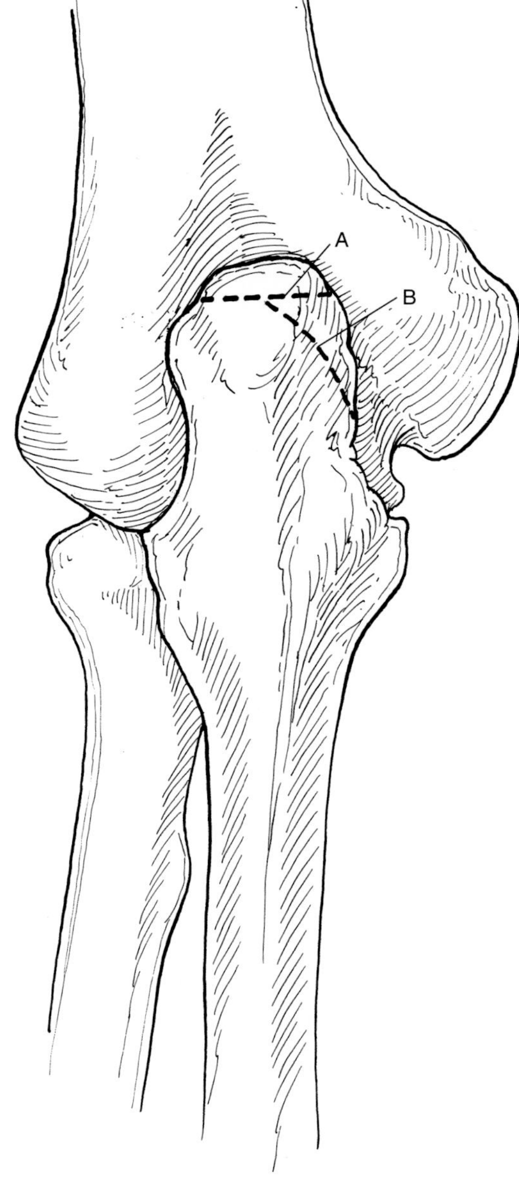

FIGURE 61–3. Osteophytes excised from the tip of the olecranon with two osteotomies, one transverse (A) and the other oblique (B).

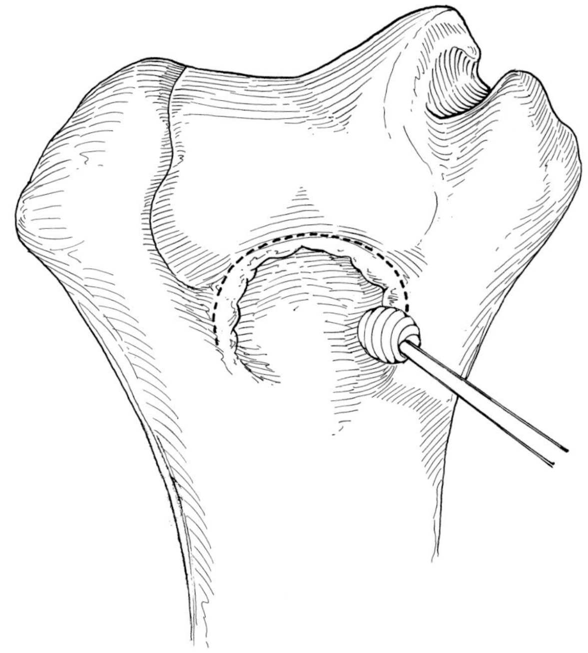

FIGURE 61–4. Osteophyte débridement of the olecranon fossa.

the capsule is excised. Anterior capsular excision is facilitated first by developing the plane between the brachialis and capsule and then by excising the capule. If additional exposure is required, the lateral collateral liagament can be released (Fig. 61–5). The brachialis and triceps muscles may need to be elevated from the humeral shaft near the joint with an elevator to improve terminal flexion and extension.

4. Closure: The extensor muscle origins reflected off the humerus are reattached with nonabsorbable sutures through drill holes in the lateral epicondylar ridge. If the lateral collateral ligament was elevated during the exposure, it is repaired back to bone through drill holes, using 2–0 nonabsorbable sutures and the Bunnell technique. The remaining wound is closed in standard fashion.

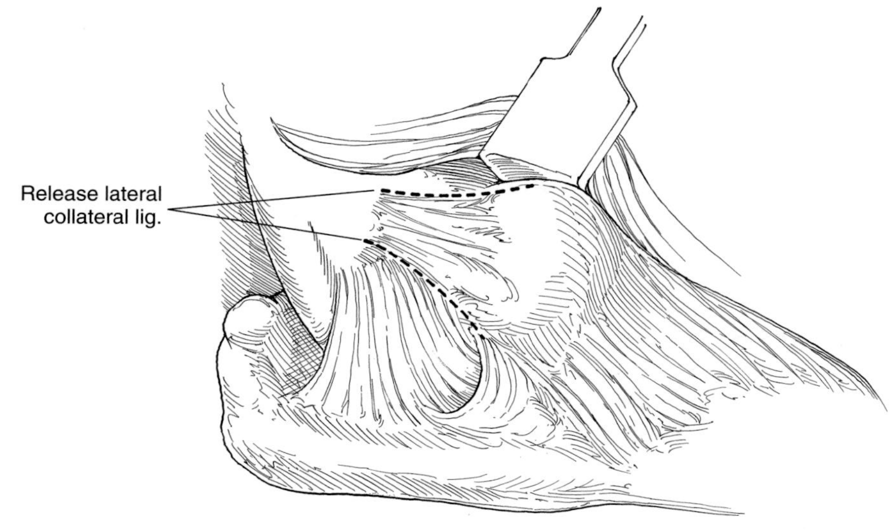

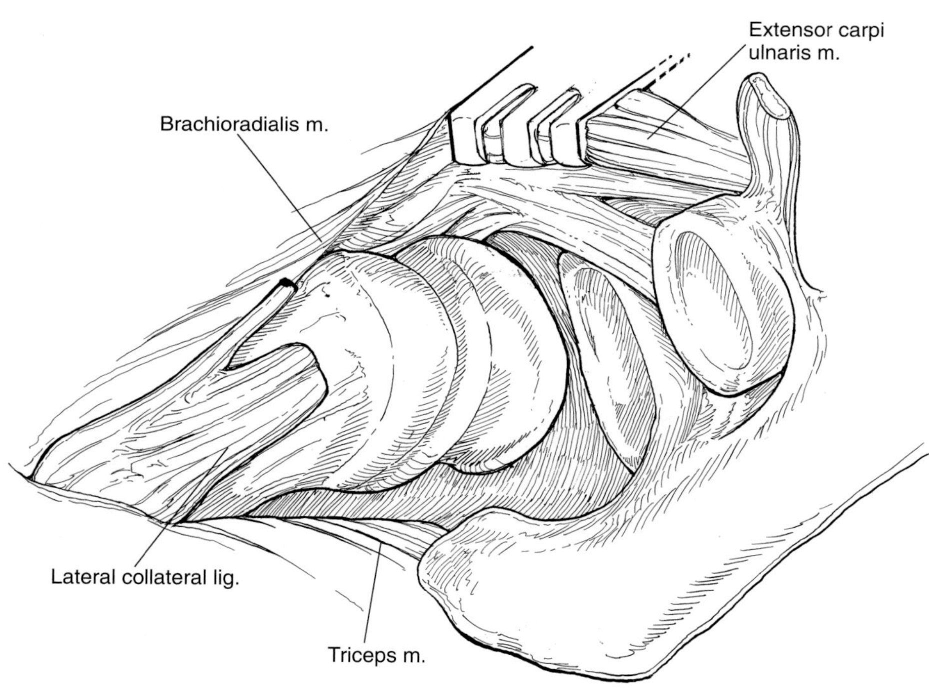

FIGURE 61–5. *A*, Extensile exposure can be achieved with elevation of the lateral collateral ligament. *B*, With the lateral collateral released and the capsule excised, the joint can be hinged open and pivoted on the intact medial collateral ligament.

POSTOPERATIVE MANAGEMENT

The elbow is rested in a splint or sling for 3 to 4 days to allow some resolution of soft tissue edema. After the period of rest, patients are encouraged to resume activities of daily living, and a physical therapy program is initiated. The therapy program is individualized to the patient's needs. The initial phase of therapy emphasizes regaining range of motion. A continuous passive motion (CPM) machine may help to restore motion in the early phase of rehabilitation, but it is not essential. Static splints are used as needed. Therapy is provided daily for the first 2 weeks and is tapered off as the patient progresses. Highly motivated patients may need little or no therapy. Patients are monitored closely for loss of motion during the first 4 weeks, and therapy is modified as indicated.

COMPLICATIONS

Nerve injury is the greatest risk associated with these procedures. Patients should be assessed carefully for nerve function during the immediate postoperative period. Recurrence of the osteophytes and joint stiffness are anticipated in most cases over time. However, the early onset of joint stiffness must be addressed with therapy. Heterotopic ossification has not been a problem, and we do not recommend prophylactic nonsteroidal anti-inflammatory medication.

RESULTS

A limited number of reports on débridement of the degenerative elbow can be found in the literature. Although the number of reported cases is limited, the findings of significant improvement are consistent. Morrey reported 90% successful results in 15 patients treated with an open technique. Similarly, Tsuge and Mizuseki reported that all of their 24 patients gained motion and pain relief with minimal complications. Ogilvie-Harris and colleagues reported significant improvement in 85% of 25 elbows treated with arthroscopic débridement; similar results have been reported by both Redden and Stanley, and Ward and Anderson.

REFERENCES

Cohen MS, Hastings H: Operative release for elbow contracture: The lateral collateral ligament sparing technique. Orthop Clin North Am 30:133–139, 1999.

Morrey BF: Primary degenerative arthritis of the elbow. Treatment by ulnohumeral arthroplasty. J Bone Joint Surg [Br] 74:409–413, 1992.

Ogilvie-Harris DJ, Gordon R, MacKay M: Arthroscopic treatment for posterior impingement in degenerative arthritis of the elbow. Arthroscopy 11:437–443, 1995.

Redden JF, Stanley D: Arthroscopic fenestration of the olecranon fossa in the treatment of osteoarthritis of the elbow. Arthroscopy 9:14–16, 1993.

Tsuge K, Mizuseki T: Debridement arthroplasty for advanced primary osteoarthritis of the elbow. Results of a new technique used for 29 elbows. J Bone Joint Surg [Br] 76:641–646, 1994.

Ward WG, Anderson TE: Elbow arthroscopy in a mostly athletic population. J Hand Surg [Am] 18:220–224, 1993

S E C T I O N V I

WRIST AND HAND

CHAPTER 62

Arthroscopy of the Wrist and Triangular Fibrocartilage Complex Injuries

INTRODUCTION

Wrist arthroscopic technique has evolved and is now standardized, although the indications and applications for wrist arthroscopy are still evolving. Diagnostic arthroscopy is a useful tool in evaluation of the painful wrist. This chapter focuses on the basic technique of diagnostic arthroscopy and selected procedures, including triangular fibrocartilage complex débridement, ligament débridement, and distal radial fracture reduction. Surgeons unfamiliar with small-joint arthroscopy are encouraged to seek additional training with cadavers in a laboratory environment before performing clinical cases. Advanced arthroscopic techniques, such as excision of ganglions and triangular fibrocartilage complex repair, are not addressed in this chapter.

RELEVANT ANATOMY

The surgeon's thorough understanding of the extensor tendon and cutaneous nerve anatomy is essential if wrist arthroscopy is to be performed safely. The dorsal cutaneous branch of the ulnar nerve and the superficial branch of the radial nerve are at risk for injury during wrist arthroscopy. The anatomy is reviewed as it relates to the arthroscopic portals.

3–4 Portal. This portal is 1 cm distal to Lister's tubercle. The extensor pollicis longus and the extensor carpi radialis brevis lie on its radial side, and the fourth dorsal compartment lies on its ulnar side. The proximal border is the distal radius, and the distal border is the scapholunate ligament. Parts of the superficial branch of the radial nerve (SBRN) are at risk for injury when this portal is made (Fig. 62–1).

4–5 Portal. This portal is bordered ulnarly by the extensor digiti minimi and radially by the fourth dorsal compartment. Proximally lies the dorsal insertion of the triangular fibrocartilage complex (TFCC) onto the radius. The distal margin is the lunate. This portal lies directly in line with the articular surface of the distal radioulnar joint.

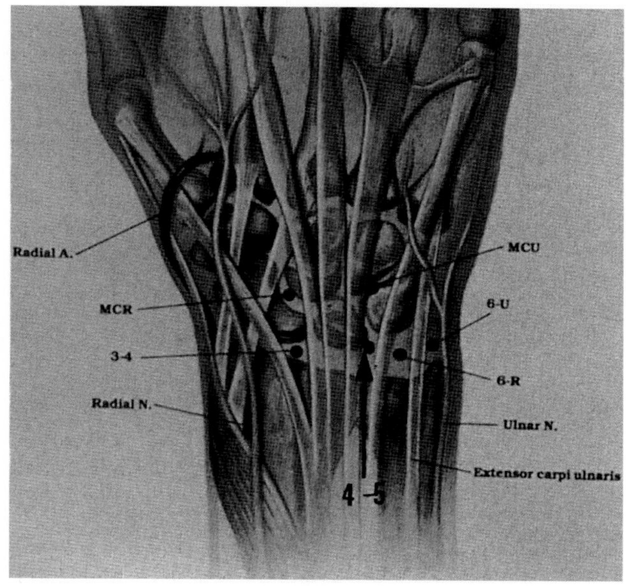

FIGURE 62–1. The anatomic landmarks for wrist portal placement. Note the locations of the superficial branch of the radial nerve and the dorsal cutaneous branch of the ulnar nerve and the radial artery relative to portal placement. MCR, midcarpal radial; MCU, midcarpal ulnar; 6-U, 6 ulnar; 6-R, 6 radial. (From Buterbaugh GA: Radiocarpal arthroscopy portals and normal anatomy. Hand Clin 10:567–576, 1994.)

6R Portal. This portal is located between the extensor digiti minimi and the extensor carpi ulnaris. The proximal border is the TFCC, and the distal margin is the lunotriquetral ligament. Branches of the dorsal cutaneous branch of the ulnar nerve may be injured when this portal is placed. On the other hand, this portal presents much less risk for nerve injury than does the 6U portal.

6U Portal. The borders of this portal are the extensor carpi ulnaris dorsally and the flexor carpi ulnaris volarly. The TFCC is the proximal border, and the triquetrum is the distal border. This portal is used infrequently because it risks injury to the cutaneous branch of the ulnar nerve.

Midcarpal Radial Portal. The margins of this portal are the extensor carpi radialis brevis radially, and the fourth extensor compartment ulnarly. The distal margin is the capitate, and the proximal margin is the scapholunate joint. The portal lies 1 cm distal to the 3–4 portal, and it lies on a line extending down the radial border of the third metacarpal. Branches of the SBRN run near the portal and are at risk for injury.

Midcarpal Ulnar Portal. The margins of this portal are the fourth dorsal compartment radially and the extensor digiti minimi ulnarly. The proximal margin is the lunotriquetral joint, and the distal margin is the capitohamate articulation. Branches of the dorsal cutaneous branch of the ulnar nerve are at risk for injury with use of this portal.

SURGICAL *TECHNIQUE*

Indications

Diagnostic arthroscopy of the wrist is indicated in the evaluation of persistent disabling mechanical wrist pain of unknown cause after an appropriate workup. Indications such as this have tremendous potential for abuse by overzealous surgeons. However, arthroscopy has evolved as the "gold standard" in the diagnosis of mechanical wrist pain. Mechanical wrist pain refers to pain associated with catching, popping, or clicking in the wrist. The pain should be completely relieved with intra-articular injection of local anesthetic. If the pain is not relieved with intra-articular injection, arthroscopy is unlikely to be beneficial. In cases in which the diagnosis is known, such as triangular fibrocartilage complex tears or scapholunate ligament tears, arthroscopy can better delineate the available treatment options by allowing accurate assessment of the severity of the problem.

Arthroscopy is contraindicated in the management of dystrophic pain. In this situation, arthroscopy is unlikely to be beneficial and may precipitate the symptoms.

Technique

1. Equipment: A 2.7-mm 30° arthroscope is used for wrist arthroscopy. A 2.0-mm 35° scope may be helpful for midcarpal arthroscopy in small wrists. However, the 2.7-mm scope functions well for radiocarpal and midcarpal arthroscopy in most cases. A 3.0-mm arthroscopic shaver and a variety of blades are recommended. Larger shavers do not fit in the joint without scuffing of the joint surface. A small joint probe is essential, and a variety of basket forceps are recommended. A traction tower greatly facilitates the procedure and is highly recommended (Fig. 62–2). Arthroscopy of the wrist can be performed with other traction techniques; however, the tower allows more freedom of positioning of the wrist.
2. Positioning: The patient is supine on the operating table with the arm extended on a hand table. A tourniquet is applied to the midarm. The arm is loosely taped to the hand table with 2-inch surgical tape. The tape is applied such that the arm can be lifted 1 to 2 inches off the arm table. The laxity of the tape assists in draping and leaves room for the base of the traction tower to slide under the arm. The application of the tourniquet in this location allows it to function as a point of counterforce during application of finger trap traction. The forearm is wrapped with Coban (self-adherent wrap, 3M Pharmaceuticals, St. Paul, MN) to limit the extravasation of fluid into the forearm. A wrist arthroscopy traction tower (Linvatec, Largo, FL) is positioned as shown in Figure 62–2. Disposable sterile finger traps are applied to the index and middle fingers. Axial traction is applied to 10 pounds. The wrist is flexed approximately 20°. The arm is exsanguinated with an elastic bandage, and the tourniquet is inflated to 250 mm Hg.
3. Radiocarpal portals: There are four radiocarpal portals and two midcarpal portals. The primary portals for radiocarpal arthroscopy are the 3–4 and 4–5 portals. The 3–4 portal is most often entered first. It is located between the third and fourth extensor compartments just distal to the radius. The surgeon can localize the portal by palpating Lister's tubercle with the thumb. The tip of the thumb can be rolled distally off the tubercle into a relative "soft spot" on the radiocarpal joint. An 18-gauge needle is inserted at the 3–4 portal site, and the joint is distended with saline. Next, to prevent cutaneous nerve injury, portals are created by incision of the skin only; then, blunt dissection is performed down to the wrist capsule. This technique is used to create all the portals. The scope sheath and blunt trocar are aimed 20° proximally and are then advanced through the capsule with a back-and-forth twisting motion. The

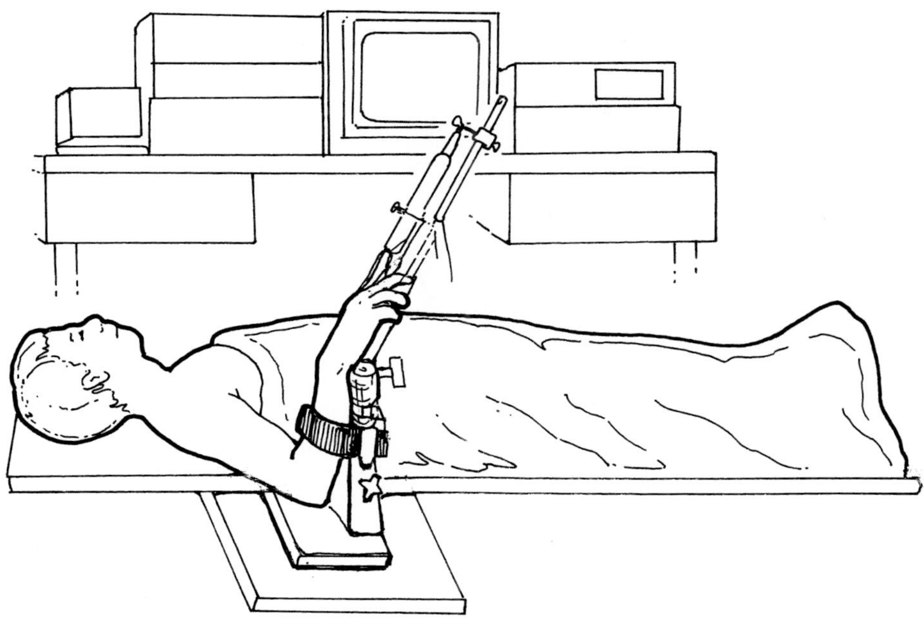

FIGURE 62–2. Illustration of operating room setup with wrist arthroscopy tower.

2.7-mm 30° arthroscope is introduced, and the saline inflow is connected to the scope sheath. The scope immediately visualizes the so-called ligament of Testu, which is a tuft of vascular synovium that lies volar to the scapholunate ligament. The scope is moved ulnarly to enable visualization of the dorsal ulnar aspect of the wrist. An 18-gauge needle is introduced at the 6U portal. The arthroscope is used to confirm proper placement of the needle. The needle is withdrawn and an outflow is established by placement of a cannula in the 6R portal. The 4–5 portal is used to insert the arthroscopic probe.

4. Radiocarpal arthroscopy
   a. The arthroscopic assessment of the joint begins on the radial aspect. The scaphoid and the scaphoid fossa of the radius are inspected. Next, the volar ligaments are visualized, beginning radially with the radioscaphocapitate ligament, which is the most radial (Fig. 62–3). Adjacent and ulnar to the radioscaphocapitate ligament is the long radiolunate ligament (Fig. 62–4). The next most ulnar ligament is the radioscapholunate or short radiolunate. However, in many patients, the radioscapholunate may be hidden from view by the overlying ligament of Testu. Some might misinterpret the presence of the ligament of Testu as signifying disease because it may be mistaken for hypertrophic synovium, and in addition, they may become disappointed with the loss of visualization that results from bleeding if this tuft of vascular synovium is erroneously débrided. This tuft of synovium marks the scapholunate ligament. If the scope is withdrawn slightly, the scapholunate ligament can be visualized and probed. However, functional assessment of the ligament is best performed from the midcarpal portal. The intercarpal ligaments in their normal state during arthroscopy appear identical to the articular cartilage; they can be identified only by the sulcus they form and their change in texture during probing.
   b. Next, the scope is rotated to view ulnarly and is advanced to view the ulnar aspect of the wrist. The lunate and the lunate fossa of the radius are inspected. The transition from the lunate fossa to the cartilage of the TFCC is subtle and often can be identified only by texture changes noted during probing. The central region and the margins of the TFCC are carefully probed to inspect for tears (Fig. 62–5). The TFCC central region should be taut such that it has a "trampoline" effect on probing. The absence of the "trampoline" effect and the presence of a loose, floating central TFCC suggest an avulsion of the TFCC insertion for the fovea of the ulnar styloid. Volar to the TFCC, the ulnolunate and ulnotriquetral ligaments are visible and are palpated with the probe (Fig. 62–6). Further visualization of the ulnar side of the wrist is optimized with the scope moved to the 4–5 portal. With the scope in the 4–5 portal, the lunotriquetral

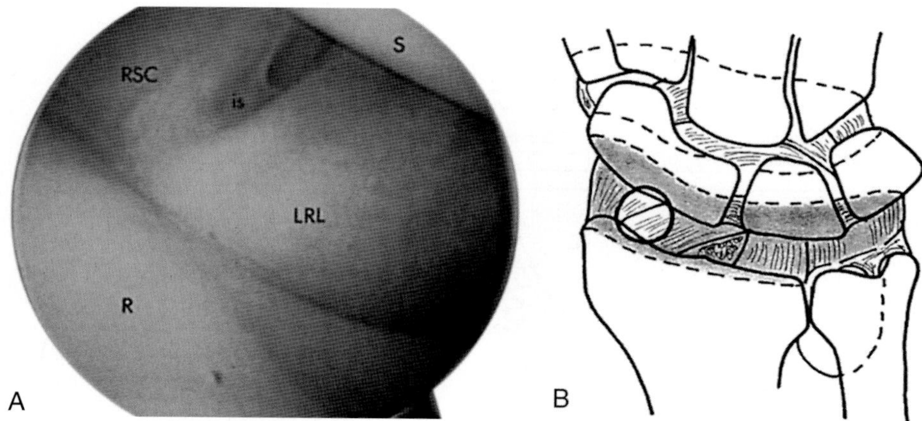

FIGURE 62–3. *A*, Arthroscopic view of the palmar radiocarpal ligaments from the 3–4 portal perspective. is, interligamentous sulcus; LRL, long radiolunate ligament; R, scaphoid fossa of the distal radius; RSC, radioscapho-capitate ligament; S, scaphoid. *B*, View area in the wrist. (From Berger RA: Arthroscopic anatomy of the wrist and distal radioulnar joint. Hand Clin 15:401, 1999.)

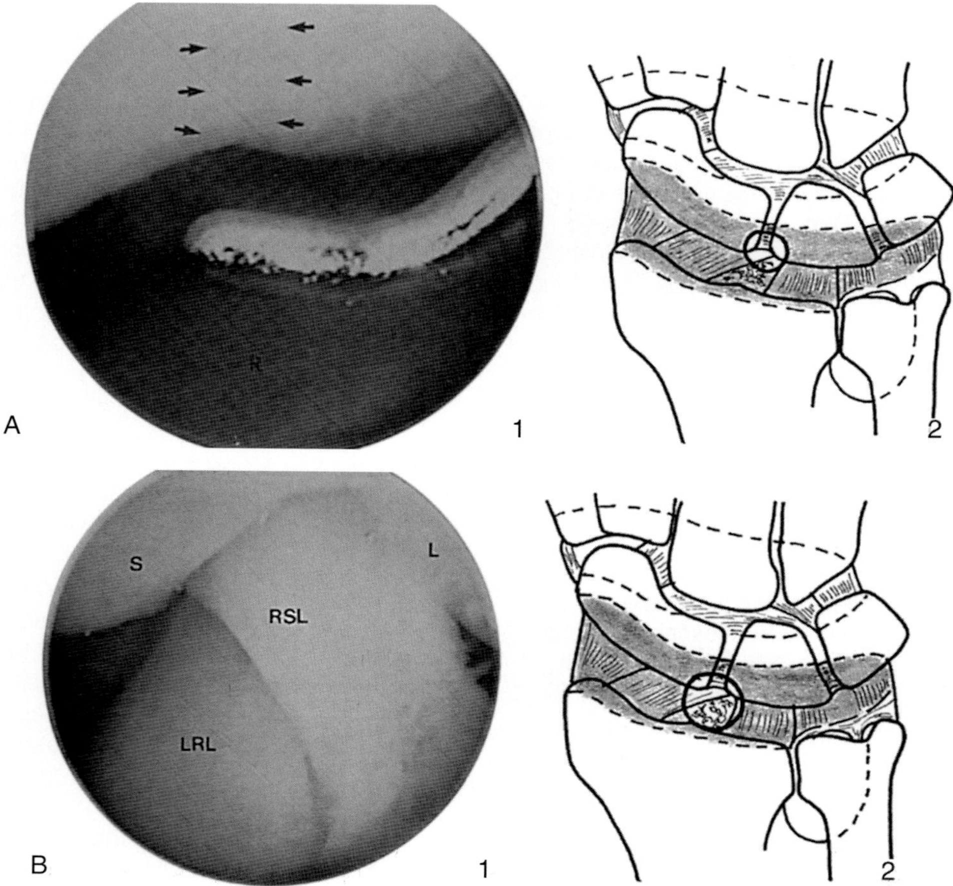

FIGURE 62–4. *A1*, Arthroscopic view of the scapholunate interosseous ligament *(arrows)* from the 3–4 portal. The distal articular surface of the radius (R) is seen in the background. *A2*, View area in the wrist. *B1*, An arthroscopic view of the radioscapholunate ligament (RSL) from the 3–4 portal. Note the vertical orientation of the RSL ligament relative to the long radiolunate ligament (LRL). The proximal articular surfaces of the scaphoid (S) and lunate (L) are visible. *B2*, View area in the wrist. (From Berger RA: Arthroscopic anatomy of the wrist and distal radioulnar joint. Hand Clin 15:402, 1999.)

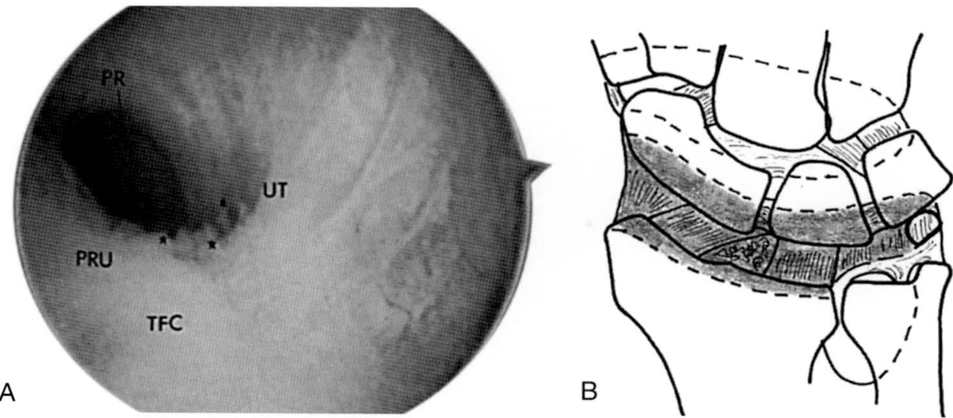

FIGURE 62–5. *A*, Arthroscopic view through the 4–5 portal of the prestyloid recess (PR) near the ulnar extent of the palmar radioulnar ligament (PRU), the ulnar apex of the triangulofibrocartilage complex (TFC), and the proximal origin of the ulnotriquetral ligament (UT). *B*, View area in the wrist. (From Berger RA: Arthroscopic anatomy of the wrist and distal radioulnar joint. Hand Clin 15:404, 1999.)

ligament is visualized and probed. This ligament is similar in appearance to the scapholunate ligament. More ulnarly, the apex of the TFCC blends into the ulnar joint capsule. Just volar to this is an opening—the pre-styloid recess. This recess is large enough in some individuals to allow viewing of the pisiform.

5. Midcarpal arthroscopy: The radial midcarpal portal is created by passing an 18-gauge needle into the joint 1 cm distal to the 3–4 radiocarpal portal. The joint is distended with normal saline and, with the standard technique, the scope sheath and the blunt obturator are placed into the joint. The radial border of the capitate is visualized first. After orientation to the capitate, the scope is passed distally to allow visualization of the scaphotrapezial trapezoid joint (Fig. 62–7). The scope is then passed proximally while the body of the scaphoid is viewed. As the inspection continues more proximally, the scapholunate joint is visualized (Fig. 62–8). At this point, the ulnar midcarpal portal is created. First, an 18-gauge needle is inserted 1 cm distal to the 4–5 portal. The ulnar aspect of the lunate is visualized during needle insertion. After the portal location has been confirmed, the portal is created with standard technique and the arthroscopic probe is inserted. Attention is directed back to the scapholunate joint. The scapholunate ligament cannot be visualized. However, probing from the midcarpal view provides an excellent assessment of the ligament's integrity. In the normal state, the scaphoid and lunate cannot be separated with a probe. Attention is directed to the lunotriquetral joint (Fig. 62–9). This joint is assessed for stability by probing. The scope is then rotated distally to provide visualization of the capitohamate articulation.

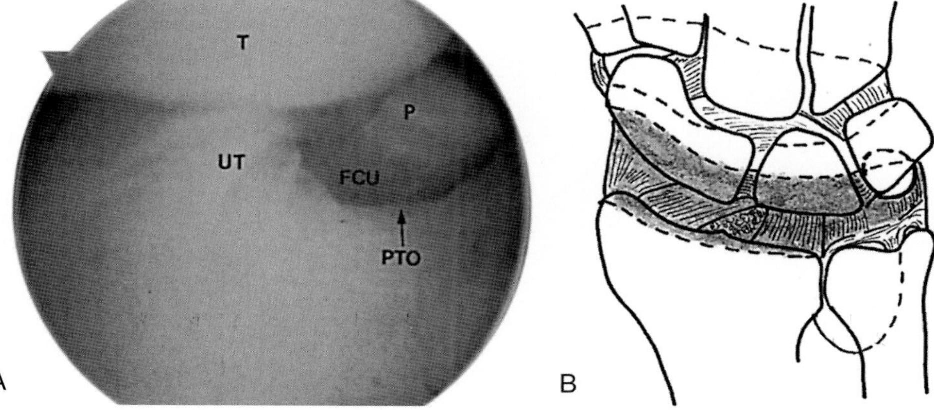

FIGURE 62–6. *A*, Arthroscopic view through the 4–5 portal through the pisotriquetral orifice (PTO) of the pisiform (P) and the insertion of the flexor carpi ulnaris tendon (FCU). TI, triquetrum; UT, ulnotriquetral ligament. *B*, View area in the wrist. (From Berger RA: Arthroscopic anatomy of the wrist and distal radioulnar joint. Hand Clin 15:405, 1999.)

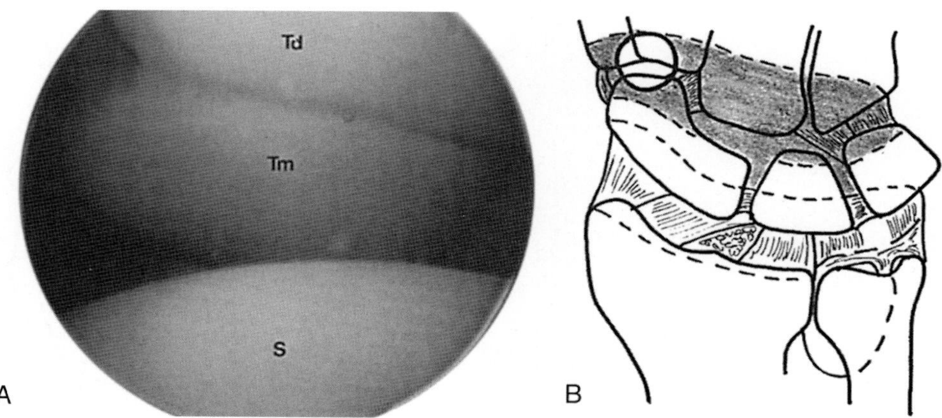

FIGURE 62–7. *A*, Arthroscopic view through the radial midcarpal portal of the scaphotrapezial trapezoid joint. S, scaphoid; Td, trapezoid; Tm, trapezium. *B*, View area in the wrist. (From Berger RA: Arthroscopic anatomy of the wrist and distal radioulnar joint. Hand Clin 15:406, 1999.)

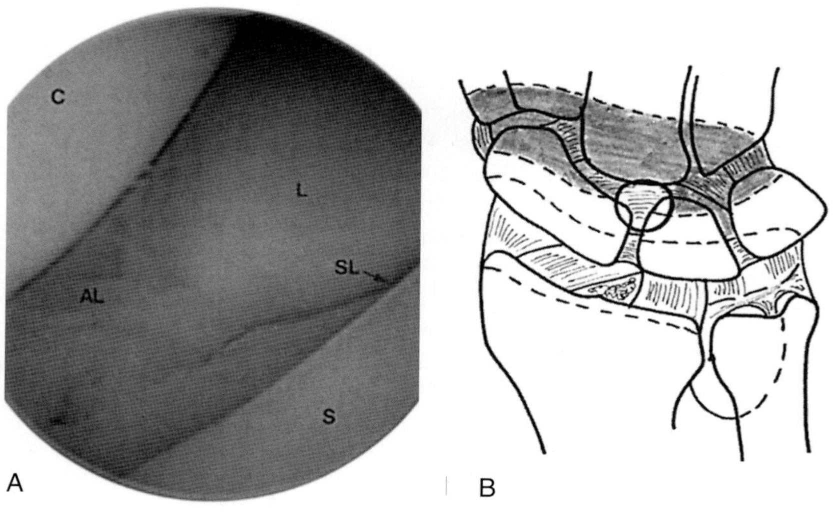

FIGURE 62–8. *A*, Arthroscopic view through the radial midcarpal portal of the junction between the scaphoid (S), lunate (L), and capitate (C). *B*, View area in the wrist. (From Berger RA: Arthroscopic anatomy of the wrist and distal radioulnar joint. Hand Clin 15:409, 1999.)

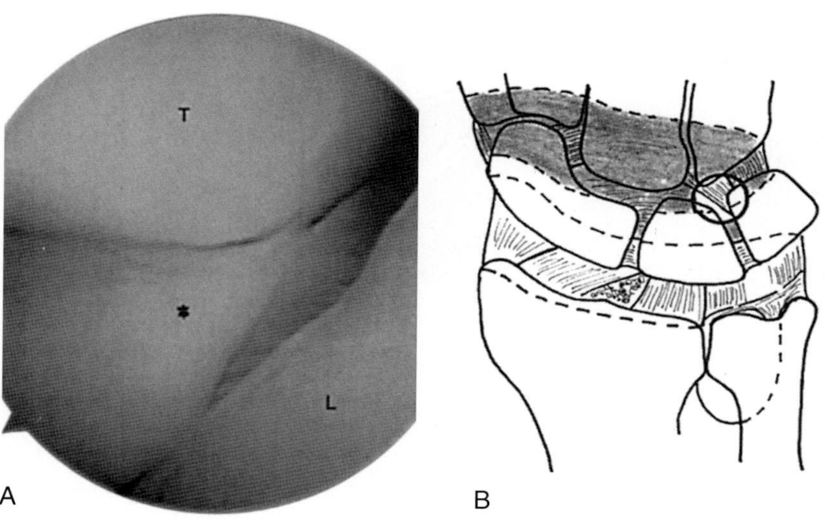

FIGURE 62–9. *A*, Arthroscopic view through the radial midcarpal portal of the lunotriquetral joint, demonstrating the projection of the synovial tissue normally seen entering the anterior aspect of the joint (*). L, lunate; T, triquetrum. *B*, View area in the wrist. (From Berger RA: Arthroscopic anatomy of the wrist and distal radioulnar joint. Hand Clin 15:409, 1999.)

POSTOPERATIVE MANAGEMENT

The majority of wrist arthroscopy is performed on an outpatient basis. At the conclusion of the procedure, the wrist and portal sites are injected with 10 mL 0.5% Marcaine (bupivacaine with epinephrine). A light dressing and volar splint are applied. The splint is discontinued in 4 to 5 days and range-of-motion exercises are started. Most patients discontinue the use of narcotic analgesics after a few days. After 2 weeks, patients are encouraged to massage the portal sites with vitamin E–based hand lotion. This assists in softening the scar and desensitizing the portal sites. Specific rehabilitation programs are dictated by the procedure performed. However, the majority of cases do not require formal physical therapy.

COMPLICATIONS

The complications of wrist arthroscopy are divided into four categories by Warhold and Ruth: (1) complications related to traction and arm position, (2) complications related to establishment of portals, (3) procedure-specific complications, and (4) miscellaneous complications associated with arthroscopy. Injury to the metacarpophalangeal or proximal interphalangeal joints can occur from excessive traction. This complication is avoided by limiting traction to 10 pounds and by using 4 finger traps to distribute the force. In addition, disposable plastic finger traps are gentler on the skin than those made of wire. The potential for cutaneous nerve injury is minimized by attention to detail when the portal is created. Furthermore, the risk of tendon injury is minimized by correct placement of the portal and incision of the skin only when the portal is placed. Finally, articular scuffing and iatrogenic chondral lesions are avoided by the use of appropriately sized instruments, gentle technique, and proper portal placement.

SELECTED PROCEDURES AND RESULTS

Ligament Débridement

Tears of the membranous portion of the lunotriquetral ligament or scapholunate ligaments may be a cause of mechanical irritation of the wrist. Ligament tears may benefit from simple débridement, which is accomplished with motorized shavers and basket forceps. In addition, recently available electrosurgical probes in small sizes allow ablation of tissue rather than excision. Tissue ablation overcomes many of the limitations of small, motorized shavers. In cases in which gross instability is absent, patients may benefit from débridement of the tear.

Weis and associates reported their experience with ligament débridement alone; they report significant improvement in 85% of patients with incomplete scapholunate ligament tears and in 100% of patients with partial lunotriquetral tears. In the acute setting, arthroscopy is useful for assessment of joint reduction. The joint is percutaneously pinned after arthroscopic assisted reduction is performed. Whipple reported success with this technique when treating scapholunate ligament (SL) ruptures. His success was better in cases with diastasis of less than 3 mm on anteroposterior x-rays.

Triangular Fibrocartilage Complex Débridement

Symptomatic central tears of the TFCC may be significantly improved with débridement. The central portion of the TFCC is excised or ablated with electrocautery. However, the peripheral margins of the TFCC must be preserved to maintain stability of the distal radioulnar joint (Fig. 62–10). The ulnar head and lunate must be inspected for evidence of ulnocarpal impaction, which is suggested by the presence of chondromalacia in these areas. TFCC débridement without ulnar shortening is unlikely to succeed if ulnocarpal impaction is the cause.

Hulsizer, Weiss, and Akelman reported relief of symptoms in 84 of 97 patients with TFCC tears treated with arthroscopic débridement. Twelve of the 13 failures obtained complete relief of symptoms after ulnar shortening. Similarly, Osterman reported that 88% of patients were satisfied with pain relief after débridement of TFCC tears; however, many patients also had partial arthroscopic ulnar head resection (2–3 mm).

Arthroscopic Reduction of Distal Radius Fractures

Arthroscopic reduction of intra-articular fractures of the distal radius has gained popularity in recent years. Recent studies have demonstrated the limitations of x-rays, which are often inaccurate in assessing displacement of intra-articular fractures. In this application, the arthroscope visualizes the reduction, which is performed with standard techniques. In addition, large Kirschner wires placed percutaneously are used to elevate depressed articular fragments. Arthroscopic reduction allows the surgeon to achieve anatomic reduction of displaced intra-articular fractures without the wrist stiffness that results from open reduction and internal fixation. Furthermore, CT is the most accurate way to assess displacement, but CT cannot be used intraoperatively. In our experience, it is best to delay this procedure for 3 to 5 days after injury. This delay allows the hematoma to organize. Arthroscopy of the wrist done before this is difficult because the unorganized hematoma mixes with the irrigation fluid and obscures the view. After 3 to 5 days, the hematoma appears as organized clot that can be removed with a motorized shaver. It is especially important that the forearm be wrapped with elastic wrap to prevent the extravasation of saline into the forearm.

Because arthroscopic assisted reduction of fractures is new, long-term results are not available. However, after

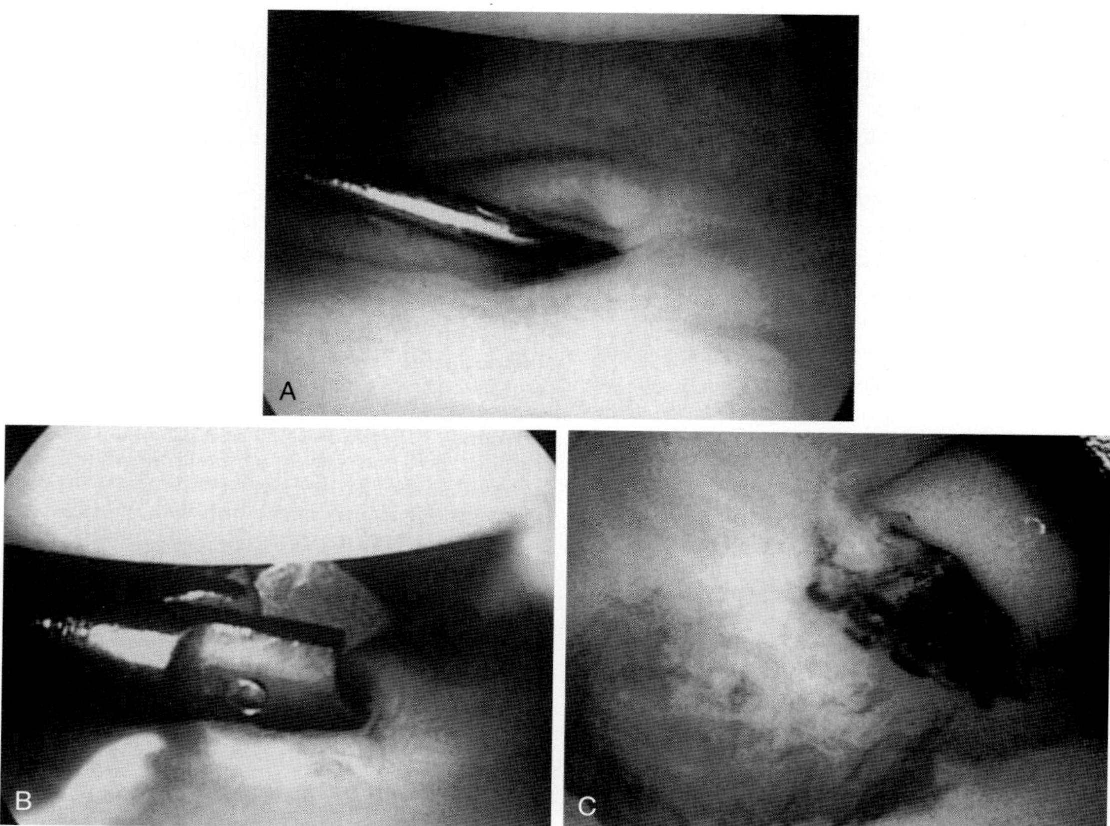

FIGURE 62–10. *A*, Transjugular fibrocartilage complex (TFCC) tear. *B*, Débridement with suction punch. *C*, Débridement completed with thermal probe. (From Dailey SW, Palmer AK: The role of arthroscopy in the evaluation and treatment of triangular fibrocartilage complex injuries in athletes. Hand Clin 16:468, 2000.)

short-term results were reviewed, several studies demonstrated that the technique is safe and effective.

REFERENCES

Abrams RA, Petersen M, Botte MJ: Arthroscopic portals of the wrist: An anatomic study. J Hand Surg [Am] 19:940–944, 1994.

Bettinger PC, Cooney WP III, Berger RA: Arthroscopic anatomy of the wrist. Orthop Clin North Am 26:707–719, 1995.

Ekman EF, Poehling GG: Arthroscopy of the wrist in athletes. Clin Sports Med 15:753–768, 1996.

Hulsizer D, Weiss AP, Akelman E: Ulnar-shortening osteotomy after tailed arthroscopic debridement of the triangular fibrocartilage complex. J Hand Surg [Am] 22:694–698, 1997.

Osterman AL, Terrill RG: Arthroscopic treatment of TFCC lesions. Hand Clin 7:277–281, 1991.

Roth JH, Poehling GG, Whipple TL: Arthroscopic surgery of the wrist. Instr Course Lect 37:183–194, 1988.

Viegas SF: Midcarpal arthroscopy: Anatomy and portals. Hand Clin 10:577–587, 1994.

Warhold LG, Ruth RM: Complications of wrist arthroscopy and how to prevent them. Hand Clin 11:81–89, 1995.

Weis AP, Sachar K, Glowacki KA: Arthroscopic debridement alone for intercarpal ligament tears. J Hand Surg [Am] 22:344–349, 1997.

Whipple TL, Marotta JJ, Powell JH III: Techniques of wrist arthroscopy. Arthroscopy 2:244–252, 1986.

CHAPTER 63

Treatment of de Quervain's Tenosynovitis

INTRODUCTION

De Quervain's disease is a stenosing tenosynovitis of the abductor pollicis longus (APL) and the extensor pollicis brevis (EPB) tendons. Athletes considered to be at risk are those who require a forceful grasp, combined with repetitive use of the thumb in ulnar deviation. Several sports that can lead to this malady include racquet sports, golf, fly fishing, and javelin and discus throwing. It has been well reported that the left thumb of a right-handed golfer and the right thumb of a left-handed golfer are susceptible to this injury owing to hyperabduction during the golf swing.

PATHOPHYSIOLOGY

The EPB and the APL tendons pass through a fibro-osseous tunnel formed by a groove in the radial styloid and overlying extensor retinaculum (Fig. 63–1). The pathophysiology of this tenosynovitis, whether it originates in the tendon sheath or in the tenosynovium itself, is unclear to date. What is clear is that the tendons pass through the tunnel and stretch as their angle increases with ulnar deviation of the wrist.

HISTORY AND PHYSICAL EXAMINATION

Patients typically complain of pain over the radial styloid that worsens with wrist and thumb motion. On examination, tenderness over the radial styloid, swelling, and, occasionally, triggering or crepitus may be present. A positive Finkelstein's test (Fig. 63–2) causes reproduction of pain with ulnar deviation of the wrist while the thumb is adducted, which is typical for this syndrome. This test is not pathognomonic for de Quervain's tenosynovitis,

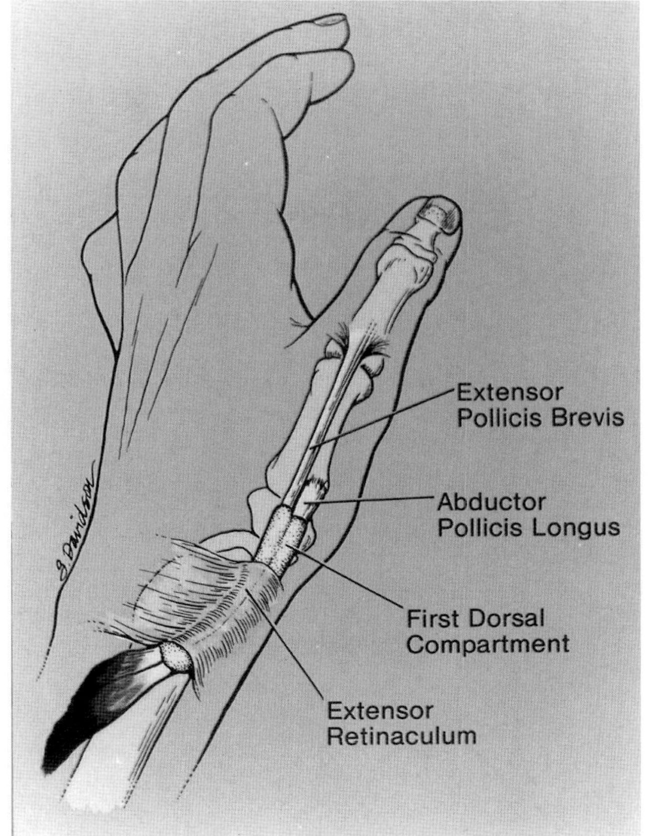

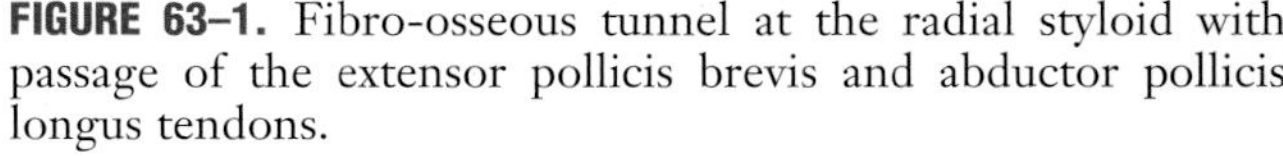

FIGURE 63–1. Fibro-osseous tunnel at the radial styloid with passage of the extensor pollicis brevis and abductor pollicis longus tendons.

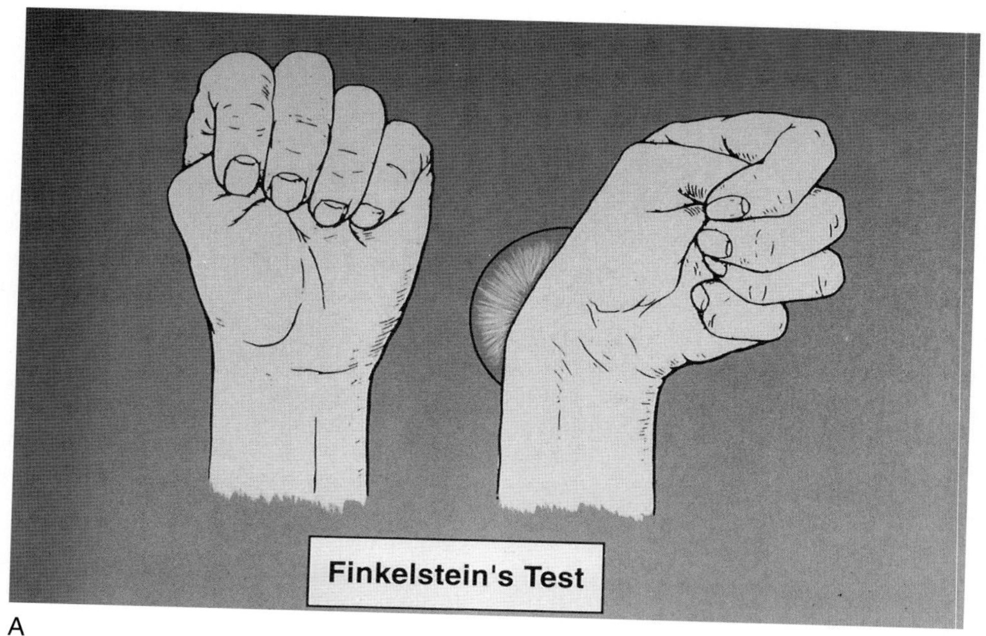

A

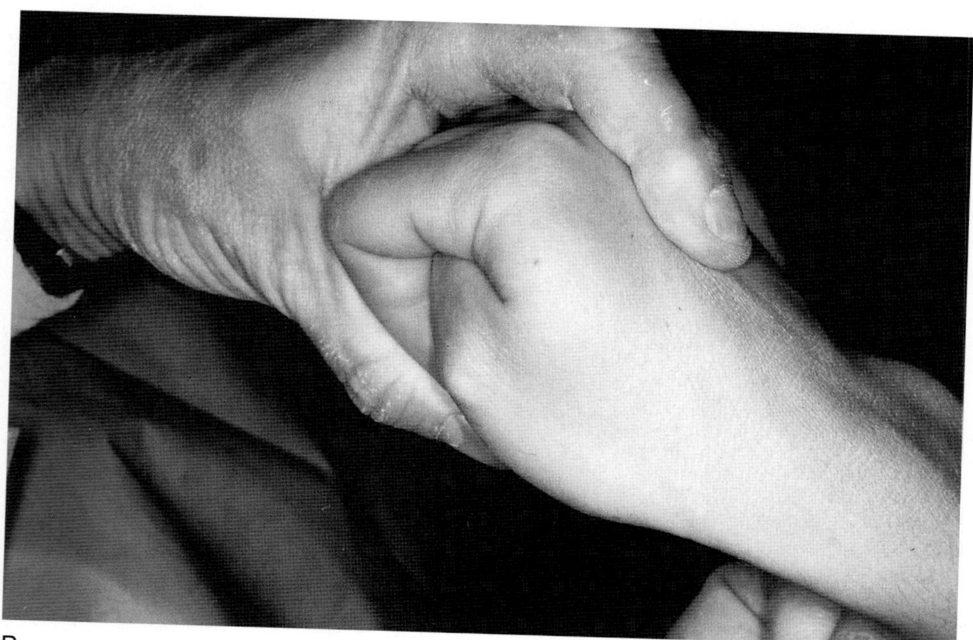

B

FIGURE 63–2. Physical examination of the wrist, demonstrating Finkelstein's test. *A*, The patient grasps the thumb. *B*, The wrist is ulnarly deviated. Reproduction of pain at the radial styloid is a positive test.

however, as carpometacarpal arthritis or underlying disease can result in a false-positive test. The differential diagnosis for pain in this region includes scaphoid fracture, flexor carpi radialis tenosynovitis, intersection syndrome, and Wartenberg's syndrome, in addition to carpometacarpal (CMC) arthritis.

DIAGNOSTIC IMAGING

A hyperpronated view or Roberts' view, along with a zero posteroanterior (PA) and lateral view of the wrist, are useful for distinguishing between the varying diagnoses listed earlier (Fig. 63–3). Roberts' view shows evidence of CMC arthritis. If all x-rays are negative and the physical examination supports the history of

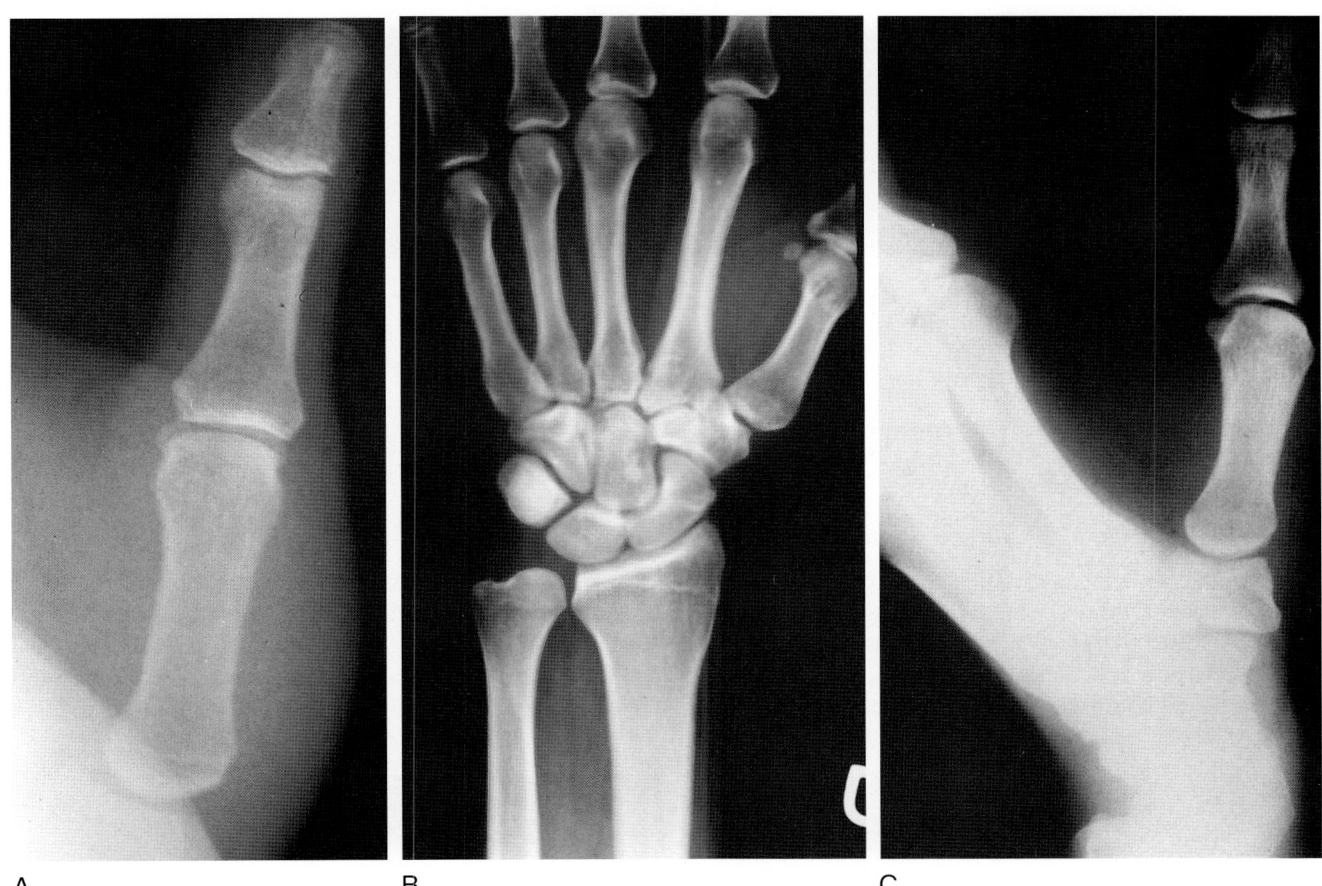

FIGURE 63–3. *A*, Roberts' view (hyperpronated). *B*, Zero posteroanterior view. *C*, Lateral view. All views are of the wrist.

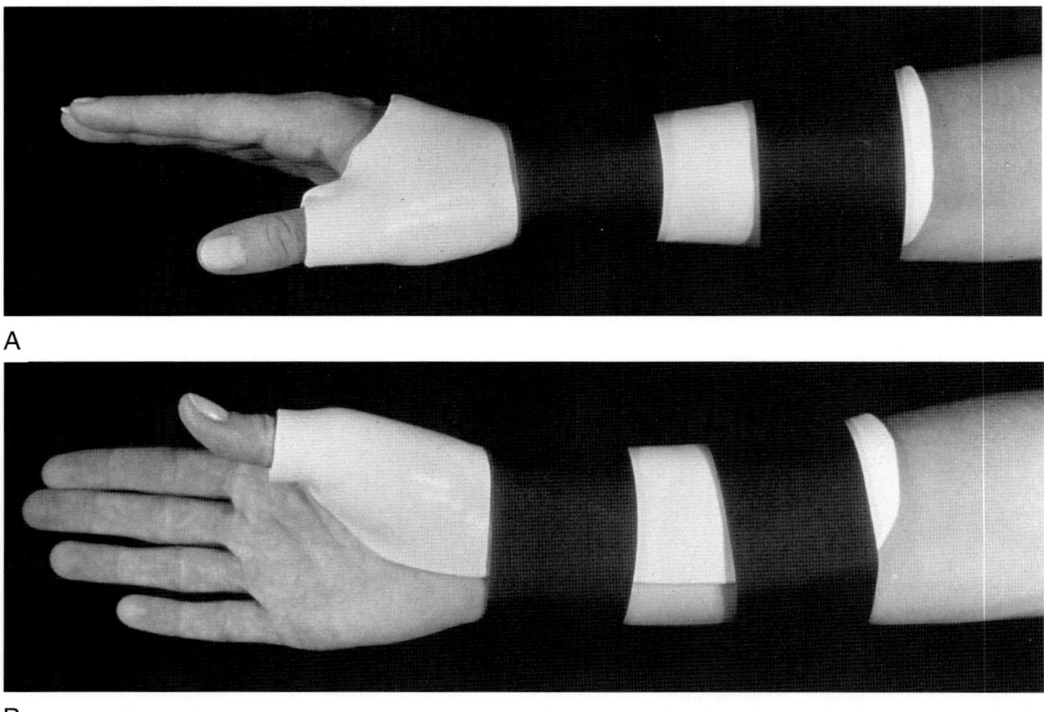

FIGURE 63–4. *A*, Posteroanterior view of the wrist in the thumb spica splint. *B*, Lateral view of the wrist in the thumb spica splint.

stenosing tenosynovitis, the diagnosis of de Quervain's can be correctly made.

NONOPERATIVE MANAGEMENT

Initial management on confirmation of the diagnosis includes a custom thumb spica splint (Fig. 63–4) made by a certified hand therapist. In addition, anti-inflammatory medications and a corticosteroid injection (Fig. 63–5) into the first dorsal compartment are important adjuvants.

RELEVANT ANATOMY AND PERILS AND PITFALLS OF SURGERY

Anatomic studies have demonstrated that a longitudinal septum may divide the APL and the EPB in 20% to 30% of patients (Fig. 63–6). This is one of the reasons for a poor response to corticosteroid injections, and it helps explain the development of recurrent symptoms. Surgical management must ensure definitive identification and release of both the EPB and the APL before closure.

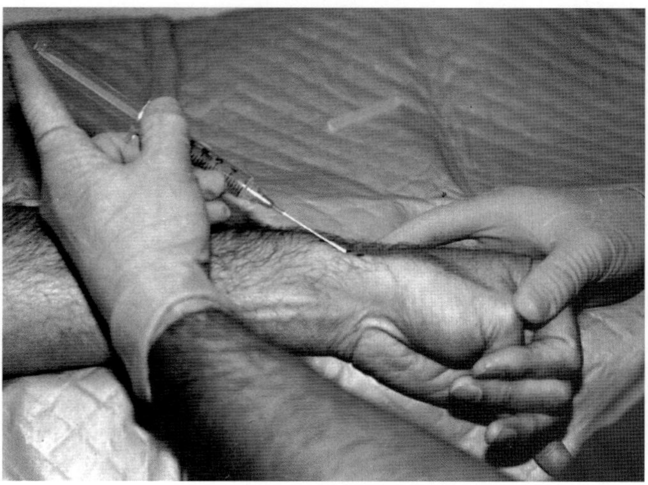

FIGURE 63–5. Technique for injection of the first dorsal compartment. Note the angle and placement of the needle.

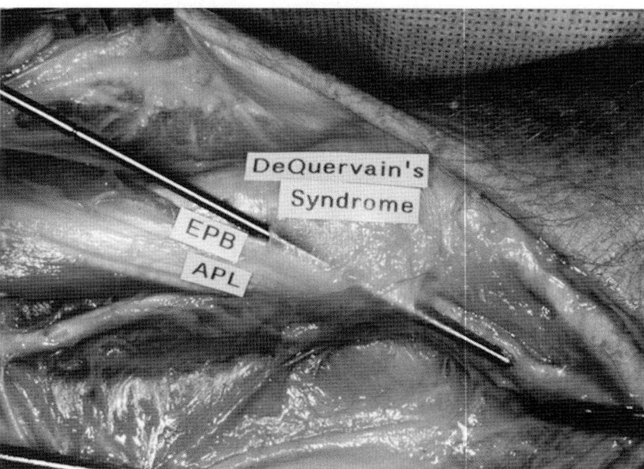

FIGURE 63–6. The septum divides the abductor pollicis longus (APL) and the extensor pollicis brevis (EPB) in up to 30% of patients.

SURGICAL TECHNIQUE

Indications

Surgical management is considered if there is no resolution of symptoms with conservative care. Surgery involves decompression of the first dorsal compartment with care taken to divide any septum present in the first dorsal compartment. Confirmation at surgery of the multiple slips of the APL (often numbering between five and seven) (Fig. 63–7) is essential, along with identification of the EPB within the depths of the wound.

Technique

1. Positioning: The patient is positioned supine with a hand table placed alongside the operating room table. A tourniquet cuff is placed on the upper arm while anesthesia (10 mL 1% lidocaine) is administered with a local field block. (Bier or axillary blocks may be performed as alternative anesthetic techniques.)

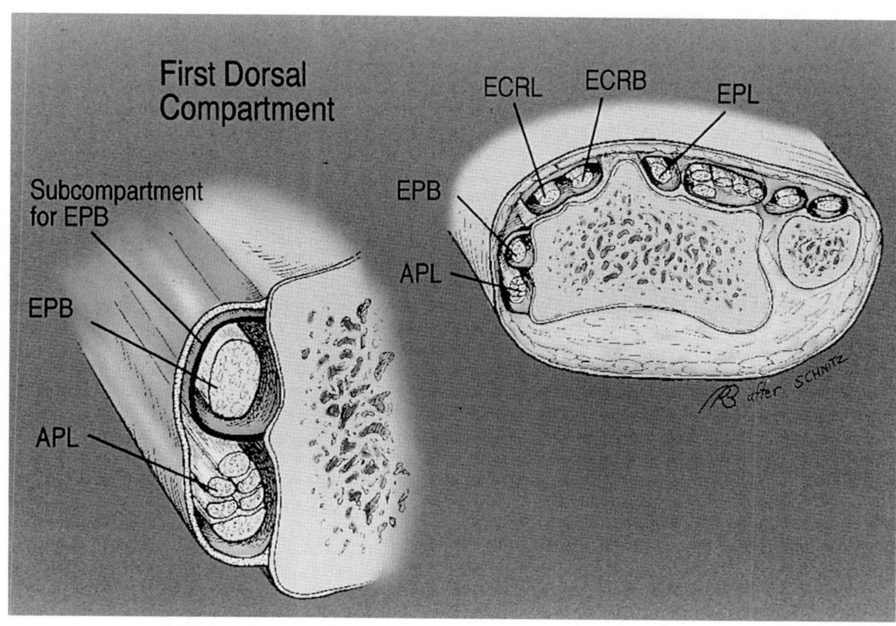

FIGURE 63–7. Illustration demonstrates the multiple slips of the abductor pollicis longus (APL) tendon. ECRB, extensor carpi radialis brevis; ECRL, extensor carpi radialis longus; EPB, extensor pollicis brevis; EPL, extensor pollicis longus.

2. Incision: A 2-cm transverse skin incision is drawn 1 cm proximal to the radial styloid, centered directly over the first dorsal compartment (Fig. 63–8).
3. The arm is wrapped with an Esmarch bandage and the tourniquet inflated to 250 mm Hg. The skin is incised with a No. 15 blade scalpel, and subcutaneous dissection is carried out with a Littler scissors, or similar blunt-tipped scissors, directly down to the level of the extensor retinaculum.
4. During dissection to the extensor retinaculum, the small branches of the lateral antebrachial cutaneous nerve are spared, if possible. Identification of the superficial radial nerve is essential; it should always be carefully dissected and protected with Ragnell retractors (Fig. 63–9).

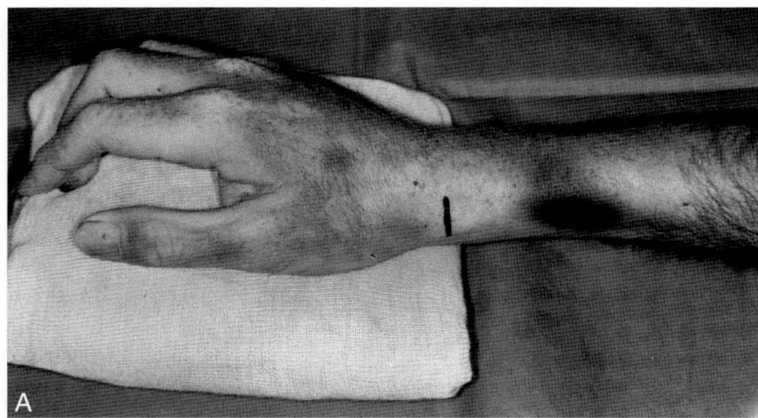

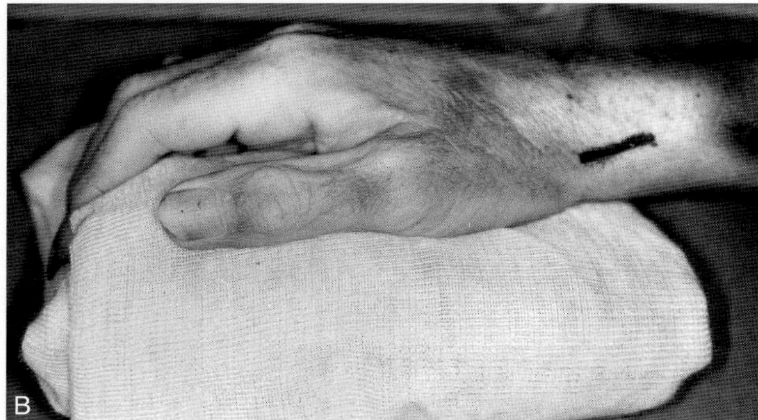

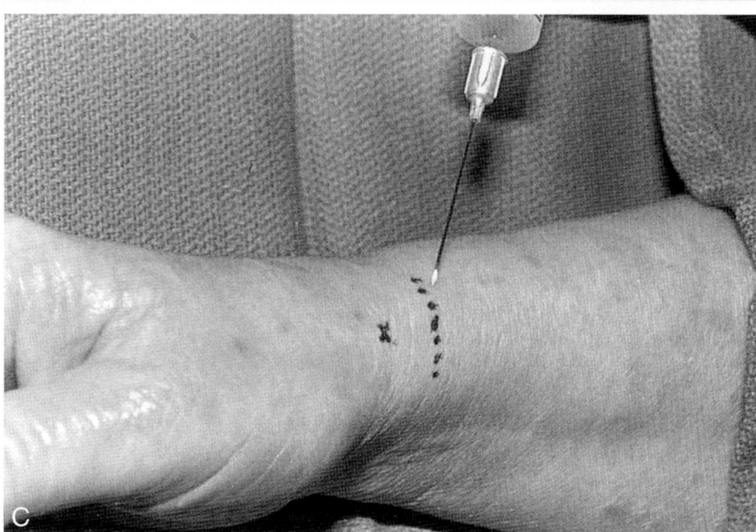

FIGURE 63–8. *A*, Cadaveric demonstration of the transverse incision for de Quervain's tenosynovitis. *B*, Cadaveric demonstration of a longitudinal incision for de Quervain's tenosynovitis. *C*, At the time of surgery, clinical picture of the transverse incision marked down 1 cm proximal to the radial styloid.

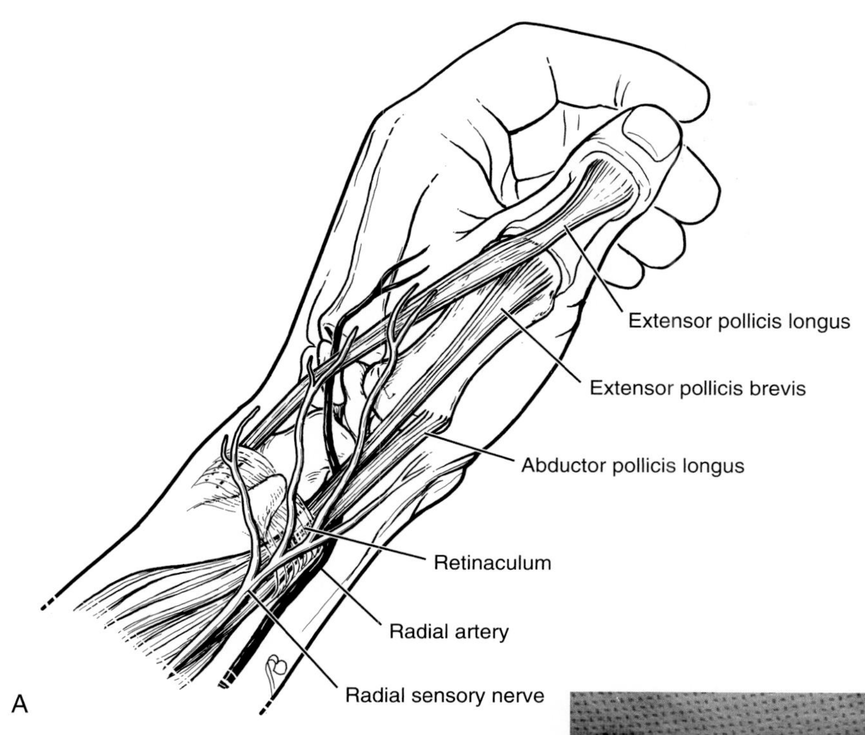

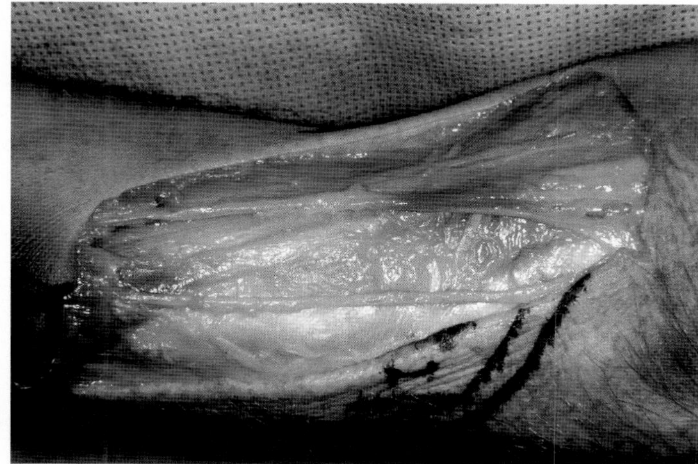

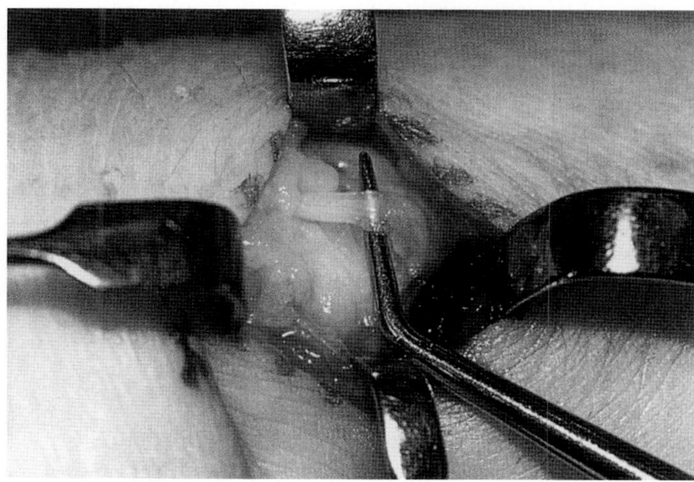

FIGURE 63–9. *A*, An artist's drawing of the superficial radial nerve in relation to the first dorsal extensor compartment. (From Bednar JM, Santarlasci PR: First extensor compartment release and retinacular sheath reconstruction for de Quervain's tenosynovitis. Atlas of Hand Clinics 4:40, 1999.) *B*, Cadaveric demonstration of the superficial radial nerve in relation to the first dorsal extensor compartment. *C*, Clinical picture at the time of surgery, demonstrating a branch of the superficial radial nerve overlying the first dorsal extensor compartment.

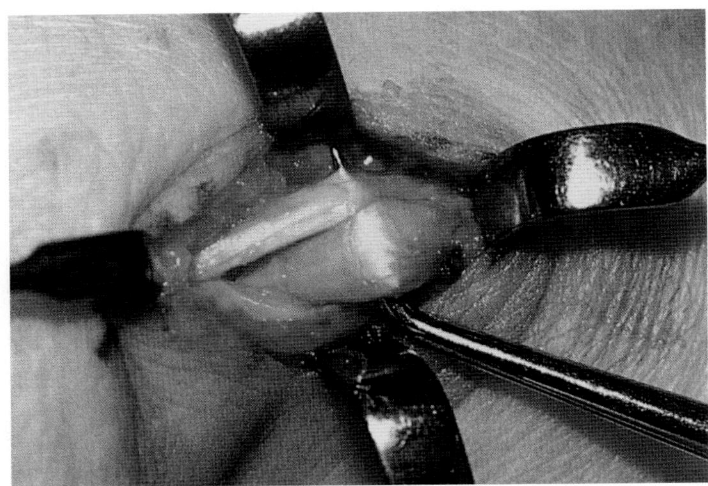

FIGURE 63–10. Complete release (proximal and distal) of the tendons during testing with blunt retraction.

5. With a 64 Beaver blade, the sheath overlying the APL and the EPB is incised in a longitudinal fashion. This is done at the dorsal margin to prevent the complication of palmar subluxation of the tendons with wrist flexion. The first dorsal compartment is inspected for multiple slips of the abductor pollicis longus and for septum that separates the APL from the EPB.
6. A Ragnell retractor is used to pull the tendons out of the first dorsal compartment as dissection is continued proximally and distally for complete release (Fig. 63–10). The APL is identified, and the EPB is pulled so that its response as a first metacarpal extender can be noted. The tendons are placed back into the sheath, and a small piece of the dorsal retinaculum is excised. A routine subcuticular closure is performed.
7. A bulky short-arm thumb spica hand dressing with a plaster splint is placed and the tourniquet is let down so that adequate circulation to all digits can be evaluated.

Note: We do not recommend the use of scissors and blind pushing to cut the retinaculum for fear of transection of the superficial branch of the radial nerve. All surgery is performed under direct observation.

POSTOPERATIVE MANAGEMENT

The patient comes back 14 days following surgery, and the bulky short-arm thumb spica dressing is removed. The wound is inspected and appropriate care is given. The patient is then given a custom thumb spica splint, which is worn for an additional 2 weeks. At 4 weeks, the patient is sent to a supervised hand therapy program to begin range-of-motion exercises. When range of motion is deemed full (at approximately 6 weeks), strengthening is begun. The patient is instructed to avoid lifting anything heavier than 5 pounds for 6 weeks. Full use of the hand is often regained at 3 months, although generalized soreness can be present for up to 6 months after surgery.

COMPLICATIONS

Complications of surgical decompression include injury to the superficial radial nerve, volar tendon subluxation, hypertrophic scarring, tendinous adhesions, and persistence of symptoms caused by inadequate decompression.

REFERENCES

Gelberman RH: Surgical management of DeQuervain disease. In Gelberman RH (ed): The Wrist, 2nd ed. Philadelphia, Lippincott, Williams and Wilkins, 2002, pp 383–392.

Green DP, Hotchkiss RN, Pederson WC (eds): Green's Operative Hand Surgery, 4th ed. New York, Churchill-Livingstone, 1999, pp 2034–2037.

Plancher KD, Peterson RK, Steichen JB: Compressive neuropathies and tendinopathies in the athletic elbow and wrist. Clin Sports Med 15:331–371, 1996.

CHAPTER 64

Treatment of Intersection Syndrome

INTRODUCTION

Athletes with intersection syndrome have pain in the dorsal radial wrist approximately 4 to 6 cm proximal to Lister's tubercle (Fig. 64–1). This syndrome is reported to occur in weight lifters, rowers, canoeists, and recreational tennis enthusiasts, all of whom are exposed to repetitive wrist motion and trauma. Swelling, tenderness, and crepitus found in this region are pathognomonic for intersection syndrome, which occurs where the abductor pollicis longus (APL) and the extensor pollicis brevis (EPB) cross over the wrist extensors (the extensor carpi radialis longus [ECRL] and the extensor carpi radialis brevis [ECRB]). This condition is called *squeakers* by many sports enthusiasts.

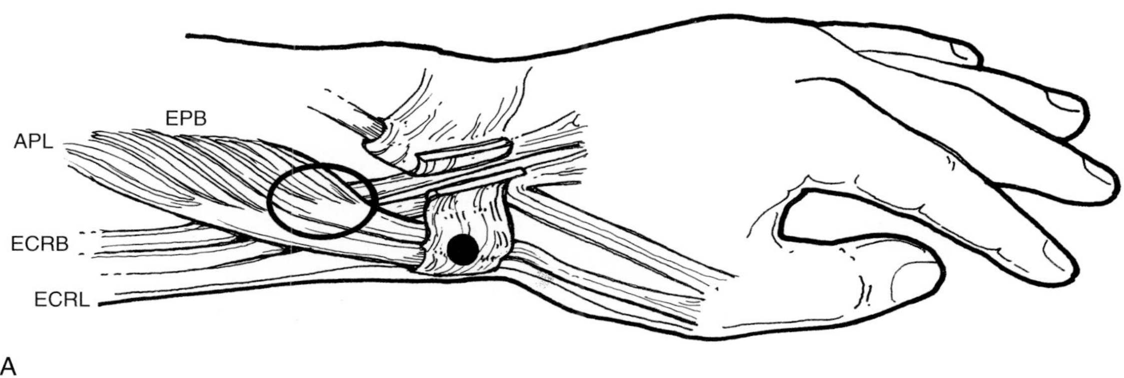

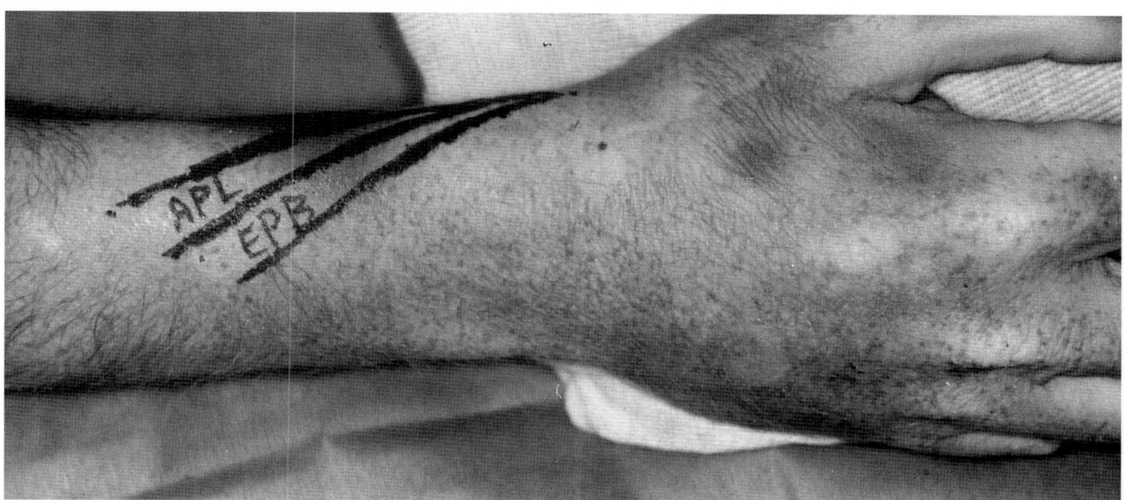

FIGURE 64–1. *A*, Intersection syndrome at a point 4 to 6 cm proximal to the wrist joint. APL, abductor pollicis longus; ECRB, extensor carpi radialis brevis; ECRL, extensor carpi radialis longus; EPB, extensor pollicis brevis. *B*, Cadaveric picture of the location of intersection syndrome.

DIAGNOSTIC IMAGING

Plain x-rays are not helpful in the diagnosis of this clinical condition. They can be used, however, to rule out any type of mass or serious bony abnormality of the forearm. The use of MRI is also unnecessary unless one suspects some type of tumor-related condition.

NONOPERATIVE MANAGEMENT

Initial treatment includes rest, splinting, activity modification, anti-inflammatory medications, and a corticosteroid injection (Fig. 64–2). A custom thermoplastic molded volar wrist splint with 10° to 20° of wrist extension is worn by the patient over 3 weeks for 24 hours a day. The patient is then weaned off the splint over the following 3 weeks. Conservative treatment is successful 95% of the time.

RELEVANT ANATOMY

Intersection syndrome, as stated earlier, involves pain in the dorsal radial wrist where the APL and the EPB cross. This occurs approximately 4 to 6 cm proximal to Lister's tubercle over the wrist extensors, ECRL and ECRB (Fig. 64–3).

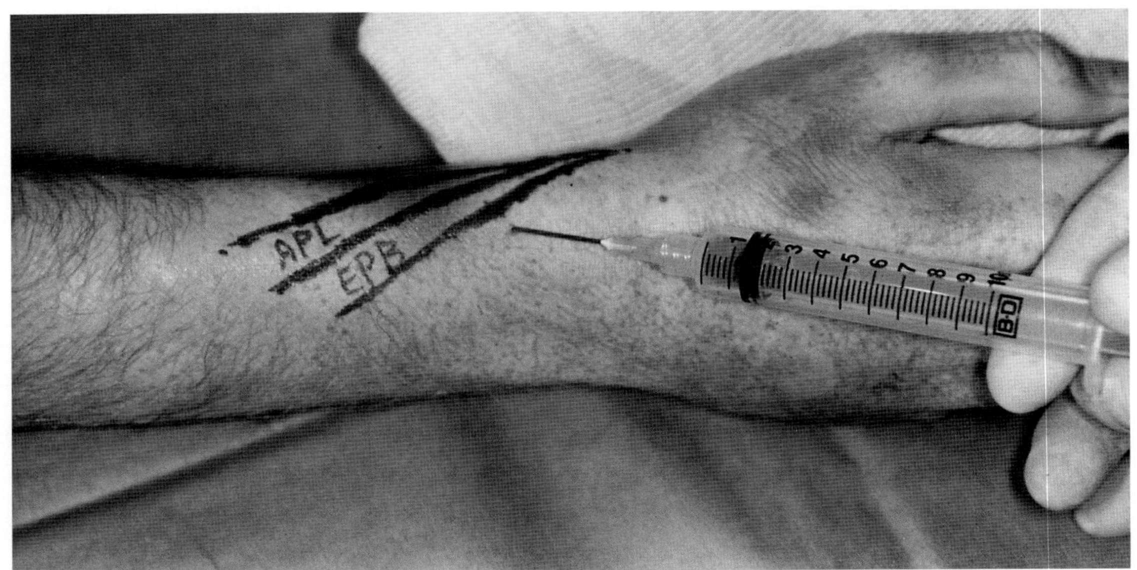

FIGURE 64–2. Injection technique for intersection syndrome. Note the location and angle of the needle. APL, abductor pollicis longus; EPB, extensor pollicis brevis.

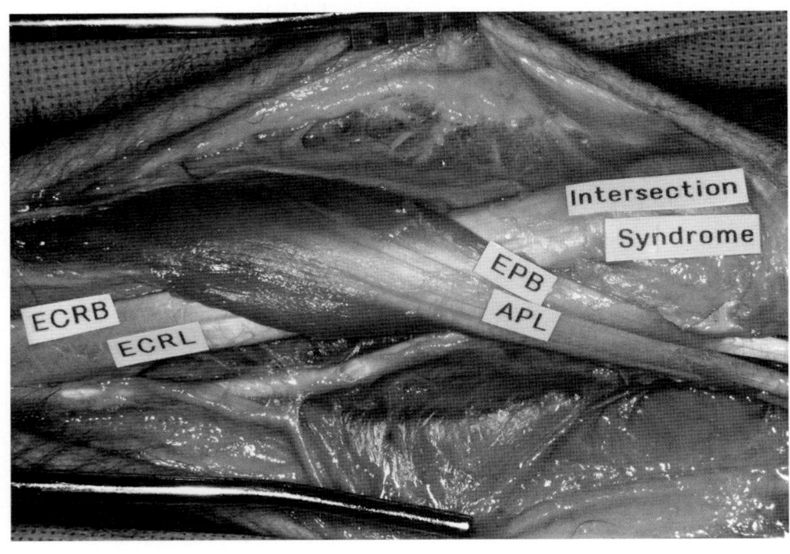

FIGURE 64–3. Detailed anatomy of intersection syndrome, demonstrating the crossing of the abductor pollicis longus (APL) and the extensor pollicis brevis (EPB) over the extensor carpi radialis longus (ECRL) and the extensor carpi radialis brevis (ECRB).

SURGICAL TECHNIQUE

Indications

Surgical treatment for resistant cases consists of release and tenosynovectomy of the second dorsal compartment, exploration of the intersection zone with débridement of any inflammatory or bursal tissue, and release of the fascial sheaths of the APL and the EPB. Conservative treatment is almost always successful, and surgical intervention should not be considered unless symptoms are refractory to splinting.

Technique

1. Positioning: The patient is positioned supine on the operating room table with a hand table placed alongside. A tourniquet cuff is placed on the upper arm, and suitable anesthesia is administered with a local field block with 10 mL 1% lidocaine. (A Bier block or axillary block may be performed according to the surgeon's choice.)
2. Incision: A longitudinal incision is marked out slightly proximal to the wrist extensors, 4 cm over the radial wrist ECRL and extending to the proximal swollen area.
3. The arm is wrapped with an Esmarch bandage, and the tourniquet is inflated. The skin is incised with a No. 15 blade scalpel, and subcutaneous dissection is carried out with Littler or similar blunt-tipped scissors, directly down to the level of the extensor retinaculum.
4. Incision of the deep fascia is performed and meticulous hemostasis maintained with a bipolar cautery. Release of the second dorsal compartment and débridement of the synovitis are performed.
5. A small piece of synovium is sent to the pathology department to investigate acute or chronic synovitis, and the intersection of the two tendons is released.
6. After subcuticular closure, a bulky short-arm thumb spica hand dressing with a plaster splint is placed. The tourniquet is let down so the health care professional can check for adequate circulation to all digits.

POSTOPERATIVE MANAGEMENT

The patient returns to the office 14 days following surgery, and the bulky short-arm thumb spica dressing is removed. The wound is inspected and appropriate care is given. The patient is then given a custom thumb spica splint, which is worn for an additional 2 weeks. At 4 weeks, the patient is sent to a supervised hand therapy program to begin range-of-motion exercises; when range of motion is deemed full, strengthening is begun. The patient is instructed to avoid lifting anything heavier than 5 pounds for 6 weeks. Full use of the hand is often seen at 3 months, although generalized soreness may be noted for up to 6 months after surgery.

COMPLICATIONS

Surgery is rare for this condition; therefore, complications are also rare. It is essential that the surgeon recognize the superficial radial nerve as it crosses in the wound so that nerve injuries of every type can be avoided.

REFERENCES

Green DP, Hotchkiss RN, Pederson WC: Green's Operative Hand Surgery, 4th ed. New York, Churchill-Livingstone, 1999, pp 2038–2040.

Peimer CA: Surgery of the Hand and Upper Extremity. New York, McGraw-Hill, 1996, p 841.

CHAPTER 65

Treatment of Carpal Tunnel Syndrome

INTRODUCTION

Carpal tunnel syndrome is the most common type of compressive neuropathy, although it is seen infrequently in the athletic population. Carpal tunnel syndrome is compression of the median nerve in the osteofibrous canal, created by the transverse carpal ligament superiorly and the carpal bones palmarly, radially, and ulnarly (Figs. 65–1 and 65–2). Carpal tunnel syndrome may be caused by direct trauma, repetitive use, or anatomic anomalies.

Sporting activities that predispose athletes to carpal tunnel syndrome include those that involve repetitive or continuous extension/flexion of the wrist, as seen in lacrosse, cycling, throwing sports, racquet sports, archery, gymnastics, and wheelchair athletics. These grip-intensive activities are known to aggravate this condition. Hypertrophy of lumbrical muscle, which is often seen in weight lifters, can also predispose one to carpal tunnel syndrome. Flexor tenosynovitis and anatomic anomalies, such as the palmaris longus placed within the carpal canal, or palmaris profundus, hypertrophic flexor digitorum superficialis (FDS), accessory lumbricalis, and a persistent median artery, can all cause carpal tunnel syndrome.

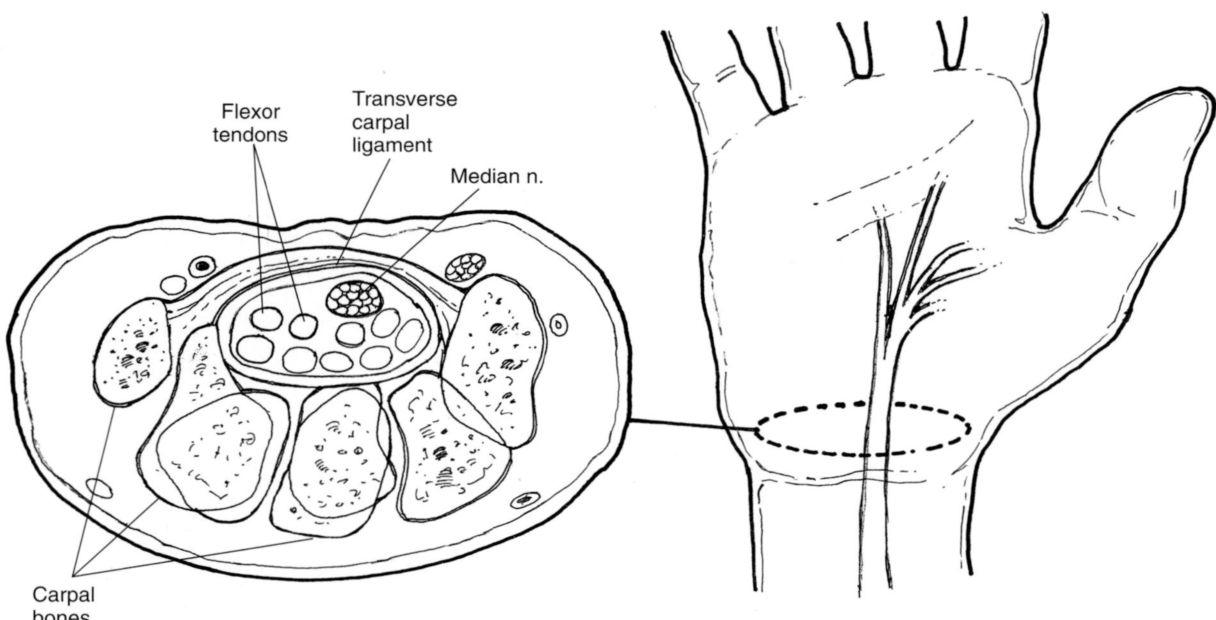

FIGURE 65–1. Drawing of cross-sectional anatomy of the carpal tunnel.

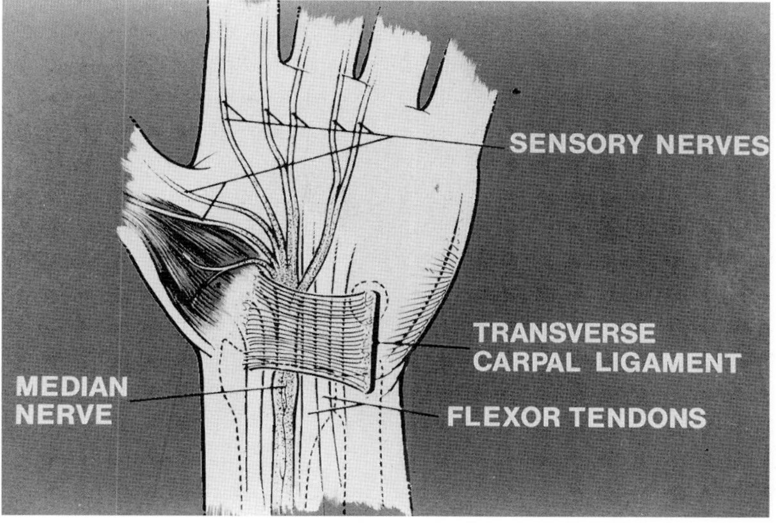

A

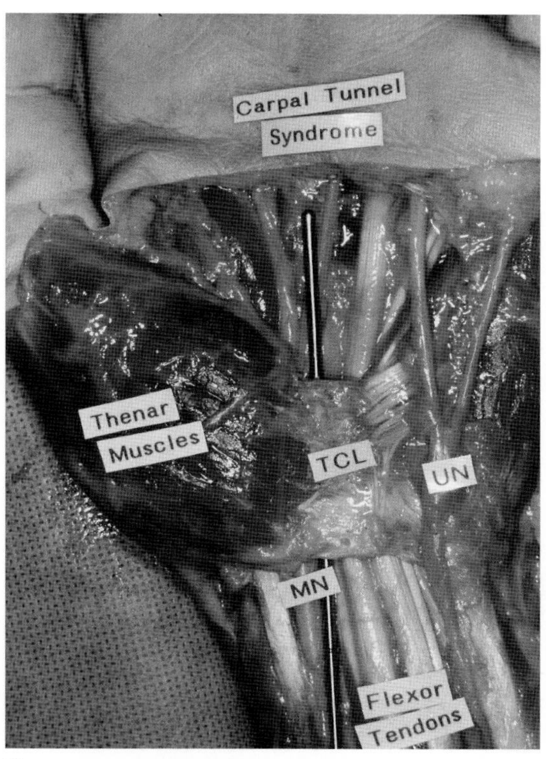

B

FIGURE 65–2. *A*, Drawing of the volar view of the carpal tunnel and its contents. *B*, Cadaveric specimen demonstrating the carpal tunnel and its contents. MN, median nerve; TCL, transverse carpal ligament; UN, ulnar nerve.

HISTORY AND PHYSICAL EXAMINATION

Patients with carpal tunnel syndrome classically have symptoms of pain and paresthesias, especially at night, in the radial 3½ digits. Athletes frequently complain of clumsiness and weakness when grip-related activities are performed.

Phalen's test on physical examination (Fig. 65–3*A* and *B*) (more sensitive) and Tinel's test (more specific) are invariably positive. Measured grip and pinch strengths are often asymmetrical except in the frequently occurring bilateral carpal tunnel syndrome. The diagnosis relies on the exclusion of more proximal lesions of nerve compression, such as thoracic outlet syndrome, pronator syndrome, and even cervical radiculopathy. Atrophy and weakness of the abductor pollicis brevis with flattening of the palmar arch are also helpful physical examination findings (Fig. 65–3*C*). Shoulder pain and upper arm pain are not uncommon and can present in 40% of patients.

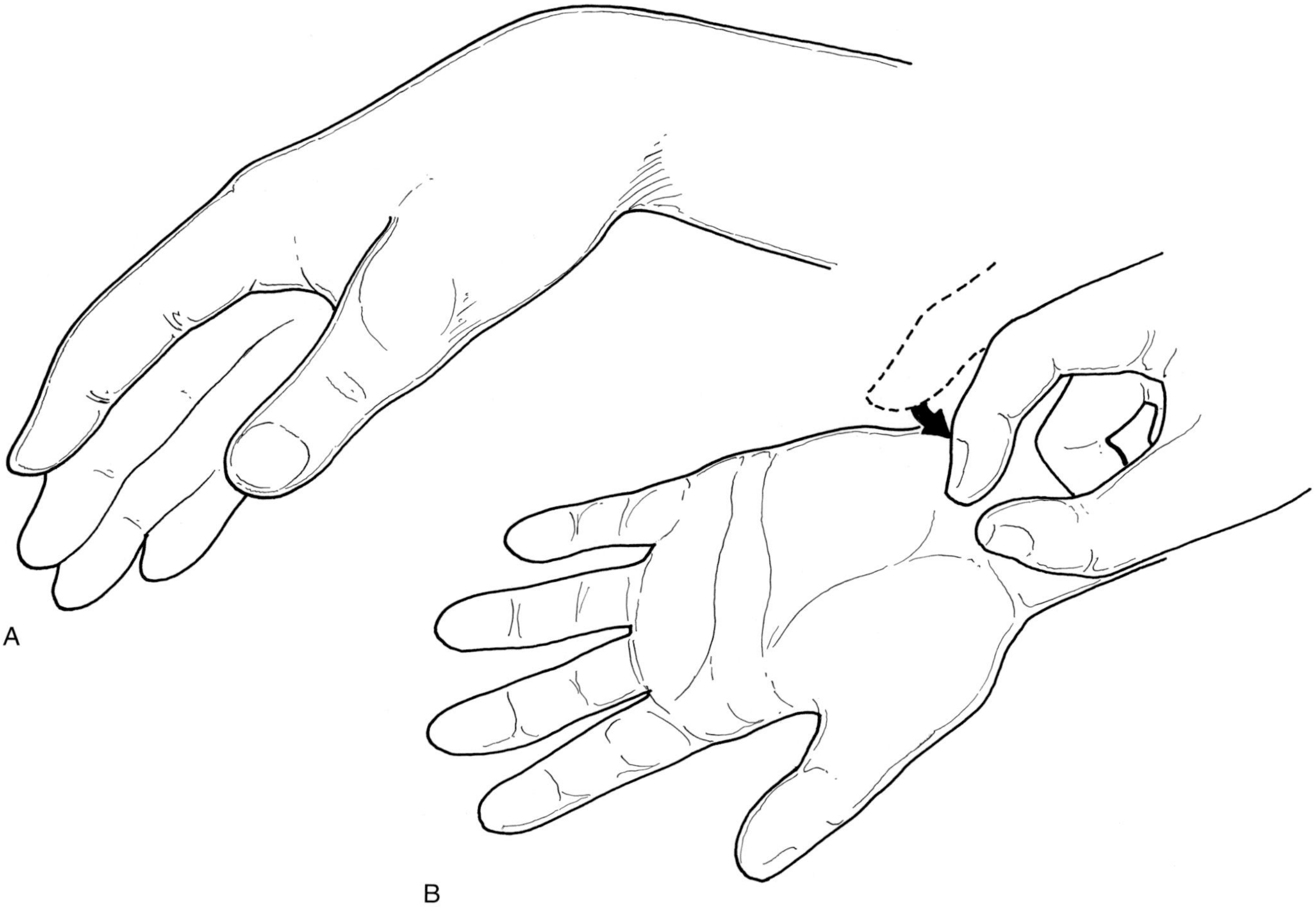

A

B

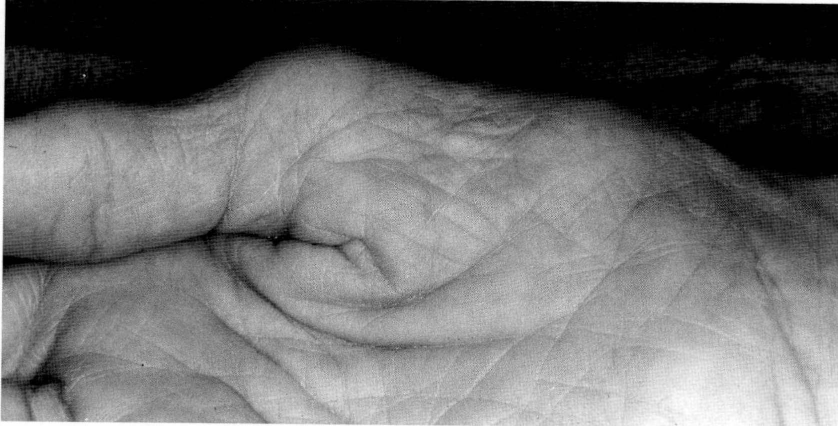

C

FIGURE 65–3. *A*, Diagram of Phalen's test. *B*, Diagram of Tinel's test. *C*, Clinical picture of thenar atrophy.

DIAGNOSTIC IMAGING AND SUPPLEMENTARY TESTING

Plain x-rays often are not helpful in the diagnosis of carpal tunnel syndrome. X-rays such as the carpal tunnel view may exclude masses in the canal as a source of the problem.

Electrodiagnostic studies often demonstrate conduction delays across the wrist and, although highly technician dependent, can still give good objective confirmation of the location and severity of median nerve compression. A distal sensory latency greater than 3.5 mm/sec, or asymmetry of conduction velocity compared with the contralateral side greater than 0.5 mm/sec, is the most consistent early electrodiagnostic finding. Abnormal values with distal motor latency greater than 4.5 mm/sec, or conduction velocity asymmetry of greater than 1.0 mm/sec, are also helpful hints for the clinician in determining the diagnosis of carpal tunnel syndrome.

Differential diagnosis of systemic disorders, such as diabetes mellitus, hypothyroidism, rheumatoid arthritis, gout, and peripheral neuropathy from underlying metabolic causes, must always be excluded. When these diagnoses are suspected, patients should be tested for a fasting blood sugar, thyroid function, rheumatoid factor and antinuclear antibody levels, sedimentation rates, uric acid levels, and red blood cell counts.

NONOPERATIVE MANAGEMENT

High-risk athletes may use padding over the heel of the hand along with protective gloves, which may lessen or alleviate carpal tunnel syndrome. The changing of hand and wrist positions with rest (at least 5 minutes every half-hour to hour) is important. Sports-specific hints for this type of athlete include the use of forearm guards, or lighter bows for archers.

Conservative treatment consists of nonsteroidal anti-inflammatory medications, custom wrist splinting by hand therapists to place the wrist in a neutral position, and activity modification. The use of off-the-shelf splints is often not helpful because one size often fits none. Recent studies have shown that the pressure inside the carpal tunnel is elevated in extremes of flexion/extension.

Corticosteroids in carpal tunnel injections may offer temporary relief in up to 85% of patients, but the lasting effect in all age groups with carpal tunnel syndrome after 1 year is approximately 20% to 24% (Fig. 65–4).

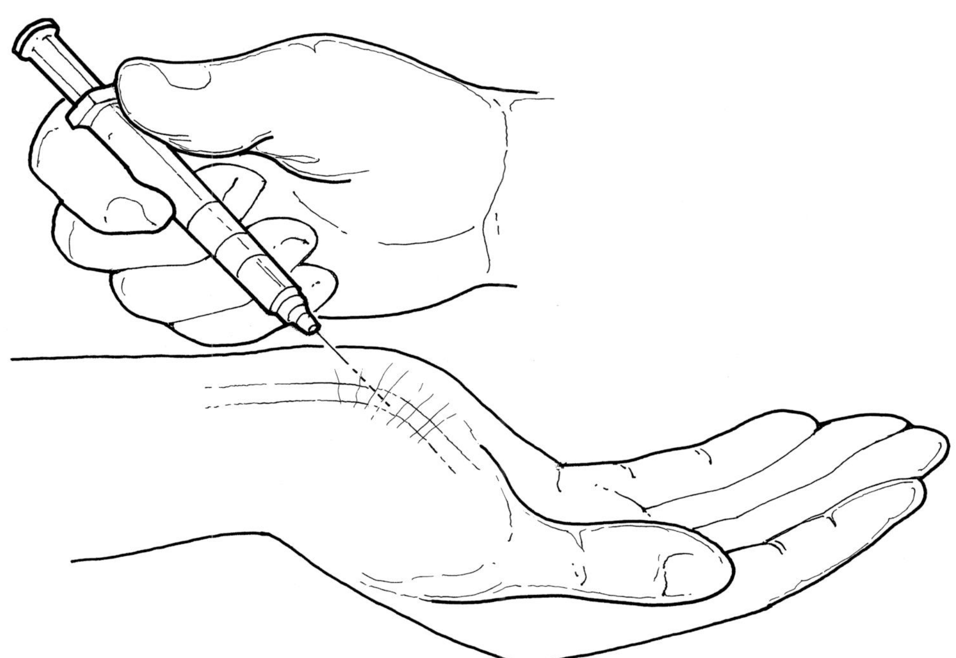

FIGURE 65–4. Injection technique of the carpal tunnel.

RELEVANT ANATOMY AND PERILS AND PITFALLS OF SURGERY

The transverse carpal ligament is a thick, fibrous band that covers the concave surfaces of the carpal bones. The radial side is attached to the tuberosity of the scaphoid and a portion of the trapezium. On the ulnar aspect, it is attached to the pisiform and hook of the hamate. It is through this tunnel that the long flexor tendons and the median nerve pass. The median nerve lies superficially to the tendons, but it is the variation of the motor branch of the median nerve that must be protected during surgical procedures so that complications can be avoided (Fig. 65–5).

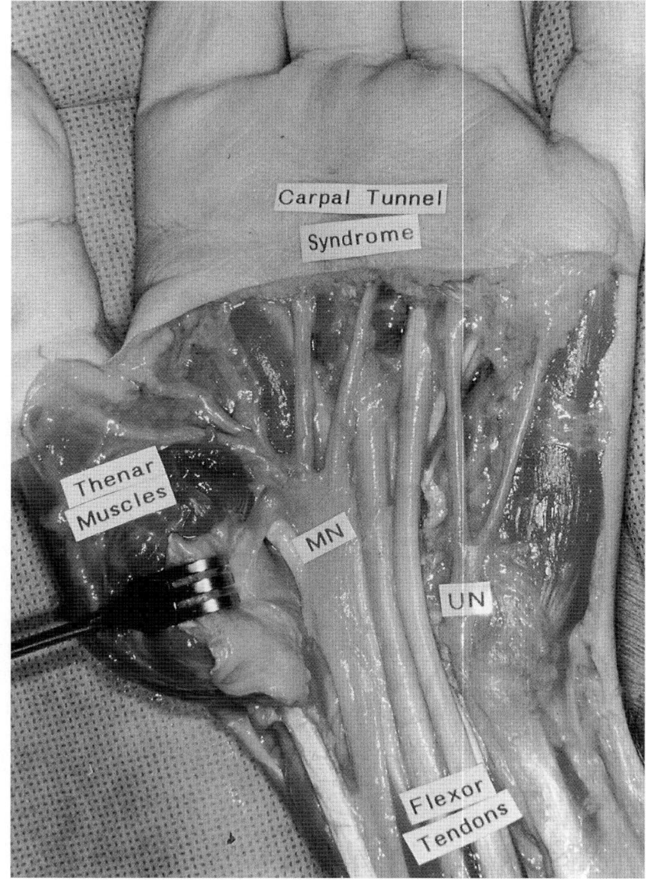

FIGURE 65–5. Cadaveric specimen with the transverse carpal ligament removed, demonstrating these structures passing beneath the transverse carpal ligament. MN, median nerve; UN, ulnar nerve.

Lanz from Germany classified the anatomic variations of the motor branch to the thenars (Fig. 65–6) into four types.

1. The most common pattern of the motor branch of the median nerve is the extraligamentous or recurrent branch. This occurs in at least 50% to 65% of patients.
2. The next most common type of motor median nerve is the subligamentous branch, in which the recurrent median nerve divides from the median nerve directly underneath the transverse carpal ligament and lies close to the main trunk of the median nerve. This type occurs in approximately 30% of patients.
3. The third most common course of the motor branch median nerve is transligamentous. In this variation, the motor branch divides from the common median nerve beneath the transverse carpal ligament and, during its course to the thenars, pierces the transverse carpal ligament somewhere between 2 and 6 mm from the distal border. Some authors believe this occurs quite frequently; others feel this is extremely rare. However, care should be taken, especially when an endoscopic carpal tunnel release or a limited open carpal tunnel release is performed.
4. The last two types of motor thenar branch variation include a branch from the ulnar border of the median nerve and a branch lying on top of the transverse carpal ligament; both are extremely rare.

The palmar cutaneous branch of the median nerve arises from the median nerve in the distal third of the forearm. This branch passes parallel to the median nerve, piercing the antebrachial fascia of the volar carpal ligament or even the transverse carpal ligament of the wrist before dividing into the medial and lateral branches of the base of the palm. This nerve and its placement on the radial side of the wrist have taught most surgeons to make their incisions ulnar to the midpoint of the wrist, or in line with the radial side of the ring finger.

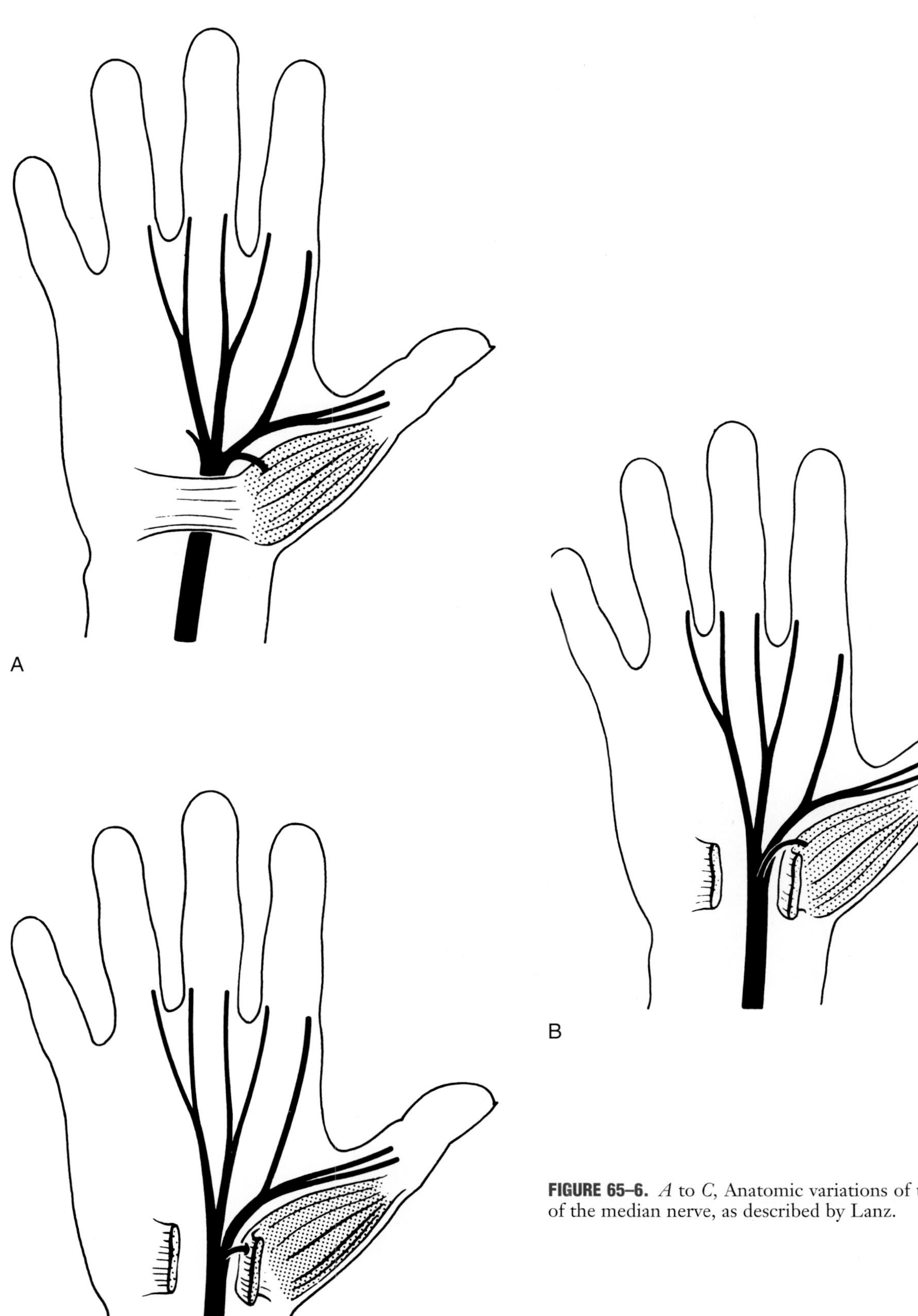

FIGURE 65–6. *A* to *C*, Anatomic variations of the motor branch of the median nerve, as described by Lanz.

SURGICAL TECHNIQUES

Indications

Numerous types of carpal tunnel release procedures can be performed. In the following section, three types are discussed—a limited open carpal tunnel release, a single-portal Agee endoscopic carpal tunnel release, and the classic open carpal tunnel release.

Surgical intervention for carpal tunnel syndrome should proceed only after conservative treatment has failed, as evidenced by electrodiagnostic studies that show moderate to severe crippling of the median nerve. Endoscopic carpal tunnel release was popularized as a less invasive method so that postoperative disability could be limited. The palmar aponeurosis in this technique is not split. Decreased scar tenderness, recovery of strength, and early return to activities of daily living and sporting activities are promoted by surgeons who use endoscopic carpal tunnel release. The limited open carpal tunnel release was introduced to decrease the perception of complications and the steep learning curve associated with the endoscopic carpal tunnel release technique, while still providing the benefits of the endoscopic carpal tunnel release technique.

Conversion to an open release is always necessary if there is resistance to blade insertion or if there is poor visualization of the transverse carpal ligament. The patient is always told of this event in all preoperative discussions.

Techniques

Limited Open Carpal Tunnel Release

1. Positioning: The patient is placed on the operating room table with the hand table adjacent. Local anesthetic (10 mL 1% lidocaine) is injected slightly ulnar to the palmaris longus in a routine carpal tunnel injection (Fig. 65–7).
2. After suitable anesthesia has been administered, the arm is wrapped with an Esmarch wrap and the tourniquet cuff inflated to 250 mm Hg. An interthenar incision is made with the use of landmarks, as illustrated in Figure 65–8. (The thenars are identified with the thumb abducted.) The thenars meet the interthenar crease in a curvilinear fashion. This marks the distal aspect of the incision; the incision is made 1.5 to 2 cm proximal to this. The incision is verified as being in line with either the ulnar side of the long finger or the radial side of the ring finger.

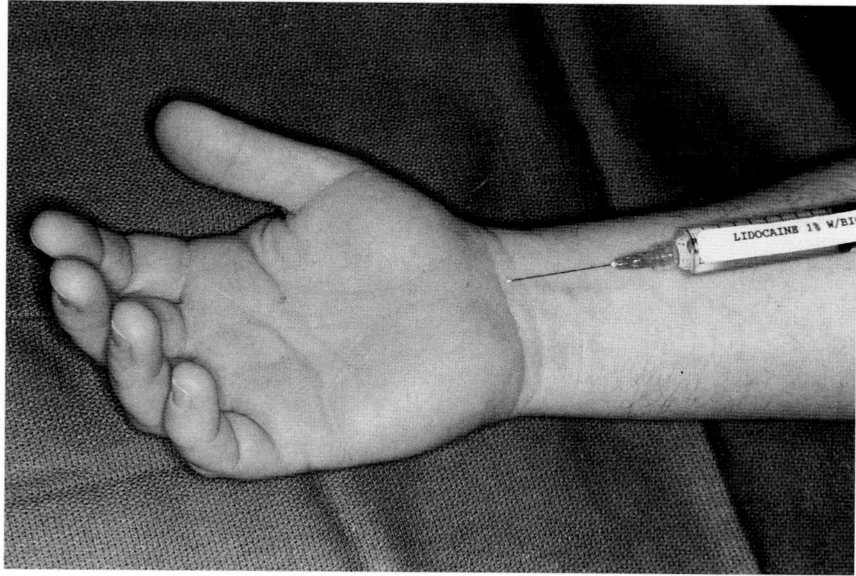

FIGURE 65–7. Local anesthetic injection of the carpal tunnel slightly ulnar to the palmaris longus.

3. With the use of a bipolar cautery, dissection is carried down through the subcutaneous tissue with meticulous hemostasis. The superficial palmar fascia is then split in a longitudinal fashion with a 64 Beaver blade.
4. A Holzheimer-type retractor is placed deep to the depths of the wound, and the transverse carpal ligament is identified. A Freer elevator is used to dissect any insertion of the abductors off the transverse carpal ligament.
5. The Holzheimer retractor is positioned in a distal fashion so that the distal aspect of the tranverse carpal ligament can be identified. Once clearly visualized, it is incised and protected with a Freer elevator. The use of Littler or blunt-tipped scissors is helpful in identifying the superficial palmar arch and the most distal aspect of the transverse carpal ligament.
6. With the Freer protecting the contents of the carpal canal and with allowance for any anatomic variance in the motor branch of the median nerve to the thenars, the Beaver blade is used to continue to separate the transverse carpal ligament into its radial and ulnar halves.
7. The Holzheimer retractor is removed then and placed proximally. The wrist is hyperextended and in neutral alignment. With the wrist hyperextended for maximum safety to the median nerve, the three instruments are used in sequential order.
8. With these instruments removed, the median nerve protector is placed; the Strickland carpal tunnel tome (Fig. 65–9) is placed in the depths of the wound under direct visualization to push gently with the wrist hyperextended through the antebrachial fascia and the transverse carpal ligament (see Fig. 65–9*A* to *E*).
9. All equipment is removed. Two Ragnell retractors are placed so that the motor branch, along with the confines of the carpal tunnel, can be identified again, and the wound is irrigated.
10. Horizontal mattress sutures (4–0 or 5–0 nylon) are placed to reapproximate the wound edges. A soft tissue dressing is placed without a splint. Tendon gliding exercises are explained to the patient in the operating room while the tourniquet is let down to demonstrate good capillary refill to all digits.

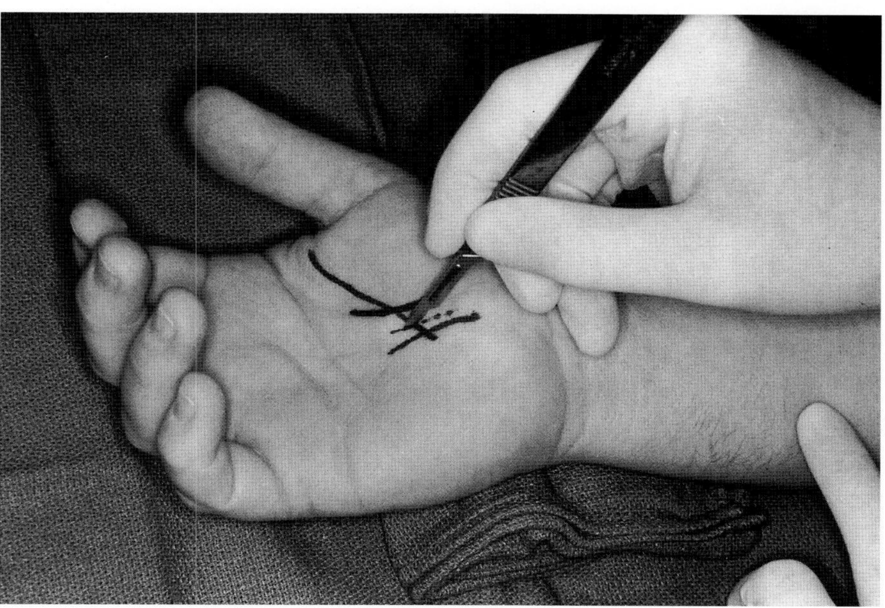

FIGURE 65–8. Incision used for the limited open technique.

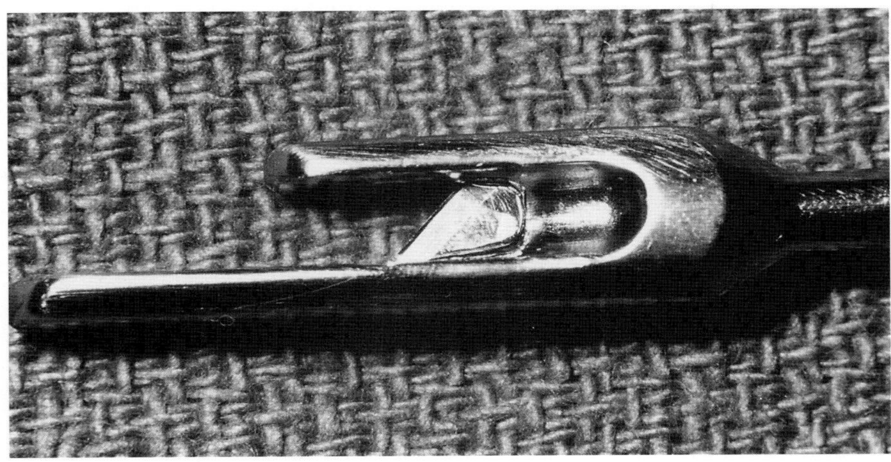
A

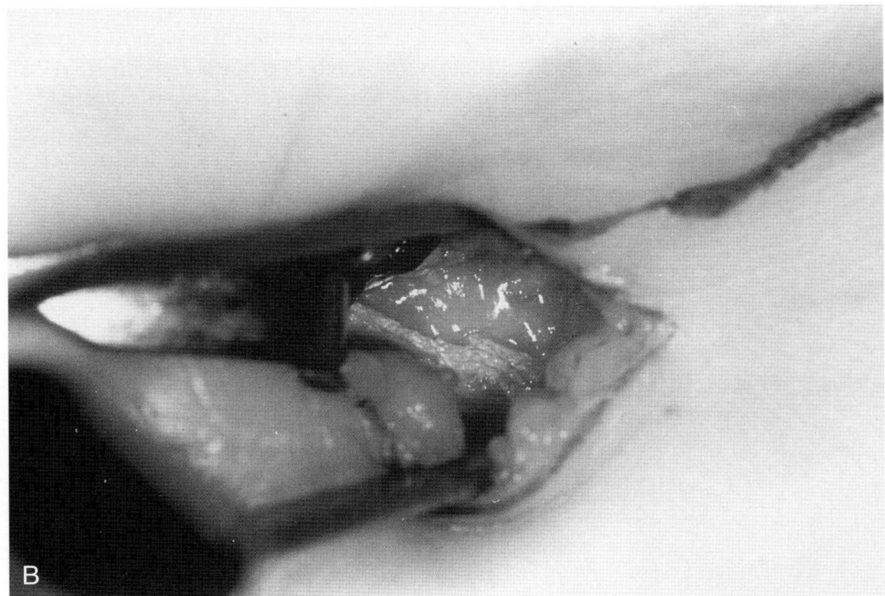
B

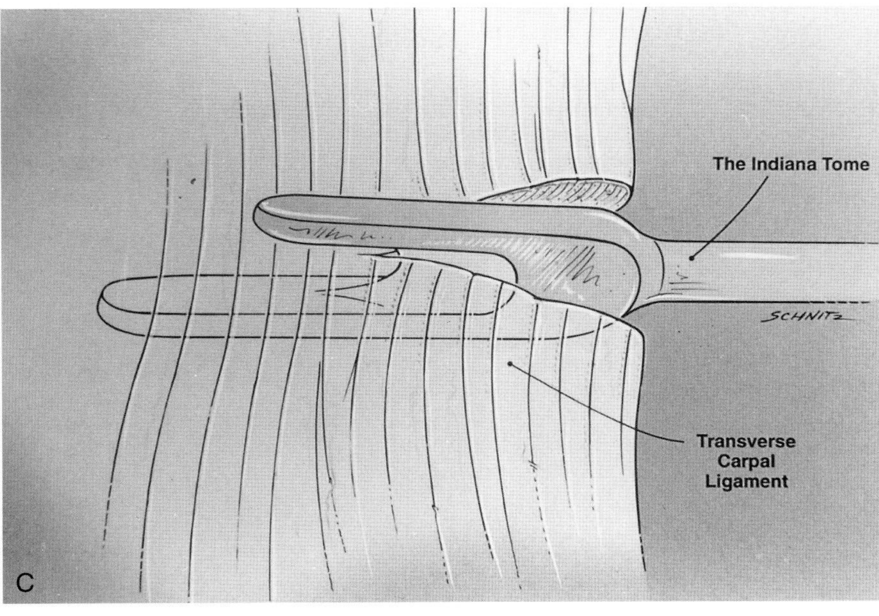

C

FIGURE 65–9. Limited open technique. *A*, Close-up of the Indiana tome blade. *B*, Exposure of the fat pad at the distal end of the transverse carpal ligament. *C*, Indiana tome blade with the transverse carpal ligament between the upper and lower skids. (*C* from Lee WPA, Plancher KD, Strickland JW: Carpal tunnel release with a small palmar incision. Hand Clin 12:276, 1996.)

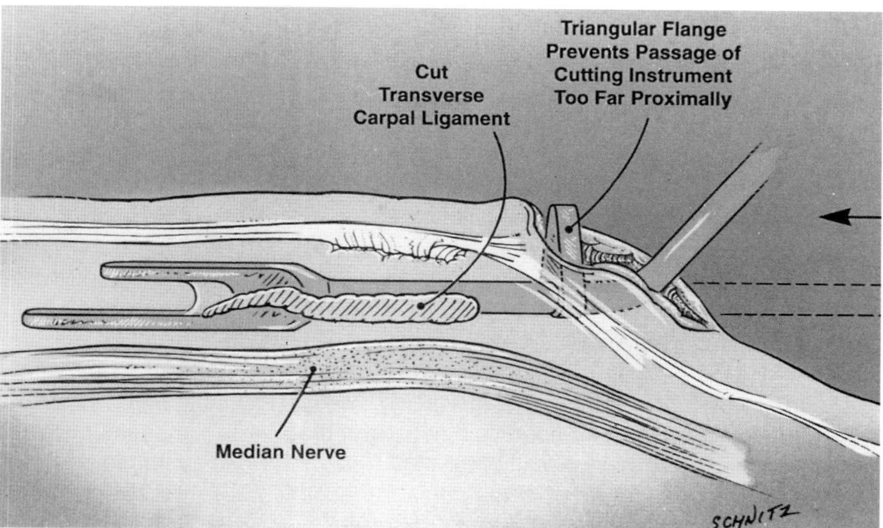

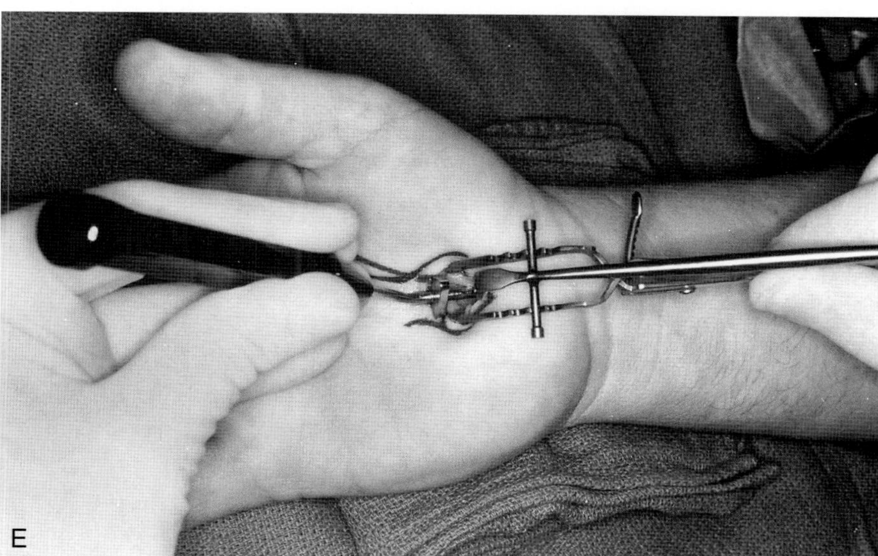

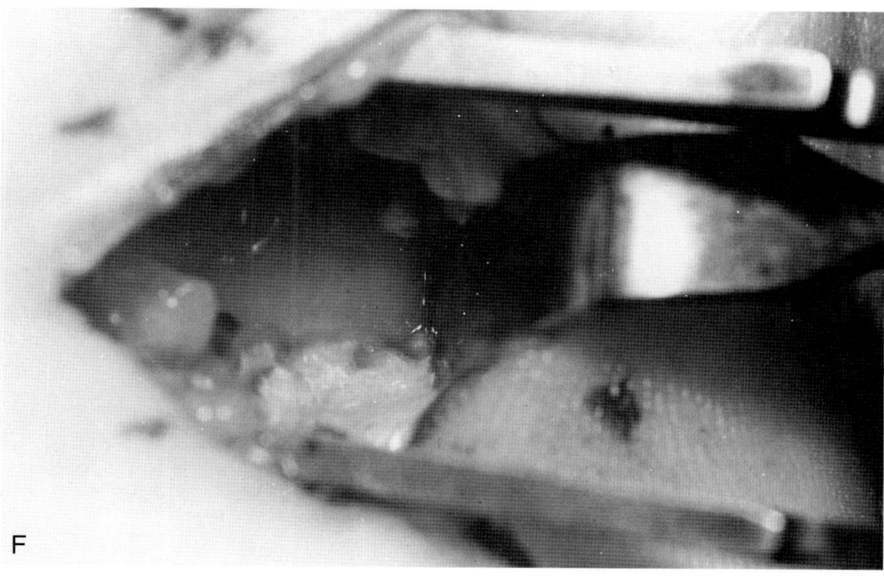

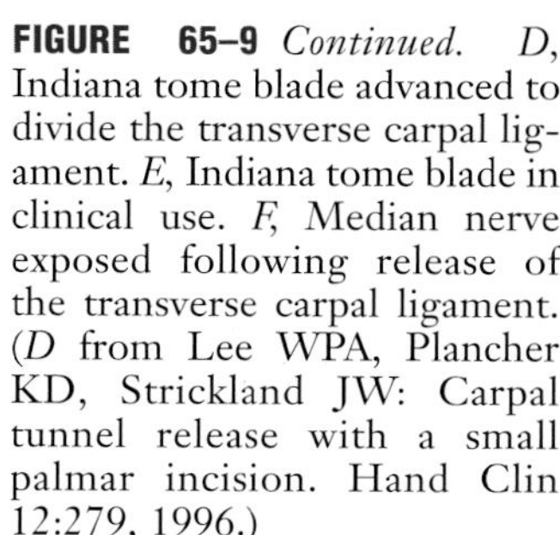
FIGURE 65–9 *Continued. D,* Indiana tome blade advanced to divide the transverse carpal ligament. *E,* Indiana tome blade in clinical use. *F,* Median nerve exposed following release of the transverse carpal ligament. (*D* from Lee WPA, Plancher KD, Strickland JW: Carpal tunnel release with a small palmar incision. Hand Clin 12:279, 1996.)

Single-Portal Agee Endoscopic Carpal Tunnel Release

1. Positioning: The patient is positioned on the operating room table with the hand placed on the hand table. General or axillary block anesthesia is recommended for this technique. Those physicians who have mastered this technique may use 10 mL 1% lidocaine injected subcutaneously across the wrist flexor crease. Care should be taken to avoid injecting fluid directly into the carpal canal, which will block adequate visualization.
2. A 1.5- to 2-cm transverse incision is made just ulnar to the palmaris longus, and subcutaneous tissues are spread bluntly to the antebrachial fascia (Fig. 65–10).
3. A 1-cm distally based U-shaped flap is made in the fascia and to the carpal tunnel (Fig. 65–11). The synovium is then removed from the dorsal surface of the transverse carpal ligament with the synovial elevator, as provided in the set. This ensures adequate visualization of the distal margin of the transverse fibers of the transverse carpal ligament.
4. This step establishes the initial path that should be in line with the ring finger access. The small hamate pathfinder is placed down the canal just radial to the hook of the hamate. Then the surgeon defines the distal edge of the transverse carpal ligament, which feels much like a washboard when this device is used.
5. The Agee carpal tunnel release system is introduced in line with the ring finger access, and observation is done with the television camera to make sure that no intervening vital structures are in view and that the distal transverse carpal ligament is well defined. The actual hand instruments must be held so that the distal aspect or cutting blade is in line with the ring finger, no matter where the proximal portion of the device is held. When the device is held in line with the forearm, the distal aspect of the device is in line with the ring finger, which limits any complications (Fig. 65–12).
6. The clinician elevates the blade and releases the transverse carpal ligament from distal to proximal by applying an upward pressure against the ligament in direct contact with the hook of the hamate and withdrawing the device. The blade is then retracted and the device is reinserted to allow the clinician to check for adequacy of release.

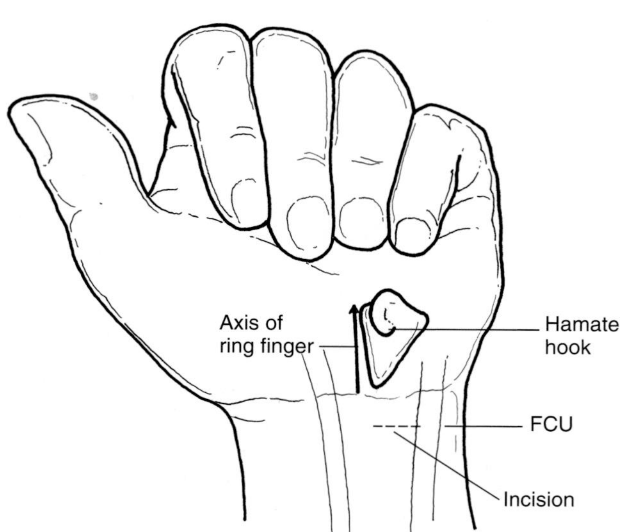

FIGURE 65–10. Incision uses for endoscopic carpal tunnel release with Agee technique.

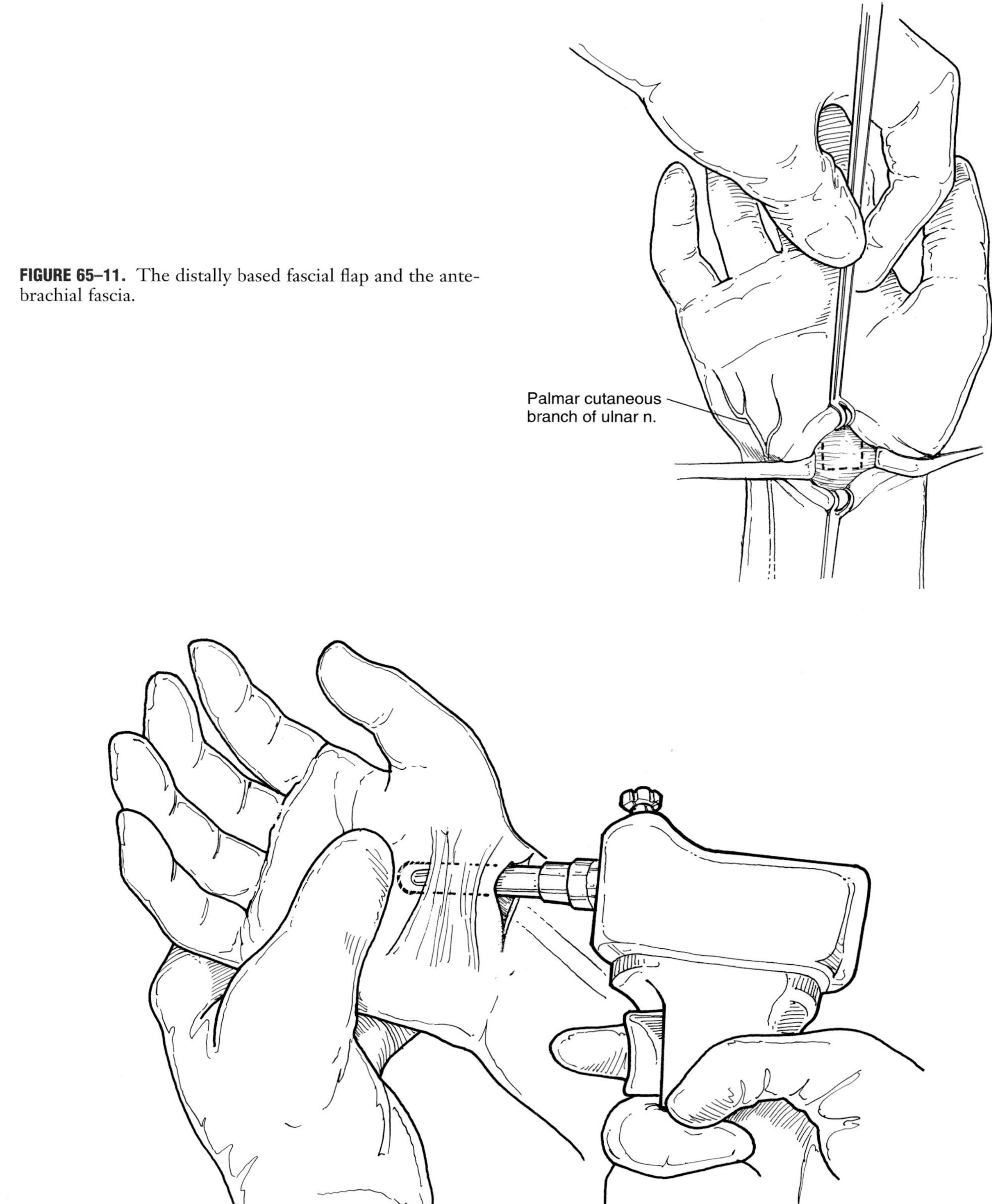

FIGURE 65–11. The distally based fascial flap and the antebrachial fascia.

FIGURE 65–12. Placement of the Agee carpal tunnel release system.

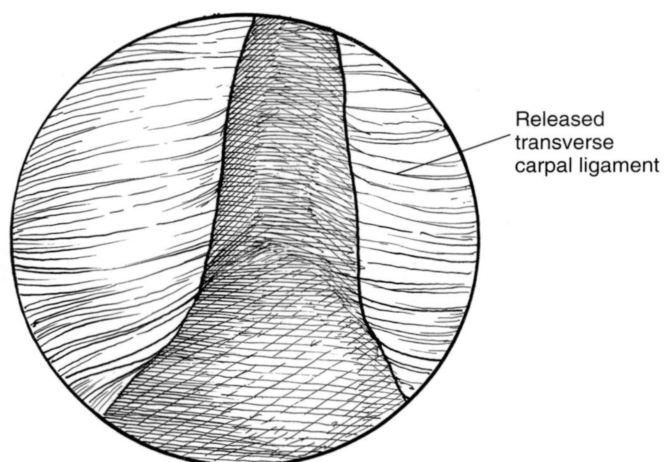

FIGURE 65–13. Complete release at the transverse carpal ligament as evidenced by visualization of the distal fat pad.

7. At times, a second pass must be performed to transect the remaining distal fibers. When complete release has been obtained through the transverse carpal ligament, a small amount of distal fat pad (which marks the distal margin of the transverse carpal ligament) can be seen coming into the field of view (Fig. 65–13).
8. A sharp or blunt-tipped scissors is then used to move proximally from this open wound and to bisect the antebrachial fascia subcutaneously for 1 to 2 cm under direct vision. The incision is closed with a subcuticular suture.
9. A light dressing is placed, and the patient is encouraged to perform activities of daily living immediately but to avoid heavy gripping, pushing, pulling, or lifting more than 5 pounds for approximately 2 to 3 weeks.

Classic Open Carpal Tunnel Release

1. Incision: The classic open carpal tunnel release is performed with an incision that ends proximally at the wrist flexor crease and is drawn in line with the radial side of the ring finger. However, any patient who has been worked up preoperatively for investigation of suspected space-occupying lesions or tenosynovectomy, or for exploration for any other anatomic anomalies, should have a conventional incision that extends proximal to the wrist crease (Fig. 65–14). Both incisions are made ulnar and parallel to the thenar crease and distal to the wrist so as to protect the motor branch arising from the radial palmar portion of the median nerve, as well as the palmar cutaneous branch passing between the flexor carpi radialis and the palmaris longus tendons.
2. Exposure: The arm is elevated and exsanguinated with the Esmarch, and the tourniquet is inflated to 250 mm Hg. An incision is made through the subcutaneous tissue to divide the superficial palmar fascia in line with its fibers. Meticulous hemostasis is obtained with a bipolar cautery.
3. The transverse carpal ligament is identified, the most distal aspect with blunt dissecting scissors and the use of a Freer elevator or equivalent device. The contents of the canal are protected as the midportion of the ligament is incised. The transverse carpal ligament is incised distally up to the fat, which marks its distal aspect as well as the superficial palmar arch. Proximally, the release is performed all the way to the wrist crease. Inspection of the carpal canal is performed with the confines of the carpal tunnel open. The median nerve is then inspected (Fig. 65–15).
4. A tenotomy scissors with the points heading toward the ulnar side of the wrist is then placed under direct visualization with the use of Ragnell retractors, and the antebrachial fascia is split.
5. Irrigation is performed and the wound is closed with 4–0 or 5–0 nylon sutures. A light, bulky dressing is placed with the wrist splints in neutral alignment. The tourniquet is let down so that the clinician can check for good capillary refill to all the digits.

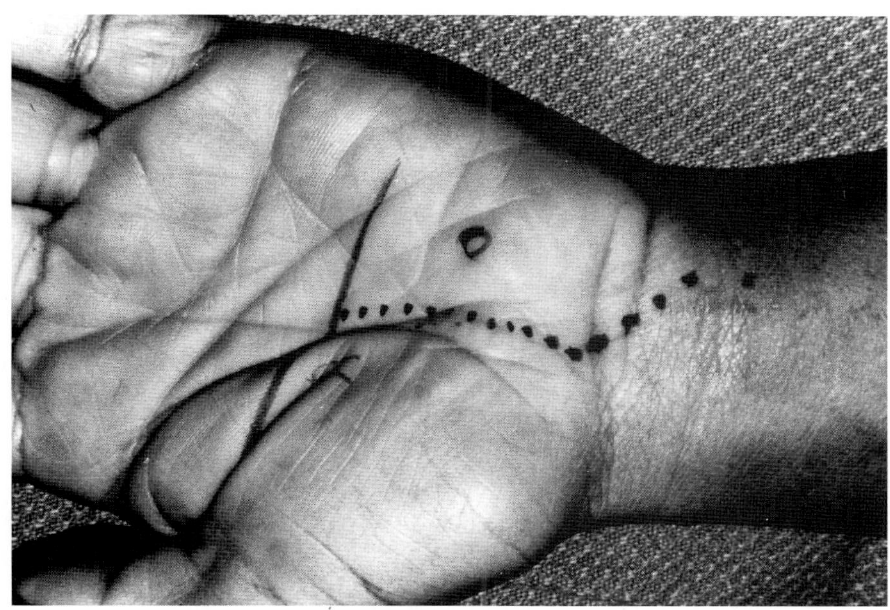

FIGURE 65–14. Classic carpal tunnel incision.

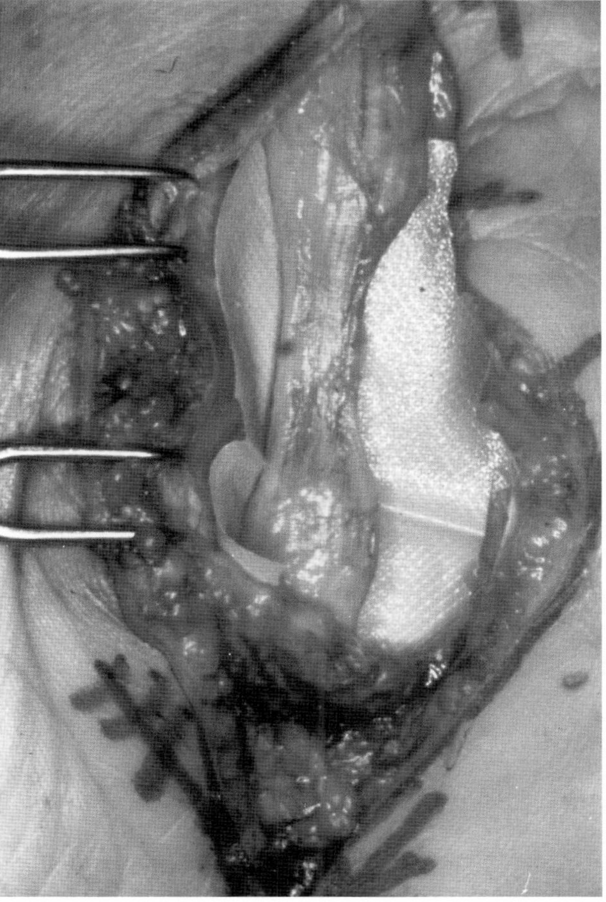

FIGURE 65–15. Hourglass deformity of the median nerve.

POSTOPERATIVE MANAGEMENT

Postoperative care consists of a period of wrist immobilization from 3 to 14 days during which time the patient is encouraged to use his or her digits. Tendon gliding exercises are taught to all patients, no matter what technique is used. The usual postoperative course often gives immediate relief of pain, but not all patients demonstrate immediate improvement in the sensibility of their fingers. If severe carpal tunnel syndrome has been present for many years, the return of sensibility may take as long as 6 months to 1 year. The disease process may be arrested, but the possibility exists that sensibility may never return.

Swelling at the base of the palm superficial to the carpal tunnel can be expected to last up to 4 months. During this period, patients may experience aching pain in the hypothenar eminence, called *pillar pain.* The use of endoscopic carpal tunnel release, as well as limited open technique, has reduced this pillar pain, which is why some surgeons have selected these techniques. At 2 weeks postoperatively, all patients have sutures removed, and at 6 weeks following surgical release, patients should have 50% of their preoperative grip strength. By 3 months, 75% to 80% of grip strength should have been regained; maximum grip strength and endurance usually do not return until after at least 6 months, or sometimes later.

COMPLICATIONS

Complications have been reported with endoscopic carpal tunnel release, including mild transient ulnar paresthesias, partial and complete lacerations of the superficial palmar arch and digital nerves, and deep motor branch injuries.

RESULTS

Nineteen percent of patients who have had carpal tunnel release never regain full strength after surgical release. Of 100 patients, 19 have a recurrence, even when successful carpal tunnel release has been obtained. Several prospective studies have compared endoscopic carpal release and open carpal release. All of these studies confirm that endoscopic carpal tunnel release is equally as effective as open release in relieving the symptoms of paresthesias and nocturnal pain. The additional advantages of quicker return to activities of daily living, quicker recovery of pinch strength, and reduced palmar scar tenderness, however, have not all been proved clinically. The limited open palmar technique has proved successful with no reported complications in a recent study by Plancher and associates. Direct comparison of all three techniques using a randomized, prospective approach is needed.

REFERENCES

Agee JM, McCarroll HR Jr, Tortosa R, et al: Endoscopic release of the carpal tunnel: A randomized prospective multicenter study. J Hand Surg [Am] 17:987–995, 1992.

Brown RA, Gelberman RH, Seiler JG, et al: Carpal tunnel release: A prospective randomized assessment of open endoscopic methods. J Bone Joint Surg [Am] 75:1265–1275, 1993.

Green DP, Hotchkiss RN, Pederson WC: Green's Operative Hand Surgery, 4th ed. New York, Churchill-Livingstone, 1999, pp 1406–1417.

Lee WP, Plancher KD, Strickland JW: Carpal tunnel release with a small palmar incision. Hand Clin 12:271–284, 1996.

Palmer D: Carpal tunnel syndrome in athletes. Op Tech Sports Med 4:33–39, 1996.

Palmer DH, Paulson JC, Lane-Larson CL, et al: Endoscopic carpal tunnel release: A comparison of the two techniques with open release. Arthroscopy 9:498–508, 1993.

Plancher KD, Perekh S: Limited open incision carpal tunnel release. In Techniques in Hand and Upper Extremity Surgery. Hagerstown, MD, Lippincott-Raven Publishers, 1997, pp 64–71.

Plancher KD, Peterson RK, Steichen JB: Compressive neuropathies and tendinopathies in the athletic elbow and wrist. Clin Sports Med 15:331–372, 1996.

CHAPTER 66

Treatment of Guyon's Canal Syndrome (Ulnar Nerve Compression at the Wrist)

INTRODUCTION

Compression of the ulnar nerve at the level of the wrist may occur as the ulnar nerve enters the ulnar tunnel or if the superficial or deep branch of the nerve is compressed. The deep branch may be compressed as it curves around the hamate hook and traverses the palm. Compression may be caused by ganglions, lipomas, anatomic anomalies, carpal fractures (most notably the hamate hook), local inflammation, or an ulnar artery thrombosis.

The predominant mechanisms in sports injuries involve direct compression or trauma. This injury has been reported widely in cyclists and is referred to as "handlebar palsy" or "cyclists' palsy."

Ulnar tunnel syndrome is also commonly seen in baseball catchers, hockey goalies, handball players, and those who play racquet sports. Distal ulnar nerve palsy can also occur as a "pushup" palsy or following fractures of the hamate hook from a missed golf shot or baseball swing. Lastly, degenerative changes in the pisotriquetral joint, causing local inflammation and inflammation of the so-called racquet player's pisiform, have also been known to create the ulnar tunnel syndrome.

HISTORY AND PHYSICAL EXAMINATION

A variety of signs and symptoms may be present, depending on whether the lesion is motor or sensory, or has mixed symptoms. The exact pattern of motor, sensory, or combined motor and sensory ulnar neve neuropathy indicates whether the location of the entrapment is at the wrist, proximal to the wrist, or in Guyon's canal before the division of the nerve into superficial and deep branches.

If the dorsal sensory branch is involved, with concomitant involvement of motor and sensory fibers of the ulnar nerve, the site of compression must be at or proximal to the origin of the dorsal branch of the ulnar nerve in the distal third of the forearm.

In some cases, the compression site is at the level of the elbow, causing patients to complain of coincident involvement of the median nerve and fixed motor deficits. While these cases are rare, they do produce characteristic lesions of the ulnar clawhand. This posture results from the unopposed action of the extensor digitorum communis, causing hyperextension of the ring finger's and small finger's metacarpophalangeal joints and hyperflexion of the proximal interphalangeal joints by the unopposed flexor digitorum profundus (FDP) (Fig. 66–1).

Anomalous motor and sensory findings may occur secondary to a Martin Gruber anastomosis. This ulnar-to-median anastomosis is seen in 15% of the population. The Riche-Cannieu anastomosis involves the deep branch of the ulnar nerve and the median nerve in the hand.

The patient's symptoms, as mentioned earlier, are due to compression, which varies with the location of the lesion. Pressure proximal to the bifurcation of the ulnar nerve results in both sensory and motor deficits. Sensation is decreased in the ring and little fingers. Intrinsic muscle weakness or atrophy may be noted. Tinel's test may cause paresthesias in the little and ring fingers. Conversely, a lesion distal to the bifurcation of the nerve results in findings that include either sensory or motor components, depending on which branch is affected (i.e., the deep motor branch or the superficial sensory branch) (Fig. 66–2).

Physical examination may reveal an Allen's test that is negative (normal), which confirms ulnar collateral circulation to the superficial or deep palmar arches. Thrombosis or aneurysm of the ulnar artery or one of its branches can be a cause of ulnar neuropathy, which may be detected when the Allen's test reveals slow circulation from the ulnar artery. Two-point discrimination should be checked, and muscle strength testing should be provided.

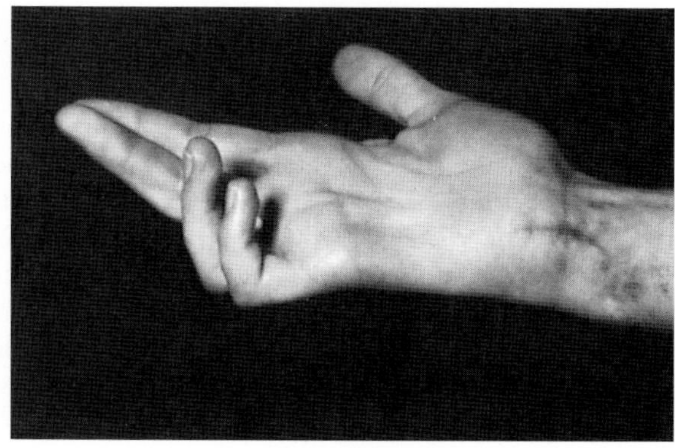

FIGURE 66–1. Ulnar clawhand deformity secondary to proximal ulnar nerve entrapment at the elbow. (From Lister G: The Hand: Diagnosis and Indications. Edinburgh, New York, Churchill Livingstone, 1993, p 150.)

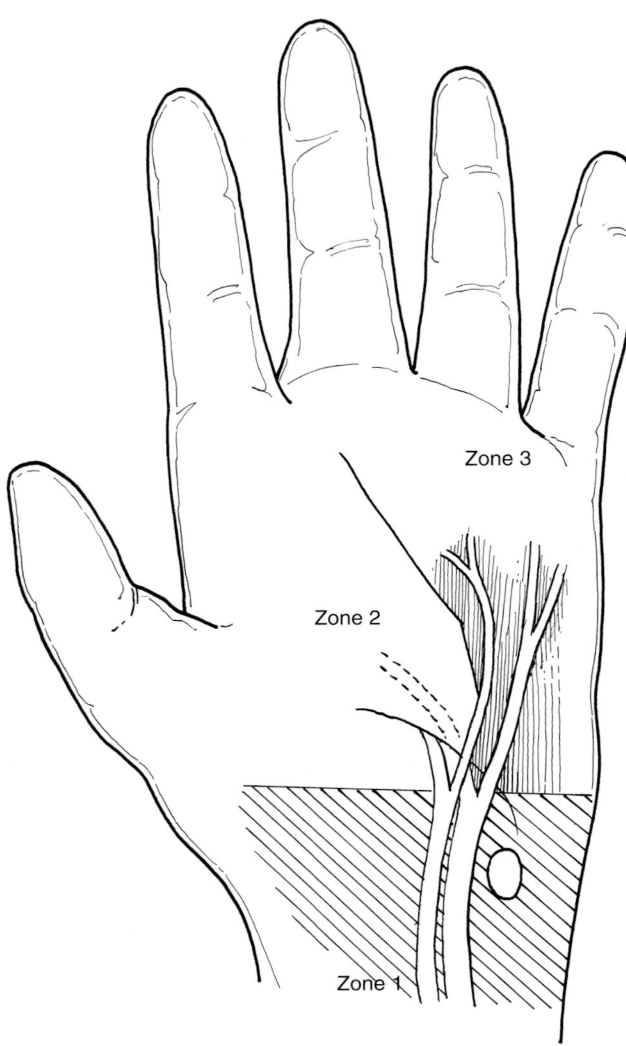

FIGURE 66–2. Illustration demonstrating the three potential zones of ulnar nerve entrapment at the wrist. Zone 1—motor and sensory involvement; Zone 2—motor involvement only; Zone 3—sensory involvement only.

DIAGNOSTIC IMAGING

Plain x-rays are important in ruling out the differential diagnosis of the hamate hook fracture. However, because plain x-rays are often negative, a CT scan of the hamate hook remains the gold standard for defining this fracture. Electromyograms (EMGs) of both ulnar and median nerves may be helpful, although most symptomatic patients exhibit normal electrodiagnostic findings. When EMGs are positive, they show denervation potentials in the interosseous muscle, with nerve conduction velocity studies showing prolongation of the motor latency to the first dorsal interossei. A difference of only 1 msec is considered significant, and these changes aid in localizing the lesion in Guyon's canal from a distal to a more proximal area of compression.

NONOPERATIVE MANAGEMENT

Treatment is initially nonsurgical, involving adjustment of hand positions on the bicycle or increased padding over the bars, mitts, or gloves. Rest, anti-inflammatory medications, local corticosteroid injections, and custom volar splinting may be of some help. When provided, injections should never be given directly into the nerve; rather, they should be placed along the canal.

RELEVANT ANATOMY

Guyon's canal is a triangular canal whose roof is formed by the volar carpal ligament. This ligament is blended with the insertion of the flexor carpi ulnaris into the pisiform bone and the distal extension of the pisohamate ligament (Fig. 66–3). The medial wall is formed by fibrous attachments to the pisohamate ligament and the pisiform itself; the lateral wall is formed by the shelf of the ligament. The ulnar nerve and artery traverse Guyon's canal; within the canal, the nerve bifurcates into superficial and deep branches, with the superficial branch passing distally in the canal. The deep branch, along with the larger branch of the ulnar artery, passes distally and deep between the origins of the abductor digiti quinti and the flexor digiti quinti minimi muscles to supply the interossei muscles of the hand. There are no tendons that traverse Guyon's canal as in the carpal canal, and the roof is relatively fibrous rather than rigid. Anatomic variations in the arrangement of the branches of the ulnar nerve are known, but these rarely cause problems.

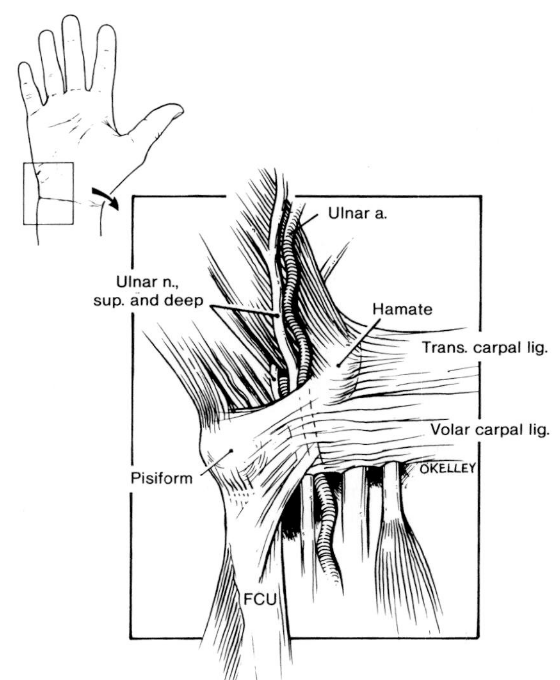

FIGURE 66–3. Anatomy of Guyon's canal demonstrating the course of the ulnar artery and nerve. (From DeLee J, Drez D, Stanitski CL: Orthopaedic Sports Medicine: Principles and Practice. Philadelphia, WB Saunders, 1994, p 1000.)

SURGICAL *TECHNIQUE*

Indications

Conservative treatment is often effective in the treatment of compression of the ulnar nerve at the wrist. Surgical treatment is indicated in patients who fail to respond appropriately to conservative treatment, or when symptoms recur after an initial treatment with custom splinting, anti-inflammatories, and modification of activities.

Technique

1. Positioning and incision: The patient is placed supine with the hand on the hand table. An incision is marked on the radial side of the flexor carpi ulnaris for 5 to 6 cm proximal to the wrist crease. This should extend in a curvilinear fashion across the crease along the line with the ulnar side of the ring finger (Fig. 66–4). Regional anesthesia (axillary block or Bier block) should be used to avoid obliteration of tissue planes with local injections.
2. Exposure: The palmar fascia is exposed proximally; it is excised to isolate the ulnar nerve proximally at the wrist and trace it distally through Guyon's canal by taking the flexor carpi ulnaris ulnarward. The pisiform bone and the pisohamate ligament are identified.
3. The motor branch of the nerve should be identified and avoided as it dives deep (dorsal). The volar carpal ligament over Guyon's canal should be incised to allow decompression of the ulnar nerve (Fig. 66–5).

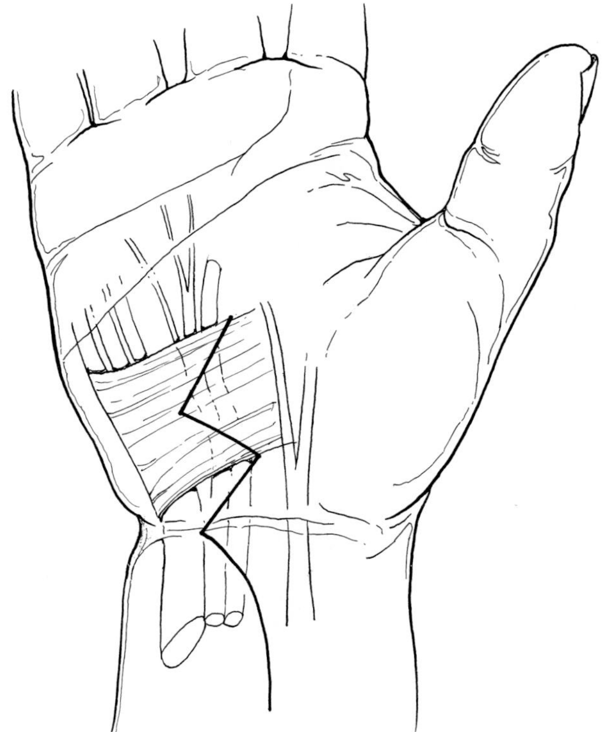

FIGURE 66–4. Skin incision for ulnar nerve release at the wrist.

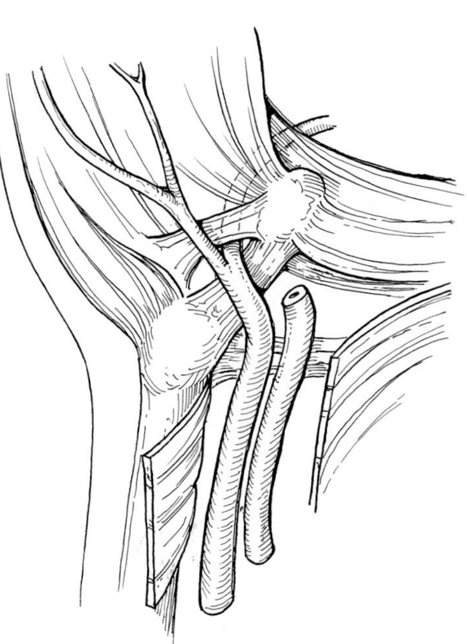

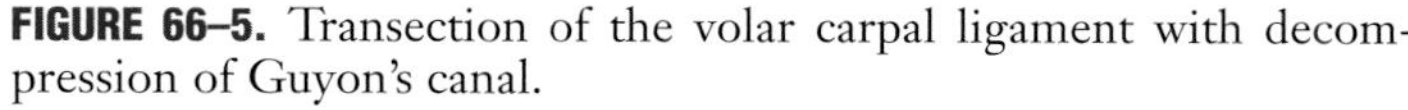

FIGURE 66–5. Transection of the volar carpal ligament with decompression of Guyon's canal.

4. Guyon's canal is explored for any masses or abnormalities, and dissection is continued up to the branch of the adductor digiti quinti minimi (Fig. 66–6).
5. With the pisohamate ligament cut, the deep branch of the ulnar nerve can be well visualized. The superficial branch and the main trunk of the ulnar nerve are visualized at the time that the volar carpal ligament is cut.
6. Closure: Closure consists of horizontal mattress sutures of 4–0 or 5–0 nylon. A short-arm bulky dressing is placed with the fingers free. The tourniquet is released to enable observation of good capillary refill.

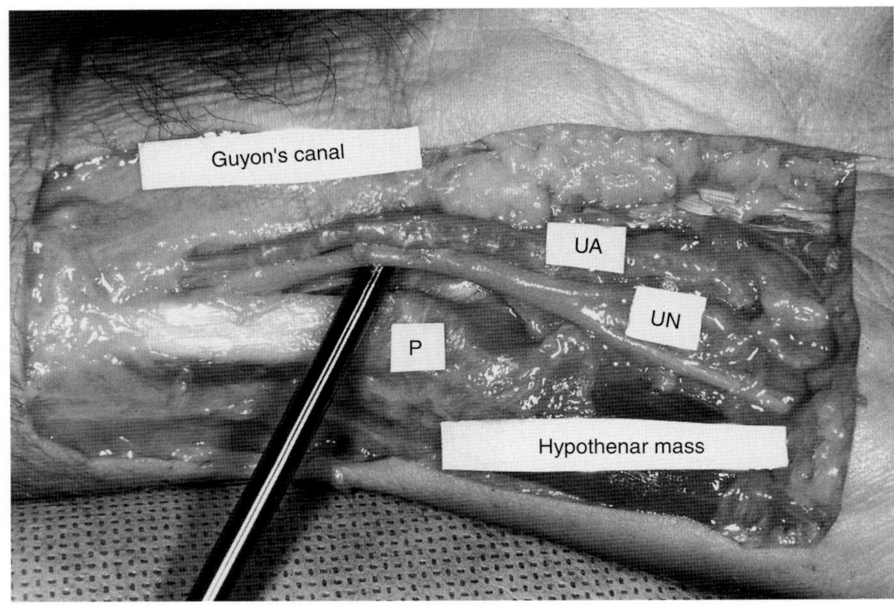

FIGURE 66–6. Cadaveric dissection of Guyon's canal. P, pisiform; UA, ulnar artery; UN, ulnar nerve.

POSTOPERATIVE MANAGEMENT

Postoperatively, the wrist is immobilized in a short-arm bulky dressing for 2 weeks, during which time the patient is encouraged to use the fingers for tendon gliding exercises. The patient returns at 2 weeks for removal of sutures, but immobilization is continued for an additional 2 weeks. However, if there has been a débridement of the hamate hook nonunion, or if an ulnar artery reverse vein graft has been placed, motion may be begun. At 4 weeks, a program of gentle range of motion of the wrist starts, and scar desensitization is begun. A strengthening program is initiated at 6 weeks and needs to be continued for an additional 8 weeks. Most athletes are able to return to sporting activities at 3 months postoperatively. Baseball catchers may pad their mitts and cyclists may pad their handlebars for several months to protect the hand from soreness in the hypothenar eminence.

COMPLICATIONS

Complications are rare with this surgery, but occlusion of an ulnar artery or reversed saphenous vein graft can occur, as well as transection of an ulnar nerve during dissection. If the latter occurs and is recognized at surgery, it should be repaired immediately.

Neuromas of the palmar cutaneous branch of the ulnar nerve have also been known to cause continued pain at the base of the palm. In addition, failure to reach Guyon's canal in the distal third of the forearm can be associated with continued entrapment neuropathy for this syndrome.

REFERENCES

Gross MS, Gelberman RH: The anatomy of the distal ulnar tunnel. Clin Orthop 196:238–247, 1985.

Shea JD, McLain EJ: Ulnar nerve compression syndromes at and below the wrists. J Bone Joint Surg [Am] 51:1095–1103, 1969.

Stern PJ, Vice M: Compression of the deep branch of the ulnar nerve. A case report. J Hand Surg [Am] 8:72–74, 1983.

CHAPTER 67

Treatment of Flexor Digitorum Profundus Avulsions

INTRODUCTION

Flexor digitorum profundus (FDP) avulsion injuries are unique to athletes. They occur when an athlete grabs the jersey of another athlete in soccer or of an offensive tight end in football; alternatively, they can occur when one catches a finger on the rim while slam dunking a basketball.

HISTORY AND PHYSICAL EXAMINATION

The ring finger is most frequently involved, although the reason for this is not totally understood.

Physical examination reveals inability to perform isolated flexion of the distal interphalangeal joint and tenderness at some point along the course of the FDP. This can occur at the finger or palm or in the wrist. A high index of suspicion is important because operative treatment is usually required for this injury; it allows for a good result only if detected soon after injury.

The finger is characteristically swollen and somewhat ecchymotic, and the local tenderness is usually more marked at the site where the FDP stump has come to sit. This commonly occurs at the proximal interphalangeal (PIP) joint, at the level of the A_4 pulley, or in the distal palm.

DIAGNOSTIC IMAGING

X-rays should be taken to reveal an avulsed fragment of bone, which at times can prevent proximal retraction of the tendon because the fragment gets caught at the level of the A_4 pulley (Fig. 67–1). Because most cases involve a tendon that ruptures directly from the distal phalanx, the correct diagnosis depends on clinical examination and loss of FDP function.

NONOPERATIVE MANAGEMENT

Nonoperative treatment is an option; however, it does not restore FDP function.

RELEVANT ANATOMY AND PERILS AND PITFALLS OF SURGERY

Three types of FDP avulsion injuries have been classified and have different implications for surgical correction:

Type I. The tendon retracts into the palm, disrupting the blood supply, and creates scar in the tendon sheath. Repair within 10 days is required, or the distal end will soften and retract.

Type II. The tendon retracts to the level of the PIP joint, where it becomes caught at the chiasm of the flexor digitorum superficialis. Early treatment is advised, but successful repair can be done as late as 3 months after injury.

Type III. FDP avulsions may involve a large bony fragment that is avulsed by the injury and now is lodged at the level of the distal A_4 pulley. Surgery can be performed up to 3 months from the date of injury.

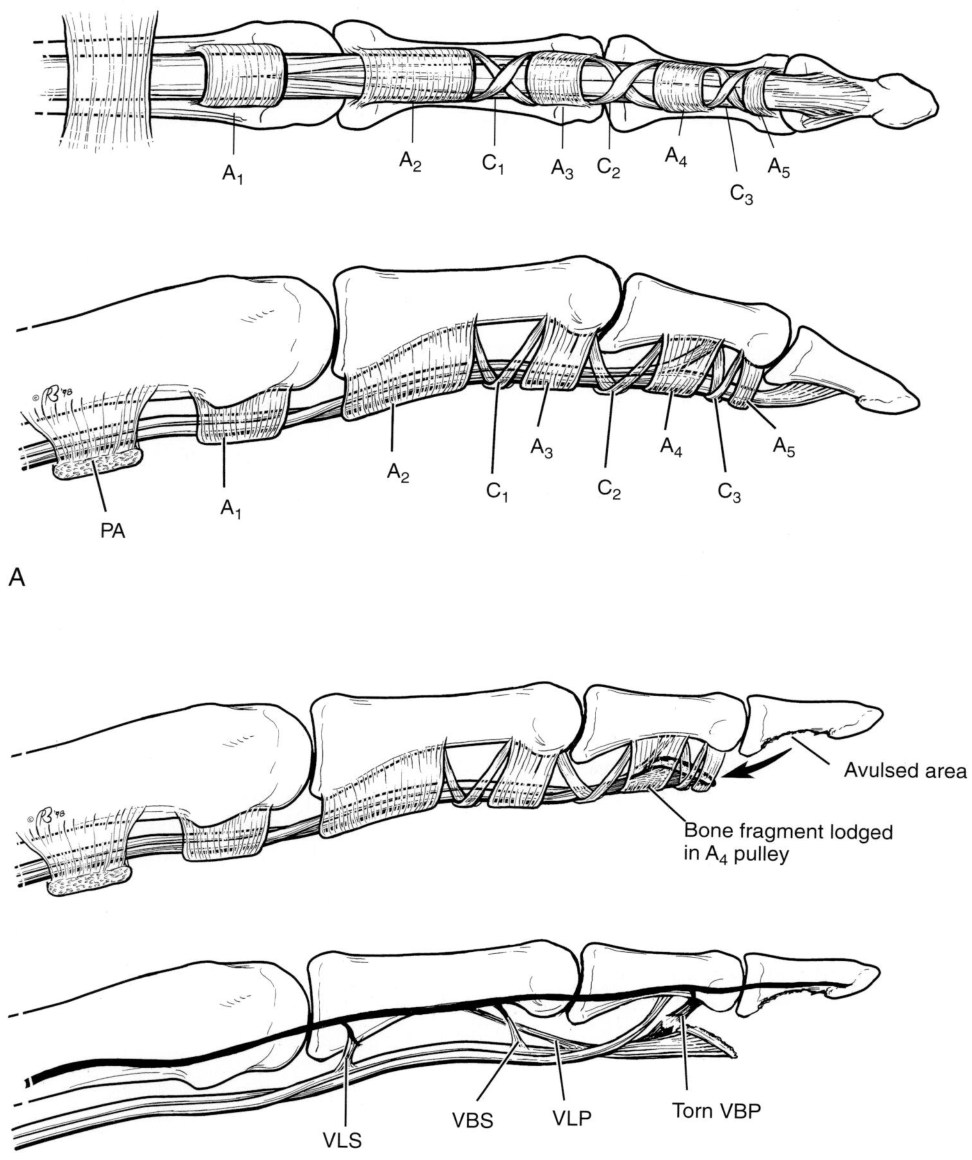

FIGURE 67–1. *A*, Volar *(top)* and lateral *(bottom)* views of the flexor tendon sheath pulley system. Note that the critical pulleys (A_2 and A_4) originate from bone. A, annular pulleys; C, cruciate pulleys; PA, palmar aponeurosis. *B*, Flexor digitorum profundus avulsion with large bone fragment lodged in the A_4 pulley. No disruption of the short vinculum is noted; the long vinculum to the FDP tendon is preserved. VBP, vinculum brevis profundus; VBS, vinculum brevis sublimus; VLP, vinculum longus profundus; VLS, vinculum longus sublimus.

SURGICAL *TECHNIQUE*

Indications

Early operative reinsertion of the avulsed type I FDP tendon is necessary to restore active flexion of the distal interphalangeal joint. The success of repair is related to the length of delay after injury, with the best results being obtained with immediate operative treatment. Surgical repair becomes more difficult after 10 days.

Types II and III injuries can be treated successfully on a delayed basis because the tendon is kept in the sheath, is bathed in synovial fluid within the sheath, and does not undergo shortening.

Although the loss of terminal joint flexion may not seem to be a major functional deficit, it does compromise strength of the hand. Athletes should not wait until the end of the season to have an FDP repaired.

Technique

1. Positioning: The patient is positioned supine on the operating table with an arm board adjacent. A tourniquet cuff is placed on the upper arm, and after the arm is exsanguinated using an Esmarch, the tourniquet is inflated to 250 mm Hg.
2. A midaxial incision is made at the tip of the finger to expose the distal insertion site of the FDP tendon. If a type I repair is necessary, a second incision is made in the palm. If a type II repair is required, the incision is made as an extension of the midaxial line. For a type III repair, the midaxial incision is extended only up to the A_4 pulley (Fig. 67–2).
3. Dissection is carried down through the skin and subcutaneous tissue, with meticulous hemostasis obtained with a bipolar cautery. The digital nerves must be identified and protected before the tendon

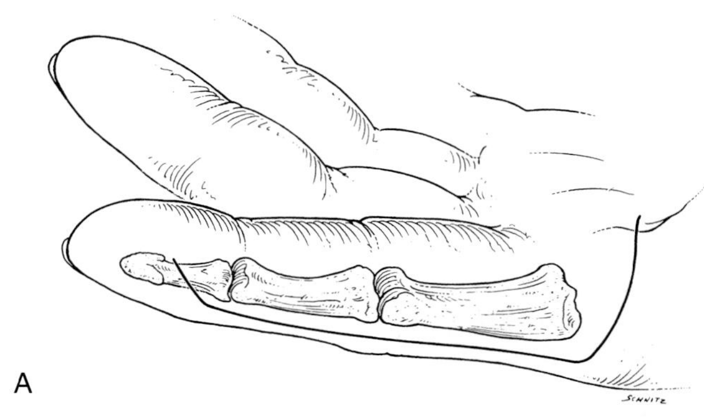

A

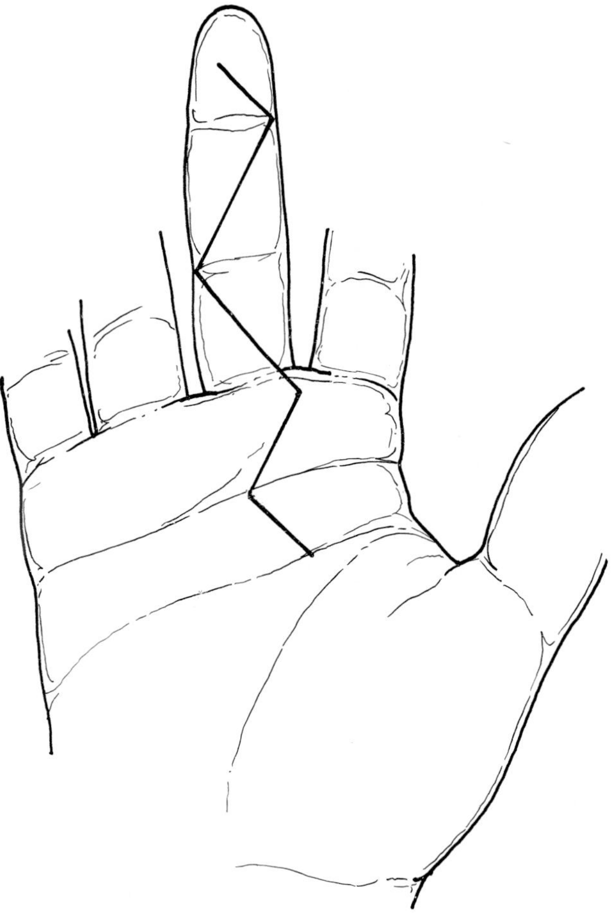

B

FIGURE 67–2. Two alternative incisions for flexor tendon surgery. *A*, Midlateral incision. *B*, Bruner incision. (*A* from Sotereanos DG, Voitz RJ, Mitsionis GJ: Flexor tenolysis. Hand Clin 1:109, 1985.)

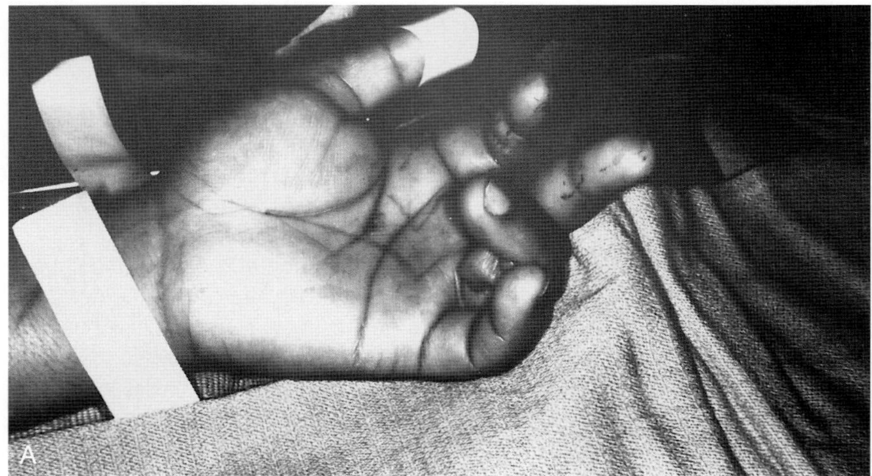

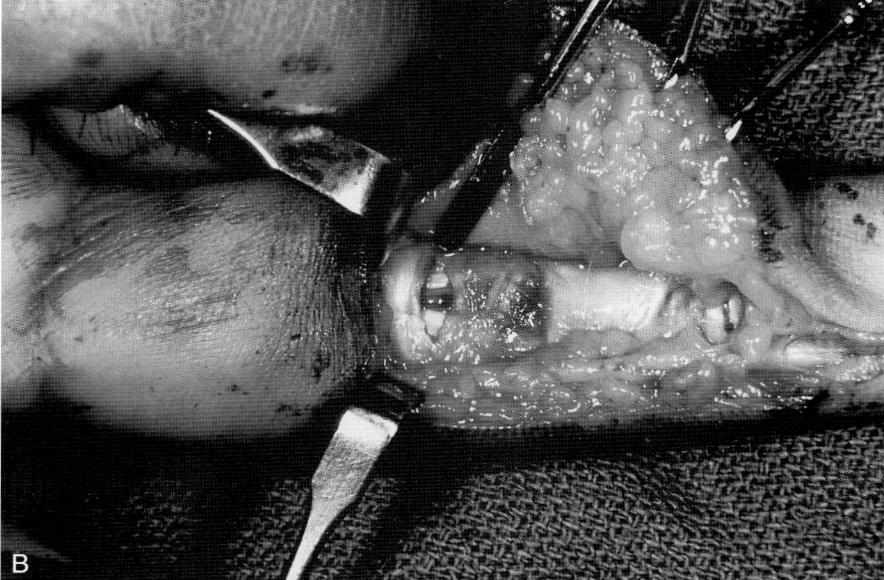

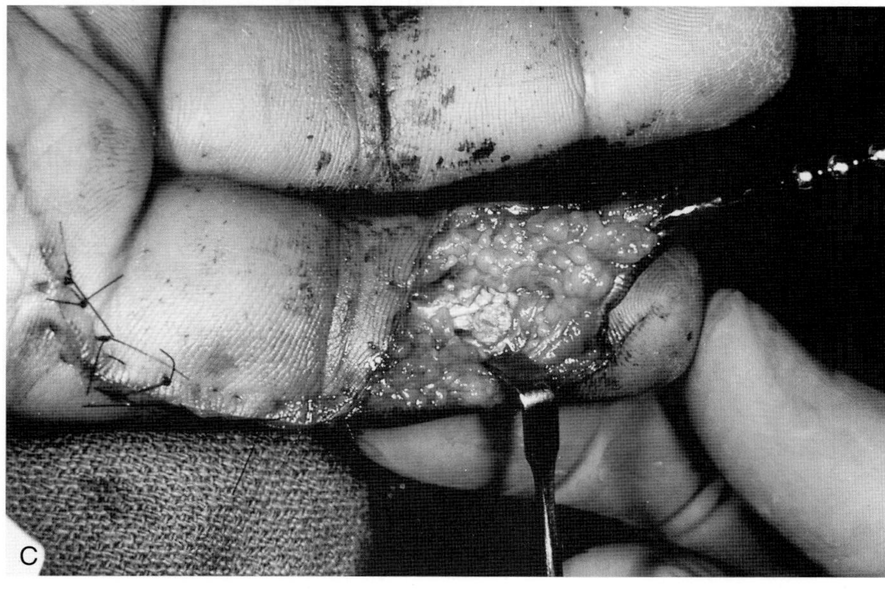

FIGURE 67–3. Illustrative case. *A*, Note the posture of the middle finger with the distal interphalangeal joint in full extension following flexor digitorum profundus (FDP) avulsion. *B*, Midlateral incision, flexor sheath exposed, flexor digitorum superficialis tendon intact, and FDP rupture beneath the A_2 pulley. *C*, FDP reattached to the distal phalanx.

sheath is entered. All pullies should be preserved during the reinsertion. It is often necessary to narrow the flexor digitorum profundus end to allow its passage beneath the distal pullies before reinserting it directly into the base of the distal phalanx. It is important to avoid damaging the flexor digitorum superficialis tendon, which should be functioning normally with this injury.

4. With the use of an atraumatic technique to avoid scarring and adhesions, the tendon is repositioned with a Carroll tendon retriever out to the distal phalanx (Fig. 67–3).
5. We prefer to use a mini-Mitek anchor drilled at the distal phalanx with the aid of a mini-fluoroscopy unit. The tendon is then laid in place, with the soft tissue of the A_5 pulley brought over the tendon to imbricate it and seal it in place.
6. An alternative to the mini-Mitek is the pullout wire and button, which has been used more commonly in the past (Fig. 67–4).
7. With the proper cascade of the digits aligned and the finger pulled into position, the skin can be sutured in routine fashion. The tourniquet is let down before the surgeon checks for good capillary refill to the digits. A soft tissue bulky dressing is placed. The patient returns several days later for extension block splinting and a proper postoperative rehabilitation program.
8. A free tendon graft may be necessary in chronic ruptures. Description of this technique is beyond the scope of this book, and the reader is referred to a hand operative textbook.

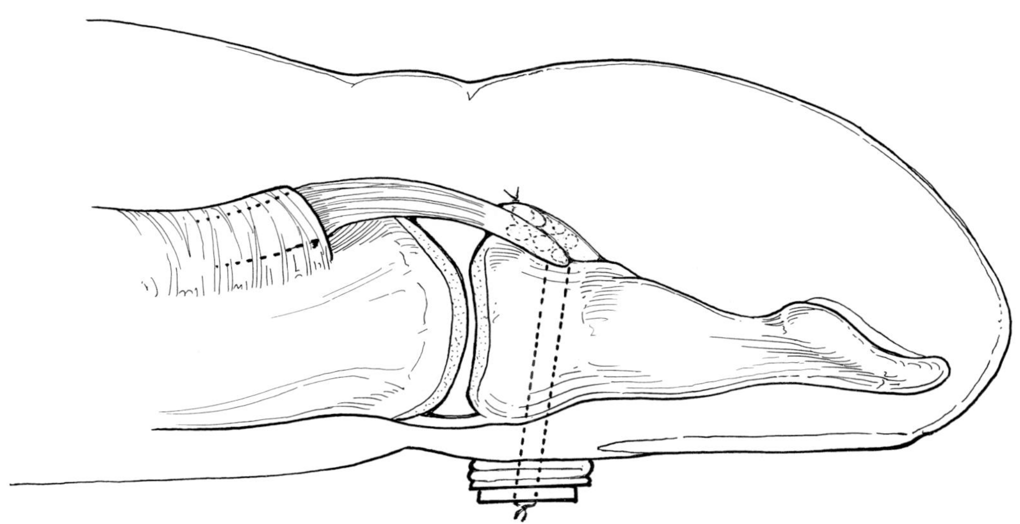

FIGURE 67–4. Pullout suture and button technique for repair of flexor digitorum profundus avulsion.

POSTOPERATIVE MANAGEMENT

The repaired tendon must be protected for at least 6 weeks. A program devised by a certified hand therapist will help prevent stresses on the repaired tendons and will help to move them early so as to improve gliding and tensile strength at the suture site. The postrepair regimens most applicable to flexor digitorum profundus avulsions are the same as those for zone I flexor tendon repairs and can be instituted during the first few days if the reinsertion is strong. Early motion programs are recommended after free tendon graft of irreparable late avulsions. The repair must be protected for at least 2 to 3 months; no athletic endeavors should be undertaken during this time.

COMPLICATIONS

It is imperative to avoid damage to the flexor tendon sheath or the intact flexor digitorum superficialis while attempting to repair the flexor digitorum profundus. If this tendon is cut and FDS function is lost, the patient's impairment is substantially worsened, and immediate surgery is required. Knowledge of flexor tendon repair is essential for the surgeon; however, it is beyond the scope of this book, and we refer you to an operative hand textbook.

RESULTS

When repair is performed in a timely fashion, athletes can often return to their sport within 2 or 3 months. It is important for them to wear some type of splint that will prevent hyperextension of the finger and re-rupture of the repair.

REFERENCES

Leddy JP, Packer JW: Avulsion of the profundus tendon insertion in athletes. J Hand Surg [Am] 2:66–69, 1977.

Robins PR, Dobyns JH: Avulsion of the insertion of the flexor digitorum profundus tendon associated with fractures of the distal phalanx. A brief review. In AAOS Symposium on Tendon Surgery in the Hand. St. Louis, CV Mosby, 1974, pp 151–156.

Smith JH: Avulsion of the profundus tendon and simultaneous intraarticular fracture of the distal phalanx. J Hand Surg [Am] 6:600–601, 1981.

Strickland JW: Flexor tendon—acute injuries. In Green DP, Hotchkiss RN, Pederson WC (eds): Green's. Operative Hand Surgery, 4th ed. New York, Chuchill Livingstone, 1999, pp 1866–1868.

CHAPTER 68

Treatment of Metacarpophalangeal Dislocation of the Fingers

HISTORY AND PHYSICAL EXAMINATION

The metacarpophalangeal (MP) joint is a condyloid joint that allows abduction, adduction, flexion, and extension with limited amounts of circumduction. The articular surface of the metacarpal head is broader on its volar surface than dorsally, which allows for the dorsal lateral aspects of both sides of its articular surface to accommodate the origin of the collateral ligaments. The overall stability of the joint largely depends on the collateral ligaments and the volar plate.

The collateral ligaments consist of two bands. The main ligament is cordlike; the accessory ligament is fan shaped and inserts into the volar plate. The volar plate of the MP joint is a thick fibrocartilaginous structure of the joint capsule that attaches distally to the base of the phalanx. More proximally, it attaches to the neck of the metacarpal with a more aerial and flexible attachment. The metacarpal volar plates are firmly attached to each other by the deep transverse metacarpal ligament, which is sometimes also referred to as the *intervolar plate ligament.*

Dislocations of all MP joints may occur in the lateral, dorsal, or volar plane; these are designated as either simple or complex (Fig. 68–1). Injuries to the MP joints are mostly caused by athletics. The patient notes an obvious deformity or complains of local tenderness and

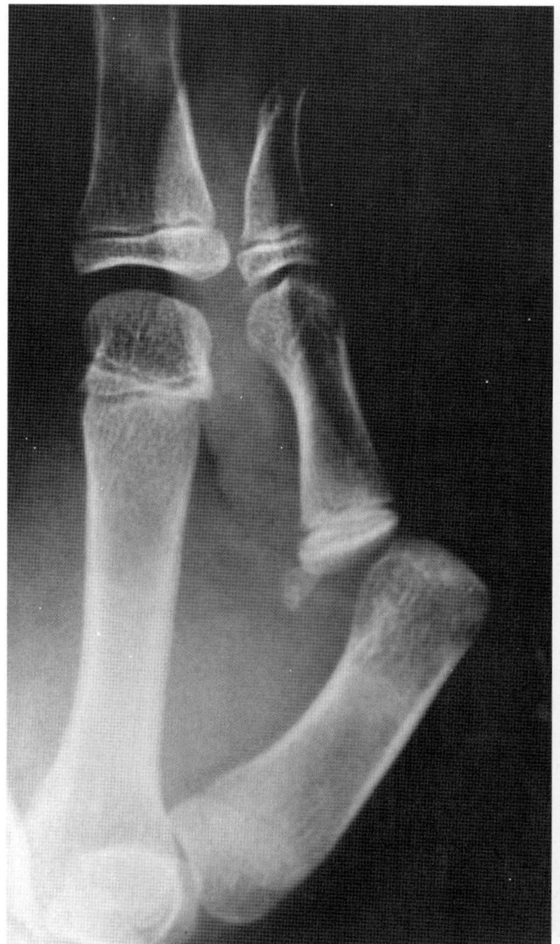

A

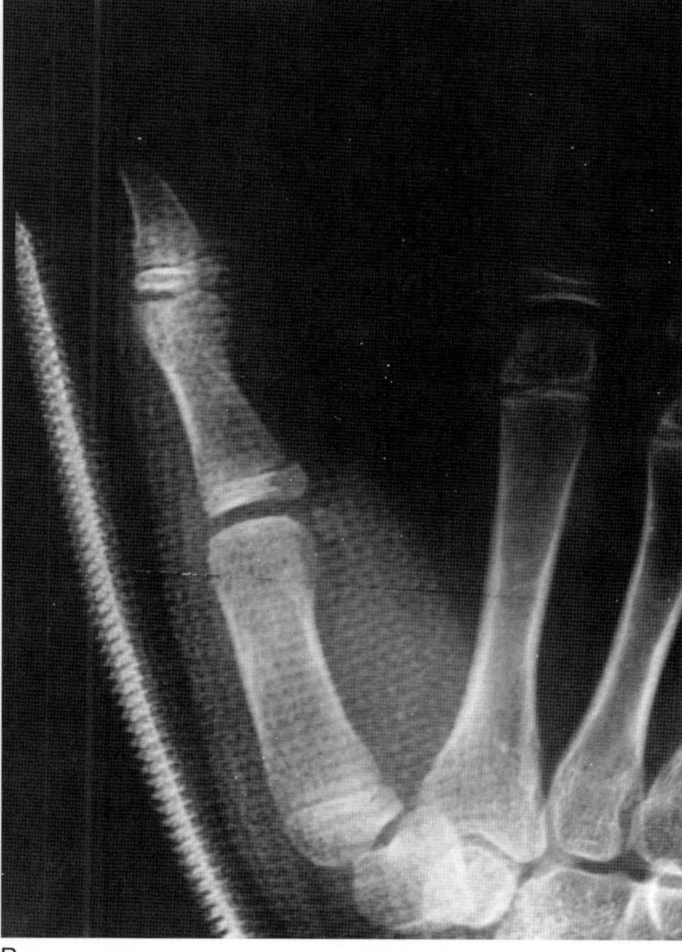

B

FIGURE 68–1. *A*, Lateral x-ray of a volar metacarpophalangeal dislocation of the thumb. *B*, X-ray after open reduction.

subtle swelling in the valley between the metacarpal heads and directly over the involved collateral ligaments. In a lateral dislocation, the normal laxity of the collateral ligament with the joint in extension does not produce pain in the direction opposite to the dislocation.

Physical examination reveals appropriate tenderness as well as deformities and lack of motion in the four planes of joint motion. Stability testing can be attempted, but this is difficult to undertake in the acute period.

DIAGNOSTIC IMAGING

X-rays are essential in the treatment of dislocations because they confirm the diagnosis in the (subtle) lateral MP dislocation. X-rays may denote collateral ligament injuries if a small fleck of bone is visible near the collateral ligament insertion. The use of Brewerton's view (a view that places the hand in a palm-up position with the x-ray centered over the MP joints and directed 30° from the ulnar side) may also reveal an MP dislocation (Fig. 68–2).

Patients with chronic MP collateral ligament injuries may show intra-articular fragments at the proximal phalanx where the collateral ligament has pulled off the bone.

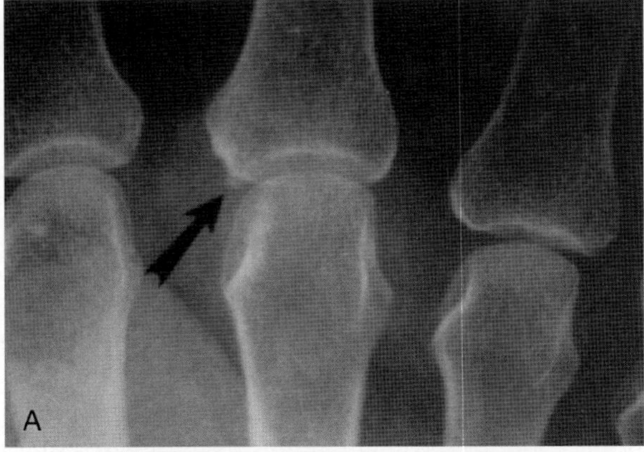

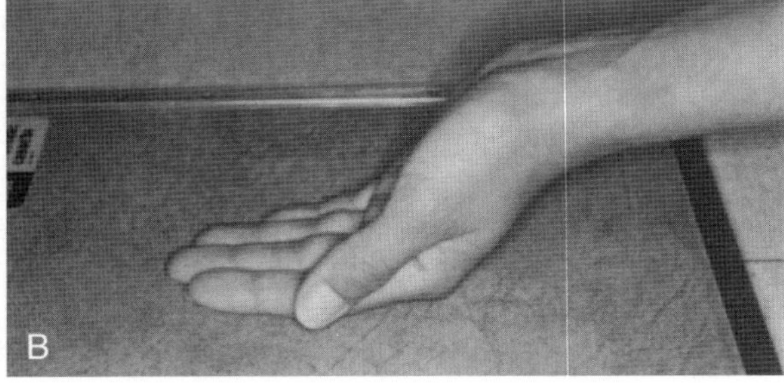

FIGURE 68–2. *A*, Metacarpophalangeal (MP) joint collateral ligament injury is occasionally associated with a small avulsion fracture *(arrow)*. B, Brewerton's view of the MP joint of the hand. The x-ray beam is centered over the MP joints and directed 30° from the ulnar side.

NONOPERATIVE MANAGEMENT

Nonoperative treatment is the mainstay for most dislocations. The initial treatment for an MP joint dislocation is closed reduction. Adequate anesthesia with a wrist block (1% lidocaine) followed by gentle longitudinal traction and hyperextension or exaggeration of the deformity, whether it be volar or dorsal, should allow for a closed reduction of the finger. In the case of a volar dislocation, sometimes hyperflexion of the MP joint and pushing the proximal phalanx back into position rather than applying traction is a successful maneuver.

Closed reduction of a dorsal dislocation requires flexion of the interphalangeal (IP) joints and wrist so as to relax the flexor tendons. The proximal phalanx is hyperextended to a position almost perpendicular to the metacarpal head; the base of the phalanx is then pushed volarly across the articular surface of the metacarpal in an effort to push the volar plate out of the way. The phalanx should maintain contact with the head of the metacarpal throughout the entire closed reduction maneuver to prevent entrapment of the volar plate within the joint. When the proximal phalanx base extends across the metacarpal articular surface and the digit is straightened and then flexed, a clunk is audible if the reduction is successful. Gentle active and passive flexion and extension confirm that the position of the joint is adequate. X-rays should be taken to confirm articular congruency with no associated fractures.

Most dislocations can be reduced in the field, although we recommend only a single attempt with a closed reduction within 2 or 3 minutes of the actual injury. If the dislocation is not reduced immediately we provide wrist or metacarpal anesthesia to prevent muscle contraction and pain, which would preclude a successful reduction. If signs of a complex dislocation (discussed later) are present, we do not perform closed reductions in the field.

The MP joint is immobilized in 50° to 70° of flexion for 7 to 10 days in a dorsal dislocation. This position allows the volar plate to relax. Active motion is begun immediately thereafter, but hyperextension is prevented by buddy-taping the involved digit to the adjacent digit. Lateral MP dislocations are immobilized with the MP in 50° to 70° of flexion, with the use of a custom "bowling alley splint" (made by a hand therapist) for 3 to 4 weeks to avoid chronic instability of the digit. The purpose of the splint is to avoid lateral stresses. Sports are interrupted for 4 to 6 weeks. Volar dislocations are kept in an intrinsic plus custom-made splint for 3 weeks. After splinting has been completed and when motion has returned, patients are allowed to proceed with unrestricted activities.

RELEVANT ANATOMY AND PERILS AND PITFALLS OF SURGERY (COMPLEX DISLOCATIONS)

The MP joint may be slightly hyperextended with the proximal phalanx lying on top of the dorsal metacarpal head and the finger partially overlapping the adjacent digit. Puckering of the volar skin (which is difficult to see in the index finger because the skin crease in the proximal palmar crease is present normally) is an important finding in this complex dislocation. This finding is apparent in the thumb and denotes an irreducible dislocation.

The complex dislocation on x-ray demonstrates the proximal phalanx and metacarpal parallel with slight angulation. The pathognomonic radiographic sign of a complex dislocation, however, is the presence of a sesamoid within the widened joint space. Normally the sesamoid resides within the volar plate; therefore, the presence of a sesamoid in the joint space should be considered an unequivocal sign of this type of dislocation. The complex dislocation occurs most commonly in the index finger, with a high incidence also in the thumb and small finger. The long and ring fingers are rarely involved, although many combinations have been described in the literature.

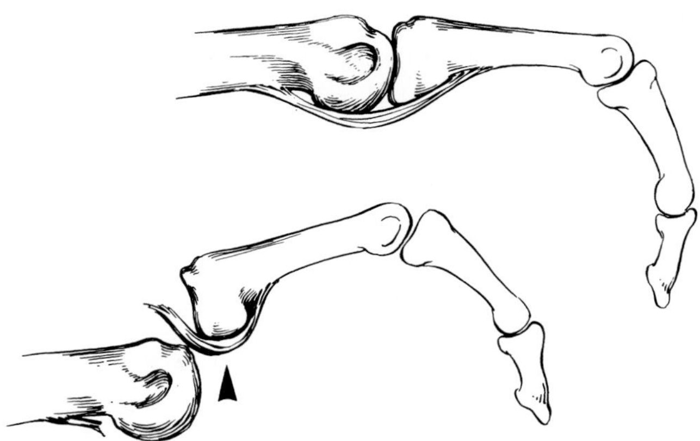

FIGURE 68–3. Artist's rendition of the interposition of the volar plate between the proximal phalanx and the metacarpal head. (From DeLee J, Drez D, Stanitski CL: Orthopaedic Sports Medicine: Principles and Practice. Philadelphia, WB Saunders, 1994, p 974.)

In irreducible dislocations, the interposition of the volar plate between the base of the middle phalanx and the metacarpal head prevents the reduction (Fig. 68–3). Failure to achieve a congruous reduction with restricted active motion is an indication for open reduction.

SURGICAL *TECHNIQUE*

Technique

Irreducible Complex Dislocations

1. Positioning: The patient is positioned supine on the operating room table with the arm placed on the hand table. There is controversy about whether a dorsal incision versus a volar incision should be made for the complex irreducible MP dislocation. We have found that the dorsal approach is easier and safer because it avoids the neurovascular bundle, which at times can be "button-holed" across the metacarpal head (Fig. 68–4).
2. Incision: The incision is made in a curvilinear fashion over the metacarpal head after the arm is exsanguinated and the tourniquet inflated. Dissection continues through the skin and subcutaneous tissue, with meticulous hemostasis obtained with the bipolar cautery.

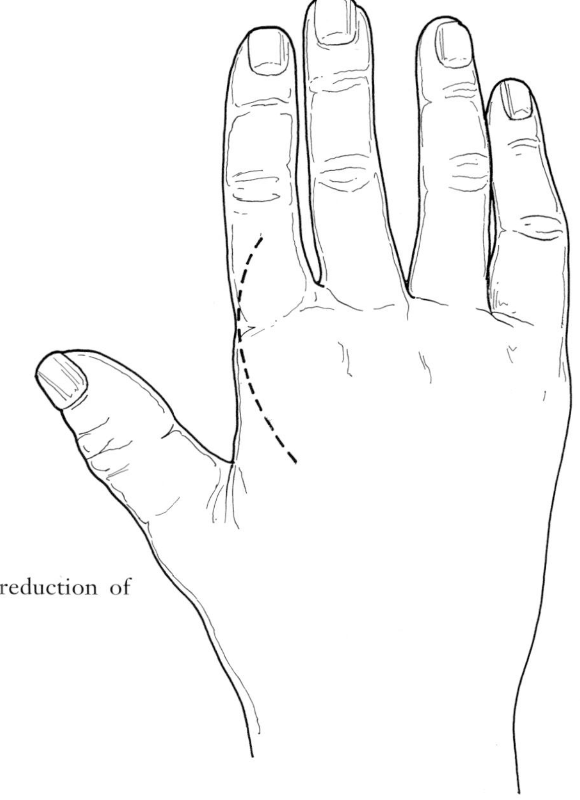

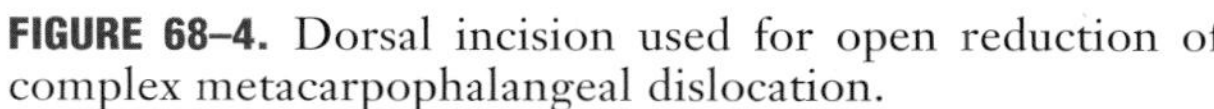

FIGURE 68–4. Dorsal incision used for open reduction of complex metacarpophalangeal dislocation.

3. Either the extensor tendon is split longitudinally in its midsection, or the sagittal band is cut, to allow for full visualization of the joint capsule. Both structures require later repair with permanent braided 3–0 undyed nylon sutures.
4. The joint capsule is cut in a transverse fashion if it is not already open, and the finger is put in longitudinal traction. The metacarpophalangeal joint is then inspected.
5. A Freer elevator or a Kutz-Kleinert elevator is placed in the depths of the MP joint to push the volar plate out of the confines of the joint; the joint is then hyperflexed to 115°. The joint is irrigated, and closure is performed in routine fashion. The finger is placed in a splint at 40° of flexion at the MP joint in a safe position, and the tourniquet is released. Inspection of good capillary refill to all digits is noted.

If the metacarpal head has been fractured, the dorsal approach allows for open reduction and internal fixation, in addition to MP reduction.

POSTOPERATIVE MANAGEMENT

Postoperatively, the hand is placed in a position of function (20° extension of the wrist, 20° flexion of the MP joint, and 45° to 50° flexion at the proximal interphalangeal joints). Gentle early active range of motion while protecting the involved digit with the adjacent digit buddy-taped is begun.

If instability was noted at the time of surgery, a dorsal extension block splint can be used to keep the finger flexed slightly for 3 to 4 weeks. After this, the finger is brought back into the extended position, and return to sports with buddy-taping of the digit is begun over the next 3 to 4 weeks.

COMPLICATIONS

Reduction and operative intervention of a complex dislocation of the MP joint require that the surgeon know the anatomy around the MP joint; these procedures rarely lead to significant complications.

RESULTS

Stiffness and swelling of the MP joint can continue for several months, but most athletes return to the playing field within 6 weeks without subsequent sequelae.

REFERENCES

Becton DL, Christian JD, Goodwin C, et al: A simplified technique for treating the complex dislocations of the index, metacarpophalangeal joint. J Bone Joint Surg [Am] 57:698–700, 1975.

DeLee JC, Drez D Jr: Orthopedic Sports Medicine: Principles and Practice. Philadelphia, WB Saunders, 1994, pp 971–975.

Green DP, Terry GC: Complex dislocations of metacarpophalangeal joint. J Bone Joint Surg [Am] 55:1480–1486, 1973.

CHAPTER 69

Treatment of Skier's/Gamekeeper's Thumb

INTRODUCTION

Skier's thumb involves acute abduction and hyperextension stress to the ulnar collateral ligament of the thumb. It is one of the most common injuries among skiers. Although the ski pole and grips have been implicated as causative factors, there is no evidence to date to show that strapless poles or special gloves decrease the incidence of injury. At the time of the fall, it is the position of the hyperextended and abducted thumb that results in an ulnar collateral ligament tear. Gamekeeper's thumb involves a different mechanism and results from a chronic injury to the same ligament.

HISTORY AND PHYSICAL EXAMINATION

The patient complains about a painful swollen metacarpophalangeal (MP) joint directly over the ulnar collateral ligament. The patient almost always states that he or she fell while skiing or performed some sport and landed on the outstretched thumb.

Evaluation is important for differentiating a partial tear from a complete tear. If the joint opens with a small amount of radial deviation or abduction stress at the MP joint, the diagnosis is obvious (Fig. 69–1*A*). We use 2 mL of 1% lidocaine injected into the MP joint to relax the muscle spasm of the adductor. A median and radial nerve block at the wrist is also possible and is often done to avoid an injection directly into the MP joint. Testing of the MP joint is done in both flexion and extension, and results are compared with those in the opposite thumb. Controversy exists about what is abnormal and what positive stress tests are, but we believe that 35° of laxity in full flexion represents a complete tear. In addition, openings greater than 15° on stress radiographs when compared with the opposite side constitute a completed ligament tear (Fig. 69–1*B*).

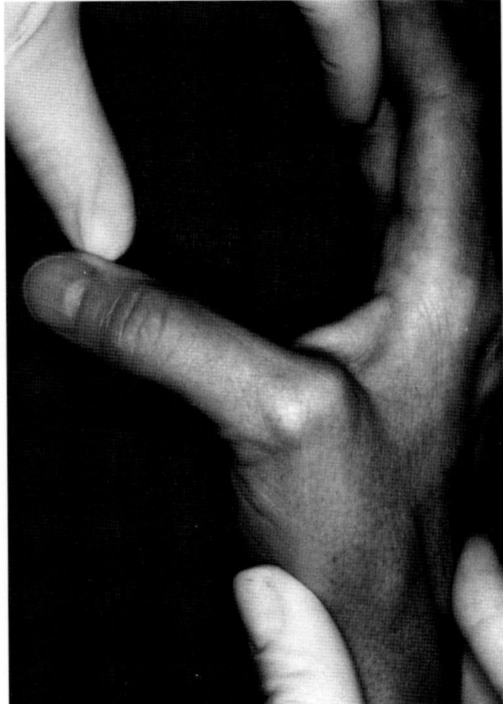

A

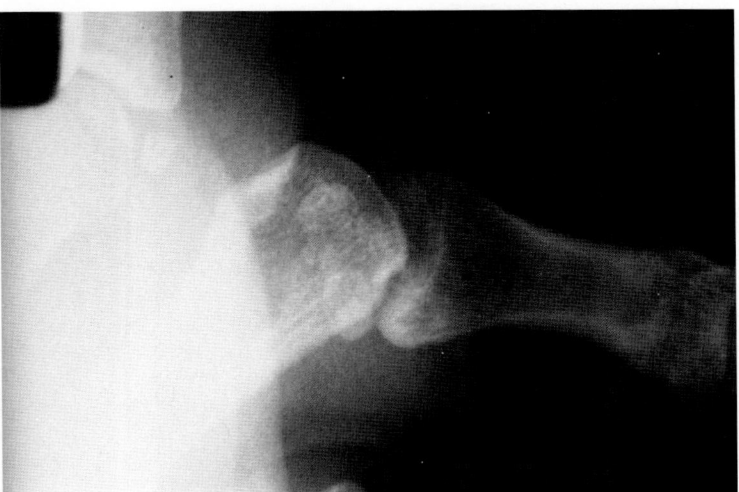

B

FIGURE 69–1. *A*, Abduction stress testing for ulnar collateral ligament tear in the thumb. *B*, X-ray stress test.

DIAGNOSTIC IMAGING

Routine radiographs are made before stress views are taken in the event that there is an undisplaced fracture of the proximal phalanx. A large intra-articular fracture involving more than one third of the articular surface of the proximal phalanx may often be seen and should be treated surgically. Roberts' view, which is a hyperpronated anteroposterior view, is the single x-ray performed (Fig. 69–2).

If no fracture is seen on the initial radiograph, stress radiographs may be taken after complete anesthesia has been administered. Films are taken with the MP joint in full extension and a radial abduction force applied to the thumb.

NONOPERATIVE MANAGEMENT

Partial tears and grade I ulnar collateral ligament tears are treated nonoperatively with a well-molded custom thumb spica splint with the MP joint in slight flexion. The patient remains in this apparatus for 4 to 6 weeks, depending on the severity of the injury to the volar plate and the extensor hood. Various types of custom splints can be constructed to allow the athlete to continue playing his or her sport while healing.

Nonoperative treatment is also indicated for grade II tears present at the time of a stress examination, if a firm end point is seen and volar subluxation is absent on lateral x-ray.

RELEVANT ANATOMY AND PERILS AND PITFALLS OF SURGERY

The Stener lesion (adductor aponeurosis interposed between the two ends of the torn ligament) may prevent adequate healing (Fig. 69–3). Stener reported that this lesion occurred with an incidence that ranged from 14% to 83%. We have found that more than 80% of skiers with complete ulnar collateral ligament tears have associated Stener lesions.

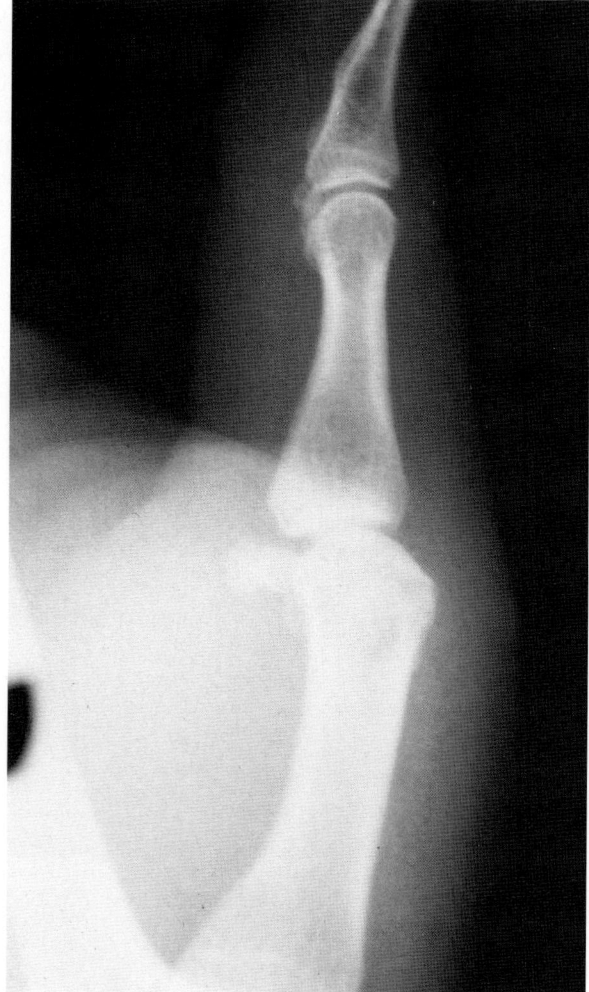

A

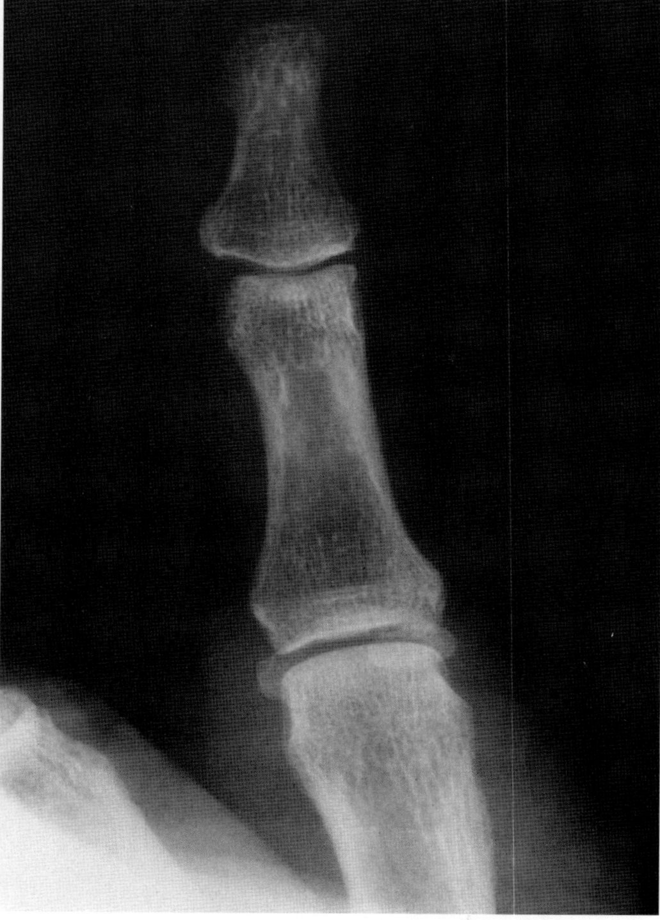

B

FIGURE 69–2. *A*, Hyperpronated (Roberts') view for assessing skier's thumb. No fracture is noted. *B*, Lateral x-ray. Note the subluxation seen with skier's thumb.

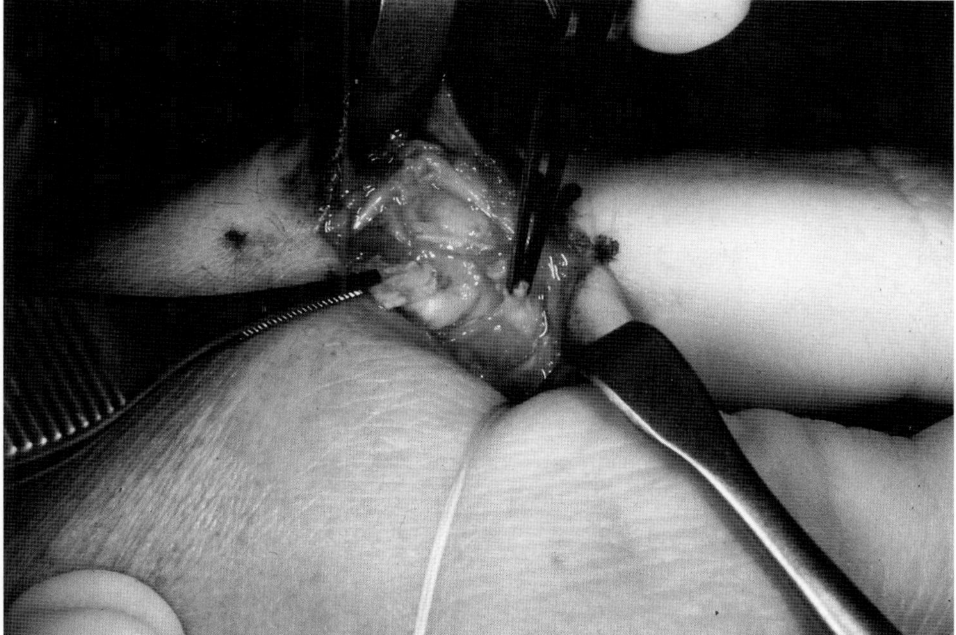

FIGURE 69–3. Stener lesion occurring in the right thumb held in forceps.

A complete rupture without a Stener lesion can also be treated nonoperatively. The Stener lesion, however, can be difficult to rule out by clinical examination or other techniques; for this reason, we prefer to operate on patients with complete ruptures. A 15-minute MRI technique with special sequences is helpful for detecting the presence or absence of a Stener lesion; use of this tool should be considered.

SURGICAL *TECHNIQUE*

Indications

Any evidence of volar subluxation of the proximal phalanx on x-ray is an indication for surgical treatment. In addition, surgery is indicated if the previously mentioned criteria are met under stress radiographs and stressing of the thumb. All patients with MRI-diagnosed Stener lesions require surgical intervention.

Technique

1. Positioning: The patient is positioned on the operating room table supine with the hand on the hand table. A tourniquet cuff is placed and the arm exsanguinated with the Esmarch wrap. The tourniquet is inflated to 250 mm Hg.
2. Incision: A small curvilinear incision is created over the MP joint to allow for access to the volar portion of the joint (Fig. 69–4). Dorsally, we attempt to identify and protect the branch of the superficial radial nerve. Meticulous dissection is done to identify the nerve to keep it out of harm's way.

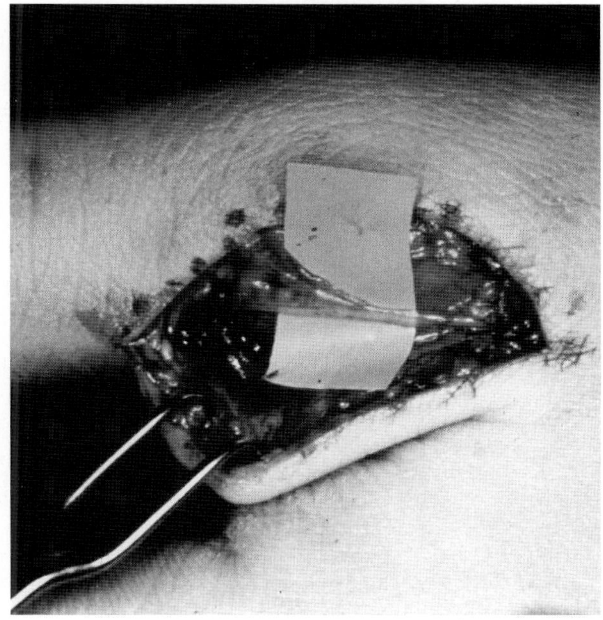

FIGURE 69–4. Incision used for approaching the ulnar collateral ligament in patients with skier's thumb. Note the dorsoulnar sensory nerve.

3. Once the adductor is exposed, the fibers are cut perpendicularly and tagged with a suture (Fig. 69–5*A*).
4. The Stener lesion is reduced, which allows identification of the collateral ligament.
5. The volar aspect of the proximal phalanx is burred; any loose bone fragments in the joint are removed as this site is prepared for a mini–suture anchor.
6. The mini-anchor with No. 2 Ethibond sutures is

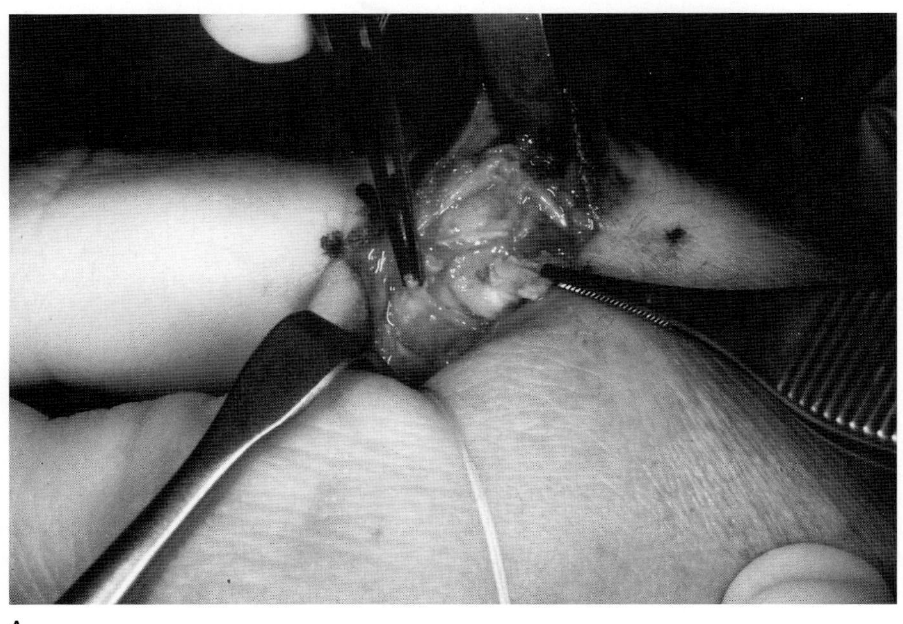

A

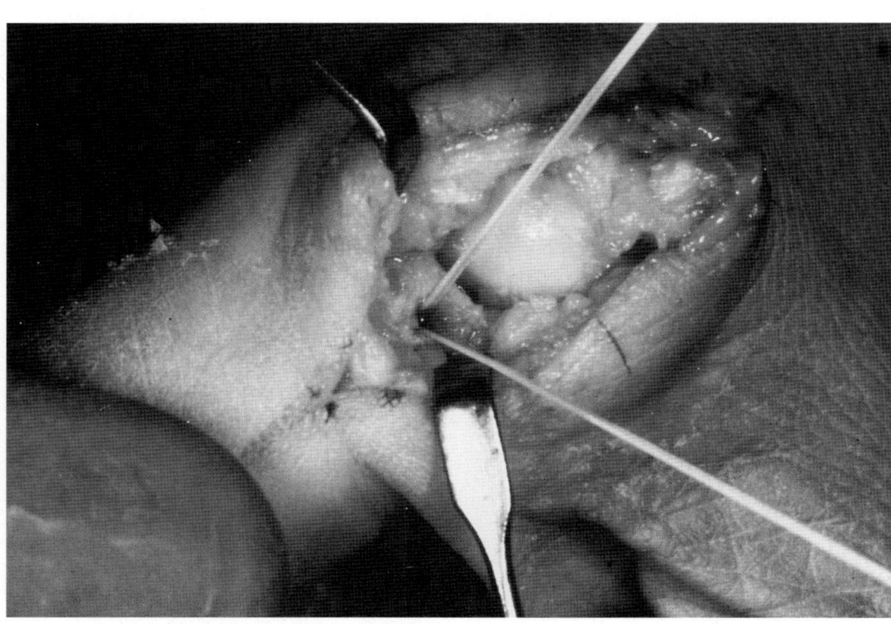

B

FIGURE 69–5. *A*, Exposure and identification of the Stener lesion. *B*, Volar aspect of the proximal phalanx with suture limbs of the mini-anchor exposed.

placed and the repair is performed while slight ulnar deviation stress is placed on the MP joint of the thumb at the time of suture tying (Fig. 69–5*B* and *C*).

7. The extensor hood and the accessory collateral ligament are also repaired, and the joint is inspected and irrigated.
8. The adductor is repaired anatomically, and the skin is closed in a subcuticular fashion with awareness of the superficial nerve (Fig. 69–5*D*).
9. A short-arm thumb spica bulky splint is placed, and the tourniquet is let down to allow the clinician to check the capillary refill to all digits.

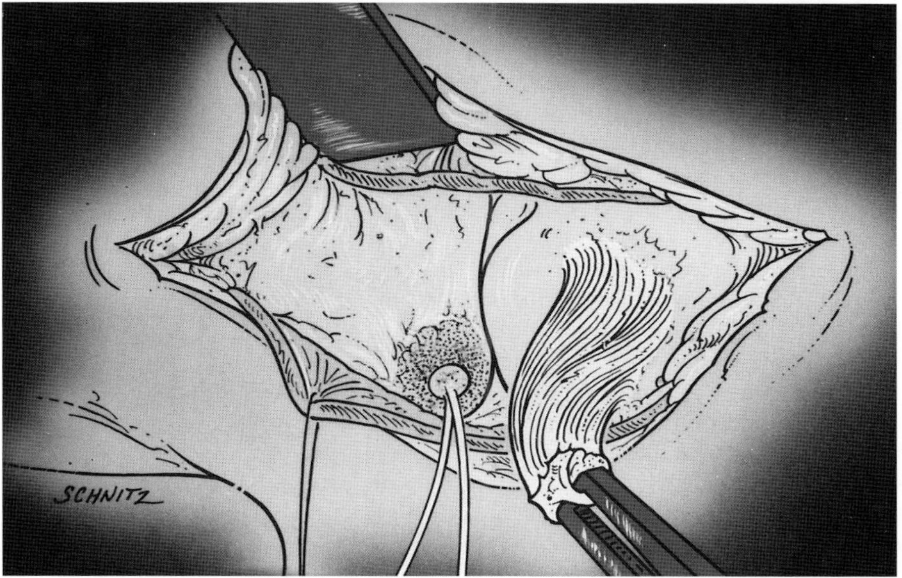

C

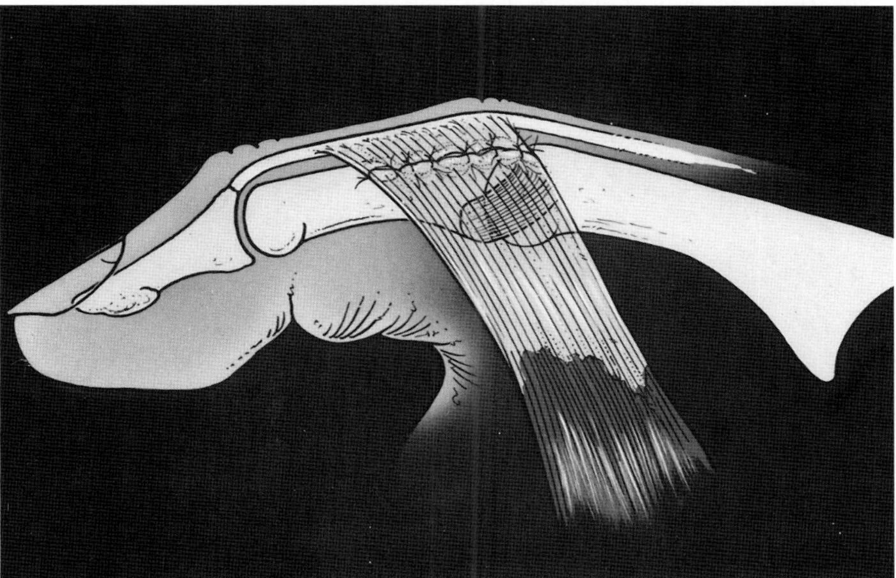

D

FIGURE 69–5 *Continued. C*, Artwork of mini-anchor of the volar aspect of the proximal phalanx with suture limbs of the mini-anchor exposed. *D*, Artwork of completed ulnar collateral ligament repair of the thumb.

POSTOPERATIVE MANAGEMENT

A short-arm bulky dressing is placed for 7 to 10 days after the repair of the ulnar collateral ligament has been completed. The thumb spica splint is removed to be replaced with a thumb spica gauntlet cast, which leaves the interphalangeal joint (thumb) free to begin motion. The cast is removed at 4 weeks, and a removable custom hand-base thumb spica splint is worn for an additional 2 weeks, as motion at the MP joint is begun in the flexion/extension arc but not in the adducted and abducted positions. At 6 weeks, stress is placed on the thumb in the adducted and abducted positions to allow for thumb apposition and strengthening. Patients usually wear their sport splint for up to 6 months after treatment for this injury.

COMPLICATIONS

Complications resulting from the treatment of skier's/gamekeeper's thumb are divided into short-term and long-term complications. Short-term complications include injury to the superficial branch of the radial nerve, wound infections, and failure of the repair. Long-term complications include loss of joint motion.

Superficial radial nerve injury is best avoided by meticulous attention to detail during the surgical exposure. Care should be taken to avoid excessive traction on the nerve, and attention during wound closure is needed to avoid incarceration of the closing sutures. Failure of the repair is an infrequent complication and it most commonly the result of noncompliance with splinting. Potential failure of the repair is one of the risk factors of an early motion protocol that does not incorporate a pin across the joint. However, it has been our experience that cooperative patients following this postoperative regimen have no problems with failure of the repair. The primary late complication is joint stiffness. Stiffness results from overprotection of the joint and failure to aggresively resume range-of-motion exercises after early ligament healing. The patient should be advised to continue stretching and range-of-motion exercises for at least 3 months following surgery. Late stiffness often results from discontinuing exercises too early in the healing process.

RESULTS

Patients who undergo surgery within 2 to 3 weeks of injury usually have excellent outcomes. Untreated partial tears with no evidence of instability on stress examination also have excellent results.

Patients with complete tears that go untreated usually develop pain, swelling, deformity, and post-traumatic arthritis. The treatment for this problem is an MP fusion; we do not repair ulnar collateral ligament tears at a late date.

REFERENCES

Heyman T, Gelberman RH, Duncan K, et al: Injuries of the ulnar collateral ligament of the thumb metacarpophalangeal joint. Biomechanical and prospective clinical studies on the usefulness of valgus stress testing. Clin Orthop 292:165–171, 1993.

Plancher KD, Ho CP, Cofield S, et al: Role of MR imaging in the management of skier's thumb injuries. MRI Clin North Am 7:73–84, 1999.

Smith R: Posttraumatic instability of the metacarpophalangeal joint of the thumb. J Bone Joint Surg [Am] 59:14–21, 1977.

CHAPTER 70

Treatment of Fractures of the Phalanges and Metacarpals

INTRODUCTION

Phalangeal and metacarpal fractures are some of the most common fractures in sports. Unfortunately, many of these fractures are often neglected or considered trivial by physicians and coaches. McCue referred to these neglected injuries as "the coaches' finger." Untreated hand fractures can lead to lifelong deformities, stiffness, and disabling pain. A majority of such fractures are treated nonoperatively. This section focuses on operative treatment of unstable fractures.

HISTORY AND PHYSICAL EXAMINATION

There are many types of fractures of the metacarpals or phalanges. The examining physician must note the resting posture of the injured hand in each case. When the fingers of the hand are flexed, a line should be drawn from the dorsal aspect of the proximal interphalangeal (PIP) joint to the fingernail. This line should converge not to a single fixed point, but rather directly to the area of the scaphoid from the radial artery to the palmaris longus. Malrotation is the most common malunion of phalangeal fractures, and it is diagnosed by examination, not by x-ray.

Deformities of the metacarpals or phalanges are often obvious. Local swelling and deformities are easy to identify. Recognition of rotational malalignment is essential (Fig. 70–1). Evaluation of the nerves and tendons, as well as motor and sensory tests, should always be performed. Open or closed injuries are noted. The color, temperature, capillary refill, and patency of collateral circulation should always be tested with an Allen's test of the wrist and digit. Satisfactory physical examination may not be possible without local anesthetic, but the block must be provided only after a careful two-point sensory examination has been completed.

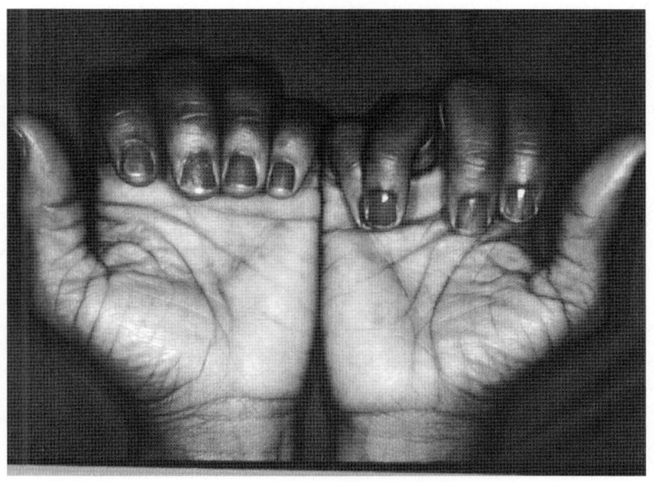

FIGURE 70–1. Clinical photo of rotational malalignment. Finger flexion readily identifies this deformity.

DIAGNOSTIC IMAGING

Radiographs are essential for evaluation of injuries in the hand, even when obvious injuries are not evident. Many significant fractures and joint injuries have been missed because x-rays were inadequate or because x-rays were not taken at all on the day of injury.

Evaluation of the metacarpals and the phalanges can be done with routine anteroposterior, lateral, and oblique films. Oblique films are especially helpful in assessing intra-articular fractures and in removing the overlap from adjacent digits. Special views for the fourth and fifth metacarpals are sometimes needed, including a lateral view with 10° of supination or 10° of pronation for the second and third metacarpals. Specialty views such as Brewerton's view (Fig. 70–2), with the hand lying flat against the cassette and the angle of the beam set at 30°, can help in evaluating metacarpal head fractures and in determinatng the presence or absence of intra-articular fragments. Before any treatment plan, either operative or nonoperative, is begun, x-rays must be evaluated; one must be able to visualize the fracture in its entirety from a joint above to a joint below the area of concern.

NONOPERATIVE MANAGEMENT

There are so many ways to treat phalangeal or metacarpal fractures that the choice of approach depends on the experience, expertise, and personal preference of the physician. No single method of treatment can be applied to all fractures of the phalanx and metacarpals, and a surgeon must be comfortable with multiple techniques. For an athlete, the choice of method will always be influenced by the season, but the potential complications must be weighed against the risks and benefits. Fracture healing will take the same amount of time no matter which method is chosen, if treatment is performed correctly.

Many fractures of the phalanges can be treated by closed reduction and cast immobilization (transverse fractures), but the fracture must be stable. Spiral oblique fractures are inherently unstable and will fall out of alignment. Soft tissue conditions with any neurovascular compromise or swelling may preclude nonoperative treatment. The preferred position for immobilization is the intrinsic plus position, with the metacarpal phalangeal (MP) joint in at least 70°, if not 90°, of flexion and the PIP and distal interphalangeal (DIP) joints in extension.

A combination of closed reduction and immobilization works well for the majority of metacarpal shaft fractures. These stable fractures can be treated with minimal or no immobilization. A proximal phalanx dorsal blocking cast can be applied with an adjacent finger held in the cast. When this hand is in the intrinsic plus position (Fig. 70–3), contracture is avoided and the intrinsics are maintained in a relaxed position. This position also effectively immobilizes stable fractures of the proximal phalanx.

RELEVANT ANATOMY

Understanding the relationship of the extensor mechanism to the hand skeleton is essential for operative management. An ideal surgical exposure preserves gliding surfaces, minimally disrupts the extensor mechanism, and provides adequate exposure for application of fixation.

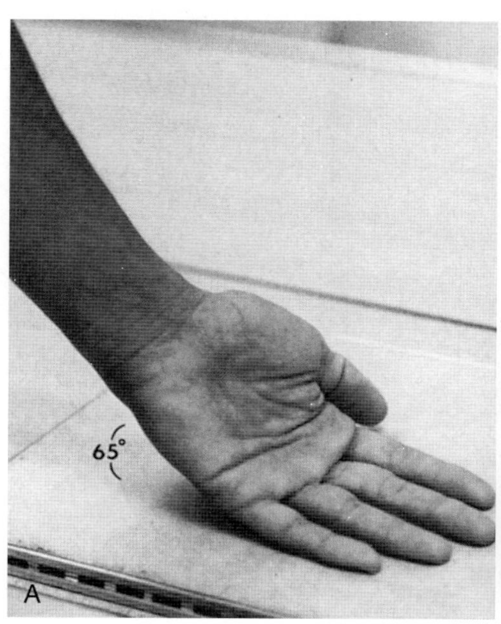

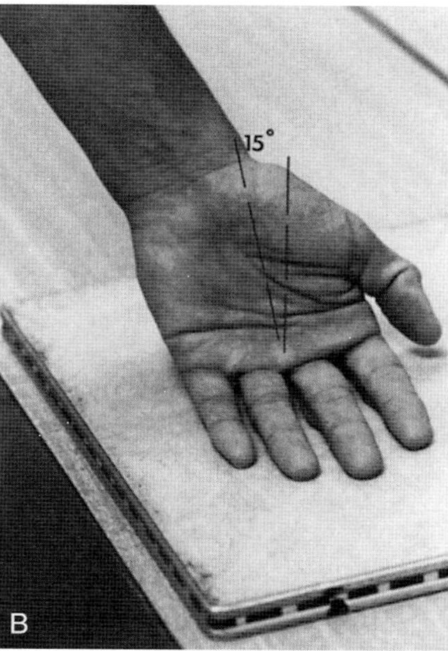

FIGURE 70–2. *A* and *B*, Brewerton's view is helpful in allowing visualization of fractures of the metacarpal head and neck. (From Berquest TH: Imaging of Orthopedic Trauma and Surgery. Philadelphia, WB Saunders, 1986, p 654.)

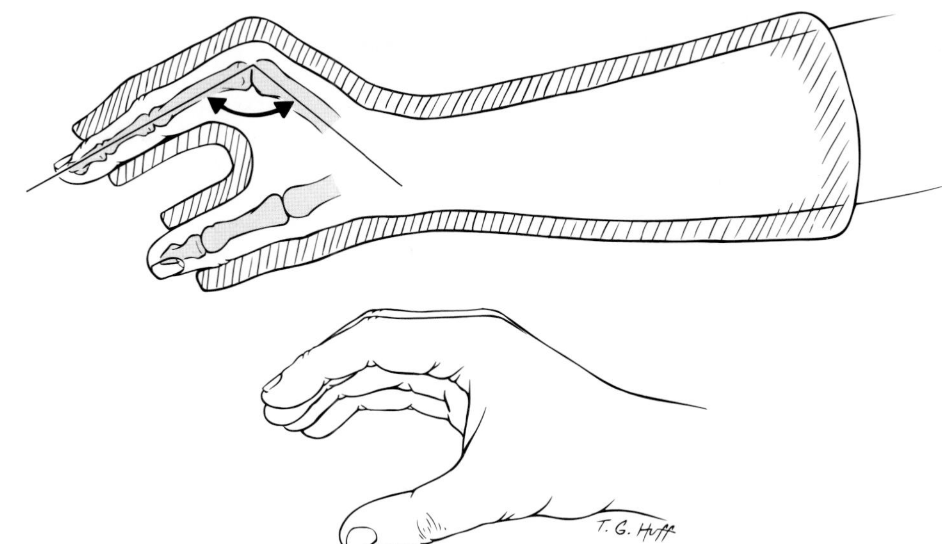

FIGURE 70–3. Intrinsic plus position cast immobilizes the hand. The fingers can be left free at the interphalangeal joints to allow range of motion, but the metacarpophalangeal joints are limited at 70° of flexion. (From Jupiter JB, Axelrod TS, Belsky MR: Fractures and dislocations of the hand. In Browner BD [ed]: Skeletal Trauma: Fractures, Dislocations, Ligamentous Injuries, 2nd ed. Philadelphia, WB Saunders, 1998, p 1233.)

The extensor mechanism covers the base of the proximal phalanx. This necessitates splitting the tendon to expose this area (Fig. 70–4). Distally, the tendon can be retracted. The sagittal band maintains the central band's position over the metacarpal head. Rupture of the sagittal band fibers results in subluxation of the tendon (boxer's knuckle). In a cross section of the finger, the flexor tendons, flexor sheath, and overlying soft tissues occupy the volar half of the digit (Fig. 70–5). The skeleton lies in the dorsal half of the finger. This relationship is import to consider during placement of percutaneous pins. The relationship of the neurovasular structures to the skeleton is best appreciated in the cross-sectional view of the finger; because of the volar location of the neurovascular bundles, the midlateral approach is ideal for most fracture exposures.

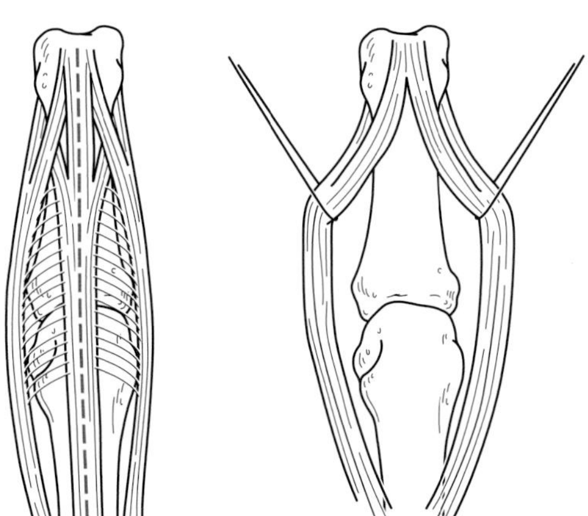

FIGURE 70–4. Dorsal exposure of the proximal phalanx through the extensor tendon–splitting approach. (From Jupiter JB, Axelrod TS, Belsky MR: Fractures and dislocations of the hand. In Browner BD [ed]: Skeletal Trauma: Fractures, Dislocations, Ligamentous Injuries, 2nd ed. Philadelphia, WB Saunders, 1998, p 1294.)

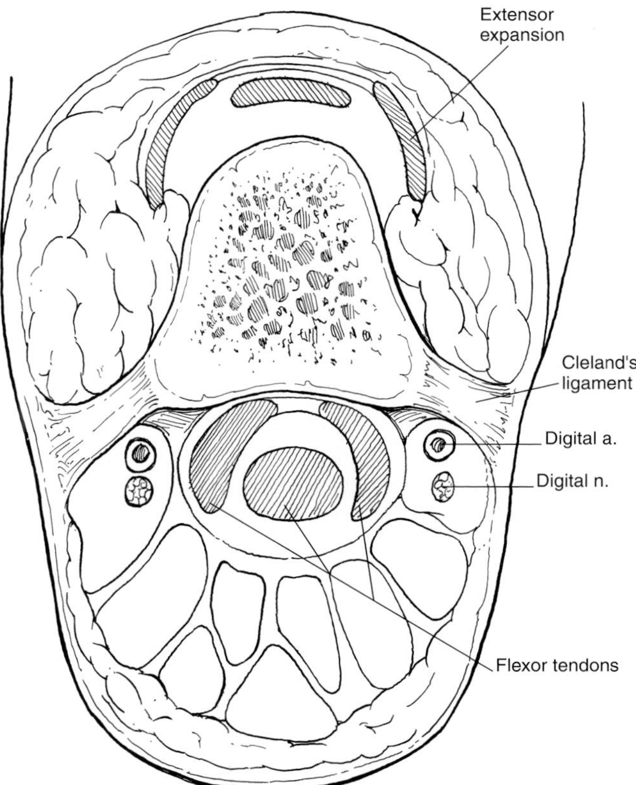

FIGURE 70–5. Cross-sectional image of the finger. Note the relative position of the bone in the dorsal half of the digit and the volar location of the digital nerves and arteries.

SURGICAL *TECHNIQUE*

Indications

The indications for operative intervention with metacarpal and phalangeal fractures include spiral and short oblique fractures that may lead to malrotation and shortening. A few millimeters of shortening is acceptable in the metacarpal but not in the phalanx. Malrotation is never acceptable. Operative intervention is required for intra-articular fractures, open fractures, fractures with bone loss, and multiple phalangeal or metacarpal fractures that occur with a neurovascular or tendon injury. Fractures associated with extensive soft tissue injury may require stable fixation to allow early mobilization. In addition, skin loss and hand fractures associated with polytrauma need operative repair.

The selection of treatment depends on many factors, some of which include fracture location, intra-articular or extra-articular deformity, angulation, rotation, shortening, open or closed injury, associated neurovascular and soft tissue injuries, and the nature of the fracture (i.e., transverse, spiral, comminuted, or oblique). Additional considerations for operative reduction or internal fixation include the surgeon's skill with the fixation device, the patient's ability to work postoperatively with an appropriate plan, and the patient's occupation.

The goal is always to avoid prolonged immobilization because of the risk of permanent deformity and stiffness, but moving fractures aggressively when fixation is not rigid can lead to soft tissue damage, infection, the need for a second procedure, and technique failure. Operative fixation must ultimately have a better outcome than nonoperative management, and the risks and benefits must always be explained to the patient.

General Concepts

Pins must be treated to avoid infection and breakage. Any pin that is loose must be removed because this can form a nidus for osteomyelitis. Multiple passes during pinning to the same area can burn bone and is discouraged; therefore, the most experienced physician should intervene rather than allowing for multiple passes in a complex finger fracture.

Rigid fixation is needed for an athlete who must go back to performance or if the fracture requires internal fixation to obtain stabilization. Interosseous wiring, tension band wiring, cerclage wiring, and mini-fragment plates and screws may be used. Plates provide the most rigid fixation. Tension band wiring and interosseous wiring are superior to Kirschner wires for rigid constructs. However, no one knows how strong the fixation needs to be in a hand fracture. Early motion with plates and screws permits an athlete to return to sports earlier than would occur without such motion, but risks not limited to infections are involved. Plates are well tolerated in the metacarpals, but they are best avoided in the phalanges.

Immobilization for longer than 4 weeks is associated with permanent loss of motion. The treatment selected and its application must achieve motion of the finger by 4 weeks (preferably, by 2 weeks).

Technique

Exposures

Phalangeal

Soft tissue handling has a profound impact on the outcome of fracture fixation in the skeleton of the hand. The ideal surgical exposure provides maximal visualization for the surgeon while preserving soft tissue gliding planes and minimizing surgical insult to the surrounding tendons. Thus, this topic is given special attention. Exposure of the phalanges for fracture fixation is done primarily from a dorsal or lateral approach. Palmar exposures are generally discouraged, except in the case of PIP joint exposure for a volar plate arthroplasty.

Skin Incision

Proximal and middle phalanx exposure is accomplished through a dorsal longitudinal incision or a midaxial incision, with the terminal aspects of the incision curving toward the midline of the digit (Fig. 70–6). The ends of the incision are incorporated into the dorsal skin creases for best cosmesis. This provides an extensile exposure of the extensor hood, as well as access to the midaxial line.

Extensor Tendon

At the middle phalangeal level, the extensor tendon can be retracted for exposure of the fracture. The periosteum should be incised at the midaxial line and raised as a flap, thereby preserving the gliding surface between the periosteum and the extensor tendon. The proximal phalanx can be exposed through a dorsal longitudinal split in the extensor tendon (Fig. 70–7). Similar to in the middle phalanx, it is recommended that the periosteum be raised as a flap to allow exposure to the fracture and preservation of a gliding surface between the fracture plane and the extensor tendon (Fig. 70–8).

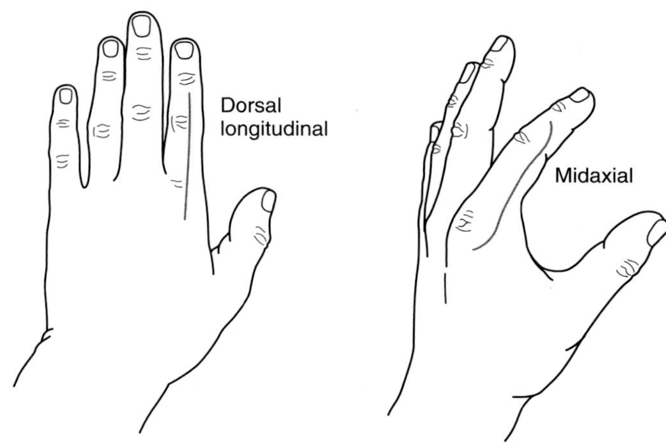

FIGURE 70–6. Illustration depicting the dorsal longitudinal and midaxial exposures used in fracture exposure for middle and proximal phalangeal fractures. Note that the midaxial incision can be curved toward the midline at its proximal and distal aspects. Incorporating these terminal curves into the skin creases over the joints results in a particularly desirable cosmetic result. (From Jupiter JB, Axelrod TS, Belsky MR: Fractures and dislocations of the hand. In Browner BD: Skeletal Trauma: Fractures, Dislocations, Ligamentous Injuries, 2nd ed. Philadelphia, WB Saunders, 1998, p 1294.)

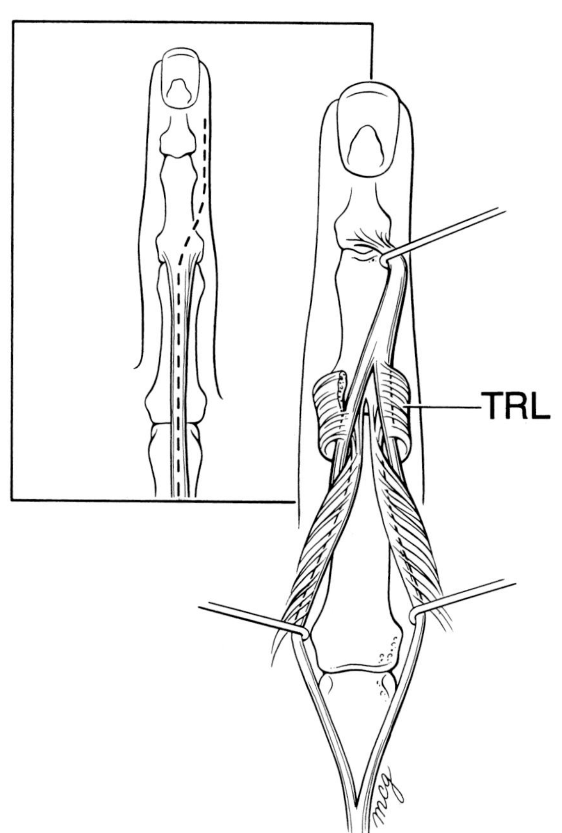

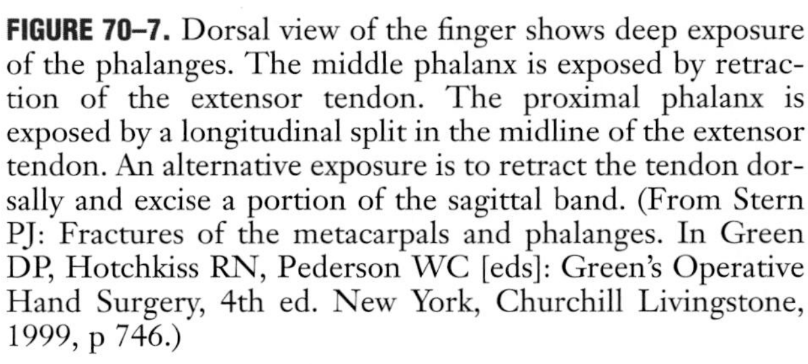
FIGURE 70–7. Dorsal view of the finger shows deep exposure of the phalanges. The middle phalanx is exposed by retraction of the extensor tendon. The proximal phalanx is exposed by a longitudinal split in the midline of the extensor tendon. An alternative exposure is to retract the tendon dorsally and excise a portion of the sagittal band. (From Stern PJ: Fractures of the metacarpals and phalanges. In Green DP, Hotchkiss RN, Pederson WC [eds]: Green's Operative Hand Surgery, 4th ed. New York, Churchill Livingstone, 1999, p 746.)

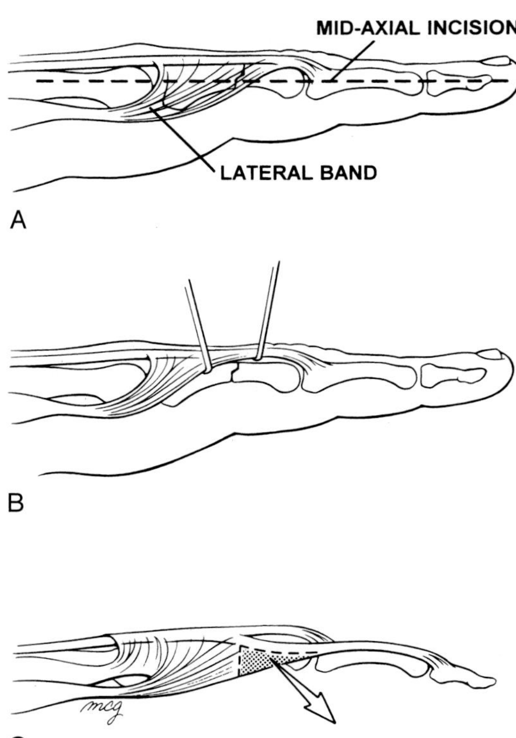

FIGURE 70–8. Lateral exposure provides excellent access to fractures of the middle and distal aspects of the proximal phalanx; however, for fractures at the base of the proximal phalanx, the dorsal tendon–splitting approach is most extensile. *A*, Midaxial incision. *B*, Lateral band retracted. *C*, A triangular portion of the distal sagittal band is excised to facilitate exposure. (From Stern PJ: Fractures of the metacarpal and phalanges. In Green DP, Hotchkiss RN, Pederson WC [eds]: Green's Operative Hand Surgery, 4th ed. New York, Churchill Livingstone, 1999, p 746.)

Exposure of the PIP joint may be achieved through the dorsal longitudinal split; an alternative is to split between the lateral band and the central slip (Fig. 70–9).

The thumb is less problematic. A dorsal longitudinal incision or a midaxial incision provides extensile exposure of the thumb. The extensor tendons in this region are relatively mobile and can be retracted for adequate exposure through the dorsal or lateral approach (Fig. 70–10). Near the MP joint, the extensor hood is divided at the insertion to the extensor tendon so that a very thin strip of the longitudinally oriented fibers of the extensor tendon is left attached to the sagittal band. This facilitates later repair.

Exposure of the metacarpals is straightforward. Skin incisions are placed between the metacarpals and are tapered toward the midline of the metacarpal on each end. This keeps the scar away from the gliding plane of the extensor tendon. The extensor tendons are mobile and are easily retracted (Fig. 70–11).

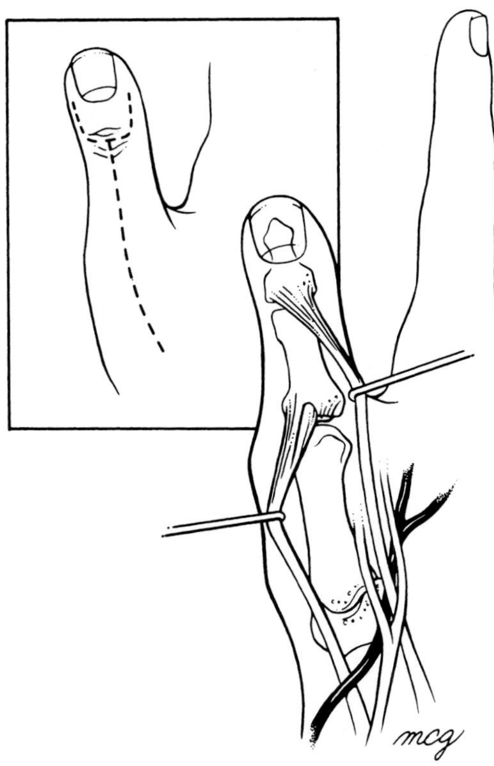

FIGURE 70–10. Exposure of the thumb metacarpal phalanges. Retractors are on the extensor pollicis longus and extensor pollicis brevis tendons. (From Stern PJ: Fractures of the metacarpals and phalanges. In Green DP, Hotchkiss RN, Pederson WC [eds]: Green's Operative Hand Surgery, 4th ed. New York, Churchill Livingstone, 1999, p 758.)

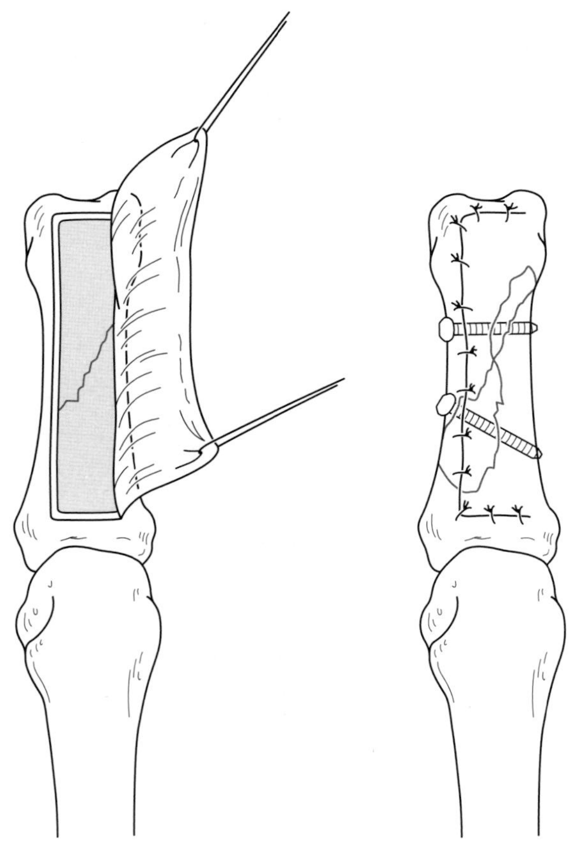

FIGURE 70–9. The periosteum is elevated in a rectangular flap and then is repaired following fixation of the fracture. This provides a gliding surface for the extensor tendon over the hardware and the fracture. (From Jupiter JB, Axelrod TS, Belsky MR: Fractures and dislocations of the hand. In Browner BD [ed]: Skeletal Trauma: Fractures, Dislocations, Ligamentous Injuries, 2nd ed. Philadelphia, WB Saunders, 1998, p 1294.)

Fixation Techniques

Kirschner Wire Fixation

Kirschner wire fixation of phalangeal fractures is the most commonly employed technique. As a rule, 0.035-inch K-wires are used for phalangeal fractures and 0.045-inch wires for metacarpal fractures. Very small fragments or fixation of fractures in small children may require the use of 0.028-inch K-wires. In general, K-wire fixation is performed with a minimum of two wires; often, three are used. Pinning fractures in distraction must be avoided. Reduction and compression of the fracture site with towel clips or pointed reduction forceps facilitates anatomic fixation. K-wire fixation of transverse fractures is performed such that the K-wires cross either proximally or distally to the fracture site to provide maximum rotation stability (Fig. 70–12). Periarticular fractures can be pinned with the K-wire passing through the adjacent joint (Fig. 70–13).

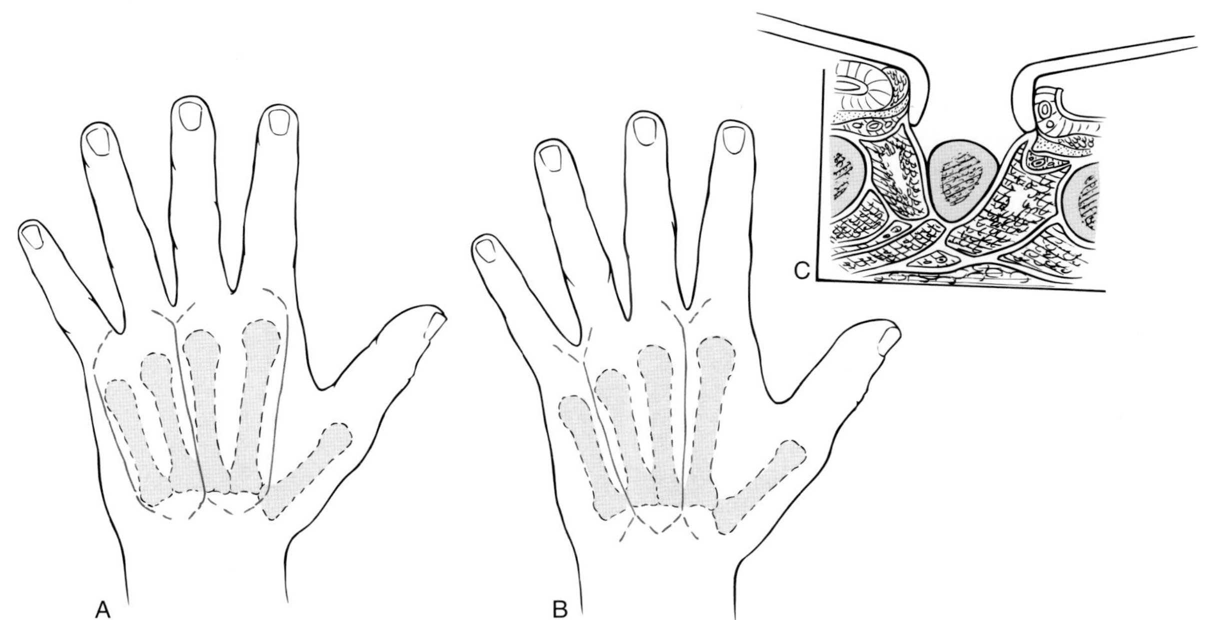

FIGURE 70–11. *A*, Incisions for individual metacarpal fracture exposure. *B*, Incisions for exposure of multiple metacarpal fractures. *C*, Reflexion of the metacarpal periosteum is performed with a flap, as was illustrated in Figure 70–9, with care taken to minimize elevation of the interosseous muscles. (From Jupiter JB, Axelrod TS, Belsky MR: Fractures and dislocations of the hand. In Browner BD [ed]: Skeletal Trauma: Fractures, Dislocations, Ligamentous Injuries, 2nd ed. Philadelphia, WB Saunders, 1998, p 1255.)

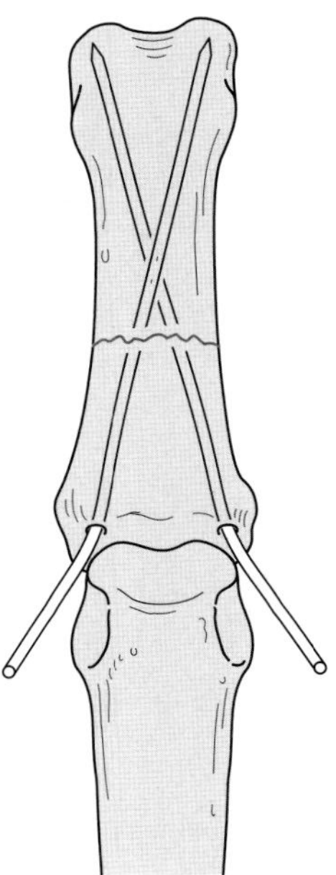

FIGURE 70–12. K-wires should not cross at the fracture site when transverse fractures are treated with axial pinning. (Redrawn from Heim P, Pfeiffer KM: Internal Fixation of Small Fractures, 3rd ed. New York, Springer-Verlag, 1987.)

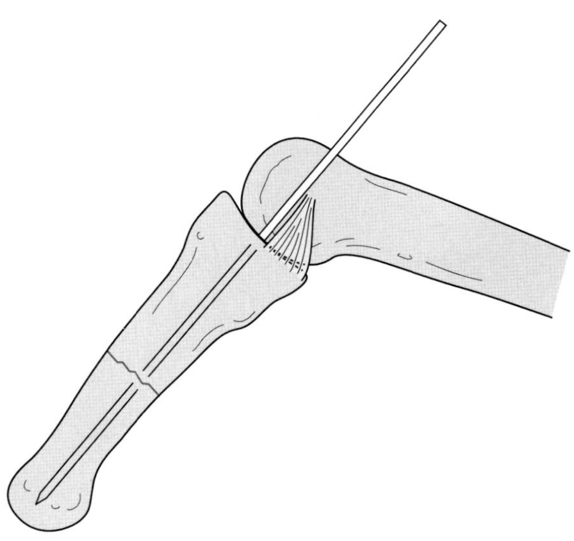

FIGURE 70–13. Transarticular pinning is useful for periarticular fractures of the proximal phalangeal base. To avoid broken pins, 0.45 K-wires are recommended. (Redrawn from Heim P, Pfeiffer KM: Internal Fixation of Small Fractures, 3rd ed. New York, Springer-Verlag, 1987.)

Pins are removed at no later than 4 weeks. We routinely remove pins at 2 to 3 weeks for simple fractures with near-anatomic reduction. Adequate soft callus has formed by this time to allow protected range of motion. Awaiting the appearance of fracture callus on postoperative x-rays unnecessarily delays the removal of pins and may result in permanent stiffness.

Interosseous Wiring Technique

Interosseous wiring provides more rigid fixation than do K-wires alone. This technique is particularly useful in unstable transverse fractures. An oblique K-wire combined with 26-gauge stainless steel wire is passed through two transverse drill holes (Fig. 70–14). This low-profile fixation is rigid enough to allow early motion, and it avoids the larger surgical exposure required for plate fixation.

Composite Wire Fixation

Composite wire fixation is particularly helpful in the management of complex fractures of the metacarpals and phalanges. This approach allows fixation of small fragments with K-wires and 26-gauge stainless steel wire looped over the ends of the cut pins. It provides rigid fixation similar to that provided by a plate. These wires should be cut off as short as possible (Fig. 70–15). This is particularly helpful in highly comminuted fractures in which screw and plate fixation is problematic. A drawback to the technique is that some component of the hardware must be removed in approximately 50% of cases; however, this is usually done in the office with the patient under local anesthesia. This technique can be combined with plate and screw fixation.

Screw Fixation

Screw fixation is used in the management of long oblique fractures. To manage fractures with screws alone, it is recommended that the length of the fracture be at least 3 times the width of the shaft. The choice of implant depends on skeletal size and fracture location. Low-profile implants are widely available now. In general, fractures of the phalanges are fixed with 1.0 to 2.0 screws, and fractures of the metacarpals are fixed with 2.4 to 2.7 screws. Self-tapping screws diminish the technical complexity of this technique.

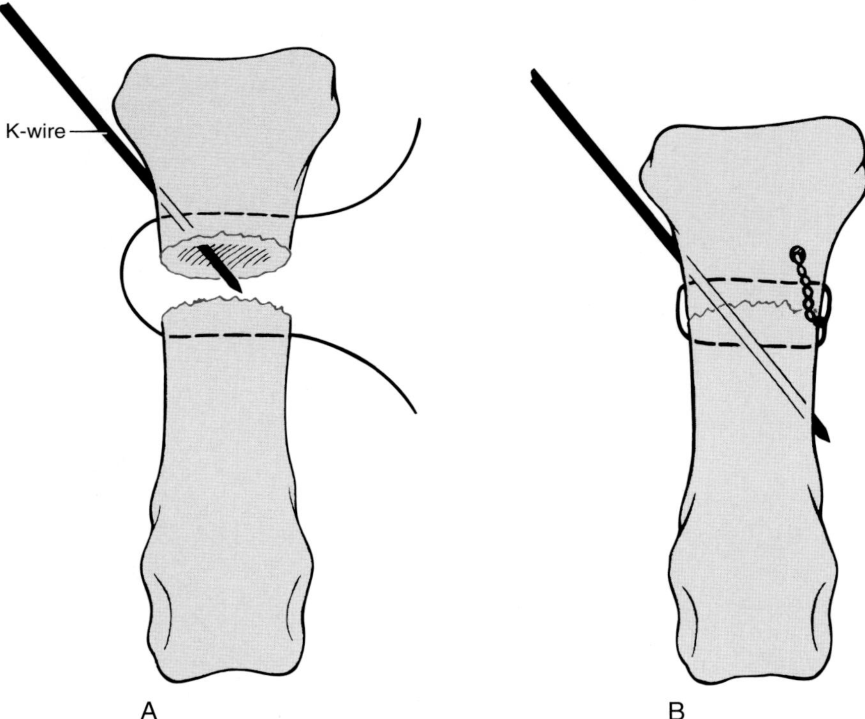

FIGURE 70–14. Illustration of interosseous wiring technique. *A*, A 26-gauge stainless steel wire is passed transversely proximal and distal to the fracture line and just dorsal to the midaxis of the phalanx. A 0.035-inch K-wire is passed obliquely into the distal fragment until the tip is in the fracture line. *B*, The fracture is reduced, the K-wire is passed into the proximal fragment, and the stainess steel wire is tightened. The twisted end can be placed into a drill hole in the cortex. (From Jupiter JB, Axelrod TS, Belsky MR: Fractures and dislocations of the hand. In Browner BD [ed]: Skeletal Trauma: Fractures, Dislocations, Ligamentous Injuries, 2nd ed. Philadelphia, WB Saunders, 1998, p 1241.)

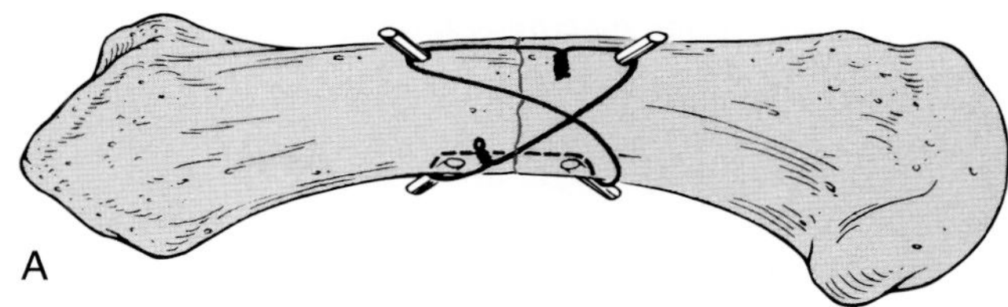

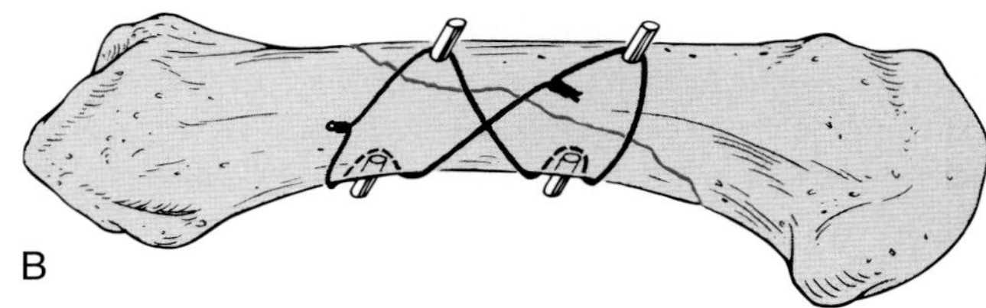

FIGURE 70–15. Illustration of composite wiring technique. *A*, for a transverse or short oblique fracture, K-wires are placed in a crossed pattern, and the stainless steel 26-gauge wire is passed around the tips in a modified figure-eight. *B*, For spiral or long oblique fractures, parallel K-wires are placed perpendicular to the fracture plane. (From Jupiter JB, Axelrod TS, Belsky MR: Fractures and dislocations of the hand. In Browner BD [ed]: Skeletal Trauma: Fractures, Dislocations, Ligamentous Injuries, 2nd ed. Philadelphia, WB Saunders, 1998, p 1244.)

Plate Fixation

Plate fixation in the hand skeleton should be infrequent and should be reserved primarily for the metacarpals. Use of plates in the fingers is discouraged because of the frequent need for removal of hardware and tenolysis. However, highly comminuted fractures may require fixation with plates to allow adequate stability for early motion (Fig. 70–16). For the phalanges, 1.5- and 2.0-mm plates are recommended. For the metacarpals, 2.4- to 2.7-mm plates are desirable. Synthes condylar plates (Synthes, Paoli, PA) are useful in the management of periarticular fractures, but they are not recommended for the novice fracture surgeon. Their application requires an extensive exposure of the joint and precise placement of the implants.

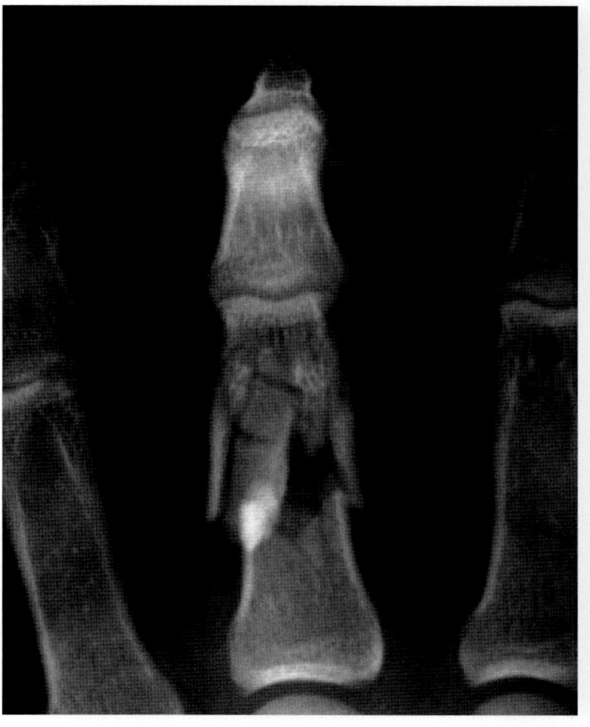

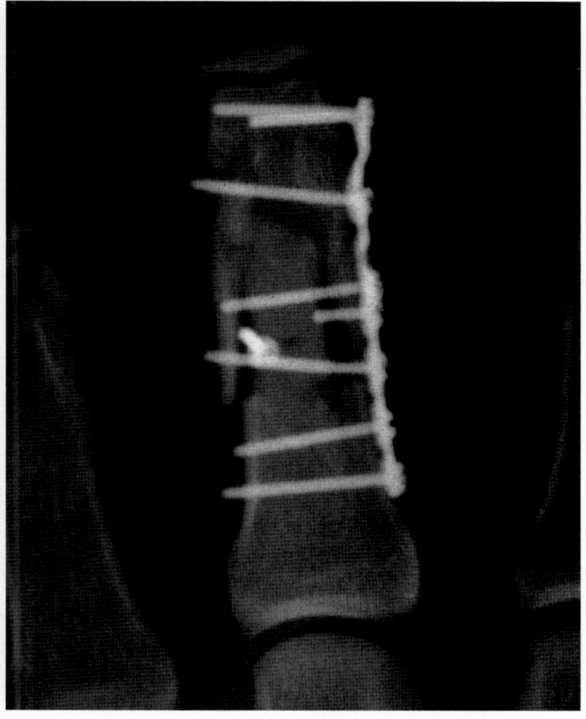

FIGURE 70–16. *A*, This highly comminuted fracture occurred from a crush injury. *B*, Rigid fixation with a plate permitted early active range of motion.

Authors' Preference for Specific Fractures

Distal Phalanx Fracture

Open treatment of distal phalangeal fractures is rarely indicated. Pinning may be required in fractures of the distal phalanx when fracture displacement occurs in association with a nailbed laceration. Stepoffs in the fracture site under a nailbed repair should not be accepted. If the fracture is unstable, anatomic reduction and pin fixation should be accomplished, along with nailbed repair. Mallet fractures with associated joint subluxation can be managed effectively with transarticular pin fixation using 0.035-inch K-wires (Fig. 70–17). In addition, the dorsal fracture fragment can be directly pinned with 0.028-inch K-wires, although this is not required in most cases. Open reduction of this injury is discouraged because the results are not better than those associated with closed pinning.

Proximal and Middle Phalanges Fracture

Fractures of the middle and proximal phalanges are primarily managed with percutaneous K-wires. Transverse fractures are pinned with longitudinally crossed K-wires. Oblique fractures are pinned with two or three transverse 0.035-inch K-wires. It is recommended that the fracture be firmly reduced and held with a percutaneous towel clip before pin placement is begun. Placement of axial pins with the finger flexed alongside an adjacent digit facilitates reduction of rotational malalignment (Fig. 70–18). Pinning in distraction is associated with high rates of nonunion and malunion. Open fractures and fractures requiring open reduction and internal fixation are particularly amenable to stabilization with interosseous wiring or composite wiring techniques. Plate application is discouraged in the middle and proximal phalanges. However, in cases of highly comminuted fractures, plates may provide the only stable fixation possible for management of the soft tissue injury.

Unstable fractures of the proximal phalanx are most often managed with percutaneous K-wires. If early active range of motion is desirable, percutaneous lag screw fixation of oblique fractures provides rigid fixation with minimal surgical trauma to the digit. Periarticular fractures at the base of the proximal phalanx can be problematic for pinning, especially when the fractures are comminuted. In treating these difficult fractures, the technique of Eaton is particularly helpful.

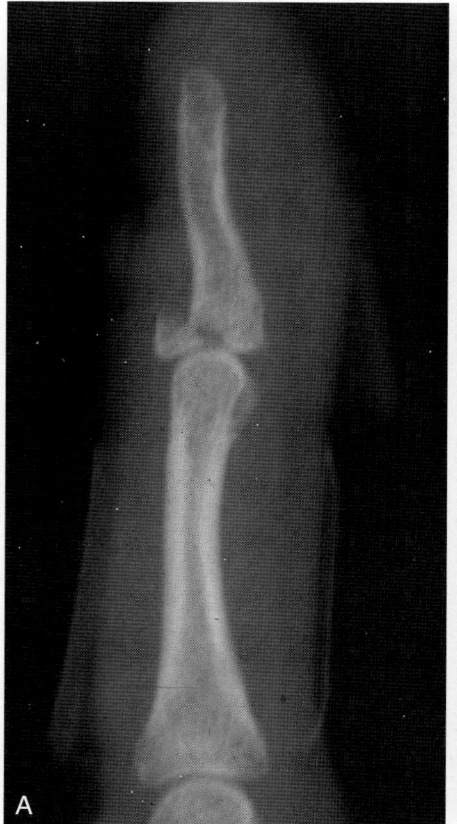

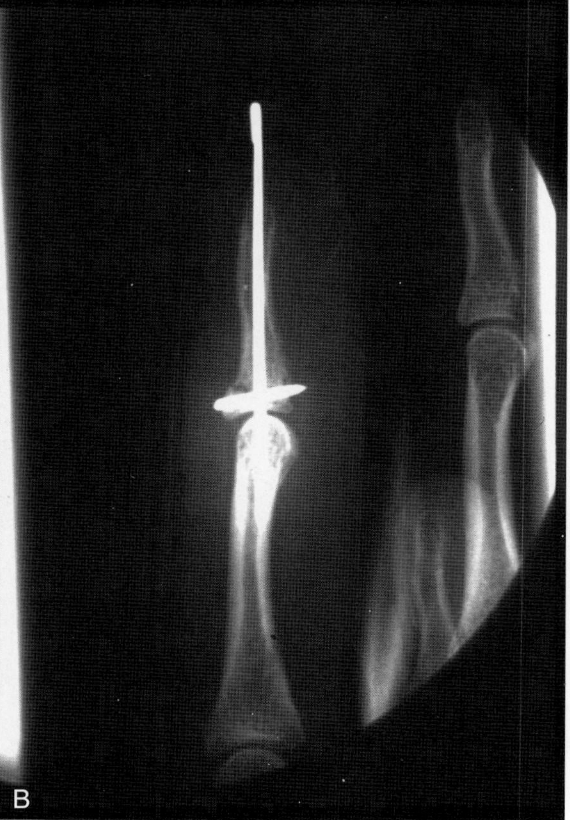

FIGURE 70–17. *A*, X-ray of a mallet fracture with joint subluxation managed with percutaneous pinning *(B)*.

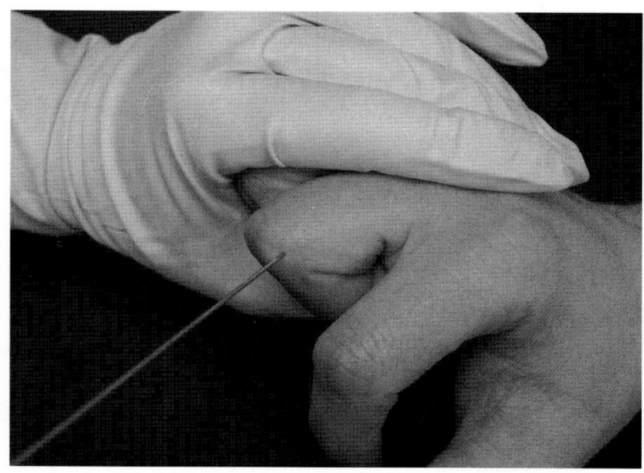

FIGURE 70–18. Axial pinning with the finger flexed and braced by an adjacent intact digit facilitates rotational alignment.

Proximal Interphalangeal Joint Fracture-Dislocation

Fracture-dislocation of the PIP joint is a particularly challenging injury. Fortunately, a majority of these patients can be managed with a dorsal blocking splint and progressively increasing range of motion over a period of 4 weeks. Fractures involving 30% to 50% of the joint may be unstable in a dorsal blocking splint. Fractures involving greater than 50% of the joint or comminution extending through the dorsal cortex cannot be managed with a dorsal blocking splint. These fractures are best managed with traction and early range of motion. A technique described by Suzuki is our preferred approach to these difficult injuries (Fig. 70–19). We find the results of this technique gratifying; as a result, we rarely perform palmar plate arthroplasty.

Palmar plate arthroplasty is indicated for PIP fracture-dislocations that cannot be managed with dorsal blocking splints. This is a technically demanding procedure that is best performed by an experienced hand surgeon, and it is not reviewed here.

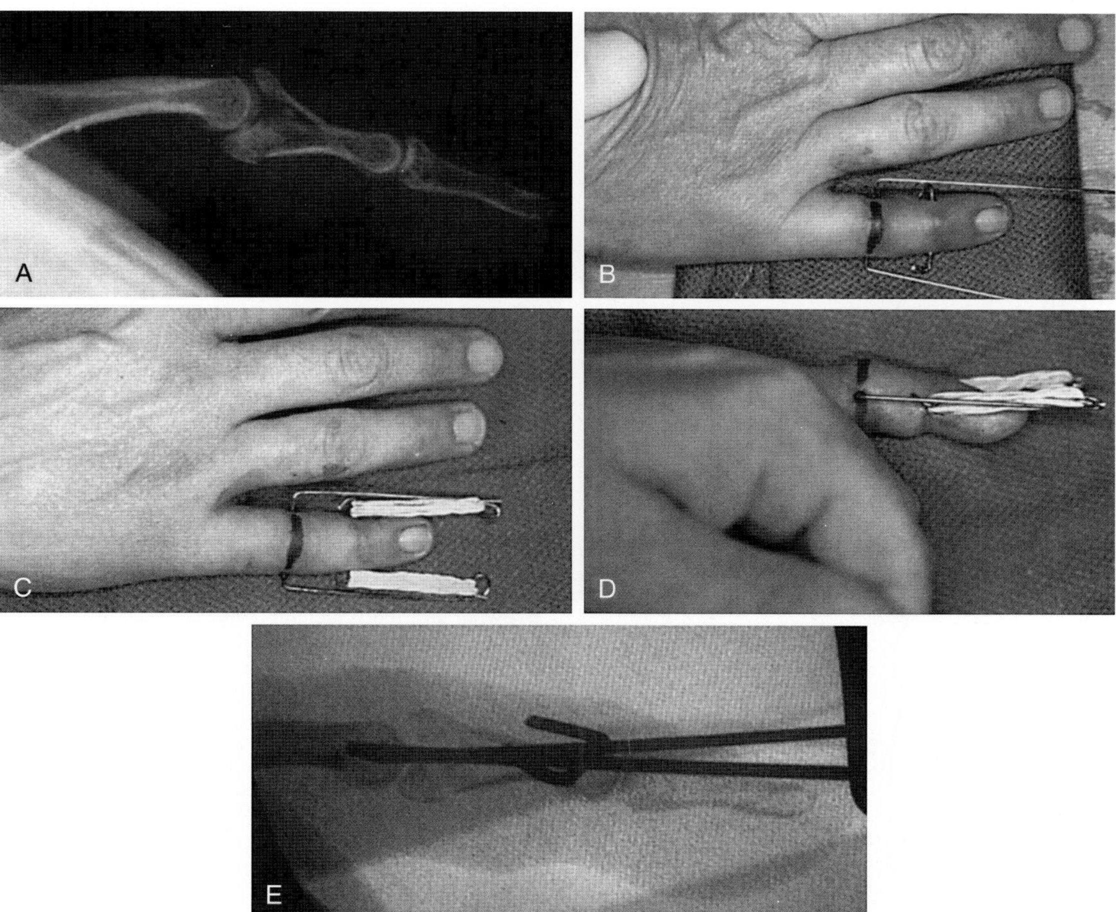

FIGURE 70–19. A comminuted fracture of the middle phalangeal base *(A)* is treated with traction technique as described by Suzuki *(B)* (see Reference section at end of chapter). Anteroposterior view *(C)* and lateral view *(D)* of final construct. Lateral x-ray showing concentric reduction of PIP joint *(E)*. The materials used here are 0.035 K-wires and dental rubber bands. Early motion is permitted, and the device is removed after 4 weeks. (From Glickel SZ, Barron OA: Proximal interphalangeal joint fracture dislocations. Hand Clin 16:342, 2000.)

Metacarpal Fractures

Metacarpal shaft fractures, like phalangeal fractures, are treated with percutaneous K-wires when fixation is indicated. Isolated single metacarpal fractures rarely require operative intervention and can be managed effectively with splints. Transverse fractures can be pinned transversely to the adjacent intact metacarpal (Fig. 70–20), or they can be pinned axially with longitudinal pins (Fig. 70–21). Surgeons who pin hand fractures infrequently find transverse pinning less difficult.

The most frequent indication for plate fixation of metacarpals is multiple metacarpal fractures. Pin fixation is the recommended treatment, and the pins are removed at 4 weeks regardless of the appearance of callus on x-rays. Plate fixation is recommended for polytrauma because the hand is likely to be bearing weight during rehabilitation. Multiple comminuted fractures are usually plated because percutaneous pinning is problematic.

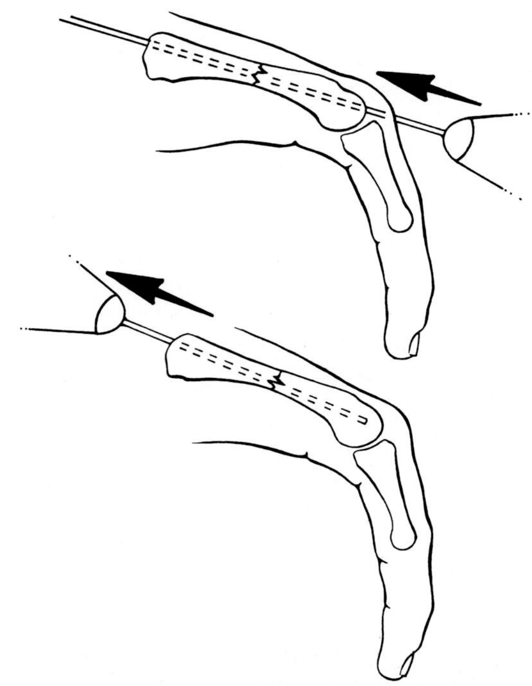

FIGURE 70–20. Axial pinning of the metacarpal fracture with 0.045 K-wires. (From Stern PJ: Fractures of the metacarpals and phalanges. In Green DP, Hotchkiss RN, Pederson WC [eds]: Green's Operative Hand Surgery, 4th ed. New York, Churchill Livingstone, 1999, p 721.)

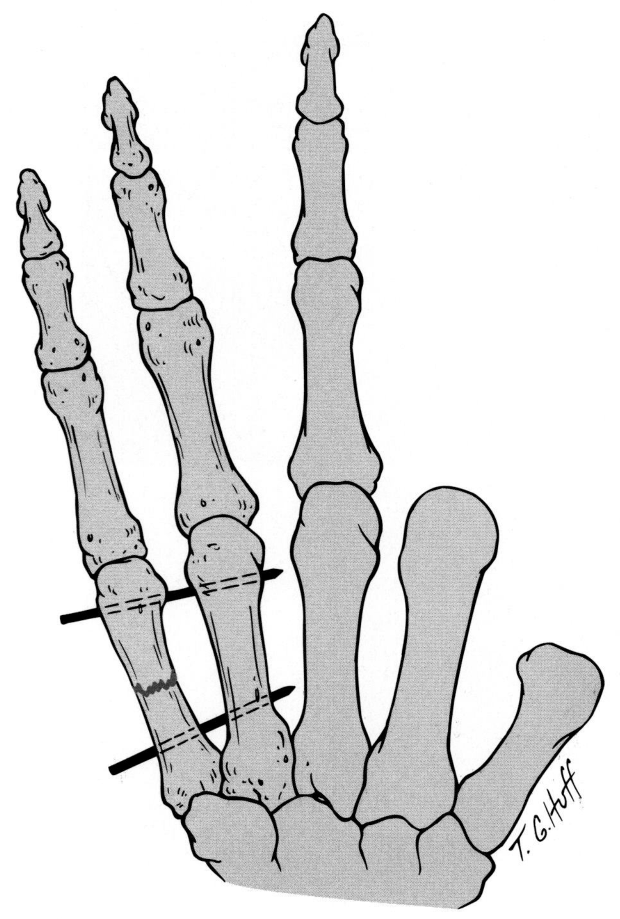

FIGURE 70–21. Transverse pinning of a metacarpal fracture to the adjacent intact metacarpal. (From Jupiter JB, Axelrod TS, Belsky MR: Fractures and dislocations of the hand. In Browner BD [ed]: Skeletal Trauma: Fractures, Dislocations, Ligamentous Injuries, 2nd ed. Philadelphia, WB Saunders, 1998, p 1257.)

POSTOPERATIVE MANAGEMENT

Early motion is desirable in the management of phalangeal and metacarpal fractures. Many factors influence the patient's ability to proceed with early range of motion. Fracture geometry, soft tissue injury, and patient reliability play major roles in decision making. As a rule, pins should be removed no later than 4 weeks in phalangeal fractures. With stable, minimally displaced fracture patterns, they can safely be removed in 2 weeks to allow early active motion. Leaving pins in longer than 4 weeks is associated with permanent stiffness of the digit.

When plate or screw fixation is performed, range-of-motion exercises are initiated after 4 to 5 days of soft tissue rest. Plate and screw fixation of the hand skeleton without the incorporation of an early active range-of-motion program results in permanent stiffness of the hand. Therefore, open reduction and internal fixation should be avoided in any patient who is unable to comply with an early active motion program.

COMPLICATIONS

Malunion and Nonunion

Malunion is a common complication of metacarpal and phalangeal fractures. The most common form is malrotation. When malunion presents a functional problem, corrective osteotomies are effective in restoring motion. Nonunion is infrequent in phalangeal and metacarpal fractures and is most often associated with percutaneous pinning of the fracture in distraction. When nonunion occurs, it is best managed with open reduction and internal fixation.

Loss of Motion

Loss of motion is the most frequent complication of phalangeal fracture fixation. Treatment of stiffness should begin with a comprehensive hand therapy program, including active and passive range-of-motion exercises combined with dynamic splinting or progressive static splinting. Tenolysis and capsulotomy of stiff joints are often helpful when therapy has failed to restore acceptable motion after 3 to 4 months.

Infection

Infection is a frequent complication of the percutaneous pinning technique; however, such infections are self-limiting and respond rapidly to antibiotics and pin removal in the majority of cases. Osteomyelitis in the hand is uncommon as a complication of pin fixation. Osteomyelitis secondary to complex open fractures can be particularly difficult to eradicate.

Tendon Adhesions

Flexor or extensor tendon adhesions may result from closed or operative treatment of phalangeal and metacarpal fractures. As with joint stiffness, a progressive therapy program should be initiated. Tenolysis may be indicated if therapy has failed to show improvement in motion after intensive treatment for 3 months or longer.

REFERENCES

Jupiter JB, Axelrod TS, Belsky MR: Fractures and dislocations of the hand. In Browner BD (ed): Skeletal Trauma: Fractures, Dislocations, Ligamentous Injuries, 2nd ed. Philadelphia, WB Saunders, 1998, p 1294.

McCue FC, Honner R, Johnson MC Jr, et al: Athletic injuries of the proximal interphalangeal joint requiring surgical treatment. J Bone Joint Surg [Am] 54:937–956, 1970.

McElfresh EC, Dobyns JH, O'Brien ET: Management of fracture-dislocation of the proximal interphalangeal joints with extension-block splinting. J Bone Joint Surg [Am] 54:1705–1711, 1970.

Stern PJ: Fractures of the metacarpals and phalanges. In Green DP, Hotchkiss RN, Pederson WC (eds): Green's Operative Hand Surgery, 4th ed. New York, Churchill Livingstone, 1999, p 711.

Suzuki Y, Matsunaga T, Sato S, et al: The pins and rubbers traction system for treatment of comminuted intraarticular fractures and fracture-dislocations in the hand. J Hand Surg [Br] 19:98–107, 1994.

CHAPTER 71

Treatment of Scaphoid Fractures

INTRODUCTION

Scaphoid fractures are common in sports. Early recognition and treatment is essential if the sequelae of nonunion are to be avoided. Treatment approaches for this difficult problem are evolving. The availability of special screws and their relative ease of insertion have broadened the indications for open reduction. A majority of nondisplaced waist fractures heal within 3 months with cast treatment. However, the amount of displacement of waist fractures is often underestimated by x-rays, and no more than 1 mm is accepted. Management of proximal pole fractures has changed in recent years. The nonunion rate for these injuries is unacceptably high with closed treatment. As a result, most surgeons favor immediate fixation of proximal pole fractures. Currently, more surgeons are using percutaneous screw fixation to avoid the problems of prolonged immobilization.

HISTORY AND PHYSICAL EXAMINATION

Scaphoid fractures, the most common fractures to affect the carpal bones, result from a fall onto an outstretched hand. Immediate pain and swelling on the radial side of the wrist are noted. Tenderness is often localized to the anatomic snuffbox or the area over the dorsum of the scaphoid. Many patients describe for the physician only minor trauma, which may mislead the physician into thinking that the injury is a minor sprain to the wrist. This type of thought process should be avoided. A finding of tenderness in the snuffbox justifies a definitive diagnosis with x-ray imaging in every case to avoid delayed diagnosis.

DIAGNOSTIC IMAGING

Localized tenderness in the anatomic snuffbox requires appropriate radiographs, including an anteroposterior (AP) view with the wrist in full ulnar deviation, an AP view in full radial deviation, a zero posteroanterior (PA) view, a true lateral view of the wrist, and a clenched-fist view. Bone scans should be used after 72 hours of injury to identify an occult fracture. A negative bone scan effectively rules out this diagnosis. MRI can diagnose a subtle nondisplaced scaphoid fracture, but it is much more costly than a bone scan. A CT scan of the scaphoid can identify a chronic scaphoid fracture and its associated humpback deformity.

NONOPERATIVE MANAGEMENT

Nonoperative treatment is indicated in acute fractures in which a stable fracture pattern is noted. Scaphoid fractures in the skeletally immature patient are best treated nonoperatively, unless there is considerable deformity and displacement. In the presence of severe osteopenia or stiffness of the wrist, nonoperative treatment is recommended. Fractures of the scaphoid tubercle and incomplete fractures of the scaphoid have an excellent prognosis.

Nondisplaced fractures can be treated with immobilization; however, the position and type of immobilization required with nonoperative treatment are controversial topics in the literature. Many surgeons, including the authors, support the use of a long-arm thumb spica cast for 6 weeks, followed by a short-arm thumb spica cast for 6 weeks. In athletes with nondisplaced fractures of the wrist, a wrist splint has been used effectively to immobilize the patient and to allow play in contact sports.

Small proximal pole fractures of less than 10% of the total length of the scaphoid need to be treated through an operative approach because they carry the highest risk of aseptic necrosis and nonunion.

RELEVANT ANATOMY AND PERILS AND PITFALLS OF SURGERY

The vascular supply of the scaphoid plays a prominent role in the high incidence of scaphoid nonunion (Fig. 71–1). The middle and distal thirds of the scaphoid receive their blood supply from the radial artery. The proximal pole receives no direct vascular supply; instead, it gets its blood supply from interosseous vessels that pass in a retrograde fashion from the waist of the scaphoid. The radial artery and the superficial palmar branch of the radial artery pass volarly, and along with the dorsal carpal branch of the radial artery, they supply blood to the tubercle or the most distal aspect of the scaphoid. The proximal pole of the scaphoid, which is covered by hyaline cartilage and has a single ligamentous attachment to the deep radial scapholunate ligament, has negligible or nonexistent independent blood supply.

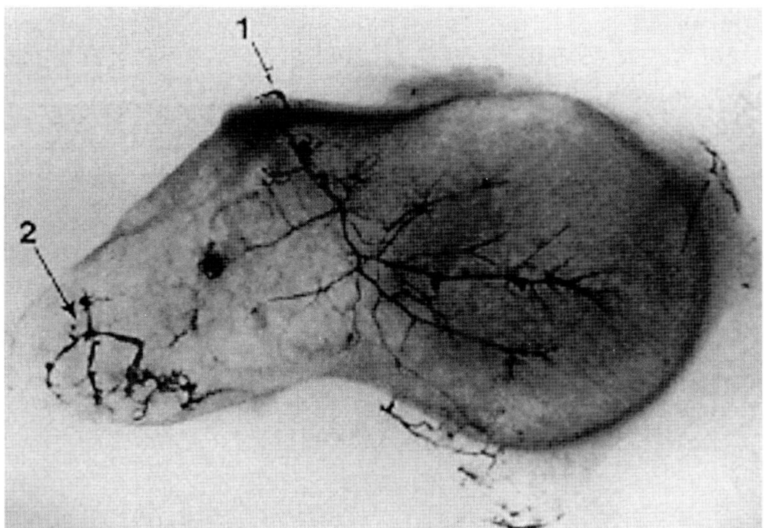

FIGURE 71–1. Vascularity of the scaphoid. 1, Dorsal scaphoid branch; 2, volar scaphoid branch. (From Gelberman RH, Panagis JS, Taleisnik J, Baumgaertner M: The arterial anatomy of the human carpus: Part 1: The extraosseous vascularity. J Hand Surg [Am] 8:367–375, 1983.)

SURGICAL *TECHNIQUE*

Indications

Scaphoid fractures displaced more than 1 mm require accurate closed or open reduction. Failure to reduce these fractures anatomically results in a high rate of nonunion. Open reduction can be accomplished by a volar approach with fixation using K-wires, Herbert screws, or Acutrak screws. Use of the latter two is technically demanding, but they have the advantage of providing compression, which allows early mobilization. When fractures of the scaphoid are associated with a dorsal intercalated segmental instability (DISI) deformity, a dorsal approach may be necessary to reduce and pin the lunate along with the scaphoid fracture, or an intercalary graft that is applied through a palmar approach may be needed. Simple transverse fractures of the waist of the scaphoid are stabilized through a standard palmar approach. If comminution is present, bone graft is used. Oblique fractures are extremely unstable; a compression screw and supplemental parallel K-wires are needed for a satisfactory reduction. Small proximal pole fractures carry a high nonunion rate, even with good internal fixation; a dorsal approach is advised.

Displaced scaphoid fractures and perilunate fracture-dislocations require an extended palmar approach to decompress the carpal canal and repair the palmar ligaments. An additional dorsal approach may be required if there is any associated ulnar carpal instability. Operative intervention is used in scaphoid fractures that show no evidence of healing after 6 months; bone graft and internal rotation fixation are used at that time with a volar approach and accurate reduction.

Technique

Kirschner wires, Herbert screws, and Acutrak screws have each increasingly allowed for better compression of the scaphoid and for limited wrist immobilization with plaster, depending on the surgeon's ability to attain a stable and rigidly fixed scaphoid.

Scaphoid Waist Fractures

Positioning and Exposure

1. The patient is positioned supine on the operative table with a well-padded tourniquet placed on the upper arm. General or regional anesthesia is selected. The ipsilateral iliac crest is prepared and draped in the event that a bone graft is required. Herbert has recommended that right-handed surgeons sit at the axilla when operating on the left wrist and that surgeons operating on the right wrist sit on the opposite side of the table. The incision is centered over the scaphoid tubercle. The distal limb of the incision is curved gently toward the base of the thumb in the carpal metacarpal (CMC) joint; the proximal limb extends for 2 cm along the radial border of the flexor carpi radialis (Fig. 71–2*A*).
2. Dissection is carried down through the subcutaneous tissue so that the palmar branch of the radial artery can be identified; this is normally ligated and divided across the palm just proximal to the tubercle of the scaphoid (Fig. 71–2*B*).
3. The sheath of the flexor carpi radialis (FCR) tendon is incised and the tendon is retracted ulnarward to

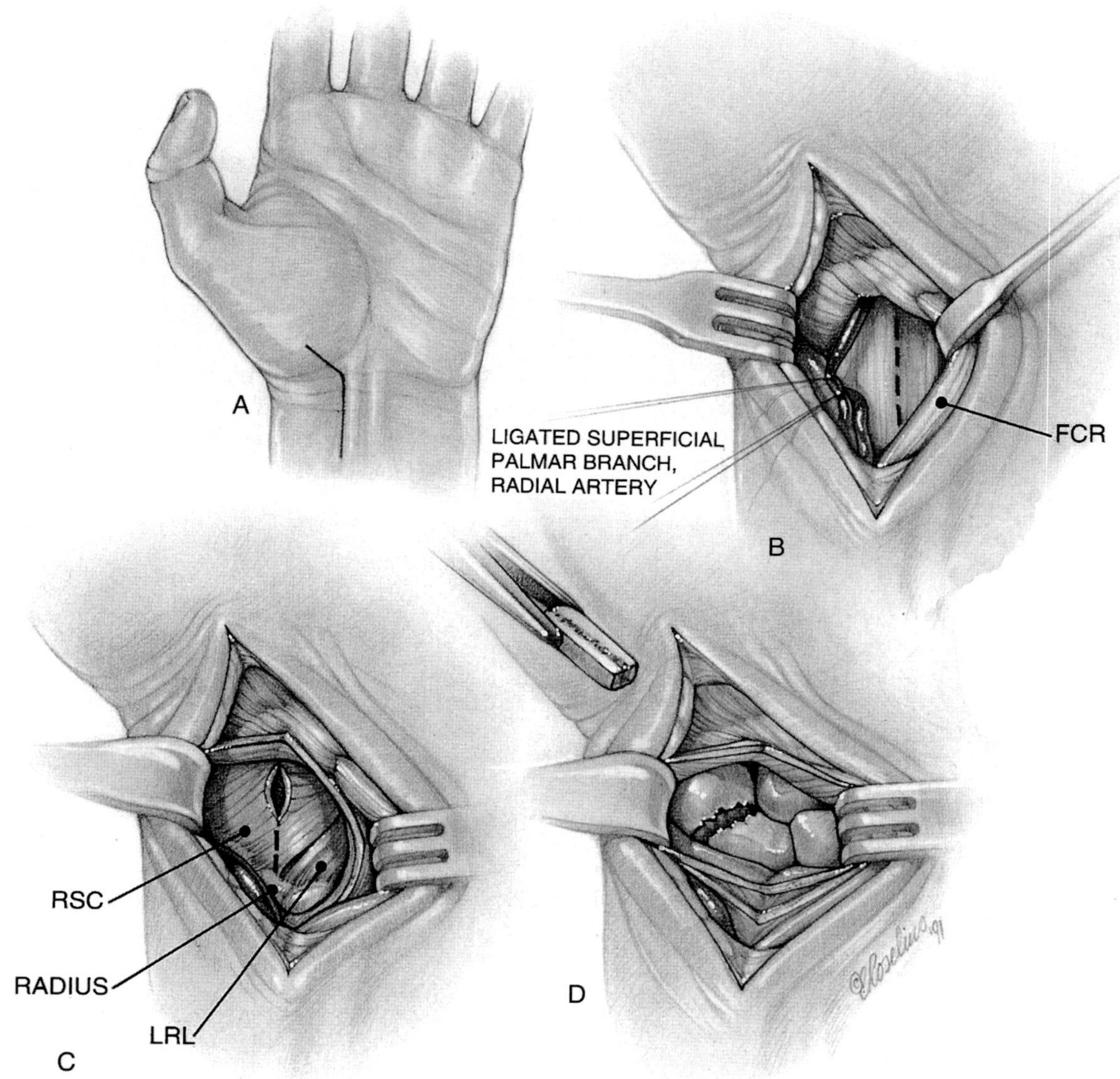

FIGURE 71–2. Volar surgical exposure of the scaphoid. *A*, The incision. *B*, The flexor carpi radialis (FCR) tendon is retracted to expose the volar capsule. *C*, The volar capsule incised *(dashed line)*. The radioscaphocapitate (RSC) ligament and the long radiolunate (LRL) ligament are incised in this approach. *D*, The scaphoid waist is exposed. (From Amadio PC, Taleisnik J: Fractures of the carpal bones. In Green DP, Hotchkiss RN, Pederson WC [eds]: Green's Operative Hand Surgery, 4th ed. New York, Churchill Livingstone, 1999, p 827.)

expose the anterior capsule of the wrist over the scaphoid bone. The incision is deepened distally, dividing the origin of the thenar muscles in line with the fibers over the palmar surface of the trapezium. The proximal portion of the incision is split. This represents the radiolunate ligament and continuation of the capsule (Fig. 71–2*C*).

4. With the proximal pole of the scaphoid well visualized (Fig. 71–2*D*), insertion of a small self-retaining Holzheimer retractor (provided in the Herbert screw set) allows for excellent visualization of the entire palmar surface of the scaphoid. The joint between the scaphoid and the trapezium is identified, and the joint capsule is incised by sweeping the knife blade around the radial aspect of the tubercle of the scaphoid. Dissection is never carried too proximally or too deep, so that damage to the radial artery can be avoided as it passes through the scaphotrapezial spiral groove.
5. With the use of fine dental picks or appropriate small

hand instrumentation, the soft tissue is cleared from the fracture site. All synovium that is trapped within the bone fragments is cleared, and the wrist is manipulated so that the instability and displacement at the fracture site can be assessed. Accurate reduction of the fracture is then carried out, with care taken to correct any rotatory, angulatory, or translocation deformity. A percutaneous K-wire is placed to hold the reduction.

6. This wire is inserted into the tip of the tubercle at the most ulnar border, directed proximal and dorsal to the apex of the proximal pole. After the K-wire has been placed, the decision is made as to whether a second K-wire should be placed more radially, or whether a Herbert screw or an Acutrak screw should be placed.

Fixation

Herbert Screw

1. The Herbert screw jig is used as a clamp around the scaphoid to hold the reduced fragments and to compress during instrumentation. The calibration of the jig is checked to ensure that the drill meets the tip. With treatment of a right wrist, the jig is held in the right position. The radial carpal joint is opened up by firm distraction of the hand, allowing the surgeon to position the hook on the dorsal aspect of the proximal pole of the scaphoid. The bow of the jig is firmly clamped in the distal pole of the scaphoid (Fig. 71–3).

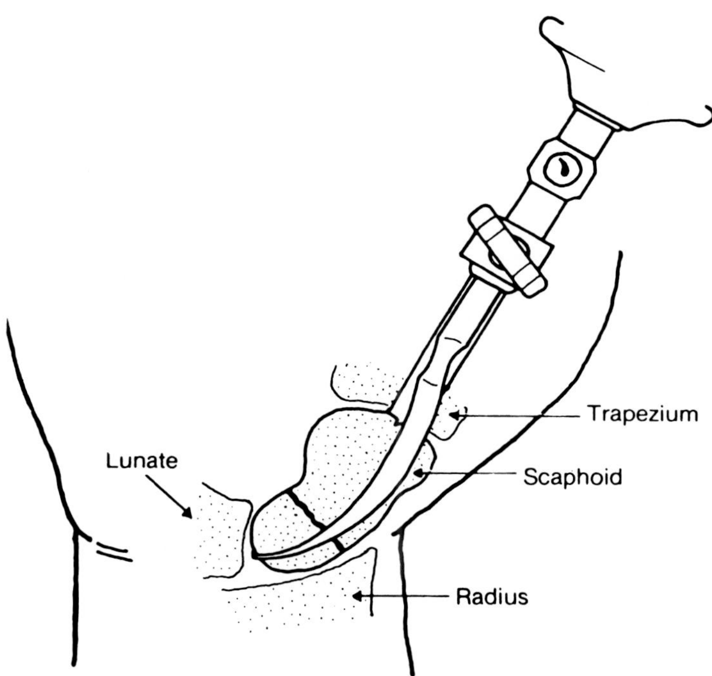

FIGURE 71–3. Diagram showing the positioning of the Herbert jig on the scaphoid. (From Amadio PC, Taleisnik J: Fractures of the carpal bones. In Green DP, Hotchkiss RN, Pederson WC [eds]: Green's Operative Hand Surgery, 4th ed. New York, Churchill Livingstone, 1999, p 823.)

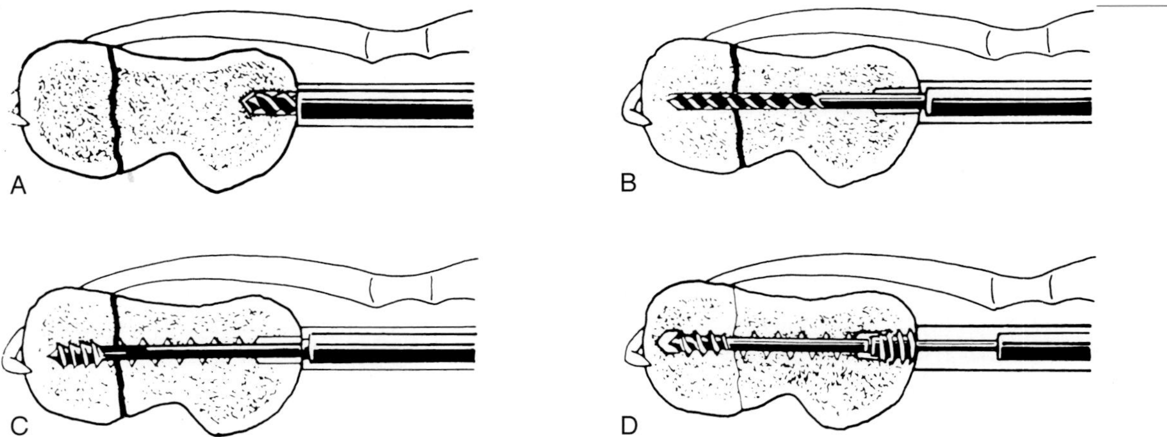

FIGURE 71–4. Diagram showing the stages of instrumentation for Herbert screw fixation. *A*, Larger pilot drill hand drilled. *B*, Long small drill hand drilled. *C*, Tap. *D*, Screw inserted below the articular surface. (From Amadio PC, Taleisnik J: Fractures of the carpal bones. In Green DP, Hotchkiss RN, Pederson WC [eds]: Green's Operative Hand Surgery, 4th ed. New York, Churchill Livingstone, 1999, p 823.)

2. Verification with the C-arm in the AP and lateral planes is completed to ensure that the screw is firmly seated within the substance of the scaphoid. The surgeon controls the jig with his or her left hand while carrying out the drilling with the right hand. The proximal pole is drilled. The distal pole is drilled and the appropriate screw length is inserted into the jig to the end of the screwdriver. The radial carpal joint is then distracted, the jig is removed, and the C-arm is brought in to verify appropriate placement of the screw. Both drills are removed in a clockwise direction to clear loose bone fragments. A tap is inserted in its full depth and is removed in a counterclockwise direction (Fig. 71–4). At this stage, with the jig removed, the head of the screw lies just beneath the surface of the bone; the screwdriver is carefully reinserted to make one or two additional turns to bury the screw, thereby increasing compression at the fracture site. The temporary K-wire, when used, is then removed, except in patients with a very oblique fracture, for whom it should be left in situ.
3. The palmar wrist capsule is repaired with an interrupted 3–0 Surgilon suture, and the cut ends of the radiolunate ligament are reapposed (nonabsorbable suture, 3–0 or 4–0).
4. A firm short-arm bulky thumb spica dressing is placed for adequate protection during healing, and the tourniquet is let down to check for good capillary refill through the digits.

Acutrak Screw

The mini–Acutrak screw may also be used for internal fixation of scaphoid fractures. This is a completely threaded screw with variable pitch threads. It is a cannulated system. The fracture site is first secured after reduction with a K-wire. Next, the guide wire is introduced across the fracture site at the intended site for the screw, and its location is checked under fluoroscopy. A cannulated depth gauge is used to measure screw length. The guide wire must then be advanced through the far cortex. With the mini–Acutrak drill, the path for the screw is drilled by hand, advancing slowly. A screw that is one size smaller than what was measured is then inserted over the guide wire. This is to ensure that the head of the screw is fully buried below the articular surface. A jig is also available with the Acutrak system; this may be used if desired.

Proximal Pole Fractures

1. Proximal pole fractures are approached through a dorsal approach with the use of a free-hand method. The fracture is actually reduced and is held with a 0.045-inch K-wire. The wrist is hyperflexed to allow placement of a guide wire. The wire is placed just radial to the edge of the scapholunate ligament insertion on the scaphoid. The wire is directed as though it would come out the tip of the thumb. This places the guide wire in the center of the scaphoid (Fig. 71–5).

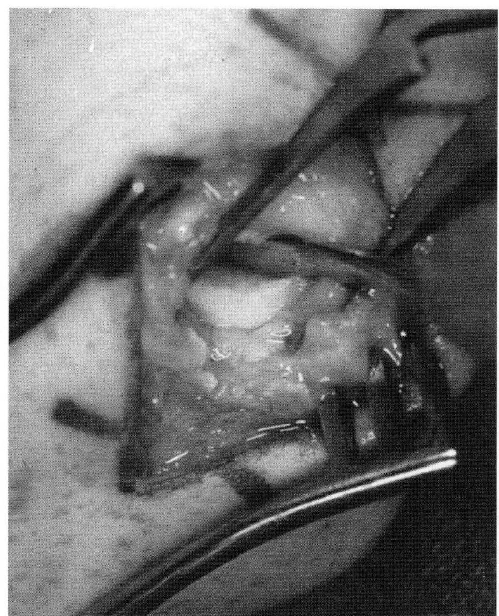

FIGURE 71–5. Clinical photo of limited dorsal exposure of the proximal pole of the scaphoid. An elevator is in the fracture site.

2. Throughout the procedure, firm manual compression is applied to the fracture via the drill guide until the screw has been tightened. A screw of 16 or 18 mm is usually long enough. It is tightened so that it is deeply buried beneath the articular surface. Intraoperative radiographs are used to check for accurate positioning of the screw, and the capsule is closed in a routine fashion for any dorsal approach to the wrist (Fig. 71–6).

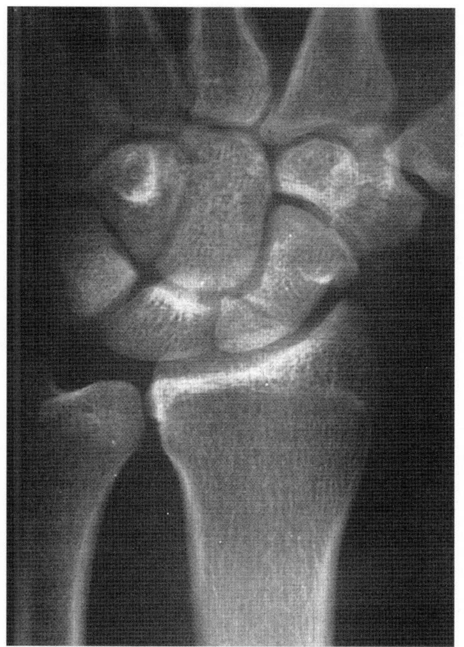

A

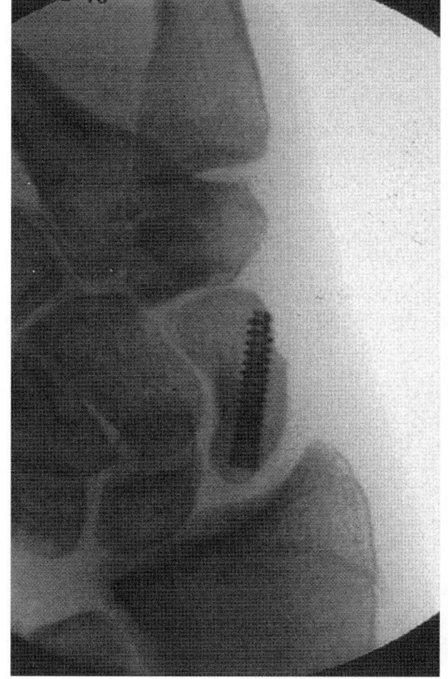

B

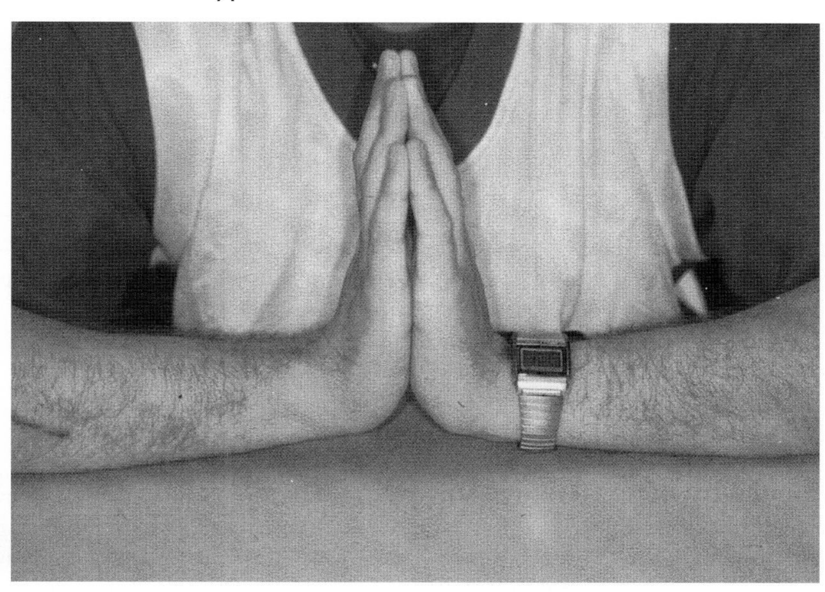

C

FIGURE 71–6. *A*, Minimally displaced proximal pole scaphoid fracture. *B*, X-ray after Acutrak screw is inserted from a dorsal approach. *C*, Clinical photo 8 weeks after surgery. Excellent motion is possible when the volar capsule is not violated.

Arthroscopic-Assisted Internal Fixation

Arthroscopic-assisted internal fixation is technically demanding and is used only in select cases of displaced but reducible fractures. Finger-trap traction is applied to the thumb. This maneuver reduces many fractures. Diagnostic arthroscopy of the radiocarpal joint is performed through standard 3–4 and 4–5 portals. Fracture hematoma is evacuated; the joint surface and ligamentous injuries are assessed. Midcarpal portals are then established. The ulnar midcarpal portal provides the best view of the scaphoid fracture.

Fracture reduction is performed if necessary via direct manipulation of the distal pole and percutaneous manipulation of the proximal pole. A small volar incision is made just radial to the flexor carpi radialis. Blunt dissection is carried down to the joint capsule; the radial artery and palmar cutaneous nerve are protected. A guide wire is placed across the reduced fracture, and a cannulated screw is then placed over the wire (Fig. 71–7).

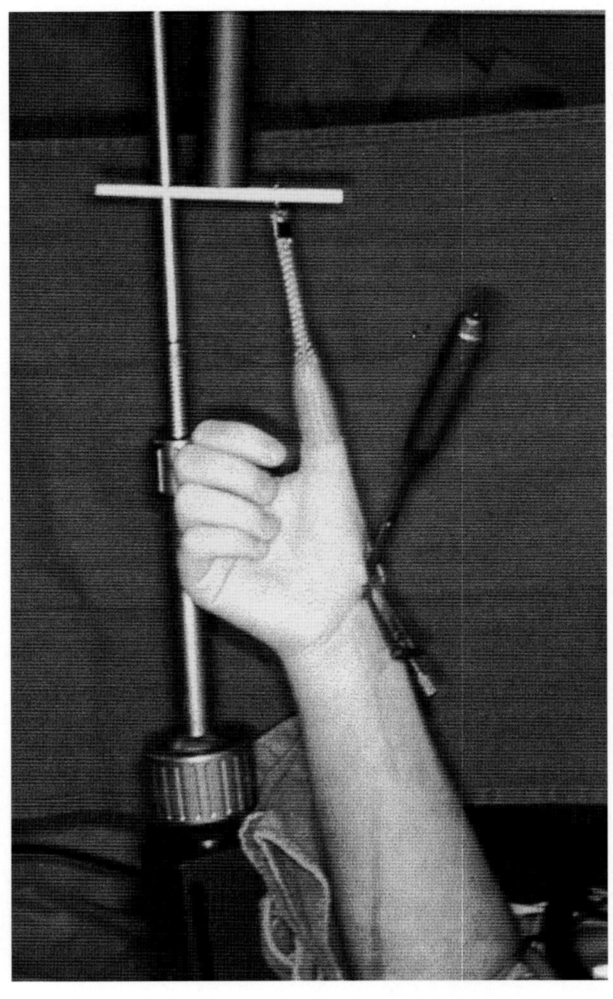

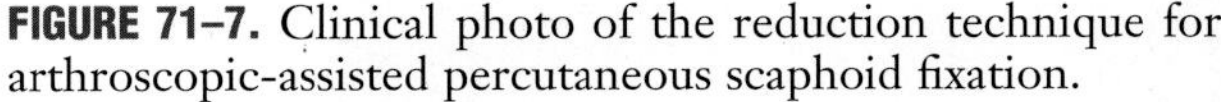

FIGURE 71–7. Clinical photo of the reduction technique for arthroscopic-assisted percutaneous scaphoid fixation.

COMPLICATIONS

Scaphoid nonunion can occur; various techniques have been used to alleviate this problem, including open wedge grafting with iliac crest bone graft and vascularized bone grafting. Post-traumatic radiocarpal arthritis may result despite the successful healing of the scaphoid. Proximal row carpectomies have been advocated for chronic ununited fractures of the scaphoid, for radioscaphoid arthritis, and for treatment of patients who do not wish to accept a long period of immobilization. Partial arthrodesis (scaphocapitate fusion or scaphoid-trapezium-trapezoid [STT] fusion) has been advocated for nonunion of the scaphoid. Allografting has been advocated by some for treatment of dorsal avascular fragments.

Infection or disruption of normal cartilaginous surfaces within the wrist joint, caused by lack of care when the intricate jigs are used, should be avoided. Care is taken throughout the procedure to avoid damage to the palmar cutaneous branch of the median nerve. Joint stiffness or loss of fixation may result from inappropriate postoperative immobilization in plaster or fiberglass.

RESULTS

Nonunion is rare following good internal fixation; Herbert has reported a personal series, wherein acute unstable fractures treated by primary internal fixation had less than a 1% chance of nonunion. Range of motion may be limited after extensive surgical exposure. Our limited experience with percutaneous fixation techniques shows promise for restoration of full wrist motion in the majority of cases.

REFERENCES

Adams BD, Blair WF, Reagan DS, et al: Technical factors related to Herbert screw fixation. J Hand Surg [Am] 13:893–899, 1988.

Gelberman RH, Menon J: The vascularity of the scaphoid bone. J Hand Surg [Am] 5:508–513, 1980.

Herbert TJ, Fisher WE: Management of the fractured scaphoid using a new bone screw. J Bone Joint Surg [Br] 66:114–123, 1984.

Rettig AC, Kollias SC: Internal fixaton of acute stable fractures in the athlete. Am J Sports Med 24:182–186, 1996.

Rettig ME, Raskin KB: Retrograde compression screw fixation of acute proximal pole scaphoid fractures. J Bone Joint Surg [Am] 24:1206–1210, 1999.

Slade JF, Grauer JN, Mahoney JD: Arthroscopic reduction and percutaneous fixation of scaphoid fractures with a novel dorsal technique. Orthop Clin North Am 32:247–261, 2001.

CHAPTER 72

Treatment of Hamate Fractures

HISTORY AND PHYSICAL EXAMINATION

Fractures of the hamate usually occur at the hook, and the diagnosis is often missed. In athletes, this injury occurs as a direct result of force from a bat, a racquet, a club, or a ball that is being caught. Patients complain of pain localized to the hamate hook over the hypothenar eminence, as well as pain over the dorsal aspect of the fourth ray (Fig. 72–1).

Some patients come into the office with a rupture to the flexor tendon of the ring or little finger or with numbness and tingling in an ulnar nerve distribution. These symptoms represent chronic injuries that have not been properly diagnosed.

DIAGNOSTIC IMAGING

A carpal tunnel view is necessary to demonstrate the fracture radiographically, although CT scans can aid in the diagnosis when it is not clear on plain films (Figs. 72–2 and 72–3).

NONOPERATIVE MANAGEMENT

Nondisplaced fractures of the body of the hamate are less common than hamate hook fractures and can be associated with dorsal dislocations of the fourth and fifth metacarpals. These fractures can be treated in a cast for

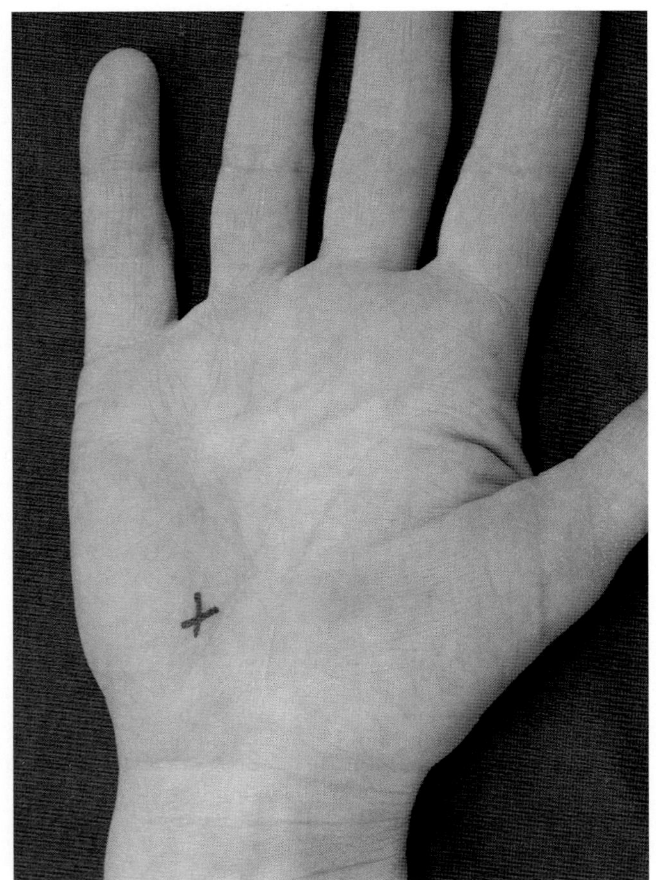

FIGURE 72–1. Clinical photo of the palm. The X indicates the usual point of tenderness in a hamate hook nonunion.

4 to 6 weeks. The lateral x-ray is taken in 30° pronation to ensure that the metacarpal-hamate articulation is not subluxed. If it is subluxed, closed reduction and percutaneous pinning are indicated. Hamate hook fractures can heal with prolonged immobilization. However, many athletes are unwilling to accept a long period of inactivity.

RELEVANT ANATOMY AND PERILS AND PITFALLS OF SURGERY

The deep branch of the ulnar nerve in its course must be reviewed before any type of surgery is begun. The nerve, which is in contact with the hamate on the distal side of the hook, must be identified and protected during the exposure.

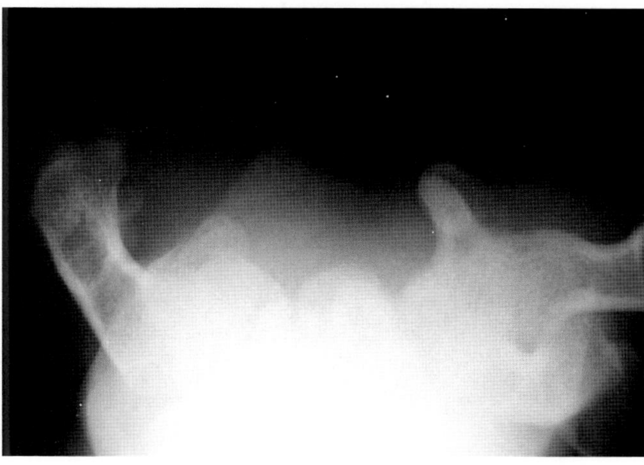

FIGURE 72–2. Carpal tunnel view of a normal hamate hook.

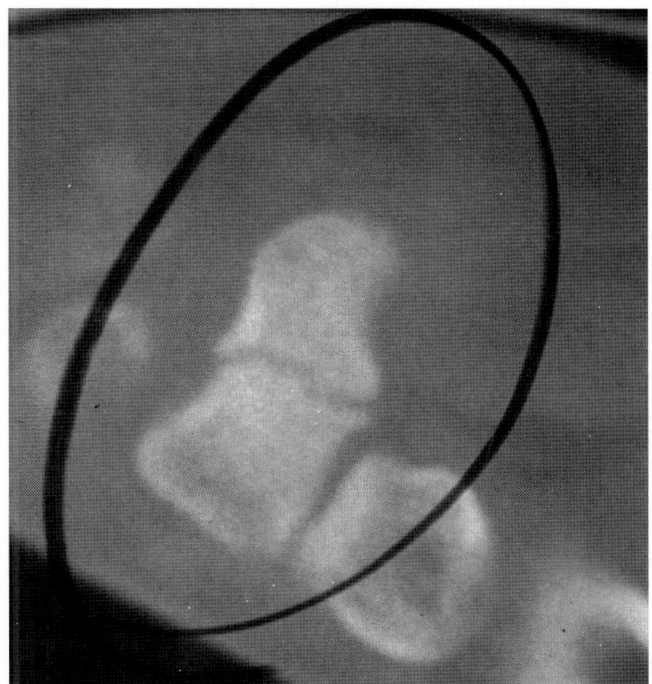

FIGURE 72–3. CT scan of nonunion of the hook of the hamate.

SURGICAL *TECHNIQUE*

Indications

Healing of acute hamate hook fractures is rare, even with open reduction and internal fixation; therefore, excision of the hook through the fracture site is an effective way to allow athletes to return to sports in 6 weeks. Displaced fractures of the body of the hamate should be reduced and pinned with K-wires, or they can be fixed with fluoroscopic guidance and screws.

Technique

1. The patient is placed supine with the hand on the hand table, and an incision is marked out as for an extended carpal tunnel exposure. Incisions zigzagging over the hypothenar eminence frequently result in hypersensitive scars and are discouraged (Fig. 72–4).
2. The palmar fascia is exposed proximally to isolate the ulnar nerve above the wrist and trace it distally through Guyon's canal by taking the flexor carpi ulnaris ulnarward (Fig. 72–5).
3. The hamate hook is identified, and the transverse carpal ligament is released from the hamate hook. A rongeur is used to remove it. A small file is used to smooth off any sharp edges, and the wound is closed. The flexor digitorum profundus is isolated and identified before wound closure is performed.

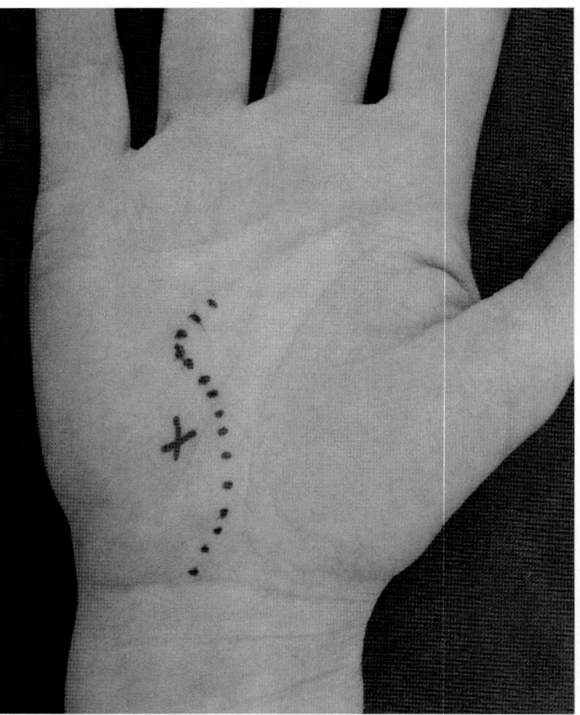

FIGURE 72–4. Clinical photo of incision line for hamate hook excision.

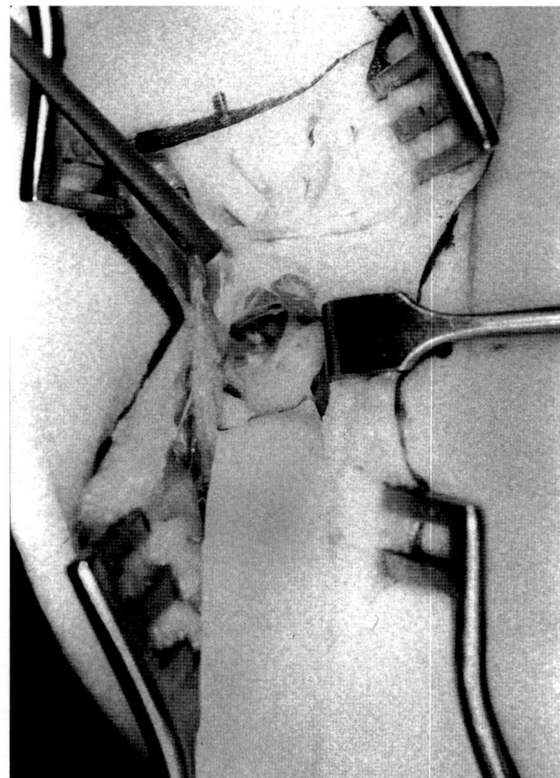

FIGURE 72–5. Hook of the hamate exposed. Vessel loop retracts the ulnar artery and nerve.

RESULTS

Excision of the hamate hook significantly improves symptoms in most cases. A majority of athletes return to full function within 6 weeks. For this reason, few surgeons show enthusiasm for open reduction and fixation for acute displaced fracture of the hamate hook. Residual scar tenderness may delay return to full function, but this is usually temporary when appropriate incisions are used.

COMPLICATIONS

Complications from this injury occur infrequently. Late recognition has resulted in flexor tendon rupture to the ring and small fingers. Surgical complications are related to injury of the median or ulnar nerve. Specifically, the deep motor branch of the ulnar nerve is at risk for injury. Incisions that pass directly over the glabrous skin of the hypothenar eminence may result in tender, painful scars. This is best avoided by using a midpalmar incision such as that used for an extensile carpal tunnel release.

REFERENCES

Bishop AT, Beckenbaugh RD: Fracture of the hamate hook. J Hand Surg [Am] 13:135–139, 1988.

Egawa M, Asai T: Fracture of the hook of the hamate: Report of six cases and the suitability of computerized tomography. J Hand Surg [Am] 8:393–398, 1983.

Hartford JM, Murphy JM: Flexor digitorum profundus rupture of the small finger secondary to nonunion of the hook of the hamate: A case report. J Hand Surg [Am] 21:621–623, 1997.

Parker RD, Berkowitz MS, Brahms MA, et al: Hook of the hamate fractures in athletes. Am J Sports Med 14:517–523, 1986.

Whalen JL, Bishop AT, Linscheid RL: Nonoperative treatment of acute hamate hook fractures. J Hand Surg [Am] 17:507–511, 1992.

CHAPTER 73

Treatment of Scapholunate Dissociation and Acute Ligamentous Disruption

HISTORY AND PHYSICAL EXAMINATION

Patients often complain of pain over the scapholunate interval with a history of trauma that has usually occurred within 3 weeks of their visit to the office. Pain over the snuffbox, tenderness, and pain with radial and ulnar deviation can occur. Typically, the mechanism is a hyperextension injury to the wrist with concomitant forearm pronation and intercarpal supination.

Physical examination focuses on the involved wrist as well as the contralateral side, which is used as a reference for baseline measurements of range of motion and ligamentous laxity. Palpation of the scapholunate joint is performed, with tenderness noted through this area, especially at the dorsal aspect approximately 1 cm distal to Lister's tubercle. The Watson, or scaphoid shift, test is used to determine whether there is abnormal motion and mobility of the scaphoid. On occasion, a painful snap or clicking is elicited during this test, which is often diagnostic of the condition. The scaphoid shift test is performed with the examiner's thumb on the tubercle of the scaphoid. The patient's hand is passively moved from ulnar to radial deviation with a counterforce that opposes the palmar flexion of the scaphoid tubercle as it attempts to ride out of the scaphoid fossa. Pain on this maneuver is indicative of a scapholunate ligament tear.

DIAGNOSTIC IMAGING

Routine radiographs, including standard posteroanterior (PA), zero PA, lateral, radial deviation, ulnar deviation, and oblique views, as well as an anteroposterior (AP) supinated clenched-fist view, are necessary to help the clinician in diagnosing this condition. Scapholunate instability usually includes the following classic radiologic features:

1. Scapholunate gap. The intercarpal distance between the scaphoid and the lunate on the AP radiograph is often increased (Fig. 73–1). A gap greater than 3 mm (the Terry Thomas sign) is considered diagnostic of the scapholunate dissociation. This increase in the scapholunate intercarpal distance should be verified with bilateral AP supinated clenched-fist radiographs. A gap greater than 2 mm is worrisome when it is associated with a positive physical examination. In cases of dynamic instability, the clenched-fist view may widen an otherwise normal scapholunate interval (Fig. 73–2).
2. A foreshortened scaphoid. The scaphoid in a scapholunate ligament tear assumes a palmar flexed position owing to the dissociation from the surrounding bones. This appears as a foreshortened scaphoid on PA and AP radiographs.
3. The cortical ring sign (see Fig. 73–1). The flexed position of the scaphoid results in an end-on view of the scaphoid tubercle and distal scaphoid. This superimposition creates a circular cortex on the scaphoid. A cortical ring–to–proximal pole distance of less than 7 mm is considered abnormal.
4. The dorsal intercalated segment instability (DISI). The scaphoid assumes a palmar flexed and dorsally subluxed posture, and the lunate assumes an extended and palmar subluxed posture. The capitate lies in a flexed position. The scapholunate angle is defined by many to have normal values that range from 30° to 60°, with an average of 47°. Angles greater than 80° are considered an indication of a scapholunate dissociation (Fig. 73–3).

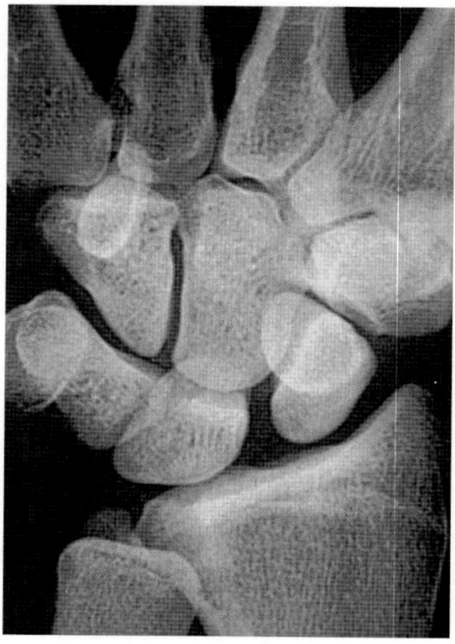

FIGURE 73–1. Rotary subluxation of the scaphoid. The scaphoid is foreshortened. The scapholunate gap is widened, and the scaphoid has a cortical ring appearance. (From Nathan R, Blatt G: Rotary subluxation of the scaphoid. Hand Clin 16:420, 2000.)

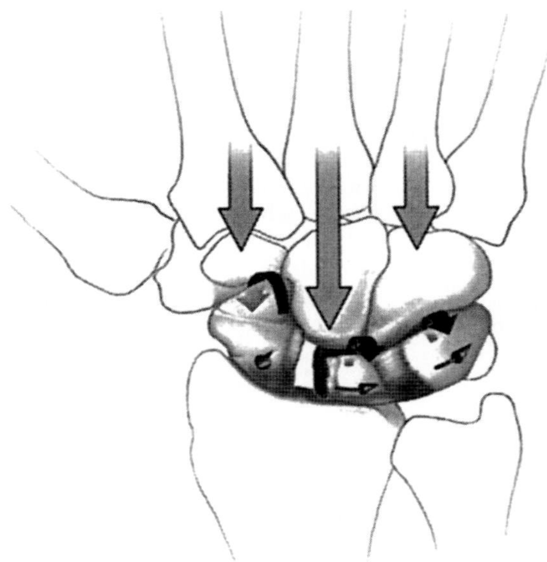

FIGURE 73–2. Dynamic scapholunate dissociation may be demonstrated with the clenched-fist view. This illustration shows how the scaphoid flexes under axial load, resulting in widening of the scapholunate interval. (From Blatt G, Tobias B, Lichtman DM: Scapholunate injuries. In Lichtman DM, Alexander AH [eds]: The Wrist and Its Disorders, 2nd ed. Philadelphia, WB Saunders, 1997, p 273.)

5. Lack of parallelism. One of the most subtle signs of scapholunate dissociation is the lack of parallelism between the opposing articular surfaces of the scaphoid and the lunate in the AP view. This finding is more appropriately seen during cineradiographics or a dynamic motion series.

6. Carpal height. Carpal height is a term used to designate the distance between the base of the third metacarpal and the distal articular surface of the radius, as measured along the proximal projection of the longitudinal axis of the third metacarpal. The carpal height ratio (carpal height divided by the length of the third metacarpal) has been found to be 0.54 ± 0.03 in the normal wrist. The suggestion of a modified carpal height ratio implies the presence of subtle carpal instability as the capitate descends between the scaphoid and the lunate.

NONOPERATIVE MANAGEMENT

Although the literature is replete with articles emphasizing the importance of early diagnosis and treatment, scapholunate dissociation unfortunately is rarely recognized early; this is especially true for isolated scapholunate dissociation. Given this information, treatment of scapholunate dissociation can be extremely difficult. Despite occasional reports in the literature suggesting that scapholunate dissociation can be successfully treated with cast immobilization, many surgeons share the opinion that it is virtually impossible to consistently maintain a satisfactory reduction with the use of casting alone. Therefore, at a minimum, closed reduction and percutaneous pin fixation is performed. In our practice, patients with acute scapholunate ligament disruptions undergo open reduction and internal fixation with repair of ligaments to avoid the natural progression to a scapholunate advanced collapsed wrist.

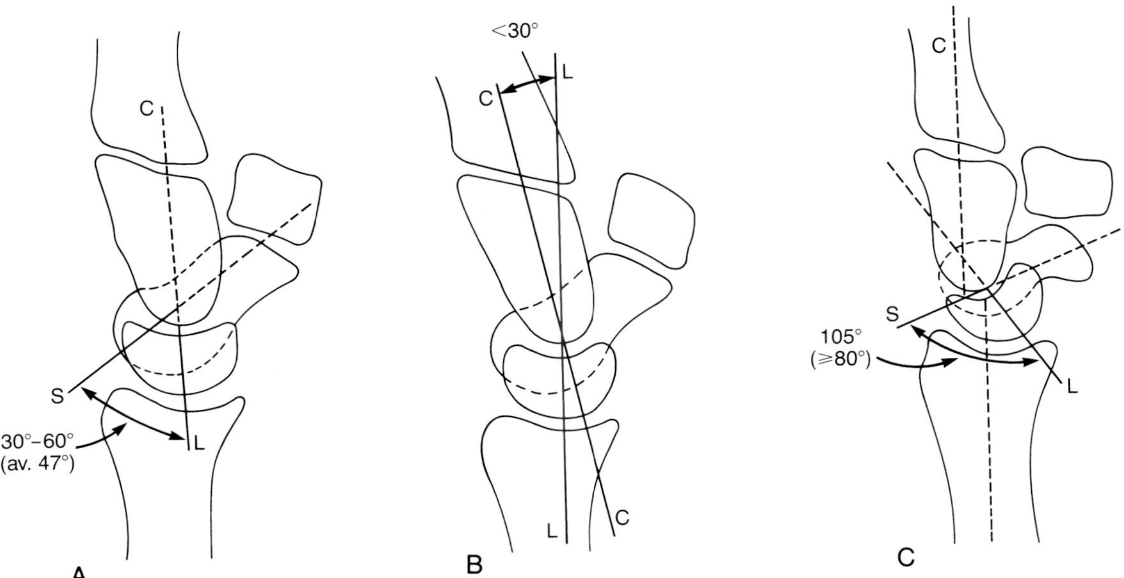

FIGURE 73–3. *A*, Normal scapholunate angle is 30° to 60°. *B*, Normal scapholunate angle is less than 30°. *C*, Scapholunate angles greater than 80° are associated with scapholunate ligament disruption. C, capitate axis; L, lunate axis; S, scaphoid axis. (From Mann FA, Gilula LA: Post-traumatic wrist pain and instability: A radiographic approach to diagnosis. In Lichtman DM, Alexander AH [eds]: The Wrist and Its Disorders, 2nd ed. Philadelphia, WB Saunders, 1997, p 105.)

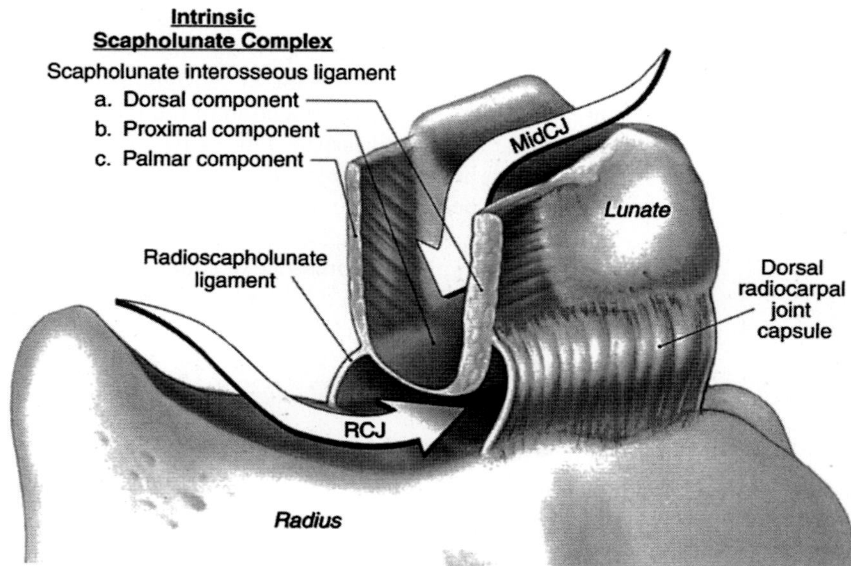

FIGURE 73–4. Illustration of the scapholunate ligament complex. The midcarpal joint (midCJ) is closed off from the radiocarpal joint (RCJ) by the membranous portion of the scapholunate interosseous ligament. (From Blatt G, Tobias B, Lichtman DM: Scapholunate injuries. In Lichtman DM, Alexander AH [eds]: The Wrist and Its Disorders, 2nd ed. Philadelphia, WB Saunders, 1997, p 270.)

RELEVANT ANATOMY AND PERILS AND PITFALLS OF SURGERY

The surgeon's understanding of the anatomy of the scapholunate interosseous ligament (SLIOL) is essential to successful surgical repair. The dorsal and palmar SLIOLs are the main load-bearing elements, and the dorsal SLIOL is the thickest and strongest. The membranous midportion of the ligament provides little strength to the SLIOL complex (Fig. 73–4). Currently, the most popular repair techniques focus on restoration of the dorsal SLIOL.

SURGICAL *TECHNIQUE*

Indications

Evidence of an acute scapholunate ligament tear by physical examination or supporting evidence from x-rays requires operative intervention.

Technique

Closed Reduction and Pinning

Several authors have recommended percutaneous pin fixation of acute scapholunate dissociations of less than 3 weeks' duration, if satisfactory alignment can be achieved in a closed manipulation. The procedure should be done under image intensification with Kirschner wires placed from the scaphoid to the lunate, as well as from the scaphoid to the capitate (Fig. 73–5). The wires are left in place for 8 to 10 weeks; protection is provided by a removable splint for an additional 4 weeks. Following this, motion is begun.

Open Reduction and Ligamentous Repair

1. The patient is placed in a supine position with the hand on the arm table. A tourniquet is placed on the upper arm, and either regional or general anesthesia is administered.
2. Manual examination of the involved wrist is performed to confirm the diagnosis, and a Watson shift test is performed. A longitudinal incision is made in line with the third ray; it continues slightly ulnarward to Lister's tubercle. The skin and subcutaneous tissue are dissected. Meticulous hemostasis is obtained with the use of bipolar cautery.
3. The extensor pollicis longus (EPL) is taken out of its sheath (by cutting through the extensor retinaculum in longitudinal and T fashion) and is retracted to the radial side of the wrist. The fourth extensor compartment is not entered; instead, it is released off the bone with a 64 Beaver blade and pulled ulnarward. The second dorsal compartment is now pulled radially and is dissected off in a subperiosteal manner. With the wrist capsule now exposed, it is opened in an H fashion with preservation of the radiotriquetral and dorsal intercalary ligaments. The proximal H flap is preserved for the dorsal capsulodesis at the time of closure (Fig. 73–6).
4. When the fourth dorsal compartment is lifted up, the terminal branch of the posterior interosseous nerve

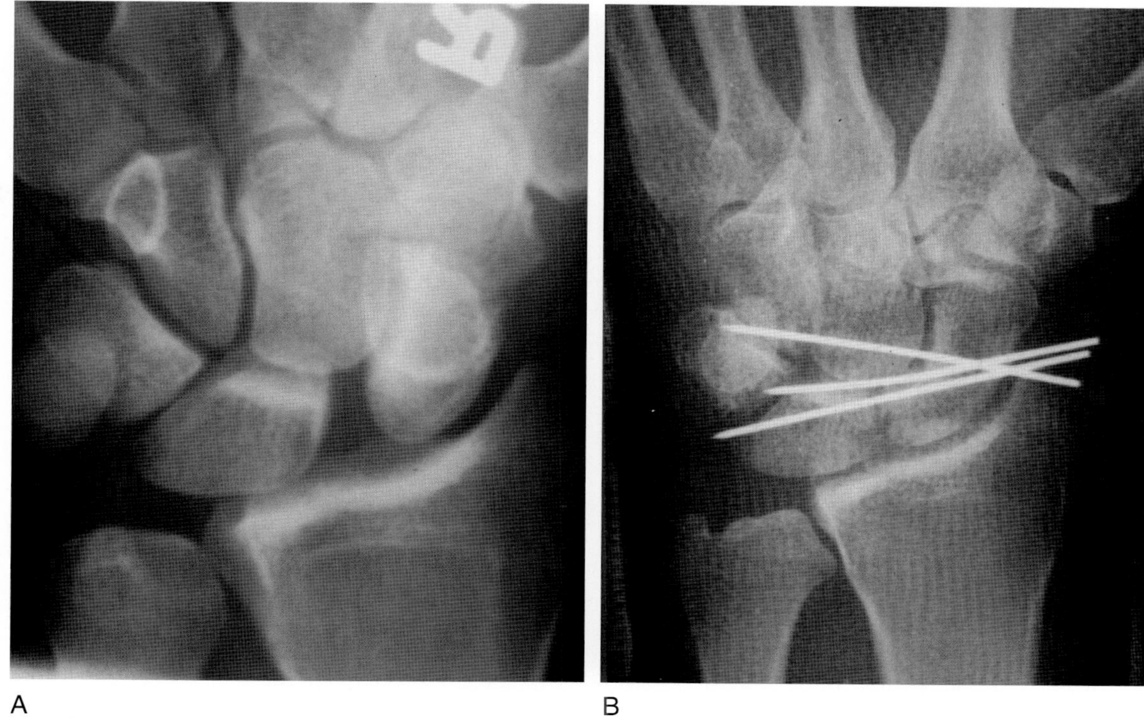

FIGURE 73–5. Acute scapholunate dissociation. *A*, Anteroposterior (AP) x-ray showing scapholunate interval widening. *B*, AP x-ray after closed reduction and percutaneous pinning.

can be seen directly under the extensor indicis proprius. Once it has been visualized and identified, a small piece is resected back to decrease pain within the joint capsule.

5. The scapholunate ligament tear is identified. The typical central membranous portion of the ligament within the scapholunate articulation is identified and freed appropriately but is left attached to the lunate. The radiotriquetral ligament is detached from the radius, and the dorsal intercalary ligament is detached from the triquetrum.

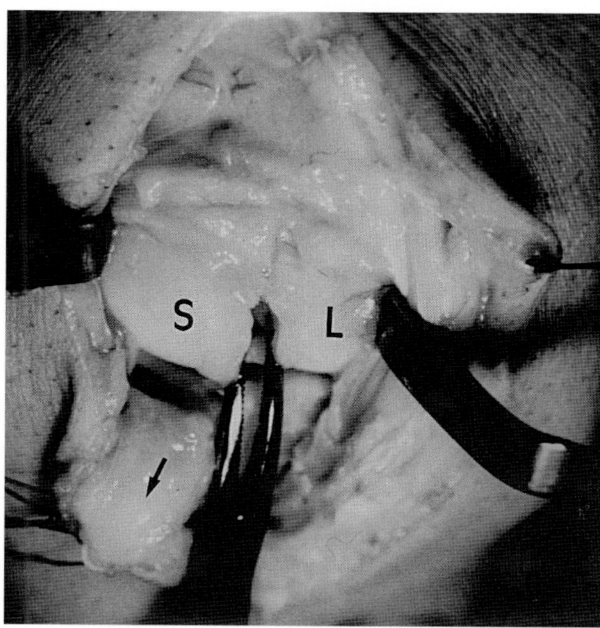

FIGURE 73–6. Clinical photo of dorsal wrist exposure. A hemostat is in the scapholunate interval. L, lunate; S, scaphoid. *Arrow* indicates the capsular flap for capsulodesis. (From Garcia-Elias M: Carpal instabilities and dislocations. In Green DP, Hotchkiss RN, Pederson WC [eds]: Green's Operative Hand Surgery, 4th ed. New York, Churchill Livingstone, 1999, p 888.)

6. K-wires (0.062-inch) are placed onto the scaphoid and the lunate as joysticks to control and reduce the relationship between the scaphoid and the lunate (which is usually in a dorsal intercalary segment instability position). The Kirschner wire in the scaphoid is placed in the most proximal portion before the scaphoid is palmar flexed. The wire in the lunate is placed in the most distal aspect because the lunate lies in a dorsiflexed position. With the joysticks holding the bones in a reduced position (under direct vision and fluoroscopic guidance), a single 0.062-inch-diameter Kirschner wire is placed to hold the relationship between the scaphoid and the lunate (Fig. 73–7). A second pin (0.062) is put in parallel to the first. A 0.062-inch pin is then placed percutaneously to fix the scaphoid to the capitate. With this reduction in place, verification using the C-arm is performed to check that the positions of the lunate and the scaphoid are now appropriate (Fig. 73–8).
7. A mini–anchor system is drilled into the scaphoid, and the sutures are tied in a horizontal mattress fashion through the avulsed scapholunate ligament. Alternatively, drill holes can be passed from the scaphoid waist to the repair site. Mattress sutures are passed through the drill holes and are tied over the scaphoid waist (Fig. 73–9).
8. A second anchor is placed slightly distal to Lister's tubercle, which has been rongeured off for a smooth surface. The dorsal intercalary ligament (attached now to the scaphoid) over the scapholunate interval is sewn into place. The fourth extensor tendon is now brought back into place after the capsule has been closed with a nonabsorbable suture. The third compartment EPL is left outside the remnants of the extensor retinaculum, and the skin is closed with a subcuticular stitch after a drain has been placed in the depths of the wound. The tourniquet is let down to verify that good capillary refill to all structures is seen. If the procedure has been done on an outpatient basis, the patient is sent home with a short-arm bulky dressing and volar splint.

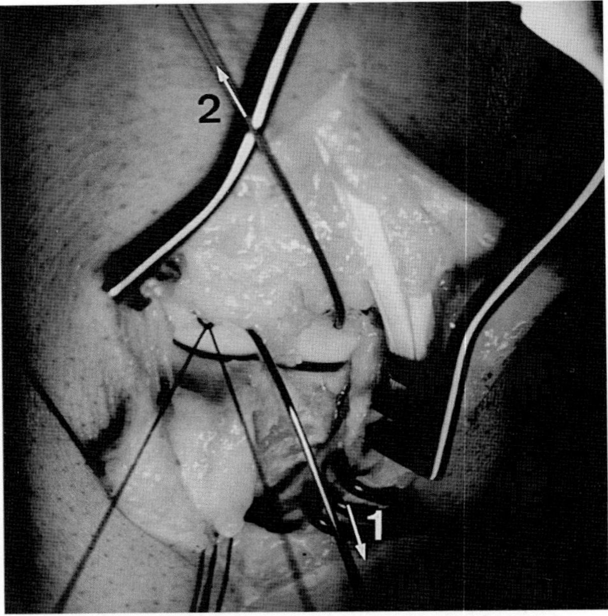

FIGURE 73–7. Clinical photo of scapholunate reduction. Joysticks are inserted into the scaphoid (1) and lunate (2) to facilitate reduction. (From Garcia-Elias M: Carpal instabilities and dislocations. In Green DP, Hotchkiss RN, Pederson WC [eds]: Green's Operative Hand Surgery, 4th ed. New York, Churchill Livingstone, 1999, p 888.)

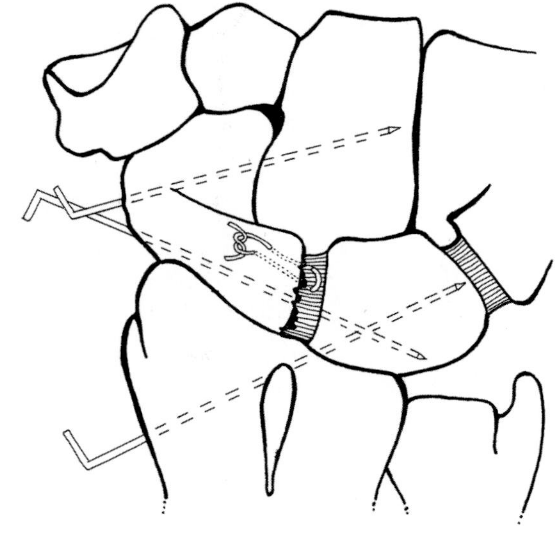

FIGURE 73–8. Illustration of K-wire placement after reduction and ligament repair. (From Garcia-Elias M: Carpal instabilities and dislocations. In Green DP, Hotchkiss RN, Pederson WC [eds]: Green's Operative Hand Surgery, 4th ed. New York, Churchill Livingstone, 1999, p 888.)

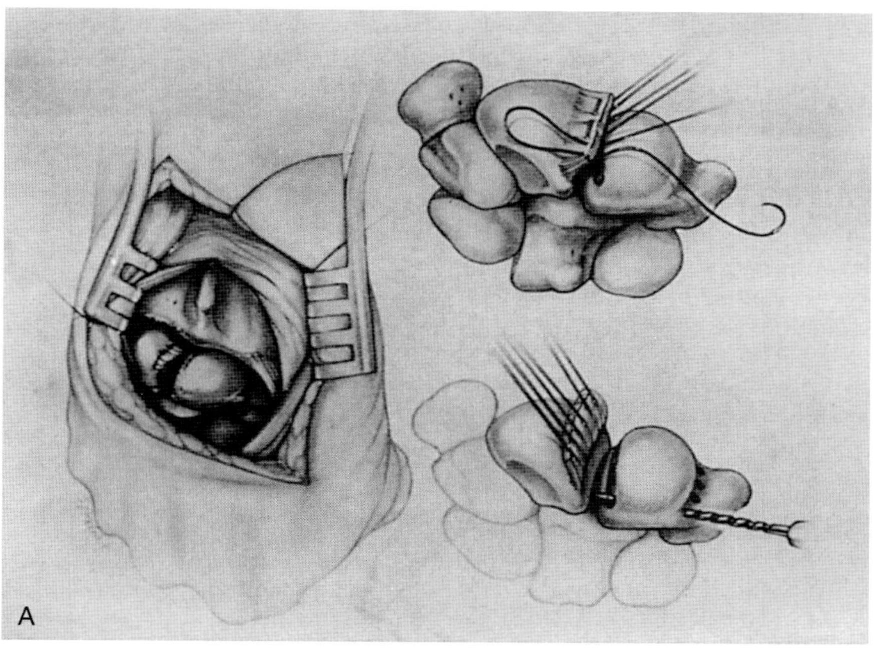

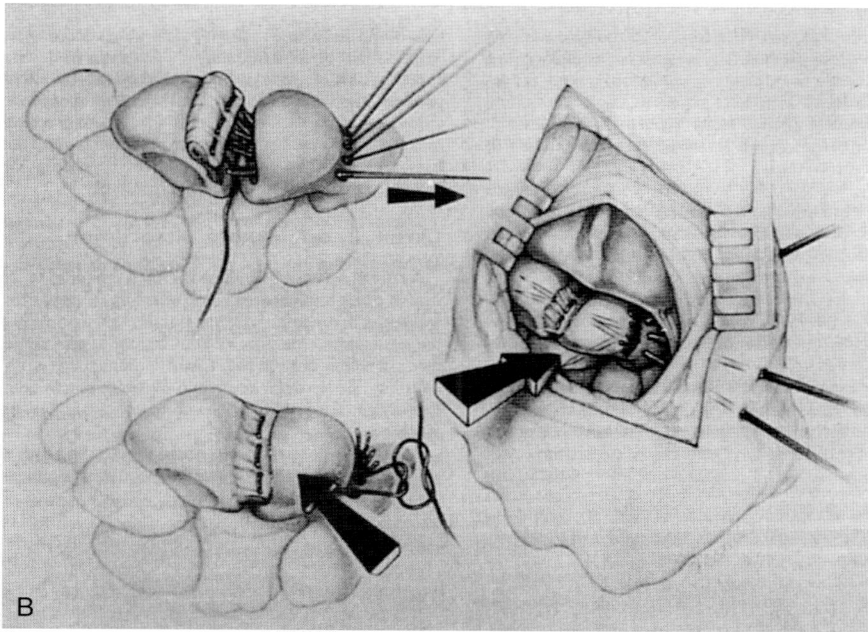

FIGURE 73–9. Illustration of scapholunate interosseous ligament (SLIOL) repair technique. *A*, Holes are drilled from the scaphoid waist to the insertion site of the ligament, and mattress sutures are placed in the SLIOL. *B*, Sutures are passed through the drill holes and tied over the waist of the scaphoid. (From Blatt G, Tobias B, Lichtman DM: Scapholunate injuries. In Lichtman DM, Alexander AH [eds]: The Wrist and Its Disorders, 2nd ed. Philadelphia, WB Saunders, 1997, p 286.)

POSTOPERATIVE MANAGEMENT

The wrist and forearm are immobilized in a long-arm splint for 2 weeks; then a Muenster cast is worn for another 6 weeks. At 8 weeks, the pins are removed (any pin that was loose was removed earlier), and a short-arm cast is placed for another 4 weeks. At 3 months, range-of-motion exercises are begun. During the period between 3 and 6 months postoperatively, the patient will have stiffness; however, activities of daily living are begun. Lifting more than 5 pounds at a time is avoided until strength is regained to within 10% of the opposite side.

An expected small-degree loss of flexion is noted in the wrist; this is caused by the dorsal scarring of the capsule and the ligamentous reefing.

COMPLICATIONS

Any increase in intercarpal scapholunate distance seen on x-ray during the postoperative period implies loss of fixation and disruption of the repair. If such an increase is noted, reexploration must be performed. Pin problems, including pin track infections, should be treated with antibiotics and removal of the pins. Wrist stiffness is expected when acute scapholunate dissociation occurs secondary to perilunate dislocation.

RESULTS

The amount of recent research on new repair techniques speaks volumes about the results of repair. The literature strongly supports efforts to repair the SLIOL. In the acute setting, closed reduction and percutaneous pinning is associated with improved outcomes. However, some patients have scapholunate widening and wrist pain. Overall, results remain somewhat unpredictable. In the subacute setting, open repair improves pain and preserves preinjury motion in the majority of cases. Historical comparisons of series are difficult to undertake because many different repair techniques have been used. A significant number of patients remain symptomatic, especially with heavy loading of the wrist.

REFERENCES

Blatt G: Capsulodesis in reconstructive hand surgery. Hand Clin 3:81–102, 1987.

Kleinman WB, Steichen JB, Strickland JW: Management of chronic rotary subluxation of the scaphoid by scapho-trapezio-trapezoid arthrodesis. J Hand Surg [Am] 7:125–136, 1982.

Kozin SH: The role of arthroscopy in scapholunate instability. Hand Clin 15:435–444, 1999.

Lavernia CJ, Cohen JS, Taleisnik J: Treatment of scapholunate dissociation by ligamentous repair and capsulodesis. J Hand Surg [Am] 17:354–359, 1992.

Taleisnik J: Current concepts review: Carpal instability. J Bone Joint Surg [Am] 70:1262–1267, 1988.

Watson HK, Ballet FL: The SLAC wrist: Scapholunate advanced collapse pattern of degenerative arthritis. J Hand Surg [Am] 9:358–365, 1984.

Weiss AP, Sachar K, Glowacki KA: Arthroscopic debridement alone for intercarpal ligament tears. J Hand Surg [Am] 22:344–349, 1997.

Index

Note: Page numbers followed by the letter f refer to figures.

D

E

F

G

H

I

J

K

L

M

N

O

T